T0344812

HANDBOOK OF APPLIED DOG BEHAVIOR AND TRAINING

Volume One

*Adaptation
and
Learning*

HANDBOOK OF APPLIED DOG BEHAVIOR AND TRAINING

Volume One

Adaptation and Learning

Steven R. Lindsay

FOREWORD BY Victoria Lea Voith

Charter Diplomate, American College of Veterinary Behaviorists
President, American Veterinary Society of Animal Behavior

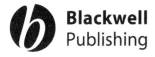

Blackwell
Publishing

Steven R. Lindsay, MA, is a dog behavior consultant and trainer who lives in Philadelphia, Pennsylvania, where he provides a variety of behavioral training and counseling services. In addition to his long career in working with companion dogs, he previously evaluated and trained highly skilled military working dogs as a member of the U.S. Army Biosensor Research Team (Superdog Program). Mr. Lindsay also conducts workshops and is the author of numerous publications on dog behavior and training.

Cover design by Justin Eccles
Text design by Dennis Anderson

© 2000 Iowa State University Press
A Blackwell Publishing company
All rights reserved

Blackwell Publishing Professional
2121 State Avenue, Ames, Iowa 50014

Orders: 1-800-862-6657
Office: 1-515-292-0140
Fax: 1-515-292-3348
Web site: www.blackwellprofessional.com

Cover image: "Three Puppies," 1790 by Okyo Maruyama. Courtesy of the Philadelphia Museum of Art.

Authorization to photocopy items for internal or personal use, or the internal or personal use of specific clients, is granted by Blackwell Publishing, provided that the base fee is paid directly to the Copyright Clearance Center, 222 Rosewood Drive, Danvers, MA 01923. For those organizations that have been granted a photocopy license by CCC, a separate system of payments has been arranged. The fee code for users of the Transactional Reporting Service is ISBN 978-0-8138-0754-6/2000.

First edition, 2000

Library of Congress Cataloging-in-Publication Data
Lindsay, Steven R.
Handbook of applied dog behavior and training/Steven R. Lindsay; foreword by Victoria Lea Voith.—1st ed.
p. cm.
Contents: v. 1. Adaptation and learning.
ISBN 978-0-8138-0754-6

1. Dogs—Behavior. 2. Dogs—Training. I. Title.
SF433.L56 1999
636.7¢0887—dc21 99-052013

Printed in United States of America

SKY10081532_080924

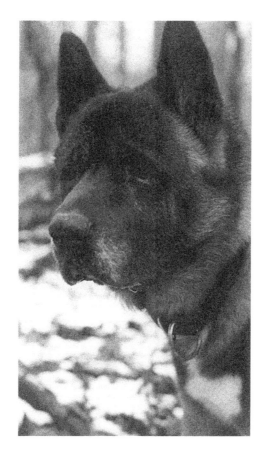

Dedicated with affection
and respect to my dog,

Yuki,

whose gentle and sincere
ways have revealed the virtues
of the human-dog bond in
ways that words alone will
forever fail to express.

Contents

Foreword

THIS IS A monumental work arising from the love of dogs and the pursuit of knowledge. Cynophiles, academics, animal behaviorists (with and without institutional degrees), literate dog owners, and anyone who has ever wanted to know something specific or just plain more about dogs are indebted to Steve Lindsay for this labor of love.

This treatise is an encyclopedia about dogs: in-depth reviews and interpretations of the literature pertaining to the dog's history, physiology, behavior, and interactions with people, and explanations and evaluations of training procedures, management strategies, and problem-solving techniques. This book is not limited to a review of the literature about dogs but also discusses basic scientific disciplines and discoveries with other species that pertain to understanding dogs. It is obvious that Steve Lindsay has thoroughly read and analyzed every publication he has referenced—an increasing rarity in today's press. The summaries of research papers or theoretical discussions will suffice for some readers, but others will be compelled to obtain the original works and read them.

Very practical and important aspects of this book are Steve Lindsay's training, treatment, and management strategies regarding dog behavior. Steve's broad experiences in the dog world have enabled him to integrate valuable components of a variety of training and management procedures. The techniques are explained very thoroughly and in sufficient detail that an educated person should be able to understand and implement them. His approaches are designed to achieve a satisfying human-dog relationship from the perspective of both species.

This handbook will help dog owners and many, many canine behavior consultants/counselors and trainers. It will also stimulate further discussion, observation, research, and analyses, ultimately leading to more knowledge about dog behavior and human-dog interactions. I consider it the most valuable publication about dogs since Scott and Fuller's classic text *Genetics and the Social Behavior of the Dog,* published in 1965.

VICTORIA LEA VOITH, DVM, PhD

Charter Diplomate of the American College of Veterinary Behaviorists
President, American Veterinary Society of Animal Behavior

Acknowledgments

MANY PEOPLE deserve acknowledgment for their contributions, but none more so than the dog owners who have given me the privilege and responsibility of helping them to train their dogs or to assist them in resolving a behavior problem. I feel a special debt of gratitude to William Carr, Scott Line, and Victoria Voith. Dr. Carr graciously gave freely of his time to read and discuss the entire manuscript. His knowledge and expertise helped to clarify a number of important areas of relevant research, especially developments in comparative psychology and the study of olfaction. Dr. Line reviewed the entire text and provided useful suggestions for its improvement. Dr. Voith has been a source of sustained encouragement for the project since its inception, giving me valuable guidance and advice. A special thank you is due to Christina Cole for her unselfish help and support. I am grateful to John Flukas, whose editorial advice has been consistently constructive and helpful. Finally, I thank Gretchen Van Houten and the great staff at Iowa State University Press for their assistance and patience in preparing the manuscript for publication.

Introduction

Before you can study an animal, you must first love it.

KONRAD LORENZ (Fox, 1998)

THE DOG has occupied an enduring place in our cultural heritage as an icon of interspecies cooperation and faithfulness. Speculation about the origins of this unique relationship continues to inspire lively debate and discussion, but nothing definitive can yet be said about the motivations guiding the first dog keepers to capture and tame wild or semidomesticated canids as companions and helpers. Even less can be said about the various functions these protodogs served or the methods used by our ancestors to train them. What is known suggests that the dog's domestication was not the result of a conscious effort or stroke of genius, but rather the outcome of a slow evolutionary process over many thousands of years. The gradual biological transformation of the wolf into the domestic dog appears to have culminated in the development of close social interaction between humans and dogs sometime during the Stone Age. What form this relationship took 14,000 years ago is not known, but it is likely that some practical implications of dogs were recognized and exploited by ancient hunter-gatherers. Most of the potential utilitarian benefits arising from domestication would have been of little use, though, if it had not been for the simultaneous development of the methods needed for managing and controlling dog behavior. The obvious necessity of behavioral control for early humans in their various dealings with dogs led the naturalist G. L. Buffon to write in the 18th century, "The training of the dog seems to have been the first art invented by man, and the fruit of that art was the conquest and peaceable possession of the earth" (quoted in Jackson, 1997).

Buffon's suggestion that dog training was "the first art invented by man" suffers from a lack of empirical evidence. Nonetheless, it is reasonable to believe that the practice of controlling and modifying dog behavior to serve human purposes springs from very ancient roots that antedate the rise of civilization. Early human association with animals as natural competitors and beasts of prey offered ample opportunity born of strife and necessity to develop an appreciation of animal habits and various methods for controlling animal behavior. Such information transmitted from generation to generation would have provided a viable cultural tradition of animal lore for the development of dog training as an art of considerable sophistication. From an early date, dogs have performed many services, such as assisting human hunters in the pursuit of game, giving alarm to the presence of intruders, pulling sledge or travois, providing warmth and comfort, as well as offering playful distraction for children. Practical uses aside, even the most casual interaction between humans and dogs would have demanded a rudimentary understanding of dog behavior and the ability to control it. Both biological changes (nature) and cultural transmission (nurture) combined to forge the primal human-dog bond—an epigenetic process that is reenacted in the life of every companion dog.

Despite the ubiquitous distribution of dogs throughout the ancient world, historical records describing their early use, breeding, and training are relatively rare and incomplete. A few ancient authors wrote at length on the subject of dog behavior, training, and management, but, for the most part, many important details about the specific methods used by ancient trainers to modify dog behavior are left to the reader's imagination. The writings of Xenophon are of particular value in this respect, but even the patron philosopher of dog and horse training provides only scant and scattered information about how dogs were trained in the distant past. Although occasional departures from this pattern can be found, very few authors took up the subject of dog behavior and training as a serious area of study, at least until fairly recent times. A turning point away from this general neglect occurred with the appearance of Darwin's *The Expression of the Emotions in Man and Animals.* Darwin's evolutionary theories and careful descriptions of dog behavior exerted a profound influence on naturalists sympathetic to his ideas, encouraging them to pay attention to dog behavior as a way to understand better the origins of human conduct. These developments played an instrumental role in the advancement of psychology and paved the way for a wider scientific and popular interest in dog behavior.

The scientific study of dog behavior and psychology was placed on an experimental foundation by the Russian physiologist Ivan Pavlov. Pavlov and his many associates crafted various experimental methods for studying associative learning processes in dogs. The result of this revolutionary research was a collection of detailed and exhaustive analyses of the functional relations controlling the acquisition and extinction of conditioned reflexive behavior. Following in the wake of Pavlov's discoveries, subsequent developments in the science of behavior and learning theory were extremely energetic and enthusiastic, with many thousands of studies being carried out and their findings published over the ensuing decades. In America, around the same time that Pavlov was making his mark on the history of psychology in Russia, Edward Thorndike was conducting a systematic study of voluntary or instrumental behavior at Columbia University. His detailed observations on how animals learn to escape from various puzzle boxes through trial and error (or, as he might prefer, "trial and success") established the study of instrumental behavior. Together,

Pavlov and Thorndike formed the intellectual and methodological foundations for the experimental study of animal behavior and learning. Most behavioral research in the 20th century can be traced back to the pioneering work of these two experimentalists.

Darwin's evolutionary approach to the investigation of animal behavior was embraced by another group of scientists, mainly composed of Europeans, who emphasized the importance of direct observation of species-typical behavior occurring under natural conditions. Their efforts set the foundations for the development of ethology. In America, comparative (animal) psychologists, who, like their European counterparts, were also interested in the evolutionary continuity of behavior across species, also took up the Darwinian banner. Unlike the early ethologists, however, comparative psychologists stressed the need for experimental methodology, thus limiting their research to a few species (mainly primates, rodents, and birds) housed under laboratory conditions.

These combined scientific efforts have produced an authoritative body of knowledge about animal behavior. Much of this information is highly specialized, sometimes difficult to access, and often only available as isolated research reports. Consequently, an important purpose for writing this book has been to draw upon these various trends in order to establish a foundation of principles and methods for understanding and managing dog behavior. The material reviewed for this purpose has been selected based on two general criteria: scientific validity and relevance for the practical management of dog behavior. In surveying the literature, I have made a conscientious effort to review the original materials. It became apparent early on that many reports and secondary texts had been either inappropriately interpreted or generalized beyond what is justifiable by the available data. I have done my best to avoid such pitfalls and to correct errors of the past where appropriate. The topics covered in *Volume One* include origins and evolution, ontogeny, neurobiology, senses, biological constraints, classical conditioning, instrumental learning, aversive control, and behavioral pathology. A concluding chapter examines the human-dog relationship, including its cultural and psychological significance. *Volume 2* (in press) covers the etiology and assessment of behavior problems, aggression, fear and phobias, separation distress, hyperactivity, compulsive behavior, destructive behavior, and social excesses.

Many of the experiments described in the following chapters were performed at a huge cost of suffering for scores of laboratory animals, including thousands of dogs, experimented upon for the sake of scientific curiosity and the advancement of our collective knowledge. It is heartening to know that, over the past decade or so, many reforms (often led by experimental scientists themselves) have taken place with respect to the way experimental animals are treated and housed. These regulatory changes would make many historically important studies very difficult or impossible to perform under the current standards of laboratory animal care and welfare. However, to ignore this significant body of scientific literature because of the suffering it has brought to laboratory animals would be tantamount to a double injury. It seems fitting that such knowledge should be applied whenever possible for the benefit of those animals whose sacrifice made it possible. Morally speaking, there are no good or bad scientific facts, but there are good and bad ways in which experiments are performed and scientific knowledge applied for practical purposes.

Finally, dog behavior problems represent a serious welfare concern. Currently, the vast majority of dog behavior services are performed by dog trainers, with a handful of veterinary and applied animal behavior consultants providing regional counseling services through veterinary schools and private animal behavior practices spread out thinly across the country. It is difficult to pin down exactly how professional services are divided between these groups, but a recent survey by the American Veterinary Medical Association (1997) suggests that a relatively small number of companion animals are referred for behavioral counseling. The report estimates that less than one-half of 1% of dog owners in the United States utilized veterinary behavioral counseling services in 1996. This is a somewhat surprising and puzzling statistic, considering that some authorities suggest that behavior problems represent a leading cause of euthanasia, causing the death of more dogs each year than die as the result of infectious disease, metabolic conditions, and cancer combined. Although this estimate appears to be inflated (see *When the Bond Fails* in Chapter 10), dog behavior problems do, undoubtedly, represent a significant source of distress and death for dogs. Obviously, cooperation between all applied animal behavior professionals is required in order to service the behavioral needs of the dog-owning public most efficiently and effectively. Animal behavior counseling, dog training, and veterinary behavioral medicine bring a variety of specific contributions and unique strengths to the practical control of dog behavior and the management of dog behavior problems. Recently, leadership from these various professional groups made the first tentative steps toward constructive collaboration by establishing various educational programs, sponsoring interdisciplinary forums, and organizing other mutually beneficial ventures. Unfortunately, however, practitioners from these various disciplines are not always familiar with the specialized knowledge and skills utilized by others working outside of their immediate domain or not sharing their academic and practical background. It is my sincere hope that this book will play a constructive role in ameliorating this situation by bridging some of these gaps and contributing to the process of professional and educational reform of dog training and behavioral counseling.

REFERENCES

American Veterinary Medical Association (1997). *U.S. Pet Ownership and Demographic Sourcebook.* Schaumberg, IL: AVMA, Center for Information Management.

Fox MW (1998). Concepts in Ethology: Animal Behavior and Bioethics. Malabar, FL: Krieger.

Jackson F (1997). Faithful Friends: Dogs in Life and Literature. New York: Carrol and Graf.

Volume One

Adaptation
and
Learning

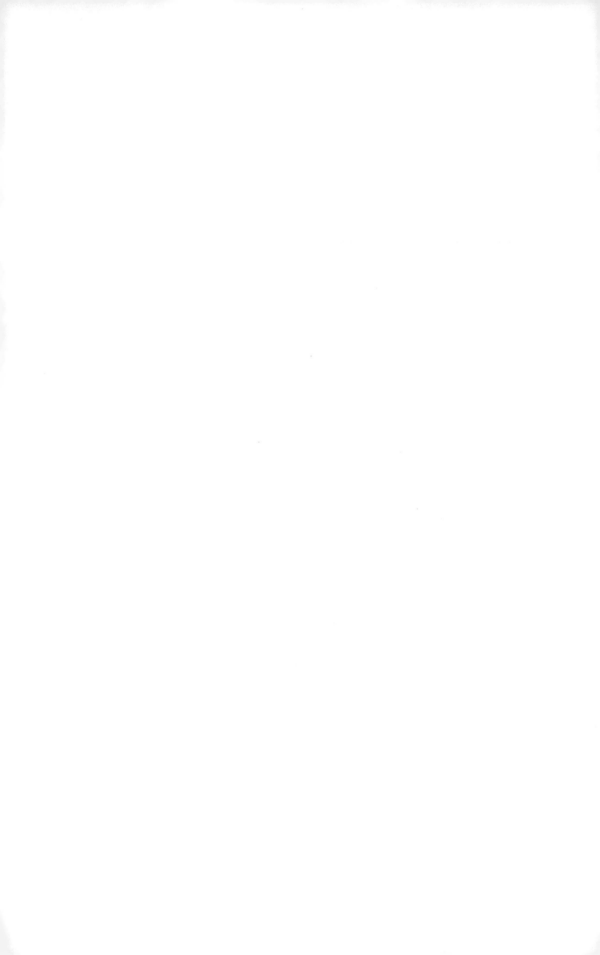

1

Origins and Domestication

For thousands of years man has been virtually, though unconsciously, performing what evolutionists may regard as a gigantic experiment upon the potency of individual experience accumulated by heredity; and now there stands before us this most wonderful monument of his labours—the culmination of his experiment in the transformed psychology of the dog.

GEORGE ROMANES, *Animal Intelligence* (1888)

U NDERSTANDING THE dog's behavior and appreciating its unique status as "man's best friend" is not possible without studying its evolution and domestication. From ancient times onward, numerous species have undergone pronounced biological and behavioral changes as the result of domestication. The purposes guiding these efforts are as diverse as the species involved.

Utilitarian interests such as the procurement of food, security, and other valuable resources or services derived from the animal were surely important incentives, but utilitarian motives alone are not enough to explain the whole picture, especially when considering the domestication of the dog.

Many theories have been advanced to explain how the progenitor of the dog was originally tamed and brought under the yoke of captivity and domestication. These theories often include colorful portraits of primitive life, motives, and purposes that rely on a number of questionable and unprovable assumptions about prehistoric existence (Morey, 1994). For example, one popular view suggests that humans may possess an ageless and universal (innate?) urge to keep animals as pets. Although this theory has some attractive features, it is difficult to defend scientifically. Certainly, dogs share an intimate place in Western society and are often treated with affectionate care in many modern primitive cultures as well (Serpell, 1986/1996); nonetheless, one cannot exclude the possibility that this so-called "affectionate" motive is a rather late cultural development. Further, although it is true that keeping pets as attachment objects is common around the world today, one cannot jump from this observation to the conclusion that a similar set of motives guided ancient people to capture and domesticate wild animals. Attitudes about animals and, in particular, dogs appear to be guided by beliefs and customs that are to a considerable extent conditioned and dependent on cultural, economic, and geographical circumstances (see Chapter 10).

Undoubtedly, a dog's life during the early stages of domestication was very different than it is today. Over the centuries, the dog's functions have evolved and changed, sometimes dramatically, depending on the assertion or absence of relevant cultural and survival pressures. In times of scarcity and need, the defining motive for keeping dogs was probably dominated by utilitarian interests; whereas, during times of abundance and well-being, dogs could be readily transformed into convenient objects for affection, comfort, or entertainment.

ARCHEOLOGICAL RECORD

Despite the difficulties, discovering when and how this enduring relationship first appeared are questions of tremendous scientific interest and importance. Authorities differ with respect to the exact historical moment or time frame, but many prehistoric sites show that a close association between humans and dogs has existed continuously for many thousands of years. Although a loose symbiotic mutualism probably existed long beforehand, the earliest archeological evidence of a "true" domestic dog is dated to 14,000 years before the present (BP). The artifact (a mandible) was unearthed from a Paleolithic grave site at Oberkassel in Germany (Nobis, 1979, in Clutton-Brock and Jewell, 1993). Protsch and Berger (1973) have collected and carbon dated canine skeletal remains taken at various sites around the world, showing great antiquity and geographical dispersion: Star Carr (Yorkshire, England), 9500 BP; Argissa-Magula (Thessaly), 9000 BP; Hacilar (Turkey), 9000 BP; Sarab (Iran), 8900 BP; and Jericho, 8800 BP. One of the most famous of these archeological finds is a Natufian skeleton of an old human (sex unknown) and a puppy buried together some 12,000 years ago at Ein Mallaha in Israel (Davis and Valla, 1978). The human's hand is positioned over the chest of the 4- or 5-month-old puppy (Fig.

1.1). One is moved by the ostensible intimacy of the two species buried together, and even tempted to ascribe a feeling of "tenderness" to the embrace binding the person and puppy together over the centuries.

The earliest remains of a domestic dog in North America were found at the Jaguar Cave site in the Beaverhead Mountains of Idaho. These bones had been previously dated from 10,400 to 11,500 BP, but radiocarbon dating of some of the artifacts revealed that they are "intrusions" of a much more recent origin, with a probable age not exceeding 3000 years (Clutton-Brock and Jewell, 1993).

DOMESTICATION: PROCESSES AND DEFINITIONS

Robert Wayne and his associates at UCLA have performed a molecular genetic analysis of the evolution of dogs and wolves, suggest-

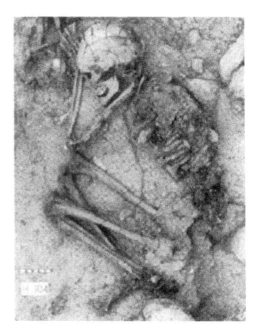

FIG. 1.1. A Natufian burial site at Ein Mallaha in northern Israel shows a human skeleton in what appears to be an "eternal embrace" with the skeletal remains of a puppy located in the upper right-hand corner. From Davis and Valla (1978), reprinted with permission.

ing that efforts to domesticate dogs may have taken place much earlier than indicated by the archeological record, putting the dog's origins back 100,000 years or more (Vila et al., 1997). The researchers argue that these more ancient efforts to domesticate dogs may have occurred without producing significant morphological change in the protodog, thus explaining the absence of dog skeletal artifacts appearing before 14,000 years ago:

> To explain the discrepancy in dates, we hypothesize that early domestic dogs may not have been morphologically distinct from their wild relatives. Conceivably, the change around 10,000 to 15,000 years ago from nomadic hunter-gather societies to more sedentary agricultural population centers may have imposed new selective regimes on dogs that resulted in marked phenotypic divergence from wild wolves. (1997:1689)

Although no physical evidence of domestic dogs living with humans before 15,000 years ago exists, skeletal remains of wolves have been found in association with hominid encampments in China (the Zhoukoudian site) from 200,000 to 500,000 years ago (Olsen, 1985).

Although contested in the past, the biological ancestry of the dog is now certain. On the basis of both genetic and behavioral studies the dog is a domestic wolf. However, considerable debate still surrounds the identity of the closest relative among wolf subspecies. Zeuner (1963) has argued that the most likely lupine progenitor is *Canis lupus pallipes* (the Indian wolf), a small Eastern variety. He bases this assumption on both behavioral and morphological considerations. The smaller Indian wolf would have been less of a threat to human encampments and would have been more readily tolerated than the larger and more aggressive northern varieties.

Olsen and Olsen (1977) have selected the Chinese wolf (*Canis lupus chanco*) as the most likely canid progenitor. They base their choice on this wolf's small size and mandible morphology, noting that the apex of the coronoid process (the uppermost part of the jaw) turns back in both the Chinese wolf and the domestic dog but not in the jaw bone of other wolf species (Fig. 1.2). Clutton-Brock

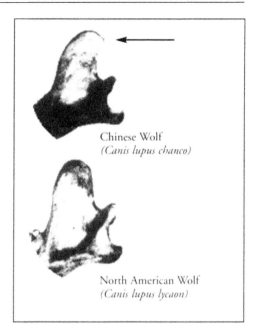

Chinese Wolf
(*Canis lupus chanco*)

North American Wolf
(*Canis lupus lycaon*)

FIG. 1.2. Note how the apex of the coronoid process (see arrow) tends to turn back. This feature is not apparent in other subspecies of wolves, coyotes, or jackals. It is a common anatomical feature found in dogs, however, suggesting that the Chinese wolf may have played an important role in the ancient domestication of the dog. From Olsen and Olsen (1977), The Chinese wolf, ancestor of New World dogs, *Science* 197: 533–535, reprinted with permission.

(1984) has identified *Canis lupus arabs* (a western Asiatic wolf) and the European wolf as the most likely ancestors of most modern European breeds, with *Canis lupus lupus* having a greater representation in the genome of Arctic and European spitz-type breeds. It is conceivable that the proliferation of domestic dogs has been genetically influenced by several wolf subspecies at different times and places, or owes its genetic past to a wolf species that is no longer existent (Fig. 1.3).

Interspecific Cooperation: Mutualism

By the end of the last glacial period, early humans' migratory activities overlapped the hunting range of competing predators, especially wolves. As nomadic people came into contact with wolves, some members of the

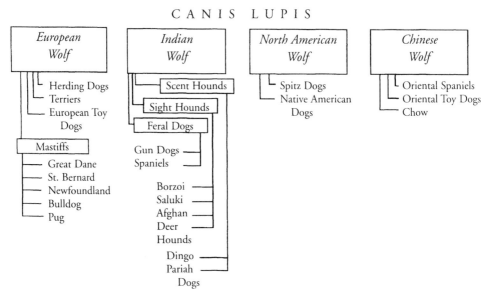

FIG. 1.3. Various subspecies of the wolf are believed to have contributed to the genome of the domestic dog. According to one theory, the dog was independently domesticated in various parts of the world, with no single site of origin. Although grouped as though from discrete origins, the breeds included here have probably undergone considerable crossbreeding over their long history of development. After Clutton-Brock and Jewell (1993).

wolf population may have been confident enough to follow closely behind these migrant hunting and gathering groups. By staying nearby, the ever-opportunistic wolves could have easily tracked animals wounded by hunters, thus securing an easy meal for themselves at least until the advancing hunting party arrived at the scene. Also, by retreating and lingering at a safe distance, wolves could scavenge on the slaughtered remains left behind (Zeuner, 1963). Juliet Clutton-Brock (1984, 1996) has speculated that such a hunting partnership may have played an important role in the development and spread of the bow and arrow as a hunting tool during the Mesolithic period, arguing that wolves or protodogs may have provided a significant advantage to early hunters by tracking and subduing large animals wounded by arrows fitted with sharp stone heads called microliths. Besides forming an effective hunting partnership, wolf-pack territories may have formed around human camps, thus providing a natural protective shield against the threat of predation by other

less friendly wolves and competing human groups. Possibly, from this mutually beneficial situation, an ecological niche was formed from which the protodog underwent novel morphological and genetic changes gradually leading to domestic dogs.

Close social contact of this kind requires that the animal in question possess a high fear threshold and a reduced tendency to flee, essential behavioral characteristics of domestication (Hediger, 1955/1968). Scientific evidence for a genetically divergent distribution of temperament traits based on relative tameness and confidence among canids has been demonstrated in the fox (Belyaev, 1979). Among farm-bred foxes, a small percentage exhibit a reduced tendency to act fearfully or aggressively in the presence of people. By breeding these less fearful individuals together over several generations, Belyaev has developed a strain of tame, human-friendly foxes (see below). Although a similar genetic basis for social tolerance has not been demonstrated in wolves, it is reasonable to assume that a certain percentage of the Pleistocene wolf population was probably less fearful and aggressive toward humans than average wolves. The adaptive value of behavioral polymorphism in wolves and its relevance to domestication have been discussed in detail by Fox (1971) and by Scott, the latter writing,

> As a dominant predator the wolf is protected from certain kinds of selection pressure, thus permitting the survival of individuals with a considerable variation from the mean. As a highly social species, wolves should be subject to selection favoring variation useful in cooperative enterprises, as a greater degree of variation permits a greater degree of division of labor. For example, a wolf pack might benefit both by the presence of individuals that were highly timid and reacted to danger quickly and effectively, and also by the presence of other more stolid individuals who did not run away but stayed to investigate the perhaps nonexistent danger. (1967:257)

Similarly, Young and Goldman reported that "wolves held in captivity have shown that in each litter there are two or three whelps that show tameness early; the remainder are absolutely intractable and often die if one attempts to train them" (1944/1964:208–209). This prosocial population would have displayed a greater tolerance for human contact or may have even been "preadapted" for domestication—especially if they were not being actively hunted or persecuted.

Mutual tolerance offered many benefits for both species. Early people who tolerated scavenging and the proximate presence of dogs enjoyed a hygienic benefit (resulting in the control of garbage and pestilence) and a protected perimeter of barking dogs, providing valuable early warning of approaching enemies. After a propitious length of time, perhaps hundreds or thousands of years, such loose symbiotic contact may have resulted in the development of a specialized ecological niche in which the most tame individual wolves began to breed in close association with people. This transitional step would have taken place gradually, requiring little or no purposeful intervention on the part of early humans. Such a pattern of scavenging around human encampments by feral and

semiferal dogs is evident in many parts of the world today (Fiennes and Fiennes, 1968). Even in large American cities, semiferal dogs satisfy the majority of their nutritional needs by scavenging (Fox, 1971; Beck, 1973). Alan Beck (1973) has observed that stray dogs satisfy most of their nutritional needs by raiding garbage cans and relying on handouts when garbage is not available. Handouts may have been an important source of food for early dogs as well. Domestic dogs exhibit a unique proclivity and skill for food begging—a behavioral attribute that would have been very useful for underfed primitive canines depending on human generosity for their survival. As the result of a growing familiarity between genetically "tame" scavengers and begging dogs, early people had many opportunities for close interaction, thereby making other social exchanges possible, including the adoption of pups.

John P. Scott (1968) has imagined that a primitive mother, having lost her own child and enduring the discomfort of lactation, may have saved a wolf puppy from the camp soup pot by adopting and nursing it as her own. If, in addition, the wolf happened to be a female, it might have chosen the camp as a suitable place to give birth, resulting in a new generation of even closer interaction and social affiliation. Although such a scenario cannot be proven, it is statistically possible, even plausible. Many examples of the suckling of domestic animals by women have been found among existing tribal cultures (e.g., the Papuan of New Guinea).

Although primitive humans' intentions and purposes for keeping dogs in close proximity are not known, a certain degree of social tolerance and mutual acceptance was clearly present in both species. In addition to various utilitarian or symbiotic benefits, early interaction between humans and dogs surely depended on a high degree of respectful deference shown by early canids toward humans. Dogs exhibiting threatening tendencies would have been quickly expelled or killed, and eliminated from the gene pool early in the domestication process. Those animals exhibiting submission behaviors and social subordination—that is, a readiness to respond to human directives—would have been more likely to survive and to reproduce under the protection of domestic conditions. Early domestic dogs that also exhibited a high degree of affection toward their captors would have been brought into even closer intimacy, enjoying added protection, better food, and other survival advantages not extended to less affectionate counterparts. As time went on, various specialized functions could have been elaborated out of this basic foundation, including all the familiar roles served by the dog today—for example, alarm barking and protection, hunting activities, herding, draft work, and companionship. Undoubtedly, at some point in the natural history of humans and dogs, interspecies tolerance and cooperative interaction became mutually advantageous, thus forging the foundation for a lasting relationship.

Terms and Definitions: Wild, Domestic, and Feral

Reports following a recent fatal wolf-dog attack exemplify some of the confused ways in which terms like domestic, wild, and tame are used. The victim, a 39-year-old mother of two, was mauled and killed as her children looked on near their Colorado home. Several authorities were asked to comment on the unusual attack. It was the first documented case in which a wolf hybrid had killed an adult person. A police detective investigating the incident said, "They [wolf hybrids] may be domesticated, but they're still wild animals subject to unpredictable behavior." Another authority, speaking for a local Humane Society, commented, "Animals like that are not tame. You can pet them but they are wild." The words *tamed* and *domesticated* are used here interchangeably, as though they mean about the same thing, roughly synonyms for *pet*. But this habit of usage is misleading. Taming is a necessary prerequisite for domestication, but taming alone is not sufficient. Many wild animals can be readily "tamed" by patient handling and socialization, but they cannot be classified as domestic animals until they have also undergone extensive behavioral and biological change resulting from selective breeding over the course of many generations. Such breeding is designed (consciously

or unconsciously) to enhance various behavioral and physical characteristics conducive to domestic harmony and utility.

The words *wild* and *feral* are also frequently used interchangeably in popular discussions. The feral dog is not simply wild, but is a previously domesticated animal that has been released or has escaped back into nature to reproduce and fend for itself. As is discussed below, dingoes exemplify many characteristic features of feral dogs, having evolved from early Asiatic dogs that escaped domestic captivity on reaching Australia several millennia ago. Since that time, dingoes have reverted to a feral existence with only temporary symbiotic affiliations with humans. Dingoes have existed under such conditions of quasi domestication for many generations without actually returning to a true domestic state.

The Dingo: A Prototypical Dog

An excellent source of ethnographic evidence outlining the general course of early domestication can be found in the enduring relationship between the Aborigines of Australia and dingoes. This symbiotic dyad provides a valuable anthropological picture of what life between primitive humans and early canids may have been like during the earliest incipient stages of domestication. In most details, dingoes differ only slightly from Asian wolves (*Canis lupus pallipes*), except for modest behavioral and morphological changes associated with quasi domestication—for example, variable tail carriage (sometimes carried in the sickle-like form of dogs), some evidence of piebald marking (especially on the feet and chest), and occasionally lop-eared examples are observed but are probably the result of European hybridization. Like wolves, dingoes do very poorly as domestic animals—even after they have been crossed with domestic dogs (Trumler, 1973). The pelage of dingoes comes in a wide variety of colors, including black, white, black and tan, brindle, and ginger tan—the most common color observed (Corbett, 1995).

Meggitt (1965) has reviewed the relevant recorded literature regarding dingoes and their varied role in aboriginal culture. He has expressed skepticism regarding the usefulness of dingoes in hunting. Some evidence suggests, however, that a cooperative hunting relationship may have existed at various times and in ecologically specialized niches like tropical rain forests. Aboriginal hunters have been known to track free-ranging dingoes on the trail of prey and taking it as their own once the quarry was caught, leaving the dingoes with scraps and offal for their efforts. Corbett (1995) reports that the Garawa tribe of northern Australia uses dingoes to track and worry wounded prey, allowing the hunters to catch up and dispatch the weakened and distracted animal. However, in other localities like the desert, camp dingoes are driven back at the outset of a hunting expedition because they are considered a hindrance rather than an aid to a hunter's prospects of finding game (Gould, 1970). Nomadic Aborigines hunt by concealment and stealth, making dingoes of limited value to such efforts. As an independent predator, dingoes sometimes hunt cooperatively in small pack units, especially when hunting large prey (e.g., kangaroos). However, they are seldom observed to congregate in such packing groups. Of 1000 dingoes sighted by Corbett and Newsome (1975), 73% were solitary hunters, 16.2% were in pairs, and only 5.1% were observed in trios.

Aborigines routinely collect puppies during the winter months from remote denning sites and rear the captured progeny to puberty. Upon reaching sexual maturity, the captive dingoes usually escape into the bush to reproduce and never return. This pattern of adoption and escape prevents the development of a true domesticated dingo, since its breeding is not actively controlled and directed by human design. It should be noted, however, that deformed or otherwise unsuitable puppies are culled and eaten, thus providing some degree of active selection. Further, it is likely that those dingoes not performing well under domestic conditions are either expelled or killed. Although Aborigines find dingo meat somewhat unpalatable, they will eat it if hungry enough. In various parts of Southeast Asia and the Pacific Islands, dogs are preferred over pigs and fowl as meat. Corbett (1995) speculates that the

first dingoes reached Australia as cargo—a source of fresh food—but, once having reached shore, some may have fled into the bush to give birth and to fend for themselves.

Apparently, some puppies belonging to Aboriginal women are purposely crippled by breaking their front legs to prevent them from wandering off. A similarly pragmatic rationale may inform the constant pampering (sometimes involving suckling) and attention that dingoes are given by their Aboriginal captors. Such caregiving interaction may establish a strong psychological "leash" of augmented affectional bonding and heightened dependency. In 1828, the explorer Major Lockyer noted the strong emotional attachment between the Aborigines and their dingo puppies. He had taken a liking for a black puppy in the possession of a native, offering him an ax in exchange for the dingo. Urged by his companions to accept the offer, the Aborigine nearly conceded to the trade "when he looked down at the dog and the animal licked his face, which settled the business. He shook his head and determined to keep him" (in Bueler, 1973:102). These sentiments were later echoed by Lumholtz (1884, in Corbett, 1995), reporting that the Aborigines treated their dingo puppies with greater attention and care than given to their children. He describes the character of this relationship and interaction in highly affectionate terms: "The dingo is an important member of the family; it sleeps in the huts and gets plenty to eat, not only of meat but also of fruit. Its master never strikes, but merely threatens it. He caresses it like a child, eats the fleas off it, and then kisses it on the snout" (1995:16). The treatment observed by Lumholtz appears to represent an exception rather than a general rule. While treated with great fondness, the camp dingoes are often maintained in poor health and fed the poorest scraps or nothing at all—forced to fend for themselves on what they can find. Meggitt (1965) points out that domestic dingoes can be distinguished from free-ranging counterparts by their starved appearance. Among Aborigines, dingoes are kept mainly as pets, as warm sleeping companions, as scavengers of garbage and excrement, and as watchdogs.

Richard Gould (1970), an anthropologist, made several interesting observations of the interaction and bonding between Aborigines and dingoes during a brief study involving a remote group who had limited or no previous contact with Europeans. The group of Aborigines in question lived in a remote and barren area of the Gibson Desert called Pulykara located in Western Australia. They existed on the meager bounty of desert fauna and flora, mainly consisting of vegetable food, although meat was preferred whenever available. Among the 10 Aborigines forming the group were 19 dingoes, 12 of which belonged to a single woman, whom Gould christened the "Dog Lady." Although the dingoes were frequently petted and fussed over, the people rarely fed them. He noted that the dingoes were not only "the skinniest dogs I have ever seen, but they were also compulsive cringers and skulkers" (1970:65), surviving on what they could find around the camp or by stealing. Paradoxically, the people expressed great sensitivity for their dingoes' plight. One woman, upon receiving a piece of candy from the researcher, covered her dingo's eyes so that the dingo could not watch her eating it.

The Dog Lady is particularly interesting because of the manner in which she pampered and cared for her dingo companions. While she rarely fed the animals, she took great pains to make them comfortable. During the day, they slept under "shade shelters" constructed out of branches and twigs that she would periodically adjust in order to keep them maximally protected from the sun. While the desert days are hot, the nights are freezing cold. The custom of the Aborigines is to sleep around a small campfire, huddled among dogs. The Dog Lady, as one might guess, had most of the pack wrapped around her, suggesting that a large motivation for keeping so many dogs was comfort against the cold desert nights. One night Gould attempted to take a photograph of the group while they slept with their dogs. The flash of the camera startled the dingoes, causing them to run away into the night. The people were left shivering without their "doggy blankets." It appears from Gould's observations that the most important utilitarian function of the camp dingoes for this particular group was that of a living blanket.

The Carolina Dog: An Indigenous Dog?

Research led by I. L. Brisbin at the Savannah River Ecology Laboratory is under way to determine whether a dingolike dog that has been discovered living in the Savannah River Reserve and other remote areas of South Carolina is an indigenous dog with an ancient lineage or a more modern counterpart that has become feral (Brisbin and Risch, 1997; Weidensaul, 1999). In either case, the Carolina dog portends to reveal important information about the nature of domestication and its reversal. Carolina dogs present a number of behavioral and ecological adaptations that are not observed in other domestic dogs, suggesting a unique evolutionary course of development. For example, females exhibit an unusual pattern of multiple estrous cycles (3/year) as young dogs, with longer periods between estrous cycles occurring as they grow older. Brisbin and Risch speculate that this pattern of reproduction is particularly adaptive under conditions where a high risk of early death exists. A young Carolina dog quickly produces one or more litters as soon as possible after reaching sexual maturity. The threat of diseases such as heart worm—a mosquito-born condition that is rampant in the South—may exert selection pressures that favor dogs who exhibit a more frequent pattern of estrous cycles. Another unusual feature exhibited by female Carolina dogs is their tendency to dig dens in which to whelp their young. Domestic dogs typically do not dig dens before whelping their young. When in estrus or after giving birth, females also exhibit the rather unusual habit of burying their feces by covering it with sand that is pushed about by their nose. Another unusual behavioral oddity found in these dogs is their avidity for digging "snout pits"—small holes dug in the shape of their muzzle. The function of such behavior has not been determined, but Brisbin speculates that the dogs may be deriving some nutritional value from eating the soil (geophagia). In addition, unlike most domestic dogs, Carolina dogs exhibit effective predatory behavior that enables them to survive independently of human protection and care. A central hypothesis that Brisbin is testing concerns the possibility that the Carolina dogs may be a vestige of primitive dogs that accompanied human migrations across the Bering land bridge. Whether the Carolina dogs possess a true dingolike genetic ancestry is a question that is being currently evaluated through behavioral and mitochondrial DNA studies.

BIOLOGICAL AND BEHAVIORAL EVIDENCE

Biological Evidence

Domestic dogs interbreed with three wild canid species: coyotes, jackals, and wolves. Charles Darwin (1875/1988) discusses at length in *The Variation of Animals and Plants Under Domestication* that the variability and diversity of the dog could only be adequately explained by postulating an admixture of several wild species represented in the canine genome. Following in the tradition of Darwin, Konrad Lorenz (1954) also argued that domestic dogs owe their genetic endowment to a combination of canid bloodlines. He believed that the dog was first domesticated from the jackal (*Canis aureus*) and only later crossed with the wolf. However, upon subsequent reexamination of the behavioral evidence, Lorenz (1975) reassessed and reformed his theory by substituting *Canis lupus pallipes* in place of the jackal. An important factor affecting his change of opinion was the

finding that jackals are much less sociable and exhibit a distinctive howling pattern not shared by dogs.

"The wolf, disarmed of ferocity, is now pillowed in the lady's lap." This speculation written by Edward Jenner in 1798 has turned out to be true. The genetic and behavioral evidence to date points uniformly to the wolf as the exclusive wild progenitor of the dog. Supporting this view is the fact that both dogs and wolves share a very similar genotype and readily interbreed. Testifying to the ease with which wolves and dogs interbreed is the growing population of wolf-dog hybrids. It has been roughly estimated that approximately 300,000 wolf-dog hybrids are currently kept as companion animals in the United States (Clifford and Green, 1991), although these numbers have been disputed and remain controversial.

Robert Wayne (1993) has confirmed the close genetic relationship between dogs and wolves by comparing the mitochondrial DNA sequences of wild canids and dogs. According to this line of research, dogs are domesticated wolves with only slight genetic alterations affecting developmental timing and growth rates: "Dogs are gray wolves, despite their diversity in size and proportion; the wide variation in their adult morphology probably results from simple changes in developmental rate and timing" (1993:220). Both wolves and dogs possess 78 chromosomes (Table 1.1). Comparisons of canid DNA sequences reveal that dogs are more closely related to wolves than to coyotes. Al-

TABLE 1.1. The diploid chromosome numbers for canids showing a close relationship between the dog, wolf, coyote, jackal, and other canids

Species	Common name	Range	Chromosomes
Canis aureus	Golden jackal	Old World	78
Canis lupus	Gray wolf	Holarctic	78
Canis iatrans	Coyote	North America	78
Cuon alpinus	Dhole	Asia	78
Lycaon pictus	African wild dog	Sub-Sahara Africa	78
Speothos venaticus	Bush dog	South America	74
Chrysocyon brachyurus	Maned wolf	South America	76
Vulpes vulpes	Red fox	Old and New World	36
Alopex lagopus	Arctic fox	Holarctic	50

Source: After Wayne (1993:219).

though coyotes can interbreed successfully with dogs and produce fertile offspring, the coyote is eliminated as a significant contributor to the dog's evolution by virtue of geographical considerations. Any possible role the coyote may have played in the origin of the dog is negated by the fact that its range is limited to North America and it is not found in any of those areas associated with the dog's earliest appearance. The DNA sequencing of the dog's genotype differs from the wolf's by only 0.2%, whereas the coyote's genotype differs by about 4%. Although the jackal may be represented to some extent in the dog's genotype, the jackal does not appear to be an important genetic contributor to the dog's evolution.

Behavioral Evidence

Another important source of evidence in favor of the primogenitor status of the wolf is the behavioral similarity between the two canids. Scott (1950) has compiled an ethogram of dog behavior derived from observations of semiferal dogs maintained in open-field enclosures and well-socialized counterparts maintained under laboratory conditions. He then compared these observations with field reports of wolf behavior. Of the 90 behavior patterns exhibited by dogs, all but 19 are also exhibited by wolves. Most of the behaviors not described at the time of Scott's ethogram have been subsequently reported by other observers (Mech, 1970; Fox, 1971). Scott's study demonstrates that the behavior patterns of dogs are very similar to those of wolves.

An interesting example of behavioral parallelism between wild canids and dogs is the *play bow*—an apparent invitation to play. Bekoff (1977) has observed that the form and function of the play bow is similar among young dogs, coyotes, and wolves. Among canids, the play bow is a stereotypic, "relatively" fixed action pattern signaling playful intentions. Another highly social and affiliative display shared by dogs and wolves is an enthusiastic greeting ceremony in which reciprocal affectionate and solicitous behavior is exchanged between pack members on return from excursions or upon waking from

sleep. The behavioral components expressed during these animated displays include facial gestures indicating pleasurable excitement and vigorous tail wagging—the canid equivalent of the human smile.

Besides the ubiquitous play bow and greeting ritual, dogs and wolves share many expressive facial and bodily movements employed to communicate threat and appeasement intentions. These behaviors occur under various social circumstances, but especially during ritualized dominance challenges and squabbles. Rudolph Schenkel (1967) has analyzed in detail the submissive behavior of wolves and dogs. His work is of considerable historical and theoretical importance in the clarification of canid appeasement displays, particularly with regard to the differentiation of active and passive submission behaviors (Fig. 1.4).

Understanding dog behavior rightly begins with a study of wolf behavior. However, a long history of domestication behaviorally segregates dogs from wolves, and one must take care not to overly generalize between the two canids in terms of their respective motivations and behavior patterns.

EFFECTS OF DOMESTICATION

Although it is doubtful that early humans consciously deliberated upon the reproductive activities of their captive dogs, there certainly existed many unconscious selection pressures. Dogs of special interest or usefulness were probably more carefully managed, fed, and protected than others, thereby enhancing their chances of survival and reproduction. Darwin (1859/1962) reported striking evidence revealing the high regard and protection that dogs enjoyed in some tribal cultures. In support of the existence of such unconscious selection pressures, he reports that the tribal people of Tierra del Fuego would sooner eat one of their old women in times of famine than one of their favorite dogs:

> If there exist savages so barbarous as never to think of the inherited character of the offspring of their domestic animals, yet any one animal particularly useful to them, for any special

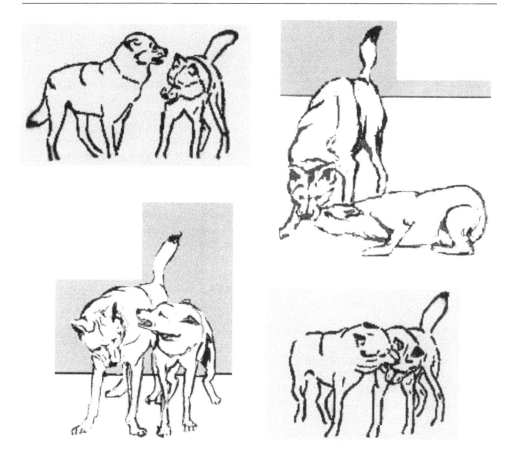

FIG. 1.4. Changes in bodily posture express relative dominance and submission. The dominant wolf can be identified by his upright tail carriage. After Schenkel (1967).

purpose, would be carefully preserved during famines; other accidents, to which savages are so liable, and such choice animals would thus generally leave more offspring than the inferior ones; so that in this case there would be a kind of unconscious selection going on. We see the value set on animals even by the barbarians of Tierra del Fuego, by their killing and devouring their old women, in times of dearth, as of less value than their dogs. (1859/ 1962:51–52)

Morphological Effects of Domestication

The effects of domestication have resulted in dramatic and extensive alterations of the wolf's morphology. The archeological remains of the dog show a number of structural changes associated with domestication, including smaller skeletal size, a short compact muzzle, crowded dentition and proportionately smaller teeth, ocular orbits set more toward the front, the cranial capacity of the skull is reduced, and, finally, the domestic dog's cranium is proportionately wider and possesses a more sharply rising stop (Morey, 1992). Over the course of the dog's domestication, the shape of its skull has been modified in two opposing directions (Fig. 1.5). In the case of bulldogs, for example, the skull has been simultaneously shortened and widened, whereas in greyhounds it has been lengthened and narrowed. Another important morphological feature differentiating dogs from wolves is the carriage of the canine tail.

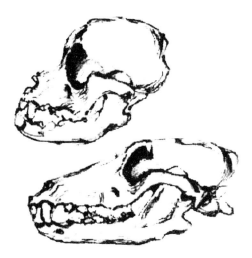

FIG. 1.5. These skulls show the opposing tendencies of shortening/widening (brachycephalic) and lengthening/narrowing (dolichocephalic) of the cranium.

Most dogs carry their tails in either a tightly curled or sickle-like shape—a tail shape that wolves never (or rarely) exhibit. The general conformation of the average dog differs considerably from that of the wolf. The wolf's general physical structure is one of harmonic cooperation between form and function. A wolf's shoulders are narrow with elbows turned inward causing the front legs to move along in a single line with the rear ones. The coordination is so accurate and refined that the hind feet follow in the tracks of the front ones. The consequence is efficient locomotion involving graceful trotting and loping movements that are not commonly observed in dogs.

An interesting physical oddity that can be found on the feet of domestic dogs but not normally exhibited by wolves is metatarsal dewclaws. Many large breeds (Great Pyrenees, St. Bernards, Newfoundlands) exhibit dewclaws on their hind feet. Some dogs even exhibit a pair of vestigial dewclaws on their hind feet; these vestigial dewclaws are attached to the feet with little more than skin. The absence of paired dewclaws in the briard is a disqualifying fault. Alberch (1986) has

pointed out that dewclaws on the hind feet are observed only among large dogs and are rarely seen in smaller breeds like the Chihauhau or Pekingese. He has proposed that large dogs may exhibit such dewclaws as the result of embryological differences occurring early in development—that is, the embryos of larger breeds have larger limb buds containing more cells than smaller breeds. This hypothesis, however, does not explain why many large breeds do not exhibit metatarsal dewclaws. Another possible explanation for extra digitation is genetic drift or founders effect stemming from the early population of dogs common to those animals exhibiting the trait.

A great deal of attention has been focused on anatomical differences between the dog's cranium and dentition and those of wild canids. This reliance is partly due to the paucity of complete dog skeletons in the archeological record. Most existent remains of the early dog are limited to the jaws and teeth. An important morphological difference between the wolf and the dog is that the latter's canine teeth appear to be proportionately smaller (Olsen and Olsen, 1977). Morey (1992) has questioned the validity of this widely held view and has proposed an alternative explanation for the observed differences. He has argued that the body size of some large breeds may have increased faster than corresponding dentition size—that is, the teeth have not become proportionately smaller, but the body has become larger. He points out that smaller dogs often have proportionately larger teeth than wolves, suggesting a similar alteration but in an opposite direction—that is, the body has become smaller at a rate faster than a proportionate decrease in the size of the teeth. It should be noted, however, that even for the untrained eye, the canine teeth of wolves are impressively large when compared with the canine teeth of average dogs. Although the dog and the wolf share the same number of teeth (20 upper teeth and 22 lower for a total of 42 permanent teeth), the dog's teeth are often crowded together in a proportionately shorter and wider jaw.

TABLE 1.2. Some behavioral differences between the wolf and dog brought about through domestication

Behavioral tendency	Wolf	Dog
General activity level	High, varies with rank	Varies with breed—hypo- or hyperactive
Exploratory behavior	High, varies with rank	Significant sensory specialization
Neophobia	Low threshold/slow habituation	High threshold/rapid habituation
Vocalization	Very common	Less common, includes barking
Group howling	Rare—threat only	Common in many situations
Barking	Absent	Common
Yelping		
Agonistic displays		
Hip slams	Common	Rare—wolflike breeds
Muzzle biting and pinning	Dominant display	Rare—wolflike breeds
Vertical tail threat display	Dominant display	Threat—tail arched
Face licking (greeting)	Common—low frequency	Common—high frequency
Secondary social bonding	Weak	Strong, except guard dogs
Trainability	Weak	Strong
Allelomimetic behavior	Strong	Strong in some breeds (hounds)
Dominance	Complex, basically linear	Common but highly variable
Fighting	Varies with rank	Varies according to breed
Sexual behavior		
Maturation	2 Years	6–9 Months
Female season	Annual estrus	Biannual estrus
Male season	Seasonal spermatogenesis	Constant spermatogenesis

Source: After Fox (1978:253–256). See references following Chapter 1.

Behavioral Effects of Domestication

Although dogs share a great many behavioral characteristics with wolves, the former have undergone a tremendous transformation in the direction of enhanced docility and affectionate dependency as well as many other behavioral changes (Table 1.2). Price has argued that these changes are probably not due to a permanent loss of behavior, but rather reflect quantitative alterations (lowering or raising) of response thresholds mediating the expression of species-typical behavior:

> With respect to behavior, it appears that domestication has influenced the quantitative nature of responses. The hypothesized loss of certain behavior patterns under domestication can usually be explained by the heightening of response thresholds above normal levels of stimulation. Conversely, lowered thresholds of response often can be accounted for by excessive exposure to certain forms of stimulation. (1998:55–56)

Whether as the result of quantitative or qualitative evolutionary changes, and despite occasional atavistic examples to the contrary, most dogs have lost the lupine carnivorous drive and predatory behavior exhibited by wild canids. Dogs appear content to eat practically whatever food they are given, even though it is often far removed from the diet which their ancestral progenitors enjoyed. Most dogs, however, still exhibit a definite preference for meat whenever it is available. Dogs tend to mature physically and sexually much more rapidly than wolves: the former become sexually active (on average) between

7 and 10 months, whereas the latter reach sexual maturity at approximately 22 months of age (Mech, 1970). There exists a great deal of variation with regard to the onset of puberty in dogs. Smaller dogs tend to reach puberty earlier than larger ones. Dogs have become polygamous and readily accept multiple sexual partners, whereas wolves tend to be more selective and monogamous. This change in sexual preference away from a single mate enables dogs to breed more freely with partners defined by *breeders*—an essential facet of domestication. Another aspect enhancing canine reproduction is the dog's biannual breeding cycle in contrast to the wolf's annual breeding cycle. Whereas male wolves are able to breed only during a short period once a year, male dogs can breed any time a female is receptive. An interesting aspect of wolf sexual behavior involves the seasonal control of spermatogenesis. At times other than the breeding season, the male wolf's testes atrophy, rendering the wolf infertile. Male dogs are not subject to such variations of testes size or fertility. Dogs are fertile all year round.

Two behavioral patterns exhibited by wolves that have become strongly exaggerated in domestic dogs are alarm barking and urinary scent marking. Although wolves exhibit both forms of behavior, they perform them far less frequently than dogs. When alarm barking does occur among wolves, it is a subdued or whispered "wuff, wuff" sound. Zeuner (1963), however, has noted that the southern Asian wolf (*Canis lupus pallipes*) has been reported to bark in a manner resembling that of the dog.

It should be noted that not all domestic dogs are equally inclined to bark. The absence of barking in dogs belonging to native American Indians was frequently noted in the journals of early observers (Young and Goldman, 1944/1964). In fact, Spanish explorers of the New World referred to native dogs as *perros mudos* (mute dogs). These native dogs, however, gradually acquired the habit of barking, presumably as the result of close daily contact with their more vocal European-bred counterparts. This observation suggests that the tendency to bark may be socially facilitated or learned. Barking definitely

has a contagious quality, as anyone who has lingered about the outside of a kennel can verify. Interestingly, European-bred dogs appear to have been affected by this "canine cultural exchange" but in a reverse way. Columbus is reported to have complained that his European-bred dogs had lost some of their valuable inclination to bark as the result of contact with the "mute" native dogs (Varner and Varner, 1983).

Even among modern breeds, the tendency to bark is marked by wide variability. Although many dogs bark a great deal (e.g., Shetland sheepdogs), others do so only infrequently (e.g., Akitas), and some nearly not at all (e.g., basenjis). The advantage of a lower response threshold for barking may seem obvious to the average homeowner, but Coppinger and Feinstein (1991) have disputed the functional and communicative value of the dog's barking behavior. They have argued that barking behavior is poorly directed, excessively ambiguous, "indecisive"—even "meaningless." They conclude that the dog's increased tendency to bark is an inadvertent symptom of domestication, that is, a paedomorphic elaboration and by-product, rather than a genetically selected tendency. Clutton-Brock (1984) has argued the opposing point of view, stating that it is likely that the dog's barking behavior has undergone "intensive selection" because of its value as an early warning that signaled the approach of intruders. Undoubtedly, considerable attention has been focused on the selection of alarm barking by dogs. A dog exhibiting such barking would naturally have been more valued as a protector than a dog not moved to bark at strange or suspicious sounds. Among trailing hounds, the melodious baying or "voice" is a highly valued breed feature that has been carefully selected for in the breeding of such dogs.

Spectrographic analysis of the dog's bark reveals that it is a composite of growling (threatening) tones and whining/yelping (distress or appeasement) tones, making the bark itself appear ambivalent or flexible with regard to intention and meaning. Coppinger and Feinstein (1991) contend that such ambivalence of meaning reduces the value of the bark as communicative signal. It may be precisely the bark's flexible ambivalence, though, that makes it so communicative and meaningful. The bark as a signal is composed of the two extremes of threat and distress on a continuum admixing these two opposing intentions and sources of meaning. To define precisely a dog's current intentions, which may, in fact, be ambivalent or expressive of any number of other graduated shades of intention, the bark leans intentionally in the direction of increasing threat or distress as required by the situation. A growling, deep-throated bark thrust forward with forceful bodily movement is clear to any intruder approaching a guard dog, just as the insecure yapping of a separation-anxious dog is clearly understood as a distress call for social contact.

Often the precise meaning of any particular segment of barking depends on the presence of additional context-related information specifying a more exact delineation of the intent motivating the barking behavior—for example, the dog barking to be let outdoors may also scratch at the door. Fox (1978) has interpreted the hypertrophy of canine barking behavior in terms of an expanding set of situations in which the bark is used as a signal. As a result, the meaning of the dog's bark has suffered in terms of specificity, making it necessary to incorporate other supplemental signals to help specify a more exact intention and meaning. These supplemental signals belong to other sensory modalities (e.g., sight, smell, and touch). Barking, from this perspective, is a general means of attracting attention to more specific communicative signals. However, this altered function of barking is far from meaningless, but significantly extends—rather than limits—the dog's ability to communicate. Barking is not an arbitrary activity, but a highly adapted communicative system used to express various intentions or states of alarm, conflict, and need.

Many dogs exhibit an almost compulsive urge to investigate and scent mark the environment with urine. Such excessive urinary scent marking is not observed among wolves. Although an urge to communicate appears to motivate the habit, the precise meaning and purpose of scent marking by dogs is not known. Scott (1967) has argued that canine scent marking does not serve a territorial

function, but rather functions more or less to communicate that the dog has been recently in the area. Overmarking may be used by a dog to personalize its surroundings, thereby making them more familiar and secure. If there is an anxiety-reducing aspect associated with scent marking, it may help to explain the often excessive character of such behavior and some common behavior problems associated with it. Recent studies involving stray and feral dogs indicate that, under "natural" conditions, scent marking and territorial defense may assume a more wolflike character among such dogs (Font, 1987; Boitani et al., 1996). Among wolves, scent marking is associated with the declaration of territorial rights or rank (Peters and Mech, 1975). Their urinary scent marking occurs most frequently during the breeding season and is the prerogative of the alpha male and female. Subordinates usually urinate by squatting.

Besides the aforementioned social and territorial functions of lupine scent marking, Harrington (1981) has found that urine marking is also employed by wolves to identify emptied caches of food. He observed wolf urine marking activity around caches that he had prepared by digging large holes and placing several chicks into them. He observed that wolves rarely (and then, perhaps, by mistake) urinated on caches containing food, whereas they consistently urinated on caches emptied of their content. The empty cache often was marked rapidly (within a minute or so) after it was emptied, usually by another wolf. Harrington speculates that such urine marking is employed to render exploitation of caches more efficient. The smell of urine signals to foraging wolves that no more food is available in the cache despite the presence of lingering food odors.

Another behavioral area where dogs significantly differ from wolves involves the display of aggressive behavior patterns. An average dog is much more docile, submissive, and trainable than a wolf. These qualities make dogs more responsive and adjustable to life in close association with humans. Although domestic dogs are not entirely free of troublesome dominance testing and even aggression, wolves, on reaching sexual and social maturity, tend to compete much more aggressively and earnestly for social status. The fighting styles of dogs and wolves differ significantly. Dogs, for instance, tend to limit their attacks to the head, neck, and shoulder. Wolves, on the other hand, make greater use of body blocks and, during damaging fights, may attack extremities—injuries to which render an opponent very vulnerable. Another important difference between wolves and dogs is the latter's social openness and tolerance toward strangers. Dogs are typically much more friendly toward strangers than are wolves, and appear to treat outsiders as members of an extended pack-family, whereas wolves become progressively xenophobic and intolerant of strangers not belonging to their immediate pack.

An important influence of domestication on the behavior of dogs is the attenuation of predatory instincts. Wolves possess a set of innate predatory behavior patterns that are readily evoked by an adequate stimulus. When presented with a prey animal, wolves respond in a species-typical manner by emitting an appropriate series of behavioral sequences, ranging from crouching, stalking, worrying, charging, pouncing, biting, and shaking. Faced with the same prey stimulus, dogs may do little more than play or tease the target animal. The *predatory response* of the wolf is so constant and uniform that the relative amount of lupine heredity expressed in a wolf-dog can be roughly estimated by comparing its behavior with a wolf serving as a control (E. Klinghammer, personal communication). The display of predatory behavior by wolf-dog hybrids is of considerable concern, especially with regard to young children who, in their awkward movements and screaming, may appear as distressed prey to a poorly socialized hybrid.

Many authorities have speculated that wolves are more intelligent than dogs, sometimes attributing this alleged difference to the fact that wolves must "work" for their living. Another line of reasoning correlates variations in proportional brain sizes with relative intelligence. Hemmer (1983/1990) has estimated that the domestic dog's brain is 25% to 45% smaller than the brain of the northern wolf (*Canis lupus lupus*), depending on several genetic and habitat (geographic and climatic)

variables. The majority of European breeds are ranked at an intermediate level, ranging between 25% and 35% smaller than the wolf. A great deal of variation exists among the various breeds, but none of the modern breeds exhibit a brain size (relative to bodily proportions) comparable to the northern wolf varieties. Although these measurements are very suggestive and statistically significant, differences in intelligence can not be directly extrapolated on the basis of brain size alone.

Although such speculation is fascinating, it may be more productive to study relative intelligence among canids by comparing their performance under controlled conditions and to discuss intelligence in terms of quantifiable learning skills and problem-solving abilities. Further, there may not exist a general intelligence factor per se, but rather a set of various talents or individual "intelligent" abilities. Frank and Frank (1983) have found that wolves perform problem solving and other insight-driven learning activities better than dogs, whereas dogs perform tasks involving rote learning and inhibition better than wolves. However, it should be noted that wolves are much more reactive to forceful handling than are dogs, the former being quick to deliver warning bites or to retreat whenever they are exposed to such treatment. Consequently, it is hard to judge from their experiment whether intelligence or reactive emotionality is being measured. Another possible factor confounding their results is the effect of competing species-typical avoidance reactions (Bolles, 1970), which are adjusted through domestication to a higher threshold in dogs than in wolves.

Other researchers have found a similar differentiation of learning abilities in wolves and dogs as that reported by the Franks above. For example, Hemmer (1983/1990) found clear differences between dogs and wolves in problem-solving abilities. In his simple test, animals were tethered in front of a short length of cord that was attached to a piece of food placed just out of their reach. By manipulating the cord, the subjects could pull the food toward themselves and eat it. Most of the dogs tested eventually solved the problem, given enough time. The wolves solved the problem rapidly, with some of them solving the problem without hesitation on their first attempt—an apparent display of insight that was not exhibited by any of the dogs. Mech reports an anecdote involving a high degree of insight learning in a wolf who had learned how to escape from his pen:

> Once a wolf has learned how to escape from a pen, for example, it is almost impossible to keep the animal in. One such escape artist I knew learned to raise a drop door in its pen by jumping to the top of the eight-foot-high pen, and grabbing with its teeth the door cable on the outside of the pen, which was exposed to the inside through a three-inch gap. By jumping up and grabbing the cable, the wolf could lift the door at the bottom of the cage. After the wolf raised the door many times, it stuck in the "up" position, and the wolf ran out! (1991:26)

Humphrey and Warner (1934) reported early efforts to train wolf-dog hybrids for police and military work. They found that the hybrids did well on leash, but became uncontrollable when they were worked off-leash. Macintosh (1975) found that dingoes are virtually untrainable in obedience. Even the intensive efforts of well-experienced police dog trainers were unable to obtain "anything resembling obedience" in dingoes.

Paedomorphosis

Many of the changes occurring as a result of domestication appear to involve the prolongation of puppylike or juvenile characteristics into adulthood. The overall outcome is a neotenization of the wild prototype—a process in which maturity is developmentally delayed and growth rates altered (Fox, 1967). In many ways, an adult dog behaves and looks like a juvenile wolf. All of these characteristics (soft coat, curled tail, skinfolds, floppy ears, and short legs) give the domestic dog a puppylike appearance when compared with the wild visage of the wolf. Among the most neotenous of the modern breeds are various Eastern "toys" like the Pekingese, shih-tzu, and Japanese spaniel. These breeds are not only socially dependent and diminutive, they are soft and cuddly to touch and can be easily held on the lap or embraced like a baby. Behaviorally, they are very receptive to the admiring attention of their human keepers and happily entertain hours of affectionate handling and petting. In addition, such toy breeds exhibit other notable infantile characteristics that invite parental care, including protuberant and tearing eyes, brachycephalism (extreme shortening of the muzzle), short legs, a "cute" curly tail, and floppy ears.

Along with the aforementioned structural changes, several behavioral changes can be detected in the direction of youthfulness. These behaviors are usually exaggerated forms of neonatal behavior topographies normally perpetuated into adult behavior and integrated into the animal's social signaling system. Zimen (reported by Fox, 1971) has compared the emergence of social behavior in the wolf and the domestic dog (standard poodle). He found that dogs exhibit a pronounced delay of social spacing, as defined by social distance and the number of direct contacts between conspecifics, in comparison to the time table followed by wolves. By 6 months of age, wolves begin to distance themselves from other conspecifics, whereas a corresponding behavior does not appear in dogs until 12 months of age. By the time wolves are 18 months old, they exhibit adult-like independence under open-field conditions, ranging far and wide from companions. Poodles, on the other hand, were never observed to split off from group members for any length of time.

On the whole, domestic dogs appear in many respects to act like 4- to 6-month-old wolf puppies. This tendency is also reflected in patterns of daily activity. Adult wolves tend to follow a crepuscular pattern of activity, being most active in the early morning and evening, whereas the young wolves exhibit a more erratic activity pattern, moving more rapidly from periods of rest to activity than the adults. Adult poodles are much more like immature wolves in this regard, being more easily aroused into spontaneous activity than adult wolves. Zimen interprets these developmental differences as a paedomorphic phenomenon resulting from the dog's domestication.

Zimen (1987) has also noted that dogs are distinguished from wolves by the ease with which dogs form social affiliations with humans. Wolves only form social bonds with humans in the absence of adult conspecifics and fear. Dogs, on the other hand, readily form such attachments, often preferring human contact over contact with conspecifics when given the choice. Zimen concludes that besides "reducing flight tendencies, domestication has thus strongly increased the motivation to seek social contact with man" (1987:290). Although wolves can be tamed and socialized to a great extent, they never attain the full range of social responsiveness that is exhibited by most domestic dogs. When the two species are compared as adults, dogs appear to be much more playful and socially flexible than wolves. Social "promiscuity" is an innate temperament feature of dogs that has resulted from many generations of unconscious selection for reduced agonistic behavior and playfulness:

> Unlike the wolf, many dogs show not the least wariness towards strange people, and immediately accept them, showing passive and active submission behaviour. This type of dog—its temperament and general demeanor—certainly resembles that of a five-week-old puppy or wolf cub trustingly accepting all comers. It is not inconceivable that this behavioural paedomorphosis, or perpetuation of infantile behaviour patterns into adulthood, and the absence of fear of strangers are the result of generations of domestication, facilitated by early socialization to a wide variety of people in different social situations. ... This "wariness", which is so characteristic of the wild temperament of the wolf, appears to have been selectively eliminated in many breeds of domesticated dog. (Fox, 1971:154)

Frank and Frank (1982) have confirmed many of Zimen's observations regarding the behavioral neotenization of domestic dogs and have contributed several interesting findings of their own. In their study, the development of the malamute and the wolf were carefully compared along several behavioral dimensions. Considerable differences between the two animals were observed in general activity and sleep-wake patterns, aggres-

sion and agonistic play, the degree of sexual dimorphism, ritualized aggression, and dominance ranking. Malamutes tended to lag developmentally behind wolf pups up until around 10 weeks of age, when the earlier motor differences disappear. Socially, the malamutes were found to be more outgoing and receptive to social contact with people than were the wolf pups. Unlike the malamutes, who actively solicited attention and contact with people, the wolf pups exhibited varying degrees of wariness, avoidance responding, and flight behavior from weeks 6 to 8 onward. In general, wolf pups exhibited a definite social preference for contact with other canids (in spite of having received greater amounts of direct socialization with human handlers), whereas the malamutes displayed a stronger preference for human contact than for canine contact. The malamutes also tended to be much more independent of the foster mother than were the wolf pups. Although the malamutes exhibited a friendly, deferential excitement toward the foster mother on her return after a brief period of separation, human handlers were met with an effusive and prolonged "greeting frenzy" not displayed otherwise.

The general activity level of malamutes during the first 6 weeks of life was much lower in comparison to that of wolves. The malamutes slept longer and more deeply than wolf puppies. The wolf pups engaged in more exploratory behavior of various kinds, ranging from "manipulating, dragging, chewing, stalking, shredding or carrying objects." An unexpected finding was the high degree of intense aggressive behavior exhibited by malamute puppies as early as 2 weeks of age and the delayed appearance of agonistic play until around week 4 or 5. Social interaction between wolf pups peaked around 8 weeks of age and then progressively declined, whereas such interaction steadily increased among malamutes through the age of 4 months. Active and passive submission behaviors were exhibited by the wolf pups during greeting rituals, begging displays, and play, but were not exhibited in response to dominance challenges by adults until after the pups were 12 weeks of age. Some sexually dimorphic tendencies were also evident in the behavior of malamutes that were not exhibited by wolf pups. Female malamutes tended to be less aggressive, less socially assertive and demanding of attention, and less competitive over food and toys. Hart and Hart (1985) have noted a similar distribution of behavior along sexually dimorphic lines in a wide variety of domestic dog breeds.

Among several highly adaptive domestic features exhibited by the malamutes, the researchers found that the dog puppies were more fastidious and careful to avoid fecal material than were wolf pups. They speculate that unconscious selection pressures may have contributed to the malamute's high degree of cleanliness. The malamutes deposited their feces well away from their immediate nesting area from 32 days onward. Also, during feeding, the malamutes were more receptive to bottle nursing and accepted the transition to solid food more rapidly. An interesting feature distinguishing the malamute from wolf pups is the former's conspicuous appearance of immaturity and marked motor awkwardness in comparison with the wolf. As previously noted, the malamutes are more quiet and "peaceful" as puppies, spending more of their time sleeping or resting. The resultant image is one of helplessness and innocence: "In a sense, man has created the domestic pup in the image of an idealized infant" (Frank and Frank, 1982:515). The authors speculate that the prolongation of these qualities in domestic puppies facilitates greater attention, protection, and nutrition from their caretakers. An important feature of prolonged immaturity, vulnerability, and dependency is the establishment of a strong affectional bond between the "parent" and the animal, thereby forming a secure foundation for a lasting relationship along with many significant biological advantages. Interestingly, Frank and Frank (1982) note in this regard that the wolf foster mother showed a definite preference for the easier to manage and "cuter" malamutes. She washed them more frequently, spent much more time with them (two to three times as much), was more protective against intruders, exhibited more distress when separated from them, and played more often and longer with them than with the wolf pups.

Coppinger and associates (Coppinger et al., 1987; Coppinger and Schneider, 1996) have studied the effects of neoteny on the evolution of working dogs. They have argued against a trait-by-trait accumulation of breed characteristics in favor of a more generalized process of biological change. According to this theory, early selective pressures were focused more on general behavioral tendencies like tameness and utilitarian function than specific physical characteristics. Apparently, these early breeding efforts were guided by a "form follows function" philosophy. Only after the functional behavioral phenotype had been well established did breeding efforts turn to the refinement of appearances and conformation to type. These behavioral phenotypic changes were largely the result of neotenization. Typically, traits that are associated with tameness (playfulness, dependency, and care seeking) in adult domestic dogs are traits exhibited by juvenile and adolescent wolves. A factor of considerable importance in the process of neoteny is the timing of sexual maturity. There appears to be some linkage between precocious sexual maturity in dogs and the retardation of adult wolflike behavior patterns. An important result of early sexual maturation is the concordant appearance of loosely organized, playful patterns of behavior that resist articulation into phylogenetically functional motor sequences as expressed by adult wolves. These loosely organized neotenic behavioral patterns make domestic dogs much more receptive to training and socialization than are wolves. According to Coppinger's theory, working dogs (sled dogs, livestock-guarding dogs, and herding dogs) are distinguished by their relative degree of neoteny. For example, without the attenuation of aggressive tendencies and the simultaneous potentiation of a playful willingness to pull, sled dogs would not prove to be very effective workers. In the case of sheepdogs, livestock-guarding dogs must be protective but not aggressive toward the sheep in their care. Guarding dogs are considered to be more neotenous than herding dogs, who display some predatory elements like showing "eye," "stalking," and "chasing"—that is, more adult wolflike predatory traits. Although herding dogs exhibit predatory motor sequences, they do not culminate in actual biting or killing.

THE SILVER FOX: A POSSIBLE MODEL OF DOMESTICATION

The process of behavioral and physical paedomorphosis has been observed experimentally in the selective breeding of silver foxes carried out by the Russian geneticist D. K. Belyaev and his associates at the Institute of Cytology and Genetics in Siberia (Trut, 1999). Belyaev (1979) speculated that the dog's early domestication proceeded "unconsciously" by selecting and breeding captive animals that exhibited a high tolerance for fear and a minimal tendency to behave aggressively toward humans. To test this hypothesis, Belyaev initiated a long-term genetics project in which foxes were selectively bred for tameness. The project has been ongoing for 40 years and has produced over 40,000 foxes. An important early finding was that ordinary farm-bred foxes exhibit a wide variability with regard to their response to human contact. He has estimated that approximately 30% of the farm-bred population is extremely aggressive, 20% fearful, and 40% aggressive-fearful, whereas the remaining 10% exhibit a quiet (neither fearful nor aggressive) exploratory behavior toward people. The foxes belonging to the quiet group are by no means tame or safe to handle, however.

The breeding program involved carefully selecting only those foxes that exhibited a prosocial "tame" response to human contact and handling. After fewer than 20 generations of selective breeding, tame foxes began to appear that exhibited striking physical and behavioral alterations in comparison to randomly bred counterparts (Fig. 1.6). Tame foxes are not only tolerant of human contact, they actively solicit and appear to enjoy social interaction with human handlers. Tame foxes engage in various doglike behaviors, including hand and face licking, solicitous jumping up, vigorous tail wagging, and excited vocalizations (e.g., barking)—all reminiscent of domestic dogs. The physical appearance of tame foxes has also undergone dramatic paedomorphic and doglike changes that include

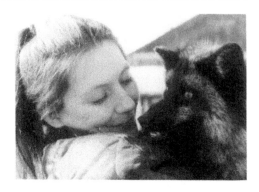

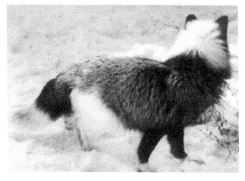

FIG. 1.6. Tame foxes are affectionate and invite contact with human handlers. Among several physical characteristics that distinguish tame foxes from farm-bred counterparts is a piebald pelage. (Photos courtesy L. N. Trut, Institute of Cytology and Genetics).

lop ears, a turned-up tail (a doglike characteristic not observed in wild foxes), and the development of piebald pelage. Such white spotting is commonly seen in a variety of domestic species and is highly correlated with tameness. Little (1920) has discussed the hereditary basis of piebald spotting in dogs, concluding that it may be a "mutational" change rather than a gradual one occurring as the result of selection pressures.

In addition to behavioral and morphological changes, Belyaev's tame foxes also underwent several concurrent physiological alterations. For instance, tame female foxes exhibit significant deviations from the norm in terms of their sexual readiness and behavior, becoming sexually receptive earlier in the year than is the custom among wild foxes. Endocrine studies have demonstrated that gonadal hormone activity in tame foxes is altered, perhaps underlying and guiding the observed behavioral changes. As is commonly observed among most domestic dogs (but not wild ones), some tame foxes actually produce offspring twice a year. In spite of increased receptivity, however, as many as 30% to 40% of the females fail to reproduce successfully. Tame females either fail to actually produce offspring or display disturbances in maternal behavior, including a tendency to neglect their young or to kill and eat them (infantiphagia). Hediger (1955/1968) has noted similar degenerative effects in the maternal behavior of other domestic species. Another seasonal activity affected by domestication is molting. Tame foxes exhibit a protracted period of shedding—a destabilizing effect that may be genetically linked to the disruption of estrous cycles.

Several neurophysiological concomitants of domestication have been isolated in tame foxes. Belyaev's associates have found significant alterations of the relative reactivity of the hypothalamic-pituitary-adrenocortical (HPA) system of tame foxes in comparison to wild counterparts. By comparing the reactions of tame and wild foxes to emotionally provocative experiences, they have determined that the tame foxes are less reactive to stressful experiences than are wild ones. Also, interesting changes have been found in brain areas associated with the expression of emotion. Serotonin levels in the brain tissue of tame foxes are significantly higher than in wild counterparts. Popova and colleagues (1991) confirmed these early findings, having isolated significant alterations throughout the serotonergic system in the brains of domesticated foxes. Serotonin has been shown to be an important neuromodulator providing inhibitory regulation over stress-related behavior and aggression. Popova and colleagues have speculated that many of the behavioral and physiological changes (e.g., polyestrous tendency and reduced HPA system reactivity) observed in tame foxes may be causally linked with alterations in these serotonergic systems.

Selection for tameness among silver foxes has also produced changes in catecholaminergic systems. For example, tame foxes exhibit an increase of norepinephrine and dopamine activity in critical brain centers associated with the expression of defensive behavior. Dygalo and Kalinina (1994) have demonstrated a significant increase of tyrosine hydrolase activity in the brains of tame foxes in comparison to wild controls. Tyrosine hydrolase is the rate-limiting factor determining the amount of dopamine and norepinephrine that can be produced by the brain. The authors conclude that variations observed in the production of this essential enzyme is caused by a genetic alteration of the catecholaminergic system itself—a direct result of selective breeding for tameness. Similar comparisons have not been made between dogs and wolves. This line of research is of great importance for a better understanding of the mechanisms controlling defensive behavior at the neural level and may ultimately lead to productive insights into the etiology and management of canine aggression and fear-related behavior problems.

SELECTIVE BREEDING, THE DOG FANCY, AND THE FUTURE

Whether consciously or unconsciously, selective breeding has been going on for many thousands of years, resulting in the genetic engineering of as many as 400 distinct dog breeds worldwide. Most of these breeds have been bred with some specific intention in mind, frequently a practical function like hunting, shepherding, and guarding. The earliest known breeds appear in the historical record around 3000 BP in Egypt. They are of a greyhound type and were probably specialized hunting hounds used for coursing game. The Assyrians had developed a much larger mastiff-type dog useful for hunting in dense cover.

Origins of Selective Breeding

According to Clutton-Brock (1984), the Romans were the first to breed dogs systematically on a large scale and to keep detailed records about the various breeds they kept. The Romans knew that selective breeding could affect physical appearance and behavior. By this time, all of the major breed types were well established (e.g., guard, hunting, coursing, shepherd, and lap dogs) and it was recognized that training was needed to properly fit form to function. The Greeks had also applied themselves to the selective breeding of dogs long before the rise of the Romans. Already in Homer's *The Odyssey* (Fitzgerald, 1963) clear distinctions are made between working dogs and pets. In the famous dialogue between Odysseus and Eumaisos, the hero (concealing his true feelings at the moment in order to maintain his disguise) comments on the topic as he looks upon his dying dog:

> I marvel that they leave this hound to lie
> here on the dung pile;
> he would have been a fine dog, from the look
> of him,
> though I can't say as to his power and speed
> when he was young. You find the same good
> build
> in house dogs, table dogs landowners keep
> all for style. (1963:320)

Not only had the Greeks understood the importance of selective breeding at an early date, they had also recognized the danger of breeding that displaces function for the sake of appearances.

By the 5th century BC, various breeds had been developed for specific hunting tasks and purposes. Xenophon, a student of Socrates, wrote an important essay around 380 BC on hunting and hunting dogs, entitled *Cynegeticus* (1925/1984). The tract gives one a rare glimpse into the breeding and training of Greek hunting dogs. For hunting hare and driving the quarry into nets, the Castorian and vulpine breeds were favored. Deer hunting required bigger and stronger breeds like the Indian hounds (mastiff-type dogs). For wild-boar hunting, a variety of dogs were employed in a mixed pack, including the Indian, Cretan, Locrian, and Laconian breeds. The vulpine breed, as its name implies, was believed by Xenophon to be the result of crossbreeding a dog with a fox. Clearly, great care was taken to keep these breeds unadulterated. Xenophon describes the use of a wide surcingle (girth strap), apparently used to prevent undesirable matings:

> The straps of the surcingles should be broad, so as not to rub the flanks, and they should have little spurs sewed into them, to keep the breed pure. (1925/1984:401)

Merlin (1971) has speculated that another function of this piece of equipment was to protect dogs from injury when hunting dangerous game like wild boar.

In the *Republic*, Plato (1961) outlines a concise description of the selective breeding process:

> Tell me this, Glaucon. I see that you have in your house hunting dogs and a number of pedigreed cocks. Have you ever considered something about their unions and procreations?
> What? he said.
> In the first place, I said, among these themselves, although they are a select breed, do not some prove better than the rest?
> They do.
> Do you then breed from all indiscriminately, or are you careful to breed from the best?
> From the best.
> And, again, do you breed from the youngest or the oldest, or, so far as may be, from those in their prime.
> From those in their prime.
> And if they are not thus bred, you expect, do you not, that your birds' breed and hounds will greatly degenerate?
> I do, he said. (*Rep*, 5:459a)

Information about dog breeding in the remote past is scant and unreliable, but certainly strong selection pressures were at work over the course of the dog's domestication.

The rise of breeding for the sake of appearances alone is a relatively new phenomenon in the history of dogs, coinciding with the appearance of organized dog showing and efforts to standardize the various breeds. This new emphasis and interest appeared shortly after the banning of dog fighting and bull baiting in England in 1835—an event closely associated with the founding of the Royal Society for the Prevention of Cruelty to Animals in 1824. With the loss of these traditional forms of canine "entertainment," the public turned its attention toward other venues for the enjoyment of dogs.

These various cultural changes moved dogs out of the hands of the lower working classes and placed them (after a transition of "proper" breeding) on a "higher" social level. The Victorian bourgeoisie adopted the dog as a newfound status object with which they could proudly display their refined taste in the form of breeding and pedigree (Ritvo, 1986). Along with this preoccupation with status came an effort to standardize the various breeds—a process based largely on appearances, with an inevitable neglect of function. Unfortunately, it is hard to separate fact from fiction with regard to the history of these various breeds, since many of their historical origins appear to be fanciful 19th-century fabrications. According to Ritvo (1987), most of the modern breeds as they are recognized today are little more than 100 to 150 years old. She notes that even the early breed standards were written almost from scratch. This observation reflects the tremendous influence that the Victorian-era dog fancy had on the development of modern dogs, especially with respect to their appearance. Clearly, though, most of the common breeds associated with purebred dogs were already well established as working dogs prior to this time, as one can readily observe in V. Shaw's histories, descriptions, and engravings included in *The Illustrated Book of the Dog,* published as a serial between 1879 and 1881.

Of course, many efforts to breed for physical appearances had occurred long before the 19th century, but never to an extent comparable to the contemporary efforts involving so many diverse breeds. In China, for instance, the Pekingese was carefully managed under the protection and patronage of the Manchu emperors. The original stock was bred with an eye toward both form and function, producing a dog of exquisite beauty, vigor, and intelligence; these animals frequently lived full and healthy lives for up to 25 years, in spite of their genetically induced physical deformities (Tuan, 1984).

Undoubtedly, appearance has always played an important role in the selection process, but it was rightfully subordinated to the far more important goals embodied in utilitarian function, health, and temperament. Many experienced breeders have lamented the genetic fact that form and function rarely interact in felicitous proportions—good working dogs are more often than not "ugly" according to breed standards of beauty. With an eye set rigidly on the arbitrary appeal of appearances and beautiful form, the qualities of intelligence and function inevitably degrade over time. Konrad Lorenz expresses a similar conclusion in *Man Meets Dog*:

> It is a sad but undeniable fact that breeding to a strict standard of physical points is incompatible with breeding for mental qualities. Individuals which conform to both sets of requirements are so rare that they would not even supply a foundation for the further propagation of their breed. ... I know of no "champion" of any dog breed which I should ever wish to own myself. It is not that these two differently directed ideals are basically opposed to one another. It is hard to understand why a dog of perfect physique should not be endowed with equally desirable mental attributes—but each of the two ideals is, in itself, so rare that their combination in one and the same individual becomes a thing of the grossest improbability. (1954:93)

The first organized dog show took place during the summer of 1859 in Newcastle-upon-Tyne, England (Davis, 1970). By 1873, the British Kennel Club was organized to regulate the breeding and exhibition of purebred dogs. Shortly thereafter, the American Kennel Club (AKC) (1884) was formed in Philadelphia as the ruling body over affiliated breed clubs in the United States. The first organized dog show in the United States was sponsored by the Westminster Kennel Club in 1877. The original purpose of the AKC was stated to be the "protection and advancement" of purebred dogs, but many critics have questioned whether the AKC really has fulfilled these promises. Whatever deserving faults and shortcomings, without the organized international efforts of dog fanciers and organizations like the AKC, a great many currently well-established and flourishing breeds might have otherwise gone extinct over the past century.

Prospects for the Future

Breeding carried out under the stewardship of responsible breeders has undoubtedly resulted in the genetic improvement of dogs in the dual directions of appearance and performance—if not in health and biological fitness (see below). Unfortunately, dogs bred by such breeders are registered on an equal basis with dogs bred indiscriminately by dilettantes and uncaring pet merchants. With the advent of large shopping centers, multibreed pet stores followed, carrying a variety of breeds for sale under a single roof. The public setting of these stores took advantage of high foot traffic and the impulsive buying habits evoked by the sight of a lonely puppy curled up behind a window. To stock these stores with puppies in sufficient variety and quantity at the lowest possible prices, the store buyers sought inexpensive wholesale sources to meet a burgeoning market. This excluded established breeders since they are usually unwilling to deal with pet retailers, or since the cost of acquiring well-bred puppies would make resale only marginally profitable. Consequently, an "industry" of commercial puppy breeding erupted (mainly in the Midwestern section of the country) producing puppies in great numbers and frequently under appalling conditions with little regard for established breeding practices. Unfortunately, these "milled" puppies are accepted and certified as purebred by the same registry (the AKC) as are their most carefully selected and conscientiously bred counterparts. The pet stores benefit greatly from this arrangement since registered purebred puppies are worth considerably more money on the retail market than are puppies sold without "papers."

This general situation is aggravated by a large population of dogs produced by average breeders whose aspirations may not extend much beyond the opportunity to supplement the family income. These so-called "backyard breeders" often neglect temperament, function, and appearances altogether. Using newspaper classified ads as their primary means of marketing, they can avoid the stigma of being associated with a pet store—but their "product" is rarely much better in quality. Producing dogs in such a way is much less expensive than carefully breeding them for excellence of form, function, and health. Consequently, professional breeders are frequently faced with an unfair disadvantage. Breeding quality dogs is an expensive enterprise. Although securing a profit is secondary to a love of the breed, the lament of many dedicated breeders is that it is not possible under current conditions to breed quality dogs and also to survive as a business. Of course, a great number of dedicated and responsible breeders have survived, and their efforts help to keep things in check, but their numbers may be dwindling in a marketplace where it is hard for them to compete.

The incidence of genetic disease is increasing, and the prospects for the future are dim unless coordinated efforts are orchestrated toward the combined goals of education and professional responsibility in dog breeding. Several laudable efforts are under way that may eventually help to mollify the current situation. For many years, screening has been available for the detection of several genetically transmitted diseases, especially eye disorders and hip dysplasia. Certification by the Canine Eye Registration Foundation (CERF) and the Orthopedic Foundation for Animals (OFA) should be required of all breeding stock prone to the expression of such disorders. A potentially beneficial project has been developed by Jasper Rine at the University of California–Berkeley. Rine and associates have launched an effort to map the evolution of various dog breeds. A possible eventual application of the Dog Genome Project is the identification of the specific genes involved in the transmission of behavioral disorders and genetic diseases. Another dog genome project is being led by George Brewer at the University of Michigan where DNA diagnostics are being studied and developed into a private diagnostics company. An important project for tracking genetic disease is the Canine Genetic Disease Information System (CGDIS), a computer software package developed under the guidance of Donald Paterson at the University of Pennsylvania. Finally, the Institute for Genetic Disease Control in Animals at the University of California–Davis is an open registry for dogs and other animals with genetic disease. Unfortunately, the impact of these tools will be evident only among responsible breeders (who are not the problem) and will not likely reach those who care nothing about the welfare of dogs and whose interest extends little beyond profitable merchandising of their AKC-registered purebred puppies.

There exists substantial disagreement with regard to the possible genetic transmission of temperament traits and behavioral disorders among dogs. However, mounting evidence suggests that some forms of dominance aggression are genetically transmitted. A possible case in point is the so-called "springer rage syndrome," or what may be more appropriately termed "low-threshold dominance aggression." Low-threshold dominance aggression is a behavioral disorder of the English springer spaniel that affects many otherwise loving and companionable dogs. Ilana Reisner at Cornell University (personal communication) has found evidence suggesting that this genetically transmitted behavioral predisposition may be traced to a single kennel. She is currently analyzing pedigrees and other statistical evidence from a large survey of Springer spaniel owners that may help to elucidate the exact mechanism of transmission more fully in the future. For now, however, the "popular sire effect" appears to be a highly plausible explanation. The popular sire effect occurs when a particularly desirable show dog is bred over and over again for some set of physical attributes, but who, in addition, may carry hidden in his genome an undesirable physical or behavioral trait that also gets haphazardly passed along in the gene pool as well. The opportunity for genetic disaster is particularly ominous in such cases. Given that a trait conducive to dominance aggression is traceable to a single kennel, one can reasonably infer that a small founder population (perhaps, even a single popular sire) is responsible for the trait's spread into the springer population. It is less likely that a "popular" dam acted as the primary catalyst, simply because of her limited reproductive potential.

Helmut Hemmer (1983/1990) has studied the genetic trend toward degeneracy and sensory disability in the dog. By comparing the sensory and behavioral abilities of the domestic dog with that of the wolf, Hemmer found that the dog has been "damaged" on many sensory and behavioral levels. In addition to the health costs associated with domestication, the dog's sensory abilities, along with many innate behavioral systems and mechanisms, have suffered under the pressure of artificial selection. The dog has experienced a general decline of what Hemmer has termed "environmental appreciation." Environmental appreciation refers to the sum input and organization of sensory information, that is, the animal's perceptual experience or gestalt. Various sensory mechanisms and underlying neural structures are involved, profoundly influencing the quality and intensity of the dog's perceptual experience. In short, domestication has narrowed the range and quality of the dog's senses, thereby adversely affecting the quality of its life.

While current breeding practices have undoubtedly contributed to the dog's contemporary decline in health and temperament, the effects of domestication—even when guided under the best intentions—are inherently degenerative with regard to the natural prototype being genetically modified to match human purposes. Clearly, the dog enjoys a biological advantage over its wild progenitor in terms of survival rate and raw numbers. But this reproductive success is at the cost of biological soundness and is fraught with dangers associated with overspecialization and close breeding, e.g., genetic drift and founder's effect. Over 400 genetic diseases have been isolated in the dog with about 10 new ones being described each year (Smith, 1994). The degenerative effects of domestication are a natural outcome of the dog's "protected" status, and may not be entirely attributable to breeding practices alone. Unlike wild canids, the dog's biological success or failure is not dependent on "fitness" in the broad sense demanded by nature, but by an arbitrary set of demands related to a narrow ecological niche in cohabitation with man's. Darwin reflected on these various dangers associated with domestication:

It can, also, be clearly shown that man, without any intention or thought of improving the breed, by preserving in each successive generation the individuals which he prizes most, and by destroying the worthless individuals, slowly, though surely, induces great changes. As the will of man thus comes into play we can understand how it is that domestic races of animals and cultivated plants often exhibit an abnormal character, as compared with natural species; for they have been modified not for their own benefit, but for that of man. (1875/1988:3)

The most important lesson to be learned from these trends is that breeding must be carried out with great care and attention to the whole dog, not just the way it looks.

REFERENCES

Alberch Pere (1986). Possible dogs. *Nat Hist*, 12:4–8.

Beck AM (1973). *The Ecology of Stray Dogs: A Study of Free-Ranging Urban Animals.* Baltimore: York.

Bekoff M (1977) Social communication in canids: Evidence for the evolution of a stereotyped mammalian display. *Science*, 197:1097–1099.

Belyaev DK (1979). Destabilizing selection as a factor in domestication. *J Hered*, 70:301–308.

Boitani L, Francisci F, and Ciucci P (1996). Population biology and ecology of feral dogs in central Italy. In J Serpell (Ed), *The Domestic Dog: Its Evolution, Behaviour, and Interaction with People.* New York: Cambridge University Press.

Bolles RC (1970). Species-specific defense reactions and avoidance learning. *Psychol Rev*, 77:32–48.

Brisbin IL, Risch TS (1997). Primitive dogs, their ecology and behavior: Unique opportunities to study the early development of the human-canine bond. *JAVMA*, 210:1122–1126.

Bueler LE (1973). *Wild Dogs of the World.* New York: Stein and Day.

Clifford DH and Green KA (1991). Chief: Attempted adoption of a wolf-hybrid led to tragedy. *Pet Vet*, Sept/Oct:19.

Clutton-Brock J (1984). Dog. In IL Mason (Ed), *Evolution of Domesticated Animals.* London: Longman.

Clutton-Brock J (1996). Origins of the dog: Domestication and early history. In J Serpell (Ed), *The Domestic Dog: Its Evolution, Behaviour, and Interactions with People*, 6–20. New York: Cambridge University Press.

Clutton-Brock J and Jewell P (1993). Origin and domestication of the dog. In HE Evans (Ed), *Miller's Anatomy of the Dog*, 3rd Ed, 21–31. Philadelphia: WB Saunders.

Coppinger R and Feinstein M (1991). 'Hark! hark! the dogs do bark...' and bark and bark. *Smithsonian*, 21:119–129.

Coppinger R and Schneider R (1996). Evolution of working dogs. In J Serpell (Ed), *The Domestic Dog: Its Evolution, Behaviour, and Interactions with People*, 21–47. New York: Cambridge University Press.

Coppinger R, Glendinning E, Torop E, et al. (1987). Degree of behavioral neoteny differentiates canid polymorphs. *Ethology*, 75:89–108.

Corbett LK (1995). *The Dingo in Australia and Asia.* Ithaca: Comstock/Cornell.

Corbett L and Newsome A (1975). Dingo society and its maintenance: A preliminary analysis. In MW Fox (Ed), *The Wild Canids: Their Systematics, Behavioral Ecology, and Evolution.* New York: Van Nostrand Reinhold.

Darwin C (1859/1962). *The Origin of Species by Means of Natural Selection or the Preservation of Favoured Races in the Struggle for Life.* New York: Collier (reprint).

Darwin C (1875/1988). The variation of animals and plants under domestication. In PH Barrett and RB Freeman (Eds), *The Works of Charles Darwin*, Vol 19. New York: New York University Press (reprint).

Davis HP (1970). *The New Dog Encyclopedia.* New York: Galahad.

Davis SJ and Valla FR (1978). Evidence for domestication of the dog 12,000 years ago in the Natufina of Israel. *Nature*, 276:608–610.

Dygalo NN and Kalinina TS (1994). Tyrosine hydroxylase activities in the brains of wild Norway rats and silver foxes selected for reduced aggressiveness towards humans. *Aggressive Behav*, 20:453–460.

Fiennes R and Fiennes A (1968). *The Natural History of Dogs.* New York: Bonanza.

Fitzgerald R (1963). *Homer: The Odyssey.* Garden City, NY: Anchor.

Font E (1987). Spacing and social organization: Urban stray dogs revisited. *Appl Anim Behav Sci*, 17:319–328.

Fox MW (1967). Influence of domestication upon behaviour of animals. *Vet Rec*, 80:696–702.

Fox MW (1971). *Behaviour of Wolves, Dogs and Related Canids.* New York: Harper and Row.

Fox MW (1978). *The Dog: Its Domestication and Behavior.* Malabar, FL: Krieger.

Frank H and Frank MG (1982). On the effects of domestication on canine social development and behavior. *Appl Anim Ethol*, 8:507–525.

Frank H and Frank MG (1983). Inhibition training in wolves and dogs. *Behav Processes*, 8:363–377.

Gould RA (1970). Journey to Pulykara. *Nat Hist*,

79:57–66.

Hamilton E and Cairns H (1961). *The Collected Dialogues of Plato.* Princeton: Princeton University Press.

Harrington FH (1981). Urine-marking and caching behavior in the wolf. *Behaviour,* 76:280–288.

Hart BL and Hart LA (1985). Selecting pet dogs on the basis of cluster analysis of breed behavior profiles and gender. *JAVMA,* 186:1181–1185.

Hediger H (1955/1968). *The Psychology and Behavior of Animals in Zoos and Circuses,* G Sircom (Trans). New York: Dover (reprint).

Hemmer H (1983/1990). *Domestication: The Decline of Environmental Appreciation.* Cambridge: Cambridge University Press (reprint).

Humphrey E and Warner L (1934). *Working Dogs.* Baltimore: Johns Hopkins Press.

Little CC (1920). A note on the origin of piebald spotting in dogs. *J Hered,* 11:12–15.

Lorenz K (1954). *Man Meets Dog.* Boston: Houghton Mifflin.

Lorenz K (1975). Foreword. In MW Fox (Ed), *The Wild Canids: Their Systematics, Behavioral Ecology and Evolution.* New York: Van Nostrand Reinhold.

Macintosh NWG (1975). The origins of dingo: An enigma. In MW Fox (Ed), *The Wild Canids: Their Systematics, Behavioral Ecology, and Evolution.* New York: Van Nostrand Reinhold.

Mech LD (1970). *The Wolf: The Ecology and Behavior of an Endangered Species.* Minneapolis: University of Minnesota Press.

Mech LD (1991). *The Way of the Wolf.* Stillwater, MN: Voyeur.

Meggitt MJ (1965). The association between Australian aborigines and dingoes. In A Leeds and AP Vayda (Eds), *Man, Culture, and Animals* (No. 78). Washington, DC: American Association for the Advancement of Science.

Merlin RHA (1971). *De Canibus: Dog and Hound in Antiquity.* London: JA Allen.

Morey DF (1992). Size, shape and development in the evolution of the domestic dog. *J Archaeol Sci,* 19:181–204.

Morey DF (1994). The early evolution of the domestic dog. *Am Sci,* 82:336–347.

Olsen SJ (1985). *Origins of the Domestic Dog.* Tucson: University of Arizona Press.

Olsen SJ and Olsen JW (1977). The Chinese wolf, ancestor of new world dogs. *Science* 197:533–535.

Peters RP and Mech DL (1975). Scent-marking in wolves. *Am Sci,* 63:628–637.

Plato (1961). *Republic.* In E Hamilton and H Cairns (Eds), *The Collected Dialogues of Plato.* Princeton: Princeton University Press.

Popova NK, Voitenko NN, Kulikov AV, and Avgustinovich DF (1991). Evidence for the involvement of central serotonin in mechanism of domestication of silver foxes. *Pharmacol Biochem Behav,* 40:751–756.

Price EO (1998). Behavioral genetics and the process of animal domestication. In T Grandin (Ed), *Genetics and the Behavior of Domestic Animals,* New York: Academic.

Protsch R and Berger R (1973). Earliest radiocarbon dates for domesticated animals. *Science,* 179:235–239.

Ritvo H (1986). Pride and pedigree: the evolution of the Victorian dog fancy. *Victorian Stud,* 29:227–253.

Ritvo H (1987). *The Animal Estate: The English and Other Creatures in the Victorian Age.* Cambridge: Harvard University Press.

Romanes GJ (1888). *Animal Intelligence.* New York: D Appleton.

Schenkel R (1967). Submission: Its features and function in the wolf and dog. *Am Zool,* 7:319–329.

Scott JP (1950). The social behavior of dogs and wolves: An illustration of sociobiological systematics. *Ann NY Acad Sci,* 51:1009–1021.

Scott JP (1967). The evolution of social behavior in dogs and wolves. *Am Zool,* 7:373–381.

Scott JP (1968). Evolution and domestication of the dog. *Evol Biol,* 2:243–275.

Serpell JA (1986/1996). *In the Company of Animals: A Study of Human-Animal Relationships.* New York: Cambridge University Press (reprint).

Shaw V. (1881/1984). *The Classic Encyclopedia of the Dog.* [originally published as *The Illustrated Book of the Dog*]. New York: Bonanza (reprint).

Smith CA (1994). New hope for overcoming canine inherited disease. *JAVMA,* 204:41.

Trumler E (1973). *Understanding Your Dog,* R Barry (Trans). London: Faber and Faber.

Trut LN (1999). Early canid domestication: The farm-fox experiment. Am Sci, 87:160–169.

Tuan Yi-Fu (1984). *Dominance and Affection: The Making of Pets.* New Haven: Yale University Press.

Varner JG and Varner JJ (1983). *Dogs of the Conquest.* Norman: University of Oklahoma Press.

Vila C, Savolainen P, Maldonado JE, and Amorin IR (1997). Multiple and ancient origins of the domestic dog. *Science,* 276:1687–1689.

Wayne RK (1993). Molecular evolution of the dog family. *Trends Genet,* 9:218–224.

Weidensaul S (1999). Tracking America's first dog. *Smithsonian,* 29:44–57.

Xenophon (1925/1984). Cynegeticus ("On Hunting"). In EC Marchant (Trans), *Xenophon: VII Scripta Minora.* Cambridge: Harvard University Press (reprint).

Young SP and Goldman EA (1944/1964). The Wolves of North America. Parts I and II. New York: Dover (reprint).

Zeuner FE (1963). *A History of Domesticated Animals.* London: Hutchinson (reprint).

Zimen E (1987). Ontogeny of approach and flight behavior towards humans in wolves, poodles and wolf-poodle hybrids. In H Frank (Ed), *Man and Wolf: Advances, Issues, and Problems in Captive Wolf Research.* Boston: Dr W Junk.

2

Development of Behavior

Organization is inseparable from adaptation: They are two complementary processes of a single mechanism, the first being the internal aspect of the cycle of which adaptation constitutes the external aspect.

J. PIAGET, *The Origins of Intelligence in Children* (1952)

DOG BEHAVIOR is determined by many interdependent biological and experiential factors. Although dogs are biologically prepared to develop in specific ways and to exhibit a limited set of potential traits and behavior patterns, the expression of these tendencies is flexible and subject to the general laws of learning. Even this adaptive *variability*, though, is ultimately limited by biological constraints. Besides the influence of genes and their biological expression, behavior is guided and modified by the influence of experience. The actualizing effect of the environment interacting with an animal's genetic potential or genotype yields its unique physical and behavioral phenotype. In contrast to the genotype, which remains outside the direct influence of learning, the phenotype results from the actualizing influences of the surrounding environment interfacing with the biologically mediated genome. These environmental circumstances can exercise either a beneficial or a destructive influence over the course of a puppy's development. General adaptation is continuously refined or rendered progressively dysfunctional depending on the type of experiences involved. Every moment offers the potential for constructive learning and adaptation or the reverse, especially in the case of an impressionable puppy.

If the environment provides a puppy with insufficient or inadequate experience for the development of a particular behavioral system, the innate behavior patterns and tendencies expressed by that system will atrophy or develop abnormally. The behavioral organization of the dog is a complex unity wherein various components are hierarchically integrated with one another at various levels. The proper functioning of one system of behavior depends on the support and adequate functioning of other systems. Early experiences are particularly influential in this regard. Puppies provided with poor socialization or deprived of environmental exposure often develop lifelong deficits and dysfunctional behaviors. A puppy isolated early in life from other puppies and humans will not only fail to establish satisfying social contact with conspecifics or enjoy companionship with people later in life (such puppies are extremely fearful of any social contact), they will also exhibit widespread behavioral and cognitive disabilities, as well. Isolated puppies exhibit poor learning and problem-solving abilities and are extremely hyperactive or rigidly inhibited, are emotionally overreactive and unable to encounter novel social or environmental situations without extreme fear and avoidance, and are socially and sexually incapacitated. Nearly every behavioral system is adversely affected, leaving the puppy encased within an autistic shell of fear, insular despair, and perpetual confusion.

The foregoing scenario is extreme and rarely observed outside the laboratory, but it does underscore the importance of early experience on the development of dog behavior. Although the vast majority of puppies are not exposed to such complete isolation, many do incur varying degrees of early social and environmental deprivation. Puppies bred under careless conditions where they are reared like livestock by irresponsible and ignorant breeders are topical cases in point. Such puppies are often exposed to the most appalling conditions and cruel treatment. When they come into homes, they are already heavily burdened, exhibiting many of the following conditions: patterns of extreme hyperactivity, intense precocious aggressiveness, and fearfulness toward humans and other dogs. They are often prone to separation anxiety, orally fixated (focusing on personal belongings as well as hands), coprophagous, and they are frequently difficult to house train. With supportive training involving intense remedial socialization, graduated environmental exposure, and endless patience, such puppies can regain some degree of composure and develop into reasonably well-adjusted companion dogs. Even after undergoing the best training available, though, such puppies will never reach their full potential.

Responsible breeders provide their puppies with daily environmental enrichment and preliminary training, including ample social experiences and constructive activities (e.g., house training), that prepare them for an easy transition into their future homes (Monks of New Skete, 1991). Experienced breeders can detect, through a keen eye and various temperament tests, the general emotional disposition of their puppies and thereby place individual puppies in homes consistent with their respective needs. Puppy temperament tests should not be employed to predict adult aptitudes or the potential exhibition of adult behavior patterns but should be used as tools to isolate and quantify a puppy's various strengths and weaknesses at the time of testing. Many behavioral indexes associated with temperament evaluation are flexible and subject to change during a puppy's development (Scott and Fuller, 1965), making temperament tests indicative rather than predictive. Puppy tests are excellent tools for evaluating training progress and for objectively assessing areas that may need additional remedial work. Finally, professional breeders should provide their clients with an information packet covering puppy care and basic training, as well as phone numbers for trainers, obedience clubs, and other relevant support professionals. Most breeders are dedicated to their breed and are willing to share their knowledge and valuable experience to help a new puppy owner through those challenging first few weeks of intensive training and care. Ideally, a breeder and a trainer should work together as a team helping an ill-prepared owner through the sometimes onerous vicissitudes of puppy rearing and training.

Learning plays a significant role in the development of puppies. Understanding how learning impacts development is an important first step in the study of dog behavior. The most influential research on this topic was carried out at the Jackson Laboratory in Bar Harbor, Maine, under the supervision of J. P. Scott and J. L. Fuller. These pioneering efforts paved the way to a fuller understanding of the general processes of ontogeny and, in particular, the development of social behavior. A central purpose of this work was to evaluate the extent and differential influence of genetic versus experiential factors on the development of behavior. With this goal in mind, they chose dogs from several distinct breeds possessing differing attributes and behavioral tendencies, and then experimentally studied their reactions to various environmental manipulations and stressors. Their study clearly demonstrates that different breeds exhibit specific inherited strengths and weaknesses when coping with environmental pressures. However, the most important result of their study was the discovery of several critical or sensitive periods for the social development of dogs. Their work was reported in a seminal text for breeders and trainers entitled the *Genetics and the Social Behavior of the Dog* (1965). Another important source of information regarding the development of puppies (especially neonatal and transitional processes) needs to be credited to the valuable work of Michael Fox. He is the author of many texts, but the most noteworthy in this regard is *Integrative Development of Brain and Behavior in the Dog* (1971).

THE CRITICAL OR SENSITIVE PERIOD HYPOTHESIS

During development and growth, dogs undergo a process of progressive biological organization and simultaneous behavioral differentiation. This ontogenesis is marked by several more or less distinct sensitive or critical periods for the development of various psychosocial functions. The onset and offset of these stages of development are biologically defined, making the animal susceptible to the crucial experience or its absence for a limited period. Within these sensitive stages, a short *optimal period* appears to occur during which appropriate stimulus contacts and experience are rendered maximally effective and beneficial to developing dogs. Scott (1962, 1968a) has argued that the critical periods of social development are defined by irreversible organizing processes reflected in growth and emerging behavioral complexity. Any system that has become well organized and stable is naturally more difficult to reorganize—that is, "organization inhibits reorganization"

(Scott, 1962), unless, of course, the system in question is organized to be flexible to reorganization. According to Scott's hypothesis, behavioral organization can be modified only while it is under the active influence of the original processes of organization, that is, during susceptible critical periods for such activity and change occurring early in an animal's life.

One of the most important functions of the critical period is the formation of social attachments and bonding (Scott, 1968a). In dogs, primary socialization begins around 3 weeks of age. Before week 3, the mother is the puppy's primary social object. With the onset of the socialization period, she begins to leave the litter alone to fend for themselves for longer periods. The result is increased social bonding and attachment between littermates, and the formation of a protopack organization anticipating more adult patterns of canine social behavior (Scott, 1958). These social imprinting effects have received a great deal of experimental attention in a variety of animal species (Sluckin, 1965; Hess, 1973).

Many other behavioral tendencies and appetites are *imprinted* at an early age in puppies. Marr (1964) has found that puppies (3 to 4 weeks of age) can be strongly imprinted to a simple visual stimulus (a white circle against a dark background) by associating its presentation with varied stimulation, like flashing lights and rocking. Stimulated puppies (petted, rocked, or flashed) spent significantly longer time on the platform in contact with the visual stimulus than did controls, suggesting enhanced approach and *attachment* to the stimulus object as the result of varied stimulation. Some sort of learning obviously has taken place, but it is not conclusively an imprinting process. Marr's results could just as easily be interpreted in terms of other learning paradigms, like classical or instrumental conditioning.

Besides the formation of enduring attachments with people, dogs can also form strong interspecific attachments with other animals through imprinting or imprinting-like processes. Cairns and Werboff (1972), who carried out an experiment to investigate social attachment in 4-week-old puppies that had been exposed to sustained contact with adult rabbits, found that puppies housed with rabbits quickly developed social attachments with their cohabitants and exhibited a lasting preference for contact with them. These changes occurred after a very brief period of exposure (within 24 hours of cohabitation). When separated from their rabbit cohabitants, the puppies emitted intense distress vocalizations and escape efforts aimed at regaining contact with the removed rabbits—behaviors consistent with separation-distress reactions exhibited as the result of the loss of contact with conspecifics. Similarly, Fox (1971) reared Chihuahua puppies from 25 days to 16 weeks of age with kittens and a mother cat. Cat-reared puppies displayed a strong preference for kittens over contact with other puppies. The controls (reared with other puppies) exhibited a sustained and active interest (with tail wagging) in viewing their reflection in a mirror located in the testing area. In contrast, cat-reared puppies spent much less time in contact with the mirror. After reaching 16 weeks of age, the cat-reared puppies were once again reunited with conspecifics and subsequently underwent 2 weeks of remedial socialization. Testing found that the cat-reared puppies had recovered most of their species-specific behavior patterns, demonstrating that the socialization effect is to some extent reversible. Also, cat-reared puppies exhibited a pronounced new interest in the mirror, as suggested by increased vocalization scores, activity levels, frequency of contact, and duration of contact with the mirror. During earlier observations, no sustained contact or tail wagging was observed in the presence of the mirror. Following the 2-week period of remedial socialization, however, the cat-reared puppies repeatedly approached the mirror, wagged their tails, and even sat looking at themselves in the mirror—sometimes pushing against it with their nose. Fox speculates that the cat-reared puppies were previously unresponsive to their reflection in the mirror because they lacked the necessary socializing influences needed to form an adequate species identity with which to recognize themselves:

These observations lead to the conclusion that socialization influences the development of species and self-identity. Cat-raised dogs, having had no experience with their own species, were consequently nonreactive to their own reflections, but became more reactive as they were subsequently socialized with their own species. (1971:259)

In other studies, dogs have served as objects of attachment and imprinting involving species other than humans. Mason and Kenney (1974) found evidence among rhesus monkeys that the socialization effect was not irreversible. Monkeys reared under various social conditions were exposed at different ages to cohabitation with spayed female dogs. All the monkeys exhibited a pronounced initial fear of the dogs but quickly recovered with the aid of a series of graduated exposures carried out by the experimenters. Within several hours, most of the monkeys approached and began to cling to the receptive dogs. Both the monkeys and the dogs made frequent contact, played together, exhibited care-seeking and caregiving interaction (mutual grooming and anogenital licking), rested together, and exhibited every sign of enjoying each other's companionship. When separated from their dog companions, the monkeys exhibited separation-induced pacing, distress vocalization, and escape behavior—just as they would if separated from conspecifics with whom they had been socialized and attached. Similar cross-species attachment behavior and attachment reversal (upon resocialization with conspecifics) has been exhibited by lambs reared in cohabitation with adult female dogs (Cairns and Johnson, 1965).

A practical application of cross-species socialization is found among livestock-guarding dogs. Breeds like the Anatolian shepherd, the shar planinetz, komondor, and maremma have a long Eurasian tradition in the performance of this important shepherding task. From early in the socialization period, these dogs are reared with sheep and fed on ewe's milk. Such dogs form a strong social affiliation with sheep—an affiliation that inclines the dogs to protect their adopted species from predators and human intruders alike. Efforts have been under way for some years now to introduce livestock-guarding dogs for the protection of sheep against the predation of coyotes and wolves in many areas of the United States (Coppinger and Coppinger, 1982).

EARLY DEVELOPMENT AND REFLEXIVE BEHAVIOR

The ontogeny of a dog's social behavior unfolds according to a genetically programmed timetable (Scott and Fuller, 1965; Fox, 1971). These early developmental processes exercise an enduring influence over the behavioral adjustment of dogs. During a brief period from 3 to 16 weeks of age, an average puppy will probably learn more than during the remaining course of its lifetime, forming a lasting emotional and cognitive schemata of the social and physical environment. Furthermore, these early experiences format the general outline and organization of how and what the dog is prepared to experience and learn in the future. It therefore behooves conscientious breeders and puppy owners to gain a working understanding of these developmental processes and the various methods used to influence them in the most efficient and beneficial ways. A puppy's early development is divided into four more or less well-defined periods: the neonatal period (birth to 12 days), the transitional period (12 to 21 days), the socialization period (21 to 84 days), and the juvenile period (84 days through sexual maturity).

Neonatal Period (Birth to 12 Days)

Just before birth, hormonal changes occur that cause puppies to undergo sexual dimorphism. Male puppies are exposed to a surge of testosterone, forming the foundation for malelike behavior later in life. Prenatal androgen secretions are believed to play a role in the formation of hardwired neural tracts associated with maleness. Some evidence suggests that female puppies may be affected by this androgenizing effect as well (Knol and Egberink-Alink, 1989). Female mice embryos located between males in the uterus appear to be influenced by the presence of vagrant

testosterone carried in amniotic fluids, although it is not certain whether such a hypothesized osmotic mechanism is involved. Perhaps a similar effect holds for female dogs, but this possible hormonal influence has yet to be shown experimentally. The influence of cross-sexual prenatal androgenization may help to explain the display of malelike behavioral tendencies (e.g., male-directed aggression and leg-lifting behavior) by some female dogs. Another potential neuroendocrine influence on prenatal development involves the mother's emotional state (Thompson, 1957). If gestating rats are exposed to intense fear-eliciting stimulation, the resulting offspring are unstable and more emotionally reactive than controls gestated without such exposure.

A puppy is born within an allantoic sac and attached to the mother by an umbilical cord (Fig. 2.1). The cord is chewed through, the placenta removed and eaten, and the puppy thoroughly licked clean and dried. Besides cleaning the puppy, the mother's licking stimulates reflexive muscular movements and breathing. At birth, a puppy is unable to control its body temperature and is very sensitive to changes in ambient temperature. A near-constant temperature is maintained by its keeping in close physical contact with the mother and littermates. However, a puppy that becomes too warm will move away to maintain an optimal temperature (Welker, 1959). The neonate exhibits intense distress vocalizations when separated from littermates and placed on a cold surface. Fredericson and colleagues (1956) proved that such distress was not due to loss of contact comfort but the result of temperature changes experienced by the puppy. They found that neonates placed on heating pads were content and able to go to sleep without maternal or sibling contact. Dunbar and colleagues (1981) observed that a mother will readily retrieve distressed offspring that have become separated from the litter group through the first 5 days but after that will stop doing so.

From a neurological and sensory perspective, newborn puppies are both deaf and blind and thus virtually insulated from the external world. However, many primitive sensory and behavioral systems and reflexes are present at birth that assist puppies in nursing

Neonatal Period

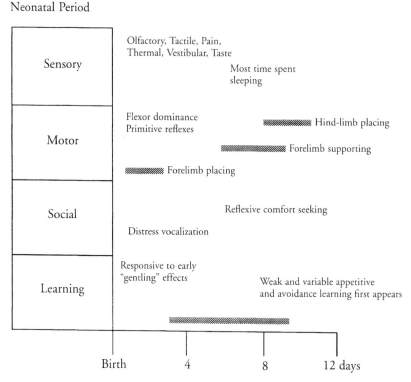

FIG. 2.1. The neonatal period is associated with reflexive activities aimed at optimizing nurturance and contact with the mother.

and keeping in contact with the mother (Table 2.1). Among these sensory capacities are sensitivities to pressure, movement, taste, and smell. Withdrawal from painful stimulation can be seen shortly after birth. Some forms of neonatal learning have been observed in the laboratory. For instance, Fox (1971) found that if the breasts of a nursing mother are coated with anise oil during the first 5 days of feeding, the exposed puppies subsequently exhibit an orienting response to a Q-tip soaked in the oil. On the other hand, puppies not previously exposed to the smell of anise oil on their mother's breasts exhibited a strong withdrawal response from it when similarly tested. This experiment indicates that some form of rudimentary learning is present in the neonatal puppies—a topic that is discussed in greater detail later in this chapter.

Most of a neonatal puppy's time is spent sleeping, with the remaining time devoted to nursing. When sleeping, a puppy exhibits extensive twitching and nervous movements over its entire body. Electroencephalogram (EEG) studies have demonstrated that waking and sleeping states exhibit nearly identical patterns of low brain activity (Fox, 1963). Urination and defecation must be elicited by the mother for the first 2 weeks or so by rhythmically licking the anogenital area. Such licking usually occurs just prior to feeding, serving to both wake the puppy for nursing and to elicit elimination (Grant, 1986). A puppy's general motor activities at this stage of development are limited to swimlike crawling movements predominately involving the front legs. Guided by tactile, olfactory, and gustatory senses, a puppy reflexively orients and locates the mother's teat. Forelimb-placing movements are seen after 2 or 3 days, and efforts at forelimb support begin between days 6 and 10. Hind-limb-placing responses are seen after 8 days. Flexor muscles are dom-

TABLE 2.1. Reflexive behavior observed in neonatal puppies

Neonatal Reflexes	S	R
Magnus	Elicited by turning the neonate's head to one side	The action causes an extension of the forelimbs and hind limbs on the side toward which the head is turned. Limbs on the opposite side tend to flex.
Crossed extensor	Elicited by pinching the webbing of the hind foot	The leg on the side pinched flexes while the opposite leg extends.
Negative geotactic	The puppy is placed on a surface that is tilted up.	The puppy reorients by twisting in the direction of the elevated side.
Rooting	The hand is cupped around the puppy's muzzle.	Forward movement is elicited as long as the puppy maintains contact.
Photomotor	A bright light is flashed into the closed eye of the puppy.	A blink is elicited; not operative until day 2 or 3.
Reflexive elimination	Elicited by gently dabbing ano-genital area with a wet cotton ball	Reflexive urination and defecation

Source: After Fox (1971).

inant over extensors for the first few days, followed by a much longer period of extensor dominance and the emergence of unsteady walking in the transitional period. Nonnutritive sucking actions can be elicited early in the neonatal period, with a peak occurring around days 3 to 5 and gradually declining over the first 3 weeks. Early forced weaning causes a distortion in this pattern, causing puppies to suck much more actively on fingers or sometimes on littermates (Scott et al., 1959). Scott and colleagues (1959) observed that, among 500 puppies that were left with their mothers through 10 weeks of age, none exhibited the body-sucking habit exhibited by prematurely weaned counterparts. Puppies that are weaned too early (before day 15) may be prone to develop adult oral and motor compulsions involving sucking and kneading directed toward blankets and other soft objects.

Although neonatal puppies are developmentally insulated from the environment, some external influences may have long-term effects on learning, emotionality, and general adaptability. Early neonatal handling involving as little as 3 minutes a day and exposure to various mild environmental stressors, like changes of ambient temperature and move-

ment (gentling), may have positive impacts on a puppy's resistance to disease, emotional reactivity, and mature learning and problem-solving abilities (Morton, 1968). Denenberg (1964), who has reviewed a considerable body of literature regarding neonatal stimulation and its effect on adult emotionality in rats, concludes that the degree of adult emotionality exhibited by the animal is conversely proportional to the amount of infantile stimulation experienced prior to weaning (Fig. 2.2). Animals left undisturbed during neonatal development were found to be consistently more emotionally reactive as adults. Levine and colleagues (1967) exposed rats to an early differential handling/stress regimen in which an experimental group was removed from the litter and placed in a can with shavings for 3 minutes per day for the first 20 days of life. The control group was composed of animals left undisturbed during the same period. Once mature (80 days), the rats were exposed to an open-field situation, a test that reveals general reactivity and fearfulness. The behavior of the two groups was observed, especially general activity and defecation frequency, and all the animals tested were subsequently evaluated in terms of adrenocortical response. Previously handled rats were found

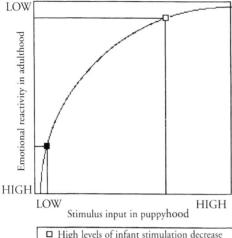

Emotional reactivity in adulthood

LOW — HIGH (y-axis)

LOW — HIGH (x-axis)

Stimulus input in puppyhood

□ High levels of infant stimulation decrease emotional reactivity in adulthood

■ Low levels of infant stimulation increase emotional reactivity in adulthood

FIG. 2.2. Hypothesized curve correlating the relative amount of early stimulation and the degree of emotional reactivity observed in the adult. After Denenberg (1964:341).

to be more active and defecated less than controls during testing, suggesting that they were less fearful and inhibited under the novel conditions. Handled animals also appeared to habituate more quickly to the test situation over several days of evaluation, rendering them more adaptable than controls. Nonhandled animals consistently exhibited higher levels of corticosteroids than handled ones, further confirming the latter's lower stress reactivity under the conditions of the test.

In other experiments performed by Levine (1960), handled rats exhibited a more precise and adaptive adrenocortical response pattern when exposed to stress induced by shock. Although both handled and nonhandled rats exhibited similar blood levels of adrenal steroids before stimulation, the handled rats showed a much higher level within the first 15 minutes following shock than the nonhandled group. The nonhandled group, though achieving the same blood levels eventually, did so only after a long poststimulation delay. Further, steroid levels in the nonhandled group were maintained at a higher

level over a much longer period than in the handled group. According to Levine, the fast hypothalamic-pituitary-adrenal (HPA) system response in the handled animals is more consistent with the proper functioning of the animal's emergency-stress system. During stress activation, an animal's emergency resources should be fully mobilized in the moment when they are needed most, followed by a rapid decline and denouement phase. As noted above, the nonhandled animals tended to react slowly to aversive stimulation with a prolongation of the stress reaction. This physiological response to stress exhibited by nonhandled animals may eventually result in various psychosomatic effects: stomach ulcers, immunosuppression, and sometimes death from adrenal exhaustion.

The aforementioned research suggests that early handling exercises a lasting influence on the activity of the HPA system. These influences include autonomic changes as reflected in reduced emotionality and increased stability. It is, therefore, possible that early handling may exercise a potentially pronounced effect on the animal's basic temperament and future trainability.

Fox and Stelzner (1966) performed a series of experiments with puppies from birth to 5 weeks of age to evaluate the effects of early handling on development. The puppies were exposed to various stimulus extremes, including cold, flashing lights, noises, and vestibular stimulation (rocking on a tilting board). The results indicate that the stressed puppies performed better in problem solving (perhaps because of reduced emotional reactivity) and were socially dominant over controls not exposed to the earlier stress-inducing experiences. Several physiological concomitants were also observed. Stressed puppies exhibited a precocious EEG pattern, produced five times more adrenal norepinephrine, and displayed a heart rate indicative of stronger sympathetic tone. A practical application of early handling stress was carried out by the U.S. Army's Superdog Program (Biosensor). Immature puppies were exposed to slow, refrigerated centrifuging to produce handling stress. To my knowledge, no published studies have been written concerning these experiments, and the potential benefits of such treatment remains conjectural, although anecdotal reports indicate "extremely promising results in terms of later stress—resistance, emotional stability, and improved learning ability" (Fox, 1978:165). Some amount of handling stress should be part of a breeder's normal rearing practice to compensate for the absence of naturally occurring stressful changes in the whelping area. Conditions in the average kennel may be too artificial, insular, and protective for optimal psychological and physical development. Not all research findings uniformly support the belief that early exposure to stress is beneficial. For example, recent research involving rats reported by Nemeroff (1998) suggests that the distress evoked by briefly separating rat pups from their mother and littermates is sufficient to exert permanent adverse effects over neural circuits mediating stress reactivity and emotional arousal (see Chapter 3 for discussion). Consequently, there may be developmental periods when stressful exposure is particularly beneficial and others (e.g., early in the socialization period) during which small amounts of stress may produce pronounced and lasting detrimental results.

Although neonatal learning abilities are limited by the range of a puppy's sensory abilities, conditioned appetitive and avoidance responses have been established between days 3 and 10. For example, Stanley and colleagues (1963) conditioned neonates to respond differentially with increased approach and sucking or repulsion and avoidance of sucking depending on whether milk or a quinine solution was presented through an artificial nipple. Stable escape-avoidance responses toward cold-air stimulation have also been achieved. Stanley and colleagues (1974) placed neonates in a plastic tub with one side covered with cloth while leaving the other side exposed plastic. Neonates were placed on the cloth side and stimulated with a flow of cold air directed onto their shoulders. Tested puppies readily escaped stimulation by moving away from the cold air and crossing into the safety of the uncovered side of the plastic tub. Subsequent tests demonstrated that the puppies responded to the cloth side as an avoidance stimulus causing them to move

into the plastic side of the tub, apparently anticipating and avoiding the presentation of the cold-air stimulus. Stanley and coworkers (1970) also demonstrated that neonates can readily learn a simple discrimination task involving approach to cloth versus wire tactile stimuli, depending on whether the respective substrates provided milk. A subsequent study (Bacon and Stanley, 1970) demonstrated that these tactile substrate discriminations could be reversed (making the positive stimulus negative and vice versa). Furthermore, they found that the ability to learn such reversals improved with experience, suggesting that the puppies might be acquiring a learning set or "learning to learn." The foregoing results led the investigators to conclude that neonatal learning, though functionally limited, follows a pattern not dissimilar to the learning of adult dogs.

Developmentally, neonatal puppies move rapidly from primitive "vegetative" functioning to more complex modes of seeking-avoiding behavior. Determining how this process proceeds is an important ontogenetic problem. Schneirla (1959) has proposed that this process includes two interwoven ontogenetic phases involving approach-withdrawal (A-W) behavior. Early neonatal A-W behavior is differentially evoked depending on the intensity of the eliciting stimulus. Low-intensity (weak) stimulation tends to elicit approach behavior, whereas high-intensity (strong) stimulation elicits withdrawal. As puppies develop, these earlier patterns of responding are further elaborated into more complex and informative types of responding to environmental stimulation. Approach behavior becomes *seeking* or, in the terminology of learning theory, positively reinforced behavior and withdrawal behavior become *escape and avoidance* or negatively reinforced behavior. These two broad categories form the foundation of instrumental learning in dogs.

Of particular interest in this regard is the suggestion by Schneirla (1965) that approach behavior (relaxed-preparatory activity) is mediated by parasympathetic processes while interruptive withdrawal behavior (reactive-protective activity) is mediated by sympathetic processes. A-W stimulation during these early weeks may facilitate the differential "tuning" of the autonomic nervous system in the opposing directions of relaxed parasympathetic dominance or, conversely, toward reactive sympathetic dominance. The sensory and motor abilities of neonatal puppies are ontogenetically organized to facilitate appropriate A-W behavior, thus ensuring the adequate procurement of nurturance and warmth. Neonatal comfort seeking is mediated by parasympathetic arousal, including various appetitive reactions like salivation, increased production of digestive juices, intestinal peristalsis, and generalized relaxation associated with normal respiration and heart rate. Maternal caregiving and *contact comfort* facilitates both digestion and emotional attachment (Fox, 1978). Without such comfort contact and the parasympathetic stimulation that it provides, normal digestive functions and growth patterns are disrupted. Protective sympathetic reactions, on the other hand, momentarily interrupt such appetitive functions and prepare the animal for emergency action.

According to Rosenblatt (1983), the transition from A-W reactions based on stimulus intensity to more mature seeking-avoiding behavior is mediated by the modality of smell. He has argued that olfaction provides the foundation for a higher order of response organization and stimulus meaning. Earlier A-W reactions mediated by tactile and thermal stimulation, for example, are identified by odor via associative learning (contiguity) mechanisms. Such olfactory stimuli become the fundamental positive and negative incentives that neonatal puppies seek or avoid as determined by prior experience with these stimuli. Although olfaction mediates some innate (or prenatally acquired) A-W behavior toward a few odors, Rosenblatt argues that the vast majority of olfactory incentives are acquired through learning. Sensory development can be viewed as progressing from stimulation requiring direct bodily contact with the evoking stimulus (touch) to thermal orientation (stimulus gradient from cold to warm) to odors that enable a broader environmental purview and a sufficient distance from which vantage to identify and anticipate significant events. As puppies develop, this ability to scan the environment for significance and, then, to precisely localize significant events occurring at remote distances sharply improves with the appearance of functional sight and hearing.

Although neonatal puppies are capable of learning, these abilities are confined to the association of primitive stimulus events and adjustment responses. The reason for this limited ability is due (among other things) to the absence of myelinization in the neonatal brain. At birth, the only nerve tracts possessing significant myelin sheathing are those associated with taste and sucking. Also, at birth, there are evidently olfactory abilities present that become progressively developed through the neonatal and transitional period. The behavior of neonatal puppies is mainly composed of unconditioned reflexes adaptively organized to ensure adequate warmth, nutrition, elimination, and general survival needs. Most of these "vegetative" reflexes become progressively variable as puppies develop, and disappear before the onset of the socialization period (Fox, 1964a; Markwell and Thorne, 1987).

Transitional Period (12 to 21 Days)

The transitional period is marked by progressive neurological development with steady improvement in locomotor ability, the appearance of additional sensory modalities (including the opening of the eyes and ear canals), and the development of greater central control over voluntary behavior (Fig. 2.3). The righting and visual cliff reflexes appear during this period, but they are not consistent until approximately 28 days of age (Fox, 1971). Throughout this period, the behavior of puppies becomes progressively more active and independent of the influence of neonatal reflexes (Fig. 2.4). As the eyes open, puppies begin to crawl backward. Hind-limb supporting reactions are weak, and variable responses appear between 11 to 15 days of age. A puppy can support itself on all four limbs and walk unsteadily as early as day 12. Early walking efforts are poorly coordinated and associated with bobbing of the head

Transitional Period

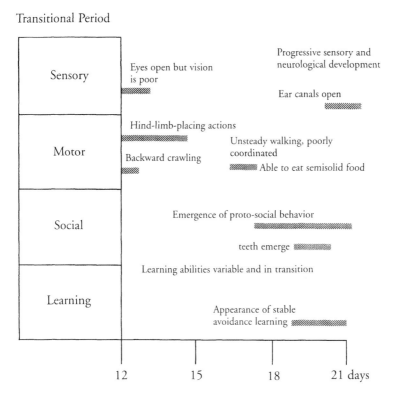

FIG. 2.3. The transitional period is associated with progressive motor and sensory development.

from side to side. As flexor-extensor balance improves, this side-to-side movement of the head disappears.

If necessary, puppies can be weaned and taught to eat gruel as early as day 16. The teeth begin to emerge late in this period. Although puppies can now eliminate voluntarily, Grant (1986) did not observe evidence of independent elimination in puppies during the 20 days of his study.

The transitional period is characterized by tremendous change and development. It is during this time that puppies begin to leave the cocoonlike protection of neonatal existence and emerge into a field of widening sensory experience. Although nursing is of great importance to puppies, an independent desire for contact comfort is also evident during this period. Igel and Calvin (1960) carried out a series of experiments with puppies between 11 to 30 days of age to determine a puppy's relative interest in nursing versus simple contact comfort. Their study duplicated an earlier experiment performed by Harlow and Zimmerman (1959) in which infant monkeys were shown to exhibit a preference for nonnutritive cloth surrogate mothers over wire "lactating" ones. Although nursing remains an important activity, the maintenance of contact comfort is of growing significance to developing puppies. The authors found that puppies spent considerably more time with nonnutritive cloth mothers than with wire surrogates that provided milk. Interestingly, the puppies exhibited a growing preference for close contact with the nonnutritive cloth mother as they grew older, suggesting the existence of an underlying developmental process mediating social bonding.

Stanley and colleagues (1970) found that neonatal puppies (2 to 7 days old) also exhibit a very strong preference for soft sub-

Neonatal and Transitional Reflexes

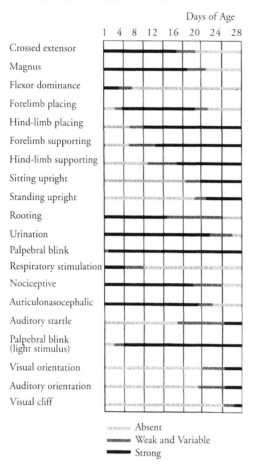

	Days of Age
	1 4 8 12 16 20 24 28

Crossed extensor
Magnus
Flexor dominance
Forelimb placing
Hind-limb placing
Forelimb supporting
Hind-limb supporting
Sitting upright
Standing upright
Rooting
Urination
Palpebral blink
Respiratory stimulation
Nociceptive
Auriculonasocephalic
Auditory startle
Palpebral blink (light stimulus)
Visual orientation
Auditory orientation
Visual cliff

⋯⋯⋯ Absent
▬▬ Weak and Variable
▬▬ Strong

FIG. 2.4. Showing the developmental changes of reflexive behavior in the puppy. After Fox (1971).

strates over wire ones. Although the neonates exhibited an initial preference for the cloth substrate whether or not it provided milk, the study demonstrated that the provision of milk only in association with the wire surrogate gradually reversed this initial preference. When the cloth substrate did not provide milk, the neonates became progressively attracted to the wire "mother" to satisfy their nutritive needs, indicating that nutritive needs are more important to neonates than are contact needs at that age. This is consistent with the aforementioned findings of Fredericson and colleagues, who found that

neonatal puppies are content without direct contact with the mother or littermates as long as they are kept warm. Further evidence that the dog's social response undergoes progressive development is provided by Gantt and colleagues (1966), who were unable to detect a consistent cardiac response to petting in puppies at 2 weeks of age. In fact, they were unable to detect stable cardiac deceleration in puppies under 3 to 4 months of age. The so-called *effect of person* and the calmative qualities associated with petting are not evident in puppies until the close of the socialization period.

Although stable avoidance learning is not consistently obtained before 3 to 4 weeks of age (Fuller et al., 1950), studies have traced the development of such learning during the transitional period. For example, Cornwell and Fuller (1961) found that puppies as young as 15 days of age could learn a reliable (50%) conditioned avoidance response to a puff of air paired with shock. They observed that avoidance learning progressively improves, reaching a 90% reliability by day 19, thus generally confirming earlier studies involving avoidance conditioning in puppies (Fuller et al., 1950; James and Cannon, 1952). Although conditioned avoidance responses can be established, they are developmentally limited to a narrow range of sensory modalities that are functional at the time, making puppies unsuitable candidates for significant early behavior modification or training. With the onset of the socialization period at around 3 weeks of age, dramatic developmental improvements occur in a puppy's ability to learn.

With the close of the transitional period, puppies experience a rapid increase in the amount of social and environmental stimulation that they must process and enter into a long period of adjustment to the environment. Fox (1966c) has compared the general course of puppy development with other altricial species and humans, finding that a similar sequence of developmental events exists for both humans and dogs. The ontogenetic expression of behavior moves steadily from primitive adaptations and reflexive organization to the culminating emergence of higher behavioral integration. The crucial step in this transition from a reflexive organization to social awareness and identity takes place during the next several weeks collectively known as the critical or sensitive period of socialization.

SOCIALIZATION: LEARNING TO RELATE AND COMMUNICATE

The developmental period extending roughly from 3 to 12 weeks of age is the most influential 9 weeks of a puppy's life. This period is associated with the development of many social behavior patterns and a great deal of learning about the environment. Much of what is learned during this early period is lasting, providing a foundation for many adult behavior patterns and problems (Fox, 1968), appetites and aversions, social affinities and responsiveness (Scott, 1958), sexual behavior (Fox, 1964b), patterns of active and passive agonistic behavior, play behaviors (Fox, 1966c), packing (allelomimetic) behaviors (Scott, 1968b), reactions to separation and other emotionally provocative situations (Pettijohn et al., 1977), approach-avoidance patterns (Fox, 1966c), the development of dominate-subordinate relationships (Scott and Fuller, 1965), patterns of exploratory behavior and general activity levels (Thompson and Heron, 1954; Wright, 1983), functional fear and avoidance responses (Melzack and Scott, 1957), general learning and problem-solving ability (Fuller, 1967; Lessac and Solomon, 1969), and trainability (Pfaffenberger and Scott, 1959). Virtually every functional behavior system is strongly impacted by the kind of treatment a puppy receives during this period.

Primary Socialization (3 to 5 Weeks)

Prior to week 3, puppies are somewhat socially insulated and only minimally aware of conspecifics. However, with the advent of increased sensory and motor abilities, an extraordinary new interest in social interaction takes place between 3 and 5 weeks of age. A constellation of interrelated behavior patterns and emotional tendencies appear at this time,

heralding a lively social awareness and responsiveness (Fig. 2.5). Puppies begin to exhibit more intense signs of distress (e.g., vocalizations and physical efforts to secure contact) when briefly separated from the mother and littermates. Kinship recognition and preference is evident from an early age. Puppies (20 to 24 days) undergoing acute separation distress exhibit a pronounced preference for bedding saturated with the odor of littermates over that of nonlittermates (Mekosh-Rosenbaum et al., 1994). Allelomimetic (group coordinated) activity and social play begin to appear around this time, with the litter behaving like a miniature pack. Playful aggressive and sexual encounters occur frequently between littermates. Various predatory components appear during play, including stalking, pouncing, and shaking. These behaviors are exhibited toward littermates as well as inanimate objects that invite such curiosity and treatment. Additionally, a great deal of sparring takes place between siblings, but the dominant-subordinate roles are unstable, with social status shifting from moment to moment. Puppies spend large amounts of time mouthing and biting each other but appearing to take care not to bite too hard. This period may be a sensitive one for the acquisition of *bite inhibition* or a soft mouth. Some puppies that have been weaned too early in this period tend to bite more vigorously and harder than the norm (Fox and Stelzner, 1967). This inhibitory effect over hard biting may stem from feedback reactions from the mother if a puppy bites too hard while nursing, or from reactions elicited during playful jousting with littermates.

This period is especially important for the development of a stable emotional temperament and affective tone. Many social and emotional deficits observed in adult dogs are believed to result from removing puppies too early from the mother and littermates. Although scientific studies are lacking, ample anecdotal reports and case histories reveal very pronounced effects resulting from early weaning or insufficient socialization with conspecifics. Behavioral sequelae commonly observed as the result of such treatment include emotional rigidness, overreactivity, and

Socialization Period

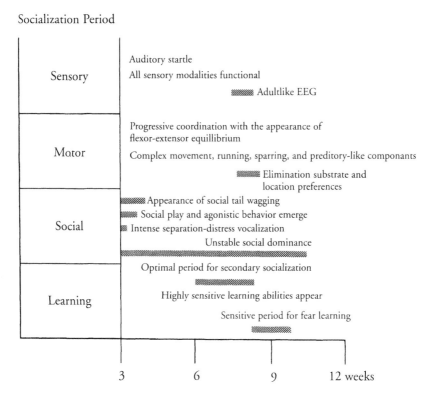

FIG. 2.5. The socialization period includes primary (3 to 5 weeks) and secondary phases (6 to 12 weeks). During this period, active social interaction, bonding, and play emerge as prominent activities occupying the puppy's time.

increased vigilance and anxiety. Such dogs are prone to develop attachment-related problems involving separation distress–evoked behaviors like excessive barking, compulsive destructive behavior, and psychogenic elimination problems. They are more likely to develop aggression problems toward other dogs as adults (Pfaffenberger, 1963). Dogs forming overly exclusive bonds with an owner may become suspicious or aggressive toward strangers, viewing them as a threat to their attachment. When not aggressive, such dogs are often overly fearful of other dogs, preferring human company over that of conspecifics. They are frequently sexually inhibited toward their own kind but may actively redirect such behavior toward their owners. Not all puppies prematurely separated from their littermates exhibit these deficits, but many do exhibit some degree of emotional

disequilibrium or deficiency.

During this period, the mother begins to leave the whelping area more frequently and for longer periods. On returning to the nest, she may regurgitate in response to the solicitous behavior of her puppies. The regurgitant feeding response is most commonly exhibited during the final stages of lactation and terminates shortly after weaning (Martins, 1949). Malm (1995) learned from breeder respondents in Sweden that the timing of the first regurgitant response is highly variable, ranging from 3 to 6 weeks of age, with the majority of mothers exhibiting the response for the first time during week 4. Further, the tendency appears to be somewhat breed dependent, with mothers belonging to some breeds being less likely to regurgitate than others. Wilsson (1984/1985), for example, found that, among 17 German shepherd mothers, none exhibited the behavior during his observations. James (1960) found that regurgitation was often elicited when the puppies attempted to nurse while the mother remained standing. In addition, the puppies exhibited begging behavior consisting of energetic jumping up and profuse licking of the mother's lips and muzzle in an apparent effort to evoke regurgitation. Rheingold (1963) reported only infrequent episodes of regurgitation by the mothers she observed. Such etepimeletic (care seeking) behavior is probably the behavioral antecedent of adult greeting ritual displays exhibited during homecomings. Fox (1971) has speculated that many adult social behavior patterns may be traced to prototypical antecedents in the dog's early ontogeny (Table 2.2). It is interesting in this regard that besides being solicitous toward the owner and guests, many young dogs and puppies may urinate during excited greetings or when leaned over or reached for, a social pattern that may be ontogenetically related to another alimentary function performed by the mother—lingual elicitation of urination. With the advent of increased motor abilities, puppies wander more widely and begin to leave the nesting area to eliminate on their own. With the emergence of this tendency,

the mother stops ingesting the feces. At this time, puppies can be taught to eat semisolid food to supplement the mother's nursing. Eating such rations is socially facilitated by group feeding. The puppies engage in intense exploratory behavior involving sniffing, pawing, digging, chewing, tearing, and picking up a wide variety of available objects. Puppies are enthusiastic and responsive to new social encounters but appear to exercise special preferences for particular individuals they know best. A striking behavioral feature appearing at this time is the development of expressive tail wagging:

> One of the outstanding changes in behavior at the beginning of the period of socialization is the tendency of puppies to respond to the sight or sound of persons or other animals at a distance. The 3-week-old puppy approaches slowly and cautiously toward a human observer seated quietly in its pen. It finally comes close and starts nosing his shoes and clothes. After this, it may start to wag its tail rapidly back and forth. The tail wagging itself appears to have no directly adaptive function, but is simply an expression of pleasurable emotion toward a social object. What effect it has on other dogs is difficult to tell, but it seems to have the same effect on human observers as the

TABLE 2.2. Comparison of puppy behavior antecedents with related adult social behavior patterns

Puppy behavior patterns	Adult behavior patterns
Anogenital presentation during reflex elimination produced by maternal licking	Passive submission displays involving rolling on the side, submissive urination
Licking and leaping directed toward the mother's mouth to elicit regurgitation	Adult greeting routine, active submission—jumping up and licking
Separation-distress vocalizations, yelping, and whining	Adult separation-distress vocalization, howling, and barking
Distress vocalizations	Passive submission vocalizations
Upward head movement, butting— nursing behavior	Social greeting—play solicitation
Competition over optimal nursing sites and food	Dominance-related behavior

Source: After Fox (1971).

smile of a child; i.e., it is a reward for the person who has initiated a social contact. (Scott and Fuller, 1965:104)

During the neonatal period, the electrical activity of the puppy brain is minimal, with only slight differences being evident between waking and sleeping states. With the onset of the socialization period at 3 weeks of age, a clear and pronounced EEG differentiation can be seen, with an adultlike EEG pattern appearing between weeks 7 and 8. These EEG changes are correlated with significant emotional and physiological concomitants associated with the socialization process. Besides the improvement in brain functions, other physiological changes reflecting emotional responsiveness can be observed. Scott (1958) identified a regular pattern of deceleration, acceleration, and denouement in the heart rates of puppies during the first 16 weeks of life. These changes in heart rate appear to demarcate the onset and offset of the critical or sensitive period for socialization, coinciding with significant changes in approach-avoidance patterns and the intensification of distress vocalization during separation from littermates. Initially, neonatal puppies exhibit a very rapid heart rate. This fast heart rate is maintained throughout the neonatal and transitional periods but then undergoes a sharp decrease after week 3 (parasympathetic dominance) and remains at that level until week 5, when it suddenly accelerates again, peaking between weeks 7 and 8 (sympathetic dominance) before gradually slowing down over the next several weeks toward adult levels. It has been speculated that the sharp dip in heart rate between weeks 3 and 5 results from the integration of corticohypothalamic neural connections and the development of increased sensitivity to emotion-eliciting stimuli and social conditioning. A sympathetic rebound between weeks 5 and 7 is followed by autonomic equilibration and fine tuning over the ensuing several weeks, with a leveling out of heart rate toward adult levels by 16 weeks of age. After week 5, puppies become progressively more cautious and hesitant about making new social contacts—a growing fearful tendency that appears to peak with the close of

the socialization period at 12 weeks. Prior to this time, puppies are virtually immune to lasting negative impressions, readily recovering from fearful social experiences without apparent effect or permanent avoidance learning. After week 5, the recovery time following aversive or fear-eliciting stimulation is significantly protracted. This pattern of development culminates in the emergence of adultlike brain activity and the appearance of a particularly sensitive period for fear imprints around 8 to 10 weeks of age (Fox, 1966c).

Scott (1967) has speculated that the development of social attachment and identification results from a combination of two primary developmental pressures. Puppies exhibit an early preference for social contact and familiar locations, becoming distressed when isolated in an unfamiliar place. Such emotional distress is immediately alleviated when contact is reestablished. This pattern of distress and relief ostensibly strengthens a puppy's tendency to maintain close contact with conspecifics and familiar surroundings and, by default, the avoidance of novelty. Intense separation reactions occurring during isolation are well developed by week 3. A simple behavioral analysis may be useful in understanding the motivational dynamics governing the phenomena involved. Contact behavior is intrinsically reinforced by relief from distress associated with isolation, presumably strengthening an underlying social bond with littermates or human companions. Scott (1967) describes an experiment in defense of this hypothesis in which 5- to 7-week-old puppies were isolated from littermates overnight and then allowed contact with human companions for 3 hours during the day. The results of this experiment indicate that the puppies exposed to overnight isolation formed stronger social attachments to human handlers than did controls, suggesting that the aversive emotions generated by isolation are closely related to the attachment process. The emotional reactions elicited by social isolation are intense drivelike affects that overshadow even hunger in priority (separation-reactive dogs are generally anorexic). Separation and isolation represent strong aversive events for puppies and dogs alike, forming the emotional basis for *time-out* procedures used in puppy training and behavior management.

A fear of strangers appears between 5 and 7 weeks of age and quickly develops over several weeks, culminating in the close of the socialization period during week 12. This developing social fear and reactive avoidance of new social contacts complements the overall solidification of previously established social contacts and bonds.

Secondary Socialization (6 to 12 Weeks)

Unlike most animals, dogs are unusual in that they must adjust to stringent interspecific demands required by domestication. These demands are far reaching, extending from toilet habits to the sharing of affection and play with an alien species—us. A dog must feel equally comfortable in the company of other dogs as well as enjoy human companionship. Such social flexibility is in large measure contingent on early exposure and experience. The process of bonding and social conditioning within the context of the human domestic environment is referred to as *secondary socialization*. For most purposes, secondary socialization begins in earnest when a puppy leaves the mother and littermates to begin life with a human family. The ideal timing for this transition is 7 weeks of age, with a relative range of −1 or +1 (6 to 8 weeks). The 7-week marker is a long-standing convention among insightful breeders and trainers, but it is also supported by various empirical observations (Freedman et al., 1961). Firstly, this period is associated with increasing irritability on the mother's part toward her young, coinciding with the decline of lactation and a growing disinterest in nursing. This disinterest is not shared by her puppies, whose appetites are as sharp as their teeth. Not surprisingly, maternal punishing activity peaks at around this time (Rheingold, 1963; Wilsson, 1984/1985). The mother's job is done both nutritionally and psychologically, making 7 to 8 weeks of age a very sensible time for final weaning and the finding of a new home for her brood. Secondly, within the litter itself, agonistic interaction between the puppies has reached a peak, and

although their aggressive play is not intended to hurt, the skills and attitudes developed by such incessant competitiveness does not beneficially serve puppies in terms of their future adaptation to family life.

In addition to the foregoing observations, experimental study of the social development of puppies reveals that several motivational parameters associated with bonding and socialization peak at about this time (Scott and Fuller, 1965). For instance, distress vocalization and reactive behavior exhibited during brief isolation from littermates reaches its highest levels at around 7 weeks of age but undergoes a rapid decline through week 10. Also peaking at this time is a puppy's willingness to approach strangers confidently and to investigate novel things with vigorous tail wagging. However, the strongest support for encouraging adoption during week 7 stems from the progressive potentiation of fearfulness and the simultaneous attenuation of social approach tendencies occurring at this time. This pattern of increasing fear and social avoidance forms a trajectory that culminates with the close of the socialization period sometime after week 12. These two opposing social dimensions (fear and attraction) optimally intersect during week 7 (Fig. 2.6). The balanced interplay of attraction and fear is fundamental to bonding and socialization in the broadest sense.

From what has been discussed, puppies appear to be developmentally prepared to experience the *most* efficient secondary socialization during a short period around 7 weeks of age. However, this does not suggest that puppies younger or older than 7 weeks are unfit or unable to benefit from socialization. The critical or sensitive period hypothesis of socialization stresses that a short period of time, or window of opportunity, exists during which optimal socialization effects can be fully realized. It does not, however, state or imply that socialization occurring outside of these developmental boundaries is not beneficial.

A reasonable objection against delaying secondary socialization until around week 7 might be based on arguments favoring an earlier starting point for socialization. Five-week-old puppies are more outgoing and less

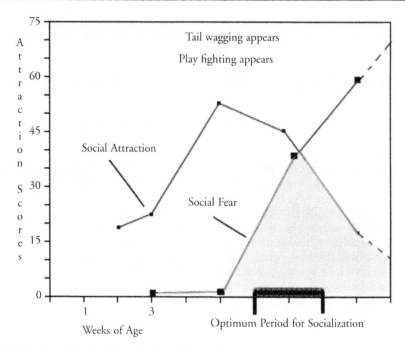

FIG. 2.6. Timing for socialization. Note that the ideal time for initiating secondary socialization corresponds to the intersection of the opposing trends of increased social fear, on the one hand, and decreasing social attraction scores, on the other. After Scott and Fuller (1965).

fearful of social contact than are 7-week-old puppies. It would appear to make sense, therefore, to initiate secondary socialization at an earlier stage in the socialization process rather than waiting. Certainly, it is a period when conscientious breeders should be providing daily and careful handling consistent with a puppy's future placement. However, there are many benefits accruing from keeping the litter intact until week 7. These factors have already been discussed in detail, but to reiterate: puppies removed from the litter too early are at risk of developing adjustment problems of one sort or another as adult dogs. Adoption is a matter of timing. Both the extreme of adopting too early (before week 6) or too late (after week 12, with the emergence of increasing social avoidance) may compete with appropriate socialization or predispose puppies to develop social adjustment problems.

Maternal Influences on Secondary Socialization

A significant factor not yet discussed is the mother's possible role as a model and facilitator of secondary socialization. The primary affectional bonds existing between the individual and the group are elaborated from the primal relationship between the mother and siblings (Harlow, 1958; Scott and Fuller, 1965); however, the mother's influence on a developing puppy in terms of her effect on secondary socialization is not completely understood, and the literature on the topic is divided. Some anecdotal reports suggest that the mother may play an important role in the regulation of aggressive behavior through the exercise of early motherly discipline. The extent of modeling and observational learning on social behavior is not well documented in dogs, but undoubtedly such learning exists to some extent. The mother's emotional tone and reactivity may encourage similar reactions in puppies via empathy, social facilitation, and observational learning, and thereby "inoculate" them with either a positive or a negative emotional bias toward people and other dogs. Her negative reactions (aggression or fear) may be the result of heredity, her own personal history with people, or a combination of both. In any case, impressionable puppies are at considerable risk of internalizing her attitudes during the socialization period and, perhaps, even before birth (Thompson, 1957). Although observational learning has not been adequately demonstrated in adult dogs (Thorndike, 1911/1965), Adler and Adler (1977) have shown that such learning does exist during puppyhood, at least. The authors emphasize the potential importance of observational learning in the acquisition of social behavior patterns. Slabbert and Rasa (1997) have demonstrated that puppies (9 to 12 weeks of age) exhibited greater trainability as narcotic detectors at 6 months of age if they were permitted to observe their mother performing searching exercises. Kuo (1967) has found that a mother exercises a strong influence on the development of food preferences in her puppies.

This is an area needing more detailed research. It is a common belief that canine progeny reflect more of the mother's emotionality than the father's, but this has not been convincingly demonstrated as a sex-linked outcome. Prenatal and postnatal influences probably exert a more significant influence in these apparent differences. Other behavioral traits are strongly encoded and resist modification by maternal and other social influences. Scott and Fuller (1965) found that many breed-specific behavioral tendencies persist in spite of cross-fostering, isolation rearing, or transferring puppies at various ages to a litter of a different breed. Similarly, McBryde and Murphree (1974) were unable to detect a significant difference between genetically nervous pointer dogs raised with their nervous mother versus those

cross-fostered with normal mothers. Finally, Wilsson (1984/1985) has proposed that maternal influences on emotionality may depend more on how the mother treats her puppies during weaning rather than on a modeling effect resulting from her reactions toward humans.

Although much remains to be learned in this area, responsible breeders should "play it safe" and choose only mothers who are exemplary in both form and temperament, not leaning toward excesses in terms of fear, aggression, or excitability. In the case where a litter is born to an unstable mother, puppies should be weaned early (Fox, 1968) and placed under the care of a more balanced foster mother, or the puppies should be hand-fed. As the study by McBryde and Murphree suggests, though, the genetic substrate of such a mating will probably not yield very much to such efforts.

Although the early effects of mother nurturance, modeling, and discipline provide a secure foundation for social development, excessive contact with the mother beyond the first few months may have a disruptive and damaging effect on a dog's development. This is particularly evident in the case of some male puppies kept under the tutelage of an excessively domineering mother for too long. Such puppies may become insecure sycophants, unable to stand on their own and develop their full potential. Another common situation that is rather problematical is when two littermates are raised together. This sort of arrangement is rarely recommended, since very often one of the puppies seems to flourish while the sibling is overshadowed and fails to achieve its potential. Pfaffenberger observed similar difficulties with dogs reared with their mother or sibling:

> At San Rafael, besides the experience of having over-aggressiveness develop in dogs who did not remain under the mother's discipline long enough, we have had some bad effects from overlong canine socialization. I cannot remember a single dog who was raised with her mother to adulthood who could be successfully trained for a Guide Dog. Where two litter

mates are raised together in the same home we have had the same results. Puppies raised in homes where there are dogs not related to them have never been affected this way by the association with other dogs. ... In the case of two litter mates raised together, one becomes a successful candidate for Guide Dog work and one fails, even if their aptitude tests were equal. (1963:125)

Play and Socialization

Play is an important aspect of dog behavior, exercising a continuous influence over social development and learning throughout the life of a dog. Bekoff (1972) notes that play serves a vital mediational role in the formation of dominance hierarchies among both domestic and wild canids. Threat and appeasement displays are highly prepared, appearing early in a puppy's life and not requiring much learning for their expression. Young puppies exhibit a large repertoire of agonistic threat and appeasement behaviors. These behaviors are often first expressed during playful sparring activities between littermates. Considering the amount of such interaction, it is safe to assume that agonistic play serves an important role in the development of social behavior in dogs. Play depends on a high degree of interactive tolerance, affection, and trust—aspects of play that help to deflect and modulate social antagonisms that arise between closely bonded group members. Playful interaction continues only as long as the players remain friendly and confident. However, play is not simply about the exchange of affection—it is an activity in which various combative skills are practiced and mastered without risk of mutual injury to playful competitors. Agonistic play is a natural way for puppies to evaluate their social standing and to explore limits. Skinner (1982) notes that the aggressive play of puppies is modified and rendered more effective by intrinsic consequences that have no real survival relevance for the puppies besides shaping more effective play. Nonetheless, these early experiences prepare developing dogs for adulthood, making them more effective and skillful when remote contingencies finally do appear that threaten to produce potentially serious consequences. In addition to facilitating agonistic learning, play has many other influential facets that profoundly affect developing puppies, especially with respect to adult social responsiveness and trainability. Eberhard Trumler emphasizes the importance of play in this regard:

The main point to remember is that the games played during the socialisation period establish once and for all who is a playmate and who is not; if his master takes no part during this period, this is a fact which, from the dog's point of view, governs his attitude in the future. The canine father, who spends much of his time as teacher and trainer, also plays with his puppies; he is adept at using a game to turn his lessons into fun. In this we ourselves can learn from the dog. Development into a good sporting dog or a performing dog which will do all kinds of tricks with genuine pleasure begins in the socialisation phase. Only at this period is the puppy susceptible to learning the joy of learning. Only if account is taken of this natural evolution can a healthy attitude to learning be inculcated and there will then never be difficulties later when something new is demanded. ... Many difficulties will be avoided if one begins, while the dog is still a small puppy, to knit the bonds of confidence and establish one's own position of predominance and command authority by means of a merry game. Then the dog will show not antipathy to the new demands which change his existence but there will be a gradual transition from playing to all those other things which a good dog should be able to do. (1973:125–126)

The role of play in training and social development is more fully discussed in Volume 2, but briefly, in the succinct words of Hediger, "Good training is disciplined play" (1955/1968:139). Play and training are not contrary things, but complementary activities. If puppies or dogs cannot be shown the play in an activity, they will not willingly perform it for long. Nothing is more motivationally important in dog training than play.

LEARNING TO COMPETE AND COPE

With the close of the socialization period, dogs enter into a long period of juvenile development and progressive independence. The remainder of the chapter addresses the emergence of a number of prominent onto-genetic changes presaging adult social behavior and environmental adjustment. The developments between weeks 12 and 21 are associated with the integration of all major behavioral functional systems, maturing sensory abilities, and learning (Fig. 2.7).

Social Dominance (10 to 16 Weeks)

A dog's tendency to form lasting social bonds is derived from the evolutionary development of the pack as the basic social organization of wolf behavior. In the context of the pack, highly aggressive, possessive, and potentially dangerous individuals are brought together in harmonic coexistence. This close interaction is not without tension and periodic disputes over food, sleeping areas, possessions, breeding privileges, and leadership. These complex dynamics require a sophisticated internal organization and various "rules" governing social exchange. To ensure efficient functioning, pack members are ranked or socially stratified along a continuum of relative dominance. This so-called peck order or dominance hierarchy not only defines status but also assigns the various roles permitted and functions required of an animal's rank in the pack order. Behaving in ways inconsistent with one's status or rank results in social tension and possibly the display of hostilities toward the offending member.

Such organization serves many biologically significant functions. For instance, to be an effective large-prey predator, wolves long ago organized themselves in a way that maximizes their effectiveness as a hunting group. Also, stratified relations of dominance and subordination provide a powerful social glue binding an otherwise aggressive species together into a working unit while simultaneously reducing

Integration Period

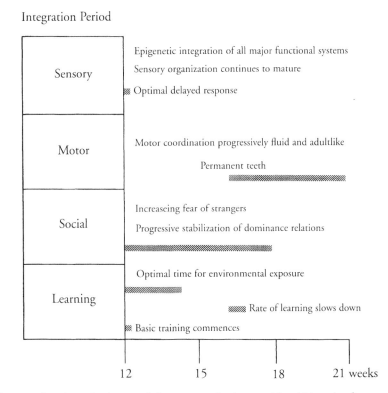

FIG. 2.7. Prominent developmental changes occurring between 12 and 21 weeks of age.

interactive tension and hostilities between members. Within the pack, there is a constant vigilance and tension pressing for the expansion of social power among members. This situation is kept in check through the exchange of ritualized threats and deferential appeasement displays. Serious dominance contests that result in damaging or lethal dominance fights infrequently occur in nature, although such fights occur more frequently among wolves (especially females) kept in captivity. Dominance is structured along sexually dimorphic lines with an alpha male and alpha female at the top of their respective hierarchies. Although the pack is usually led by the male, this is not always the case. Individual members within the pack form "political alliances" among themselves, adding further stability to the pack and complexity to the line of power. One such alliance is between the breeding pair. In essence, the union of the alpha male and alpha female brings the whole pack together in the united purpose of procreation. Social dominance yields two primary benefits to the alpha animal: status and reproductive prerogative. Within the context of the wolf pack, such positioning has tremendous value and is worth struggling to obtain and maintain, perhaps even risking serious injury when necessary.

Social competitiveness among puppies begins early, coinciding with the beginning of the socialization period. James (1955) found that, among 6-week-old puppies, dominant individuals routinely secured food first or threatened or pushed away subordinates. Actual physical attack with biting was rarely observed, indicating that at an early age more ritualized means of resolving competitive disputes are already functional. In a previous study (James, 1949), he found that a more or less stable social hierarchy develops among most litters of puppies by 12 weeks of age. He divides the hierarchy into three main parts: (1) a very *aggressive-dominant* group; (2) a midgroup (a group that may be better termed *subdominant*); and (3) an *inhibited-submissive* group. The midgroup is subordinate to the aggressive-dominant group but exhibits dominance over the inhibited-sub-

missive group. He noted that there was little antagonism among members belonging to the midgroup.

The harmonious interaction of midgroup members may be attributable to the midgroup's ample experience and exercise of both dominant and submissive behavior—that is, they more successfully ritualize their agonistic interaction. In the case of dominant-aggressive puppies, they are unable to defer, generating social tension wherever they happen to be. On the other hand, submissive puppies lack the ability to assert themselves, thus becoming the constant target of more aggressive and dominant littermates. Finally, James (1949) also observed that heated competitive interaction between dominant puppies infrequently resulted in the disputants attacking one another. Instead, a frustrated competitor was more likely to vent his hostility by redirecting it toward a submissive underling remaining at some distance away from the food bowl.

It has been frequently observed that puppies tend to eat more when fed in a social situation than when fed singly (Ross and Ross, 1949). James (1961) found that the effect of social facilitation on eating depends on the relative dominance of the puppies observed. Dominant puppies ate considerably more food in the presence of other puppies than was eaten by more subordinate counterparts. A similar dominance factor may help to explain Scott and McCray's (1967) findings concerning the effects of social facilitation on running speed in noncompetitive versus competitive situations. They determined that paired puppies ran a 200-foot course faster, but only if they were each given a food reward at the end of the run. When a competitive element was added—that is, only the winner was rewarded, the times were slightly depressed. Perhaps, under conditions of competition, the more subordinate puppy may decline to try as hard to obtain the reward. Consequently, the dominant one would not need to run quite as fast to get the food, which would explain the negative effect of competition on running speeds. Incidentally, the depressing effect of competition on running speeds was especially pronounced in cases where strong elements of competition were evident between the paired puppies.

A large portion of a puppy's interaction with littermates is of a competitive or agonistic nature. Competition may take place over the most productive teats, food, toys, sleeping areas, and, apparently, just for the fun of it. Playful dominance testing and nonspecific social quarreling is commonplace within the litter. The litter in many particulars is very similar to the pack. The latter may only be a more highly organized, purposeful, and regimented development of the former—a progression moving from a nurturing matriarchy to a stable patriarchal stratification of pack members into an organized working group.

Among wolf pups, serious aggressive efforts to establish dominance may appear as early as 30 days of age and result in a stable rank order between contestants (Mech, 1970). In the case of dogs, dominance relations between puppies are rather loosely organized and may change significantly during the early weeks of social development (Wright, 1980). A 7-week-old puppy might go to sleep content with her most recent dominance victory, only to lose it during breakfast the following day. The fluidity and instability of the dominance structure is probably responsible for the constant play fighting and agitation occupying the puppies when not sleeping or otherwise distracted. This social situation becomes progressively more organized through week 11, and by week 15 or 16 it is replaced by a stable social organization of dominant/subordinate relationships (Scott and Fuller, 1965). James (1949) also noted a stabilization of the dominance hierarchy occurring around 16 weeks of age in association with a sharp shift in dominance relations. After this time, the ranking order between the puppies remained stable into adulthood.

Although a puppy's size and sex are important determinants of social status, rank is also affected by various experiential factors, such as the quality and quantity of early social contact. Fisher (1955) found that permissively reared and indulged puppies were usually dominant over other experimental groups, including those puppies that were alternately punished or indulged during social contact, puppies whose social contact was limited to interactive punishment, and puppies that were isolated over the entire period. In comparison with these others, the indulged group was more competitive and aggressive during dominance tests; they consistently controlled the bone in spite of their often being female and smaller. Fisher noted only one exceptional case contrary to this general pattern. Of all the groups of puppies observed, the isolates were the least aggressive and competitive, having apparently lost or suffered a dramatic attenuation of the normal patterns of intraspecific agonistic behavior.

The implications of these findings are important for understanding puppy dominance testing and agonistic challenges directed toward family members. Prior to week 11, dominance positioning is more or less sham and labile, but as puppies move into month 4 and beyond, they become progressively more confident and defensive about their dominance status. Such puppies can be extremely "testy" and are often prepared for a battle of wills. As the result of previous playful fighting, dominant puppies may engage in persistent and provocative mouthing on the hands and clothing of their innocent and confused human companions, who may be of the false opinion that their puppy's oral excesses are mainly due to teething, exuberance, or affection. Precocious dominance aggression is occasionally observed among puppies of this age group. The problem with early displays of excessive mouthing or dominant behavior is that it frequently prefigures adult dominance-related problems. Further, since a dog's behavior is most flexible and malleable before 16 weeks of age, it is important that such issues be resolved by then. Many *gentle training* and massage techniques are now available to help facilitate subordination and cooperative behavior in puppies.

While young puppies may also engage in such testy behavior, their willingness to abandon the urge to dominance test and mouth makes it easier to modify or redirect. A general rule of thumb when choosing a puppy is to pick one that fits somewhere in the middle of the litter dominance hierarchy. Determining where a puppy lies within the peck order is not always easy, since dominance relations are loosely defined, especially during the early weeks. Tests devised by breeders and trainers to scan for and rate relative dominance have come under recent suspicion (Beaudet et al., 1994) although, as matters stand, testing can be useful even if the results are not entirely reliable as *fine* predictors of future behavior. There can be no doubt, however, in cases of extremes (as in overly aggressive or fearful temperament types) that such tendencies can be isolated by temperament testing performed by an experienced evaluator. Puppy testing has been used for predicting trainability in military working dogs (U.S. Army's Biosensor Research Team) and selecting guide-dog candidates (Pfaffenberger, 1963). Recently, however, Wilsson (1997) has questioned the validity of early puppy tests for predicting suitability for service-dog work. His tests carried out with 8-week-old puppies failed to detect predictive indicators for trainability when the dogs were tested again at between 15 and 20 months of age. Despite these problems, a good biweekly or weekly testing regimen may be beneficial for puppies simply because of the added attention and learning experiences it provides—contact that might not otherwise be available. These instruments are not intended to assess or predict potential temperament flaws or future performance in any particular area but are employed to evaluate a puppy's temperament at the time of testing and to define areas that may need special attention. Subsequent testing can be used to monitor a puppy's progress objectively.

Social Attachment and Separation

Puppies form very strong social attachments and become emotionally reactive and distressed when separated from littermates or the mother. For immature dogs, maintaining social contact enhances their chances of survival and is probably a strongly prepared canid trait. Sustained distress vocalization may serve to attract the attention and aid of the mother. Under conditions where help is not forthcoming, puppies (and the separation-anxious adult dogs) appear to become fixated in an unresolved state of emotional tension and progressive reactivity. The consequence of unanswered distress vocalization is escalation and perseveration. Several factors influence the magnitude of distress vocalization. Fredericson (1952) found that puppies separated from their littermates vocalized much more when confined alone, averaging 211 vocalizations per 5 minutes of observation versus 30 vocalizations when confined with a companion puppy. Another important factor is the location of confinement. Elliot and Scott (1961) found that puppies confined in a familiar area are much less reactive to separation than matched counterparts confined to a strange pen (Fig. 2.8). Furthermore, puppies tested in a familiar area appear to adjust progressively to separation from week 3 onward, whereas counterparts exposed to confinement in a strange area exhibit rising levels of distress that culminate during week 7. Comparing the two groups at 7 weeks of age shows that puppies confined to a strange pen are more than three times as reactive than those puppies confined in a familiar pen.

Pettijohn and colleagues (1977) carried out a series of experiments to compare various means of alleviating separation distress in young puppies. They compared the occurrence of distress vocalization in the presence of various stimulus conditions: food (bones, familiar food, and unfamiliar food), toys (hard toy, soft toy, and towel), dog contact (mother, unfamiliar dog, and mirror), and human contact (observer behind wire, passive handler, and active handler). The least effective stimulus condition for the attenuation of separation distress was food, with unfamiliar food being slightly more effective than familiar food or bones. Among toys, the strongest alleviation was obtained with soft objects, including a stuffed animal and a towel. The provision of hard rubber toys yielded no benefit. Interestingly, the withdrawal of the soft toys resulted in a distress surge moving above pretest baseline levels. The mirror produced a strong modulatory effect on distress vocaliza-

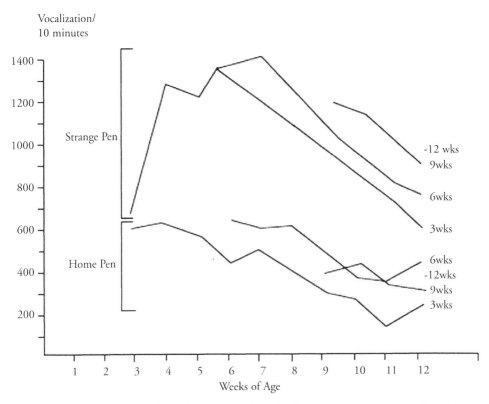

Vocalization/
10 minutes

F IG. 2.8. Distress vocalization is affected by context, with the familiar home pen producing significantly less distress than that occurring in the strange one. Note that separation-distress reactions in the strange pen peak between 6 to 8 weeks. After Elliot and Scott (1961), with permission.

tion, only slightly less so than the presence of the puppy's mother. They observed little difference in the effect of the mother versus an unfamiliar dog. The most effective attenuation of separation distress (even better than contact with the mother) was produced by both active (slightly better) and passive contact with a human handler (Fig. 2.9).

The manner in which separation reactivity and distress is handled may dramatically effect how well a puppy copes with being left alone. Care should be taken to expose the puppy gradually to increasing confinement and graduated separation experiences. Traumatic crate training, excessive confinement, long-term isolation, and dependency-producing affection rituals (excessive pampering and coddling) may contribute to the later devel-

opment of separation problems. Young puppies have a strong developmental need for close, sustained social contact with conspecifics—a need that a new owner must satisfy. The practice of having a puppy sleep in the kitchen or laundry room (often allowing the puppy to cry to point of exhaustion) is not a sensible approach, since such experiences may sensitize the puppy to react negatively when confined or when left alone. Early confinement experiences associated with high degrees of distress may potentiate unwanted separation reactions, including destructiveness, excessive vocalization, or house soiling. By exposing puppies to gradual increments of confinement and separation, they can more naturally habituate and learn to accept being left alone when that is necessary.

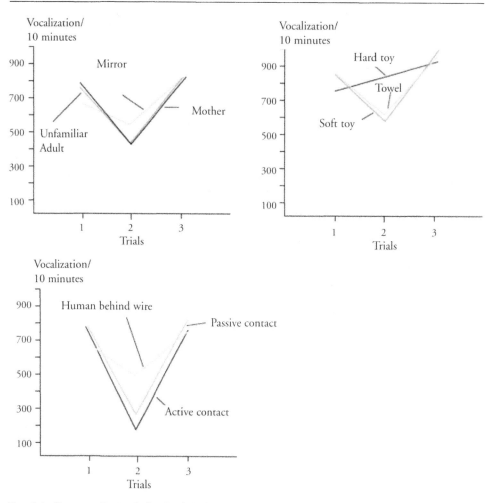

FIG. 2.9. Shows vocalization before (trial 1), during presentation (trial 2), and after withdrawal of the test stimulus (trial 3). Note that contact with a passive or active human produces more reduction of separation distress than when in the presence of the mother. After Pettijohn et al. (1977).

Puppies not exposed to separation experiences early in their development tend to become excessively reactive when they are finally exposed to it. Elliot and Scott (1961) evaluated the reactions of several groups of puppies that were exposed for the first time to separation in a strange pen at different ages beginning at week 3. The puppies were divided into four groups. Group 1 was first exposed to separation in a strange pen at 3 weeks of age—an experience that was subsequently repeated on a weekly basis through week 12. The other puppies were similarly exposed to weekly testing, but it was delayed until they were 6 weeks old (group 2), 9 weeks old (group 3), and 12 weeks old (group 4). Interestingly, puppies belonging to group 4 that were not exposed to separation until 12 weeks of age appeared to panic and were unable to cope effectively with such experiences, whereas the other groups (especially group 1) appeared to have learned how to adjust more effectively when separated from littermates—that is, they appeared to have habituated to the separation experience (Fig. 2.10). Additionally, this study also demonstrated that there exists a definite relationship between increasing reactivity to sep-

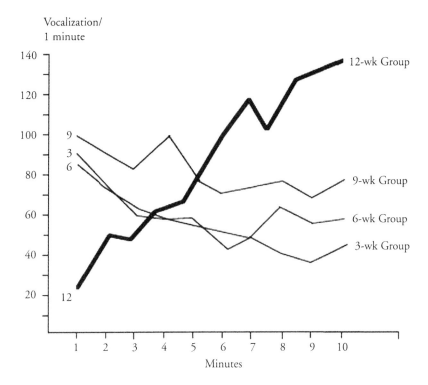

Fig. 2.10. Pattern of habituation to separation at various age groups. Note strong reaction of the 12-week group not previously exposed to separation. After Elliot and Scott (1961).

aration and the appearance of the hypothetical optimal period for secondary socialization at around 7 weeks of age. The separation re-activity of the 3- and 6-week-old puppies clearly peaked at this time (Fig. 2.8).

There appears to be no direct link between the emotions of fear (e.g., startle) with separation anxiety (Davis et al., 1977). Also, Scott (1967) concludes, on the basis of studies involving chlorpromazine, that the tranquilizer's effect on separation distress is the result of generalized sedation rather than a reduction of anxiety:

In moderate doses the tranquilizer chlorpromazine has the effect of slowing down the rate of vocalization, but larger doses do not produce a proportionate increase in the effect, which appears to be an indirect result of sedation rather than a direct effect of alleviating the emotion. Under this drug a puppy with his litter mates will be sound asleep. Placed in a strange situation, he immediately gets on his feet and starts vocalizing, at a somewhat lower rate than usual, but without a letup. Assuming that chlorpromazine has the effect of alleviating anxiety, and defining anxiety as the emotion generated by anticipation of events in the future, we can conclude that anxiety plays little part in the emotional responses to isolation in a strange place. (1967:124)

Although both fear and anxiety appear to be distinct from separation-distress reactions, punishment tends to paradoxically increase attachment behavior in young puppies (Fisher, 1955; Stanley and Elliot, 1962). Therefore, punishing a separation-anxious puppy may *indirectly* make the animal's separation distress worse, resulting in increased barking, yelping, and the exhibition of other separation-related behaviors. A similar effect has also been reported by Hess (1964), who demonstrated that attachment behavior among chicks is facilitated by the delivery of mild electric shocks presented during the imprinting process. Additionally, confining a puppy to a crate may make things worse. Despite a widespread belief to the contrary, a puppy does not appear to feel more secure when restrained in a crate. Ross and colleagues (1960) found that puppies were especially reactive to separation when restrained—whether alone or with a littermate. Restrained puppies were three times more reactive than unrestrained littermates exposed to the same conditions of isolation (Fig. 2.11). The degree of familiarity with the location of restraint also appears to play an important role. Puppies are much less separation reactive when confined in a familiar area. When puppies are restrained in an unfamiliar area, however, emotional reactivity is greatly amplified, with the frequency of distress vocalizations doubling in number (Scott, 1967). These laboratory findings suggest that the practice of confining a puppy in a remote part of the house (like the basement) should be avoided.

Although some risk exists in punishing a noisy puppy, it may be necessary to do so [e.g., a loud clap of the hands and reprimand or the toss of a shaker can (a soda can with several pennies in it)] for the sake of expediency, especially where sustained desensitization efforts have failed or have produced only modest results. Whenever possible, however, distress vocalization should be managed by shaping quiet behavior with rewards and performing a series of graduated departures. Even in cases where punishment is successful, the suppressed distress vocalization may only end up being replaced with a worse problem like house soiling or destructive behavior (Borchelt, 1984).

LEARNING TO ADJUST AND CONTROL

The foregoing discussion has emphasized the role of early socialization and attachment in the ontogeny of puppies. Puppies that fail to receive sufficient contact during the critical period of socialization may exhibit lasting deficits in their social responsiveness and general trainability. To gain the most benefit from the least effort and investment of time, it has been demonstrated that timing is of vital importance. In fact, it has been estimated that as little as *20 minutes of social contact per week* during the socialization period is sufficient to offset the adverse effects of social isolation in puppies (Fuller, 1967). With such an impact occurring as the result of minimum social contact, one can only imagine the potential benefits possible for young puppies that receive that amount of focused attention every day.

Environmental Adaptation (3 to 16 Weeks)

Of equal importance to a puppy's psychosocial development is access to a varied environment rich in diversity of objects, textures, and structures with which to interact and explore. A puppy's curiosity and excitement about the external environment emerge along with the development of the various senses and motor abilities. Nature itself provides a boundless outlet for a puppy's inquisitiveness and exploratory activity. For instance, an outdoor excursion or a playful romp in the woods provides a profusely enriched environmental experience. Nature is the most readily available resource for sensory-motor exposure and locomotor experience and experimentation, but exposure to nature alone is not enough to ensure adequate stimulation and

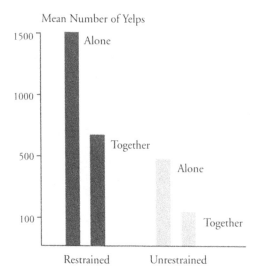

FIG. 2.11. Restraint has a pronounced potentiating effect on distress vocalization in puppies separated from littermates in a strange place. After Ross et al. (1960).

adjustment. Although the natural environment provides puppies with outlets for exploratory behavior, they must also be exposed and habituated to stimuli associated with the artificial environment within which they will spend the majority of life. This includes exposure to the sounds of traffic, everyday noises like a vacuum cleaner, and various other noisy appliances and routines.

A puppy's sensory and psychological need for environmental exposure is supported by the results of many studies on the effects of isolation on development. Thompson and Heron (1954) compared the effects of severe, moderate, and normal restriction on general activity and exploratory behavior. Their results show that activity levels and exploratory behavior significantly increased, depending on degree of restriction, but these differences gradually narrowed as a function of remedial exposure and maturity, suggesting that some of the effects of early restriction are reversible. Thompson and colleagues (1956) observed that, in addition to increasing general activity levels, severe restriction resulted in the development of compulsive whirling and tail snapping in isolates. Of 11 Scottish terriers exposed to severe restriction, eight developed the stereotypic habit of whirling. Fisher (1955) also observed similar whirling behavior exhibited by isolates while in their home cages; however, after several weeks of exposure to a nonrestricted and socially enriched environment, the whirling habit disappeared. The habit was most conspicuous among wirehaired terriers. Fox (1967) found that even short periods of partial isolation early in the socialization period produced pronounced effects on behavioral and neurological functioning. Isolates were restricted to a darkened room for 1 week (week 4) with human contact being limited to 1.5 minutes per day for cleaning and feeding. Controls were kept in a similar cage but with greater exposure and contact with other dogs. The gross behavior of isolates was different from controls along several dimensions: isolates were much more active, their behavior was disorganized, and they tended to ignore visually and tactilely interesting objects (a mirror, toy, and piece of cloth). Although both isolates and controls were attracted to a cloth item,

the isolates spent most of their time sniffing rather than biting or playing with it. When the mirror, toys, and cloth were removed, isolates were unaffected whereas controls scratched at the door or searched the testing area while whining or crying. Controls approached the mirror with tail wagging whereas the isolates took no interest in it. In general, isolates were socially withdrawn (exhibiting little vocalization or tail wagging) and did not engage in playful interaction with littermates. Further, isolates showed a preference for inanimate objects and engaged in self-play instead of making social contact with other puppies or observers. Fox also found that exposure to short-term isolation resulted in the display of tail chasing and whirling previously observed by Thompson and colleagues.

In addition to the behavioral deficits resulting from short-term partial isolation, Fox (1967) found several correlative alterations in brain-wave activity of the isolates when compared with controls. From these observations, he concluded that isolates were overwhelmed by intense arousal stimulated by the enriched testing area. He speculated that isolates suffered an increased sensitivity to sensory stimulation. The neurological locus of the dysfunction may have been "acute reticular arousal," rendering the isolate unable to filter out irrelevant from relevant input. The outcome of overarousal was a short-circuiting of the isolate's ability to select appropriate and adaptive responses to the impinging stimulation affecting them. Under the influence of remedial exposure, short-term isolates quickly recovered and appeared normal according to behavioral and EEG parameters after 7 days.

The effects of long-term isolation have also been studied. Lessac and Solomon (1969) isolated puppies from 12 weeks to 12 months of age and then compared their behavior under various testing situations with that of controls raised under the influence of social contact and environmental exposure. Isolates exhibited many "psychologically destructive, deteriorative, or debilitative effects" (1969:22). During observations of free-ranging behavior, the experimenters found that isolates exhibited sustained generalized arousal, high motor activity, diffuse emotionality, and distractibility, perhaps representing a developmental model of hyperactive-attention deficit disorder. The isolates frequently bumped into furniture and walls. They appeared oblivious to their surroundings, swept up in a vortex of "diffuse and disorganized behavior." They ignored external sounds and barked at irregular intervals independently of what they happened to be doing or attending to at the moment. While many of them raced toward the experimenter when he entered the room, they failed to make any contact. They simply raced by as though not seeing him.

In contrast, the controls, which were raised with social contact and environmental exposure, were much more focused and directed in their free-ranging activities. When they barked, the barking was directed at someone or something. They also spent a lot of time pawing at the door separating them from the experimenter. Although initially very excited, the puppies calmed down within 5 minutes. They intently sniffed and explored the test area, frequently spending as long as 90 seconds exploring a single object attracting their attention. When noises occurred on the outside of the room, they quickly oriented in the direction of the sounds. When the experimenter entered, they all approached and followed him around the room.

Two particular test situations revealed striking signs of disability involving coping mechanisms and the breakdown of previously learned behavior, especially with regard to effects associated with frustration and pain/fear reactions. Lessac and Solomon tested 12-week-old puppies on their ability to solve a simple barrier test and to learn a shock-escape/avoidance response. The experimental isolates and controls were subsequently tested at 12 months. The barrier test requires that a puppy go around a wire barrier in order to obtain meat on the other side. Puppies at 12 weeks of age exposed to this problem solved it within 50 seconds (all values are mean approximations). Testing after a year revealed that isolates languished behind the barrier for up to 130 seconds before solving the problem, while the socialized/exposed controls

solved the problem within 10 to 15 seconds—substantially bettering their scores observed at 12 weeks of age. Interestingly, Fox (1967) found that week-4 isolates were significantly slower than controls in solving this barrier test, as well. The author noted that, instead of eating as the controls did, the isolates nibbled on the meat briefly and ran off. Instead of improving over a number of trials, the isolates' ability to solve the problem appeared to deteriorate with practice.

The study also tested the isolates' ability to learn a simple shuttle-box escape-avoidance response. The puppies were placed in a box divided into two compartments divided by a shoulder-high barrier. The discriminative stimulus signaling pending shock was a 10-second darkness interval. The moment the puppy jumped the barrier, the light was turned back on and shock terminated. Shock was continued for up to 1-minute duration or until the puppy jumped over the barrier. The mean time for 12-week-old puppies to escape shock was 16 seconds. Interestingly, one of the experimental groups that had not received training at 12 weeks prior to being isolated did particularly poorly on this test, taking 45 seconds to jump the barrier while receiving continuous shock. This is in sharp contrast to the socialized control group (which also had not received training at 12 weeks), which successfully jumped the barrier in 9 seconds. In both of these tests, a strong emotional component involving frustration and pain/fear is involved. Isolates appear to possess particularly poor adjustment skills when it comes to situations charged with frustrative or fearful components.

Fuller (1967) also reported a series of experiments examining the effects of isolation on puppy behavior and has evaluated various techniques for reversing its effects (Fuller and Clark, 1966a, 1966b). Fuller exposed several groups of puppies to varying amounts of isolation to determine the causes underlying the isolation effect. Consistent with findings of Lessac and Solomon (1969), Fuller observed that isolates tended to exhibit striking emotional, sensory, and motor deficits when first exposed to an open area for observation.

However, Fuller has interpreted these findings in a somewhat different way. Lessac and Solomon viewed isolation as having a destructive, deteriorative effect on the isolate, whereas Fuller explains the isolation effect in terms of an emergence-stress response. Unlike controls that have had a chance to habituate to the complex stimuli associated with ordinary levels of stimulation, isolates when first exposed to an ordinary environment are overwhelmed by its novelty and complexity. Since they are inadequately prepared to process and respond to the stimulation, they are seized by various emotional reactions and bizarre behaviors that block more appropriate and adaptive coping behaviors. Even when puppies were raised together in pairs or permitted access to toys in their cages, the isolation effect was still evident when they were finally released from confinement.

Fuller has theorized that the behavior of isolates is precipitated by an emotional state incompatible with normal adjustment. Consequently, he carried out a series of experiments based on this simple hypothesis: if postisolation disturbances of behavior are due to excessive emotional arousal, then such disturbances could be ameliorated if the emotional reactivity of the isolated puppies was reduced. To test this hypothesis, he exposed isolates to two emotion-reducing influences: handling and chlorpromazine. Fuller found that isolates handled or given a combination of handling and chlorpromazine prior to exposure performed more like normal controls (Fuller and Clark, 1966b). Fuller and Clark conclude that isolated puppies (provided that they are not genetically hypersensitive to the effects of isolation) can recover their emotional and sensory equilibrium if exposed to appropriate handling and/or drug therapy:

> It appears that much perceptual organization can take place with minimal stimulation, and that appropriate responses can be elicited readily in post-isolates if interfering behavior is controlled. Certainly the intensity of post-isolation effects can be greatly modified by varying the conditions of emergence. Under especially favorable circumstances, forced contact with the handler, a suitable dose of chlorpro-

mazine, and a robust genotype, the post-isolation syndrome can be totally eliminated. The outlook for the experientially deprived organism may be more hopeful than recent experiments have indicated. (1966b:257)

Development of Exploratory Behavior

Socialization and environmental exposure practices should follow an age-appropriate pattern. Waiting until a puppy is 16 weeks old before letting it venture out into the real world is too late. On the other hand, exposing a puppy too early to too much stimulation may generate negative side effects, as well. Scott and Fuller (1965) found that puppies reared under semiferal conditions avoided excursions beyond 10 to 20 feet from their home boxes until they were around 12 weeks of age. Such information suggests that a puppy's readiness for environmental exploration and exposure is developmentally sensitive. Some puppies do, in fact, strongly object to leaving their immediate home environments until after they reach 12 weeks of age, yet many puppies as young as 7 weeks old happily explore new environments as long as they are in the company and safety of a human guardian.

Fox and Spencer (1969) carried out a series of experiments to determine the relative importance of experience versus age on the development of exploratory behavior. The puppies they studied were divided into two groups depending on the sort of test exposure they experienced at different ages. Cross-sectional exposure involved exposing puppies to the novel stimulus situation at various ages, some at 5, some at 8, some at 12, and some at 16 weeks of age. The second group, longitudinal exposure, had puppies exposed to novel stimulus situations at each of the above test periods. In other words, the cross-sectional group was exposed to only one test period overall, while the longitudinal group was exposed to all four test periods. The worst deficits were observed in the cross-sectional groups exposed to the test situation at only weeks 12 and 16, suggesting that early experience with novelty is crucial for the development of normal exploratory behavior. The study revealed that the longitudinal group became progressively more exploratory than the cross-sectional group over time. The puppies receiving longitudinal exposure via testing to novel stimulus situations significantly benefited in terms of their tendency to explore and tolerate novel situations and events.

Wright (1983) has studied the effects of different rearing practices on exploratory behavior and stimulus reactivity in German shepherd puppies. He tested and evaluated the differential effects of hand rearing versus litter rearing on the exploratory behavior and stimulus reactivity of puppies at 5.5 weeks and 8.5 weeks. His findings indicate that hand-reared puppies are significantly more curious, spending more time in close proximity to and examining more frequently novel objects placed in their environments. In contrast, litter-reared puppies are much more reserved and avoidant toward novelty at 8.5 weeks of age than are hand-reared counterparts. Wright concludes that rearing practices should include active handling and environmental exposure early in a puppy's life to both enhance curiosity and receptivity to novelty and to prevent the development of fearful avoidance responding:

> There are practical applications of these findings for breeders interested in increasing the chances that their pups will not develop avoidance reactions to unfamiliar aspects of their environment. First, rearing pups together, with access to large areas for locomotor activity, may not be an adequate rearing-procedure by itself. Second, handling, and the exposure to unfamiliar people, other animals and other novel stimuli (characteristic of hand-rearing) may be a more effective rearing-strategy. (1983:33)

During outdoor excursions, extra precautions should be taken to minimize risks on at least two fronts: (1) the risk of exposure to communicable disease and (2) the risk of exposure to traumatic or overly threatening experiences. The first danger can be mitigated by avoiding places frequented by other dogs and keeping the puppy's vaccinations up to date. The second caution is harder to guard safely against. As previously mentioned, there is a particularly sensitive period for the development of lasting fear impressions, extending roughly between weeks 8 and 10. For instance, if a puppy is accidentally stepped upon as a 9-week-old, he may develop a chronic fear of feet or shoes. Many adult phobic reactions in dogs may have their origins stemming from experiences occurring during this period.

Careful environmental exposure carried out systematically through gradual increments of intensity and duration allows puppies to habituate to potentially fear-eliciting stimuli without undue distress. A puppy's environment should be rich in diversity of objects, textures, and structures with which to interact and explore. A puppy's curiosity and excitement about the environment emerges as the puppy matures and develops greater confidence in the complementary directions of emotional security and physical dexterity. Owners should refrain from reassuring nervous puppies by petting and soothing words while the puppies exhibit fear, even though it seems so natural and appropriate. The provision of such emotional support is hard to resist, but it may inadvertently strengthen a puppy's fearful reaction rather than reduce it. Attempts to relax and calm puppies should be made prior to exposing them to the fear-eliciting stimulus.

An effort should be made to expose puppies to a wide variety of physical and social situations, while being careful to ensure that they are positive experiences. Techniques for reducing fear responses are discussed in great detail later, but the key to environmental exposure is a patient, gradual, and orderly progression of direct interactive exposure. It is useful to engage puppies in an activity that they have already learned and enjoy while such exposure is taking place—for example, walking quietly on the leash, playing ball or fetching a stick, taking treats of food, or receiving petting and praise. Keep the process active and moving, ever-prepared to distract puppies should they become too fearful or alarmed. In general, puppies engaged in some activity or movement tend to be less anxious and fearful than those unoccupied or standing still.

The staging of environmental adaptation experiences should include exposure to those things that are desirable for puppies to approach as well as teaching them the things and activities to avoid. Just as fears and phobias are readily established during the socialization period, appetites and potentially harmful activities are also quickly learned. Many problems can be avoided by carefully selecting chew toys that cannot be easily generalized to valued personal belongings. Giving a puppy an old shoe, socks, discarded plastic bottles, a broken chair leg, or carpet remnants establishes such objects (and similar ones) as chew toys. The consequence is to inadvertently turn the entire house into a sumptuous temptation for an orally active and exploratory puppy. In addition to the very likely possibility that oral preferences are imprinted to some extent, chewing for the dogs is both physically and psychologically satisfying. Consequently, puppies may develop a lifelong appetite and preference for items presented to them for oral entertainment early on. These acquired preferences may persist indefinitely or until they undergo aversive counterconditioning or punishment, a rather unfair outcome since the whole situation could have been prevented by more careful selection of chew toys in the first place. Prevention rests on directing oral exploration into outlets of greatest satisfaction and limiting these outlets to a small number of objects easily discriminated from personal belongings. Efforts to prevent puppies from engaging in inappropriate or destructive chewing behavior should include careful supervision and confinement. Unfortunately, crate confinement often takes the place of puppy training. Although the crate performs a useful function in puppy training, it is often used in excess or as a permanent method of daily confinement. Long-term or excessive reliance on crate or kennel confinement may have an adverse effect on the social behavior of an otherwise well-socialized puppy (Fox, 1974).

Learning and Trainability

The socialization period extends roughly from weeks 3 to 12. Throughout this period, puppies exhibit a pronounced sensitivity for the acquisition of a wide variety of social and environmental coping and adjustment skills.

If puppies are not provided with adequate social contact or exposure to an environment rich in variety during this period, their psychosocial development may be significantly compromised or impaired. Such puppies are unlikely to reach their full potential as adults and may be at risk for developing a variety of behavior problems linked with developmental deficits or trauma occurring during these early formative weeks. Controlled studies show that puppies are able learners; in fact, this period could very aptly be called the "critical period for social learning." At no other time in a dog's life is he more receptive to training based on affection and reward. EEG measures and the results of many behavioral studies demonstrate that 8-week-old puppies function at nearly an adult level in terms of learning ability. Apparently, however, as puppies mature, the ease with which they learn noticeably begins to decline by about 16 weeks of age (Scott and Fuller, 1965):

> As to basic learning capacities the puppy appears to be fully developed before the outset of the juvenile period. At about 4 months of age the speed of formation of conditioned reflexes begins to slow down. This is probably not because the nervous system deteriorates but rather because what the puppy has previously learned begins to interfere with new learning. As will be seen later there is some evidence that the behavior of the puppy begins to reach a stable organization about this age; that is, he has established the foundation for what he will learn in the future. (1965:109)

Fox performed a number of experiments to explore the developmental constraints affecting early learning in dogs. For example, in one of these influential studies, he trained puppies at various ages to run toward a handler positioned at the end of a short runway (Fox, 1966b). The puppies were divided into three age groups, ranging from 5 to 13 weeks of age. After the above preliminary training was carried out, the puppies were exposed to a mild shock that was delivered just before they reached the handler. The results from week to week were somewhat surprising and puzzling. Fox found that the 5- to 6-week-old puppies tended to "forgive" the handler between the weekly testing sessions and would approach without hesitation despite past shock experiences. On the other hand, puppies belonging to the 8- to 9-week-old group tended to be much more avoidant, with half of them refusing to approach at all. In contrast, the 12- to 13-week-old puppies tended to persevere and continued to approach the handler, apparently ignoring the threat of shock. From these results, he concluded that avoidance training prior to week 8 is not practical since the effects of such learning tend to degrade rapidly. However, waiting until the puppy is 12 or 13 weeks of age may be too late for the initiation of some forms of avoidance training. The best time to commence mild avoidance training appears to be around 8 to 9 weeks of age:

> Conditioned avoidance (electroshock on approach to human) was unstable in pups aged between 5–6 weeks, so that learning at this age cannot be reliably undertaken, for without considerable reinforcement, the learned response will disappear with age. In some pups aged 8–9 weeks, electroshock caused stable conditioned avoidance indicating this age is a sensitive period when certain traumatic stimuli have the most marked effect. Thus inhibitory training (sit, stay and house breaking) may be most easily accomplished at this time. By 12–13 weeks of age, inhibitory training is more difficult to establish for emotional attachment to man may interfere with certain inhibitory training procedures. However, leash training to heel, follow and retrieve on the basis of these findings could be commenced at this age. Thus reward training (food, or contact by stroking and vocal reward) by virtue of the close emotional bond that can be established between dog and trainer, can best be commenced at 3 months of age. (Fox, 1966b:285–286)

In another experiment, Fox and Spencer (1967) studied the development of delayed-response learning in dogs. Positive results from delayed-response testing have been strongly correlated with higher cognitive functions and working memory. To navigate the delayed-response test successfully, puppies must be able mentally to represent significant features of the stimulus situation, hold that information in memory across time, and apply it to the problem at hand. The basic experimental situation utilized by the experimenters consisted of an 8-foot (2.4-m) by 8-foot testing area containing a starting box and three other boxes uniformly distributed in the space. One compartment, the neutral box, located in the rear center of the area, never contained food. The experiment required that the various groups of puppies learn to identify the location of a piece of hidden food by relying on secondary cues provided by the handler's position. In other words, the puppies had to first learn that the hidden food could always be found in the compartment located closest to the handler. Gradually, they were exposed to increasingly difficult requirements and then tested for delayed-response abilities. The test phase of the experiment involved allowing puppies to observe the location of the handler and then blocking their view of the situation by briefly closing the starting box, at which time the handler left the testing area. Once clear, each puppy was released into the area but without the advantage of the handler's presence to help it locate the hidden food—the puppy had to remember the handler's location in order to solve the problem. The delay was gradually increased over several trials, and the puppies' performance recorded at various ages. The experiment revealed that puppies differed in their delayed-response abilities according to their age.

Interestingly, both the 4-week-old group and the 16-week-old group performed poorly on the task. The best delayed-response performances were made by puppies belonging to the 12-week-old group. The results of this study seem to provide additional support to the findings of Scott and Fuller, indicating an apparent disruption of learning abilities as puppies approach 16 weeks of age. On average, the 16-week-old puppies made far more mistakes than did the 12-week-old puppies. Fox has speculated that this negative shift in learning ability may be the result of a phasic developmental excitatory-inhibitory imbalance in which excitatory processes temporarily override inhibitory ones. As a result of such excitatory dominance, 16-week-old puppies may be less able to inhibit incorrect responses to the unrewarded box, thus making more errors than the neurally balanced 12-week-old group. These findings suggest that puppies pass through an important developmental phase or "terminal maturational processes" of increased excitability at around 16 weeks of age. It also indicates that this period may not be the best time to commence inhibitory training. This shift in ability is temporary, since adult dogs perform better in delayed response than do 12-week-old puppies.

What appear to be somewhat conflicting results concerning the puppies delayed-response abilities have been reported by Gagnon and Dore (1994). In a series of experiments exploring *object permanence* in dogs, a variation on delayed-response testing, the researchers found little difference among dogs between 8 weeks to 9 months of age with respect to their ability to locate objects that had been invisibly displaced as they looked on. Reliable evidence of object permanence was not observed in dogs that were under 11 months of age. The study suggests that a late developmental period occurring at the end of the first year is associated with cognitive elaborations involving object permanence. The researchers found that puppies between 6 and 7 months of age were unable to locate invisibly displaced objects, whereas dogs 11 months and older were regularly successful in their efforts to locate invisibly displaced objects. Dogs between 8 and 10 months of age exhibit mixed abilities with respect to object-permanence abilities. Although tentative, these results suggest the existence of a very significant change in canine cognitive abilities at approximately 11 months. Comparing these results with the earlier findings of Fox and Spencer is problematical. The two studies employ very different experimental designs and, perhaps, measure different cognitive abilities, making conclusions difficult to form regarding their significance for one another.

The quality of secondary socialization taking place after week 12 appears to have a direct bearing on a dog's trainability as an adult. Pfaffenberger and Scott (1959) carried out a socialization experiment involving guide-dog puppies. All the puppies involved were exposed to identical treatment, training, and testing until week 12. During week 12, some of the puppies were removed from the kennel situation and reared in homes under the care of 4-H Club members. Also, at this time, the usual contact between the remaining puppies and the evaluators was terminated. Of the puppies placed in 4-H homes at 12 weeks of age that had successfully passed earlier temperament and intelligence tests, 90% went on to complete guide-dog training successfully at 1 year of age. The remaining puppies were placed in foster homes over the next several weeks at different ages until week 19. The experiment revealed a striking effect: those animals that were placed into homes more than 2 weeks after the close of the socialization period (12 weeks) had a significantly higher rate of failure than puppies that had been placed in homes during week 12 (Fig. 2.12).

Pfaffenberger and Scott argued that this effect was probably due to an abrupt break in the socialization process, rather than the result of some underlying developmental change taking place during the several weeks immediately following the close of the socialization period. Provided that this supposition is accurate, it would seem to indicate that the

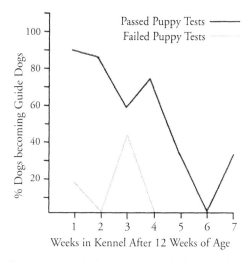

FIG. 2.12. Puppies kept in the kennel after 12 weeks of age were less likely to become guide dogs as adults. This influence was especially marked in puppies failing early "aptitude" tests. After Pfaffenberger and Scott (1959).

benefits of early socialization may be reversible in an especially negative way by abrupt cessation of socialization activities following the conclusion of the socialization period. The phenomenon observed by Pfaffenberger and Scott may be an artifact produced by the superficial socialization efforts carried out prior to week 12. From birth to 8 weeks of age, the experimental group of puppies received only minimal social contact that took place incidental to custodial care. During the period extending from weeks 8 to 12, they received a half-hour of individual contact per week associated with evaluation and various testing procedures. Although a half-hour per week of sustained socialization appears to be enough to produce a normal dog, it may not be enough to produce a puppy able to withstand the effects of abrupt partial isolation. Fox has also noted that the socialization effect is contingent on sustained social contact and may be reversed under conditions of neglect and isolation:

> Although there is an optimal period for socializing pups, there is evidence that dogs may subsequently regress or become feral. The social bond with man may be broken when well-socialized pups are placed in kennels at three or four months of age; by six or eight months they are shy of strangers and often of their caretakers if they have not been handled much. In addition, they may be extremely fearful when removed from their usual quarters. Their fearfulness is the result of a combination of institutionalization and desocialization. (1974:60–61)

This so-called *kennel-dog syndrome* is particularly evident in German shepherds, with the more independent terrier breeds being apparently less susceptible to the negative effects of prolonged kenneling (Scott, 1967).

Imprinting-like Processes and Canine Skill Learning

Imprinting is a learning phenomenon distinguished by three primary characteristics: (1) it requires a small amount of early exposure, (2) it occurs during a relatively short sensitive period, and (3) it exhibits long-lasting and durable effects. The imprinting period is usually bounded by relevant developmental processes. The learning or lack of learning experienced during this impressionable period is largely irreversible. In its broadest sense, imprinting is a process (limited by the aforementioned parameters) whereby an innately prepared species-specific tendency or pattern of behavior is brought under the control of a preferred stimulus, releasing agent, object, or situation. Although imprinting is a learning phenomenon primarily associated with social attachment and identification, its role in the development of complex behavioral patterns is worthy of speculation. Tinbergen (1951/1969) observed that Eskimo dogs in Greenland learned the territorial boundaries of neighboring packs during a fixed "critical" period associated with sexual maturity. Two of the dogs he observed began to defend territory and avoided other territories within 1 week of their first sexual encounters. Prior to this time, the dogs appeared unable to learn not to trespass onto surrounding territories in spite of repeated and severe attacks, a persistence Tinbergen attributes to developmental immaturity. Similarly, many canine skills like retrieving, willingness to stay close during walks, coming when called, and house training appear to have especially sensitive periods for their introduction and training.

For instance, a dog's willingness to fetch an object is definitely influenced by early exposure to retrieving games. If puppies are prevented from engaging in ball play until after week 14 or so, they may not show a significant interest or willingness to engage in activity later on. Although many such dogs can be eventually trained to retrieve, the process is impeded by a lack of early exposure and experience. Scott and Fuller (1965) made a valuable serendipitous discovery about the importance of early exposure for learning retrieving skills by dogs. As the result of logistical constraints, they put off retrieving tests until puppies were 32 weeks of age instead of performing them during week 9 as had been their original plan. The experimenters were surprised by the puppies' poor retrieving scores: only 11% returned the item and released it to their handlers. They also observed that the 32-week-old puppies were harder to train than those that had been introduced to retrieving earlier, at 9 weeks of age. They concluded that there might exist a critical period for learning to retrieve, "a time when the probability of executing the complete pattern is relatively high, so that reward training can be maximally effective" (Scott and Fuller 1965:219).

Incidentally, the single most reliable indicator of a puppy's general temperament and potential as a companion or working dog is revealed by the puppy's willingness to retrieve. Many "gifted" puppies perform this activity without any previous training and on the first or second try. In my experience, such puppies, all other things being equal, usually develop into excellent companions and working dogs. As an evaluator at Biosensor (U.S. Army Superdog Program), I found that the most reliable predictor among young puppies (8 to 10 weeks) for success as military dog prospects was an avidity for ball play and vigorous interest in rag play. Similarly, Pfaffenberger (1963) reports a strong link between a puppy's willingness to retrieve and later success in training as an adult guide dog. Another highly predictive indicator was a puppy's degree of tolerance toward novel (frightening) moving objects. Failure to fetch a ball or tolerate the approach of a small two-wheeled cart predicted an increased risk of failure in the guide-dog training program.

An area of interest for average dog owners regards active following and coming when called. Long walks consisting of occasional surprise maneuvers, exciting changes of pace, unexpected chase and counterchase episodes, hide-and-seek games, punctuated with occasional opportunities for ball play or stick fetching—all facilitate the learning of appropriate "staying close" skills in puppies. Such interaction strongly stimulates leader-follower bonding and other social components conducive to obedience training. If puppies are not exposed to such experiences during the socialization period, as adult dogs they are typically more difficult to train to come when called or to stay nearby on walks. In contrast, puppies exposed to off-leash walks, playful recall training, and ball play are in-variably easier to instruct in the performance of related tasks as adults.

Another behavioral tendency that appears to rely heavily on an imprinting-like processes is house training. There appears to be a narrow window of opportunity between 7 and 9 weeks of age for introducing house training most efficiently. Puppies started during this time tend to do much better and have far fewer accidents than puppies whose training is postponed until later. During this period, puppies develop location and substrate preferences away from their nesting area. Proper house training relies on directing innately programmed tendencies and patterns of behavior into appropriate outlets. If a puppy acquires a preference for eliminating indoors on the carpet or even on papers in the kitchen, it will be more difficult to redirect this activity outside later. Elimination location and substrate preferences appear to be strongly influenced during this brief period and, whenever possible, puppies should be taught to eliminate outdoors from the start, thereby skipping the confusing paper training routine. A good practice on arriving home with a new puppy is to take the puppy first thing to an outdoor area reserved for elimination; the experience will leave a lasting and beneficial impression on the puppy.

PREVENTING BEHAVIOR PROBLEMS

Much remains to be learned about the effects of early experience on adult behavior and the development of behavior problems. Growing statistical and anecdotal evidence suggests that very significant influences are at work. For example, a study by Jagoe (see Serpell and Jagoe, 1995) has detected several significant associations between pediatric illness and later behavior problems, including a higher incidence of dominance-related aggression, aggression toward strangers, fear of strangers, fear of children, separation-related barking, and abnormal sexual behavior. The author speculates that excessive and exclusive attention resulting from home medical care and reduced social contact outside of the home contributed to the development of some of these behavior problems. Given this rather compelling evidence of a relationship between early sickness and later behavior problems, it would seem advisable to offer puppy owners preventative behavioral counseling as part of the overall treatment of serious canine pediatric illness.

Hopefully, in the future, puppy socialization and training courses will become a common feature of puppy rearing—as common and routine as vaccinations are today in the prevention of communicable disease. Early behavioral training and proper socialization appear to "inoculate" immature dogs against many adult dog behavior problems such as hyperactivity, excessive fearfulness, aggression, separation anxiety, and general disobedience. Although "hard" scientific evidence is still lacking, many anecdotal reports and case histories strongly support the value of early training in the prevention of these serious problems. Unfortunately, however, many of the current rearing practices often neglect or incorrectly apply the needed training efforts.

REFERENCES

Adler LL and Adler HE (1977). Ontogeny of observational learning in the dog (*Canis familiaris*). *Dev Psychobiol,* 10:267–280.

Bacon WE and Stanley WC (1970). Reversal learning in neonatal dogs. *J Comp Physiol Psychol,* 70:344–350.

Beaudet R, Chalifoux A, and Dallaire A (1994). Predictive value of activity level and behavioral evaluation on future dominance in puppies. *Appl Anim Behav Sci,* 40:273–284.

Bekoff M (1972). The development of social interaction, play, and metacommunication in mammals: An ethological perspective. *Q Rev Biol,* 47:412–434.

Borchelt PL (1984). Behaviour development of the puppy in the home environment. In RS Anderson (Ed), *Nutrition and Behavior in Dogs and Cats: Proceedings of the First Nordic Symposium on Small Animal Veterinary Medicine.* New York: Pergamon.

Cairns RB and Johnson DL (1965). The development of interspecies social attachments. *Psychon Sci,* 2:337–338.

Cairns RB and Werboff J (1972). Behavior development in the dog: An interspecific analysis. *Science,* 158:1070–1072.

Coppinger L and Coppinger R (1982). Livestock-guarding dogs that wear sheep's clothing. *Smithsonian,* 13:65–73.

Cornwell AC and Fuller JL (1961). Conditioned responses in young puppies. *J Comp Physiol Psychol,* 54:13–15.

Davis KL, Gurski JC, and Scott JP (1977). Interaction of separation distress with fear in infant dogs. *Dev Psychobiol,* 10:203–212.

Denenberg VH (1964). Critical periods, stimulus input, and emotional reactivity: A theory of infantile stimulation. *Psychol Rev,* 71:335–351.

Dunbar I, Ranson E, and Buehler M (1981). Pup retrieval and maternal attraction to canine amniotic fluids. *Behav Processes,* 6:249–260.

Elliot O and Scott JP (1961). The development of emotional distress reactions to separation in puppies. *J Genet Psychol,* 99:3–22.

Fisher AE (1955). The effects of early differential treatment on the social and exploratory behavior of puppies [Unpublished doctoral dissertation]. University Park: Pennsylvania State University.

Fox MW (1963). *Canine Behavior.* Springfield, IL: Charles C Thomas.

Fox MW (1964a). The ontogeny of behavior and neurologic responses in the dog. *Anim Behav,* 12:301–311.

Fox MW (1964b). A sociosexual behavioral abnormality in the dog resembling Oedipus complex in man. *JAVMA,* 144:868–869.

Fox MW (1966a). Behavioral and physiological aspects of cardiac development in the dog. *J Small Anim Pract,* 7:321–326.

Fox MW (1966b). The development of learning and conditioned responses in the dog: Theoretical and practical implications. *Can J Comp Vet Sci,* 30:282–286.

Fox MW (1966c). Neuro-behavioral ontogeny: A synthesis of ethological and neurophysiological concepts. *Brain Res,* 2:3–20.

Fox MW (1967). The effects of short-term social and sensory isolation upon behavior, EEG and average evoked potentials in puppies. *Physiol Behav,* 2:145–151.

Fox MW (1968). *Abnormal Behavior in Animals,* 332–355. Philadelphia: WB Saunders.

Fox MW (1971). *Integrative Development of Brain and Behavior in the Dog.* Chicago: University of Chicago Press.

Fox MW (1972). *Understanding Your Dog.* New York: Coward, McCann and Geoghegan.

Fox MW (1974). *Concepts of Ethology: Animal and Human Behavior.* Minneapolis: University of Minnesota Press.

Fox MW (1978). *The Dog: Its Domestication and Behavior.* Malabar, FL: Krieger.

Fox MW and Spencer JW (1967). Development of the delayed response in the dog. *Anim Be-*

hav, 15:162–168.

Fox MW and Spencer JW (1969). Exploratory behavior in the dog: Experiential or age dependent? *Dev Psychobiol,* 2:68–74.

Fox MW and Stelzner D (1966). Behavioural effects of differential early experience in the dog. *Anim Behav,* 14:273–281.

Fox MW and Stelzner D (1967). The effects of early experience on the development of inter- and intraspecific social relationships in the dog. *Anim Behav,* 15:377–386.

Fredericson E (1952). Perceptual homeostasis and distress vocalization in puppies. *J Pers,* 20:472–478.

Fredericson E, Gurney N, and Dubois E (1956). The relationship between environmental temperature and behavior in neonatal puppies. *J Comp Physiol Psychol,* 49:278–280.

Freedman DG, King JA, and Eliot O (1961). Critical period in the social development of dogs. *Science,* 133:1016–1017.

Fuller JL (1967). Experiential deprivation and later behavior. *Science,* 158:1645–1652.

Fuller JL and Clark LD (1966a). Effects of rearing with specific stimuli upon postisolation behavior in dogs. *J Comp Physiol Psychol,* 61:258–263.

Fuller JL and Clark LD (1966b). Genetic and treatment factors modifying the postisolation syndrome in dogs. *J Comp Physiol Psychol,* 61:251–257.

Fuller JL, Easler CA, and Banks EM (1950). Formation of conditioned avoidance responses in young puppies. *Am J Physiol,* 160:462–466.

Gagnon S and Dore FY (1994). Cross-sectional study of object permanence in domestic puppies (*Canis familiaris*). *J Comp Psychol,* 108:220–232.

Gantt WH, Newton JE, Royer FL, and Stephens JH (1966). Effect of person. *Cond Reflex,* 1:146–160.

Grant TR (1986). A behavioral study of a beagle bitch and her litter during the first three weeks of lactation. *Anim Techol,* 37:157–167.

Harlow HF (1958). The nature of love. *Am Psychol,* 13:673–685.

Harlow HF and Zimmerman RS (1959). Affectional responses in the infant monkey. *Science,* 130:421–432.

Hediger H (1955/1968). *The Psychology and Behavior of Animals in Zoos and Circuses,* G Sircom (Trans). New York: Dover (reprint).

Hess EH (1964). Imprinting in birds. *Science,* 146:1128–1139.

Hess EH (1973). *Imprinting: Early Experience and the Developmental Psychobiology of Attachment.* New York: D Van Nostrand.

Igel GJ and Calvin AD (1960). The development of affectional responses in infant dogs. *J Comp Physiol Psychol,* 53:302–305.

James WT (1949). Dominant and submissive behavior in puppies as indicated by food intake. *J Genet Psychol,* 75:33–43.

James WT (1955). Behaviors involved in expression of dominance among puppies. *Psychol Rep,* 1:229–301.

James WT (1960). Observations of the regurgitant feeding reflex in the dog. *Psychol Rep,* 6:142.

James WT (1961). Relationship between dominance and food intake in individual and social eating in puppies. *Psychol Rep,* 8:478.

James WT and Cannon DJ (1952). Conditioned avoiding response in puppies. *Am J Physiol,* 168:251–253.

Knol BW and Egberink-Alink ST (1989). Treatment of problem behaviour in dogs and cats by castration and progestagen administration: A review. *Vet Q,* 11:102–107.

Kuo ZY (1967). *The Dynamics of Behavior Development. An Epigenetic View.* New York: Random House.

Lessac MS and Solomon RL (1969). Effects of early isolation on the later adaptive behavior of beagles: A methodological demonstration. *Dev Psychol,* 1:14–25.

Levine S (1960). Stimulation in infancy. *Sci Am,* 202:80–86.

Levine S, Haltmeyer GC, Karas GC, and Denenberg VH (1967). Physiological and behavioral effects of infantile stimulation. *Physiol Behav,* 2:55–59.

Malm K (1995). Regurgitation in relation to weaning in the domestic dog: A questionnaire study. *Appl Anim Behav Sci,* 43:111–121.

Markwell PJ and Thorne CJ (1987). Early behavioral development of dogs. *J Small Anim Pract,* 28:984–991.

Marr JN (1964). Varying stimulation and imprinting in dogs. *J Genet Psychol,* 104:351–364.

Martins T (1949). Disgorging of food to the puppies by the lactating dog. *Physiol Zool,* 22:169–172.

Mason WA and Kenney MD (1974). Redirection of filial attachments in rhesus monkeys: Dogs as mother substitutes. *Science,* 183:1209–1211.

McBryde WC and Murphree OD (1974). The rehabilitation of genetically nervous dogs. *Pavlov J Biol Sci* 9:76–84.

Mech LD (1970). *The Wolf: The Ecology and Behavior of an Endangered Species.* Minneapolis, MN: University of Minnesota Press.

Mekosh-Rosenbaum V, Carr WJ, Goodwin JL, et al. (1994). Age dependent responses to chemosensory cues mediating kin recognition

in dogs (*Canis familiaris*). *Physiol Behav,*
55:495–499.

Melzack R and Scott TH (1957). The effects of
early experience on the response to pain. *J
Comp Physiol Psychol,* 50:155–160.

Monks of New Skete (1991). *The Art of Raising a
Puppy.* Boston: Little, Brown.

Morton JRC (1968). Effects of early experience
"handling and gentling" in laboratory animals.
In MW Fox (Ed), *Abnormal Behavior in Animals.* Philadelphia: WB Saunders.

Nemeroff CB (1998). The neurobiology of depression. *Sci Am,* 278:42–49.

Pettijohn TF, Wong TW, Ebert PD, and Scott JP
(1977). Alleviation of separation distress in 3
breeds of young dogs. *Dev Psychobiol,*
10:373–381.

Pfaffenberger CJ (1963). *The New Knowledge of
Dog Behavior.* New York: Howell Book House.

Pfaffenberger CJ and Scott JP (1959). The relationship between delayed socialization and
trainability in guide dogs. *J Gen Psychol,*
95:145–155.

Piaget J (1952). *The Origins of Intelligence in Children.* New York: International University Press,

Rheingold HL (1963). Maternal behavior in the
dog. In HL Rheingold (Ed), *Maternal Behavior
in Mammals.* New York: John Wiley and Sons.

Rosenblatt J (1983). Olfaction mediates developmental transition in the altricial newborn of selected species of mammals. *Dev Psychobiol,*
16:347–375.

Ross S and Ross JG (1949). Social facilitation of
feeding behavior in dogs: II. Group and solitary feeding. *J Genet Psychol,* 74:273–304.

Ross S, Scott JP, Cherner M, and Denenberg V
(1960). Effects of restraint and isolation on
yelping in puppies. *Anim Behav,* 6:1–5.

Schneirla TC (1959). An evolutionary and developmental theory of biphasic process underlying
approach and withdrawal. In MR Jones (Ed),
Nebraska Symposium on Motivation, 7:1–42.
Lincoln: Nebraska University Press.

Schneirla TC (1965). Aspects of stimulation and
organization in approach-withdrawal process
underlying vertebrate behavioral development.
In DS Lehrman, RA Hinde, and E Shaw
(Eds), *Advances in the Study of Animal Behavior,* 7:1–74. New York: Academic.

Scott JP (1958). Critical periods in the development of social behavior in puppies. *Psychosom
Med,* 20:42–54.

Scott JP (1962). Critical periods in behavioral development. *Science,* 138:949–957.

Scott JP (1967). The development of social motivation. In *Nebraska Symposium on Motivation,*
111–132. New York: University of Nebraska

Press.

Scott JP (1968a). *Early Experience and the Organization of Behavior.* Belmont, CA: Brooks/
Cole.

Scott JP (1968b). Social facilitation and allelomimetic behavior. In EC Simmel, RA
Hoppe, and GA Milton (Eds), *Social Facilitation and Imitative Behavior* (1967 Miami University Symposium on Social Behavior).
Boston: Allyn and Bacon.

Scott JP and Fuller JL (1965). *Genetics and the Social Behavior of the Dog.* Chicago: University of
Chicago Press.

Scott JP and McCray C (1967). Allelomimetic behavior in dogs: Negative effects of competition
on social facilitation. *J Comp Physiol Psychol,*
63:316–319.

Scott JP, Ross S, and Fisher AE (1959). The effects
of early enforced weaning on sucking behavior
of puppies. *J Gen Psychol,* 95:261–281.

Serpell J and Jagoe JA (1995). Early experience
and the development of behaviour. In J Serpell
(Ed), *The Domestic Dog: Its Evolution, Behaviour, and Interaction with People.* New York:
Cambridge University Press.

Skinner BF (1982). Contrived reinforcement. *Behav Anal,* 5:3–8.

Slabbert JM and Rasa OAE (1997). Observational
learning of an acquired maternal behaviour
pattern by working dog pups: An alternative
training method? *Appl Anim Behav Sci,*
53:309–316.

Sluckin W (1965). *Imprinting and Early Learning.*
Chicago: Aldine.

Stanley WC and Elliot O (1962). Differential human handling as reinforcing events and as
treatments influencing later social behavior in
basenji puppies. *Psychol Rep,* 10:775–788.

Stanley WC, Bacon WE, and Fehr C (1970). Discriminated instrumental learning in neonatal
dogs. *J Comp Physiol Psychol,* 70:335–343.

Stanley WC, Barrett JE, and Bacon WE (1974).
Conditioning and extinction of avoidance and
escape behavior in neonatal dogs. *J Comp Physiol Psychol,* 87:163–172.

Stanley WC, Cornwell AC, Poggiani C, and Trattner A (1963). Conditioning in the neonatal
puppy. *J Comp Physiol Psychol,* 56:211–214.

Thompson WR (1957). Influence of prenatal maternal anxiety on emotional reactivity in young
rats. *Science,* 125:698–699.

Thompson WR and Heron W (1954). The effects
of early restriction on activity in dogs. *J Comp
Physiol Psychol,* 54:77–82.

Thompson WR, Melzack R, and Scott TH
(1956). "Whirling behavior" in dogs as related
to early experience. *Science,* 123:939.

Thorndike EL (1911/1965). *Animal Intelligence: Experimental Studies.* New York: Hafner (reprint).

Tinbergen N (1951/1969). *The Study of Instinct.* Oxford: Oxford University Press (reprint).

Trumler E (1973). *Your Dog and You.* New York: Seabury.

Welker WI (1959). Factors influencing aggregation of neonatal puppies. *J Comp Physiol Psychol,* 52:376–380.

Wilsson E (1984/1985). The social interaction between mother and offspring during weaning in German shepherd dogs: individual differences between mothers and their effects on offspring. *Appl Anim Behav Sci,* 13:101–112.

Wilsson E (1997). Behaviour test for eight-week old puppies: Heritabilities of tested behavior traits and its correspondence to later behaviour. *Appl Anim Behav Sci,* 58:151–162.

Wright JC (1980). The development of social structure during the primary socialization period in German shepherds. *Dev Psychobiol,* 13:17–24.

Wright JC (1983). The effects of differential rearing on exploratory behavior in puppies. *Appl Anim Ethol,* 10:27–34.

3

Neurobiology of Behavior and Learning

The possibility of understanding the central neural substrates that govern behavior is exciting not only because it deepens our understanding of humans and of all animal life, but also because it holds the promise that we may someday be able to correct imbalances in behavioral functions or restore functions lost by disease.

G. M. SHEPHERD, *Neurobiology* (1983)

BEHAVIORAL ADAPTATION depends on the coordinated interaction of many neural and sensory substrates. Together the brain and senses orchestrate what is experienced and what will be learned from experience. Considering the obvious importance of these systems and their fundamental implications for learning, it makes sense to study their various contributions to the development of adaptive behavior.

The operation of a radio is a useful analogy for illustrating the dependent relationship between behavior and the brain. The radio picks up electromagnetic waves from the atmosphere and transduces them into perceptible sound. Its ability to perform this task depends on a number of coordinated and hierarchically arranged systems, including specialized circuitry that sorts out specific radio waves one frequency at a time. This ability might be referred to as afferent selectivity. The selected signal undergoes various processes of electronic conversion and is then amplified into efferent mechanical action——the production of sound by the magnetic vibration of its speaker. Finally, the radio provides the user with several operational features with which to control the quality and quantity of sound produced, for example, tuning, volume, and tone.

To some extent, behavioral systems operate in a similar, although far more complicated, way. Environmental stimuli impinging on an animal are received as raw data by specialized sense organs. The senses afferently select and condition sensory data into sensations, relay them into appropriate neural tracts where they undergo preconscious sorting and analysis, and, finally, the input is cortically transformed into meaningful information, cognitions, emotions, and actions. This neurally processed information prepares the animal to adjust appropriately to current environmental conditions. In every degree and nuance, experience and learning are limited by neural and sensory constraints. The experiencing subject is first and foremost a biologically defined experiencer. To return to the radio analogy, the receiver converts electromagnetic waves into music, but only if it is tuned to the specific frequency carrying the relevant

"information." There is no possibility of music being produced unless the receiver intercepts and decodes this electromagnetic information and converts it into an audible dimension. If interference, defective parts, short circuits or any dysfunction whatsoever occurs within this highly organized system, the music produced will be adversely affected or, perhaps, completely lost. Similarly, neurosensory systems define the sort of input that will be received and to a large extent how it will be acted on. The neurological substrates, for example, controlling stimulus-response processing depend almost entirely on such *hardwired* mechanisms.

The operation of the radio set also metaphorically parallels the limited variability of innate behavioral systems. The mechanisms controlling signal selection, volume, and tone are all ways in which a radio can be adjusted to a listener's pleasure. Learning mechanisms are themselves biologically prepared and accessible for manipulation only under special conditions and within a limited range of variability defined by functional constraints. Training and behavior modification are largely limited to response selection (i.e., stimulus control) and the shaping of behavior (tuning), augmentation or suppression of behavior (volume + or −), and the modification of emotional states and the stimulus-response thresholds controlling them (tone control). But unlike the simple and immediate response of the radio, external control of behavioral systems requires far more persistent and skilled effort. In general, behavioral systems are reluctant to change without compelling need.

Behavioral adjustment depends on learning, but learning is possible only to the extent that an animal is biologically equipped and prepared to learn. The organization of behavior is genetically programmed to be flexible and variable but only to a certain extent and according to more or less fixed laws and parameters of change defined by the brain and senses. In essence, the brain and senses biologically define the limits of what an animal can learn and how it can learn it, while experience dictates the moment-to-moment direction of these changes. Survival depends on an animal's ability to learn from its experiences, to adjust its behavior in accordance with what it has learned, and to form a set of reliable predictions and strategies of control that enable it to encounter similar circumstances most effectively in the future.

The subject of brain anatomy and function is highly complex but very valuable for understanding the basic processes of behavior, emotion, and learning. The following discussion has been largely restricted to areas of practical significance for trainers or behaviorists working with adjustment and behavior problems in dogs.

CELLULAR COMPOSITION OF THE BRAIN

Neurons

In contrast to the simple radio receiver, the dog's brain is a profoundly complicated organ consisting of billions of neurons and interconnecting neural circuits. The neuron shares many of the same basic biological functions exhibited by other cells of the body. One notable exception to this generality is the neuron's inability to replicate. Shortly after birth, neurons stop dividing in the dog's brain and thereafter no new neurons are produced. Consequently, injuries to the brain involving direct trauma or anoxia may be very serious—and permanent—since lost neurons cannot be replaced. Although neurons may be more or less specialized, their structure and function are remarkably similar. Basically, the neuron is designed to send and receive information. These functions are facilitated by structural components called axons and dendrites. The axon is an elongated projection of the neuron that carries messages away from the cell body (efferent messages) while dendrites carry the message toward the cell body (afferent messages). Transmissions occur at locations where axons form connections with other neurons. These points of transmission are called synapses.

The synapse is a narrow cleft between the transmitting axon and the receiving dendrite. This gap is bridged by the secretion of various chemical neurotransmitters released by

the neuron when it is appropriately stimulated. Excitatory and inhibitory synapses compete for dominance over the target neuron. Depending on whether inhibition or excitation is dominant, the neuron either remains quiet or is excited, evoking an axonal depolarization or action potential. As the result of excitation, an electrical charge moves rapidly down the length of the axon to the presynaptic terminal. Once arriving at the presynaptic terminal, the charge triggers the release of specific neurotransmitters into the synaptic cleft, thereby stimulating adjacent dendrites belonging to target neurons. Movement of this electrical charge is accelerated by a thin insulating substance called myelin that covers the length of the axon. The foregoing cycle of excitation, depolarization, and release of neurotransmitters is repeated in countless neurons until the signal completes its circuit.

Glial Cells

The majority of cells composing the brain are glial cells. Besides providing structural support for neurons and their interconnections, the glia serve many additional functions. An important glial function is to absorb vagrant neural substances (including neurotransmitters) and to dispose of cellular debris associated with injury or the death of neurons. Astrocytes are star-shaped cells that perform these "housekeeping" functions. Astrocyte activity is especially intense at the sites of brain injury. Another very important function of glial cells is the production of myelin sheathing and the formation of the blood-brain barrier.

Myelin is a fatty substance that insulates the axon. It is produced by specialized glial cells called oligodendrocytes (brain axons) and Schwann cells (peripheral nerves). The myelin sheath is discontinuous, having small gaps or nodes of Ranvier regularly spaced about a millimeter apart from each other. The action potential produced by the chemoelectrical excitation of the neuron moves rapidly along the axon by jumping from node to node. Myelin sheathing significantly increases the speed at which the neural impulse is able to travel. At birth, many brain and peripheral axon fibers lack functional myelination (Fox, 1966). Myelination follows a developmental course in which necessary functions like ingestion are myelinated at birth, whereas fibers associated with less immediately vital functions like hearing and vision are incompletely sheathed. The optic nerve, for instance, is only slightly sheathed with myelin at birth but attains adultlike myelination by about 3 weeks of age, whereas sensory tracts associated with taste and smell are well myelinated at birth in the dog.

Neurons are protected from substances in the blood by a cellular layer composed of astrocytes that surrounds blood-bearing capillaries. Additionally, capillaries in the brain are not as freely permeable as those of other parts of the body and do not allow the passage of large molecules across their walls. The net result is selective transport of only certain necessary nutritional molecules (e.g., glucose and amino acids) and dissolved gases like oxygen and carbon dioxide. Interestingly, portions of the hypothalamus are not protected by the blood-brain barrier (the portal blood supply),

due to its homeostatic and bioregulatory functions, which require direct monitoring of blood content (Reese, 1991).

HINDBRAIN AND MIDBRAIN STRUCTURES

The dog's nervous system is divided into two major parts: the central nervous system (CNS) and the peripheral nervous system (PNS). The CNS includes the brain proper and the spinal cord (Fig. 3.1). The PNS encompasses all nervous processes extending beyond the spine and skull, including a subsystem called the autonomic nervous system (ANS). The ANS is composed of two antithetical but complementary branches: the sympathetic and parasympathetic. The ANS is intimately involved in regulating basic bodily processes and in the mediation of the physiological expression of emotion and distress. Later in this chapter, autonomic functions are discussed in detail, since they appear to play a very significant role in the elaboration of disruptive stress and maladaptive behavior.

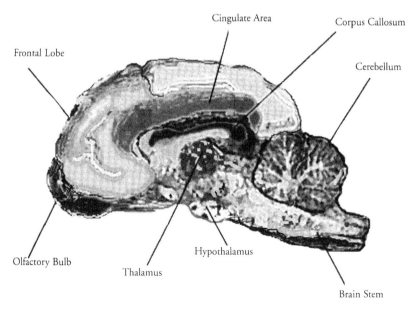

Cingulate Area

Corpus Callosum

Frontal Lobe

Cerebellum

Olfactory Bulb

Hypothalamus

Thalamus

Brain Stem

FIG. 3.1. Medial view of the dog's brain. Note the comparatively large olfactory bulb, providing the dog with the neural means to detect and analyze olfactory information.

Medulla Oblongata, Pons, and Cerebellum

The hindbrain consist of the medulla, pons, and cerebellum. The medulla is a primitive brain structure located just above the spinal cord and regulates many vital biological functions, such as the control of heart rate, respiration, gastrointestinal functions, salivation, coughing, and sneezing. Together with the pons, the medulla is an important relay site for auditory and vestibular information, gustatory sensations and associated motor reactions, and information about various visceral states. The central portion of the hindbrain contains the reticular formation, a network of interconnected neurons that is associated with wakefulness and generalized sensory arousal.

An important function of the hindbrain is the synthesis of monoamine neurotransmitters. Serotonin-producing cells are located in the raphe bodies, a narrow strip of specialized neurons in the hindbrain, extending from the medulla to the midbrain. Norepinephrine (NE) is made by a group cells in the pons called the locus coeruleus, an area with highly pigmented blue neurons (Ranson and Clark, 1959). Whereas NE is associated with wakefulness and learning, serotonin appears to play an important role in the activation of sleep and the modulation of various inhibitory processes.

The cerebellum, a brain structure associated with "automatic" coordinated movement and sensory processing, is interconnected via thalamic relays with the sensory-motor areas of the cerebral cortex. These interconnections form a complex loop of ascending projections from the cerebellum to the motor cortex and, subsequently, from the motor cortex descending back to the cerebellum via pontine nuclei. Cerebellar lesioning results in uncoordinated and awkward movement. Although the cerebellum plays a minimal role in higher conscious functions, the lateral portion of the cerebellum appears to be involved in certain cognitive and memory functions, especially in the mediation of skilled motor performances and aversive conditioned responses (Lavond et al., 1993). Interestingly, the only output from the cerebellar cortex is inhibitory, which is mediated via axons of specialized Purkinje cells. The Purkinje cells are large GABAergic neurons [the primary neural effect of GABA (gamma-aminobutyric acid) is inhibitory]. The inhibitory Purkinje cells project to highly active and excitatory subcortical nuclei, exerting a modulatory and regulatory effect on these neurons whose fibers ultimately project to higher motor brain centers.

Reticular Formation

The reticular formation is a brain stem structure extending from the medulla to the thalamus. The primary function of the reticular formation is the maintenance of a state of generalized neural arousal and alertness. Many projections leave the reticular formation and extend throughout the limbic system and cerebral cortex. This system of diffuse reticular fibers is referred to as the ascending reticular activating system (ARAS). In addition to its arousal functions, the ARAS is also believed to mediate an integrative effect on the nervous system. Electrical stimulation of the reticular formation of a sleeping dog results in the dog's arousal and awakening. On the other hand, lesioning of the reticular formation results in a permanent comatose or sleeplike state. Besides the arousal and attentional functions of the ARAS, the reticular formation also receives and gates sensory inputs, apparently mediating increased excitement and arousal resulting from peripheral sensory transmissions relayed through it. Unlike the corticothalamic relays where more specific sensory sorting, routing, and information processing takes place, the reticular formation is concerned with the general enhancement of alertness and excitability caused by these sensory inputs and the subsequent elaboration of a nonspecific orienting response to them. The auditory tract sends collateral axonal fibers directly into the reticular formation, perhaps accounting for the rapid and intense orienting responsiveness dogs exhibit toward novel sounds.

Gray (1971) has speculated that the ARAS

is especially well connected with sensory tracts associated with pain. He reports studies carried out by James Olds in which direct electrical stimulation of various portions of the ARAS (especially the periventricular areas) resulted in the evocation of escape and other pronounced behavioral expressions evidencing pain and discomfort. According to Gray (1971), the midbrain ARAS may play an important role in the arousal and activation associated with punishment or frustrative nonreward. Electrical stimulation of the midbrain reticular formation results in a direct potentiation or strengthening of ongoing behavior in a manner similar to that observed during punishment or frustrative nonreward.

Arousal resulting from activation of the reticular formation probably depends on the neurotransmitter NE. Inescapable trauma and prolonged stress result in the depletion of NE, and NE depletion is associated with learned helplessness (Seligman, 1975) (see Chapter 9). Seligman reviews some of the relevant physiological literature indicating that learned helplessness and collateral symptoms of depression may be linked to adrenergic depletion. Some disagreement in the literature exists with regard to the importance of NE and dopamine in the production of pleasure and reward. Thompson (1993) and many others attribute the brain's reward-and-pleasure system to dopaminergic activity. An important area for the elaboration of pleasure is the medial forebrain bundle (MFB)—a major ascending pathway of various neurotransmitters, including serotonergic, adrenergic, and dopaminergic fibers. Siegel and Edinger (1981) emphasize the importance of the MFB as a conduit for *adrenergic* fibers originating in the locus coeruleus and projecting into the lateral hypothalamus and amygdala. Animals stimulated with electrodes inserted into the MFB act as though they were actually eating, drinking, and copulating, that is, appearing to be rewarded by the consumption of the corresponding but absent reward item (viz., food, water, and sex). However, drugs that block dopaminergic activity also apparently inhibit the pleasure resulting from electrical stimulation of these areas (White and Milner, 1992). Animals operantly trained to perform a bar-press response for intracra-

nial stimulation of MFB sites quit when dopamine levels are reduced. According to this theory, a dopaminergic pathway exists between the MFB and the ventral tegmentum and terminates in the nucleus accumbens. Precise stimulation of the nucleus accumbens (located in the forebrain, anterior to the hypothalamus) produces all the effects observed during electrical stimulation of the MFB, suggesting that earlier studies may have confounded dopamine and NE pathways. Most authorities currently believe that reward is most likely mediated by dopaminergic systems. However, modulating NE pathways may play a significant role in the experience of pleasure and reward via enhanced alertness, mood, and feelings of well-being affected by NE activity. Low levels of dopamine in the brain result in a loss of affect and positive feelings, whereas low levels of NE result in depressed mood and a sense of helplessness (Seligman, 1975).

DIENCEPHALON

Thalamus

The thalamus coordinates sensory and emotional inputs, serving as a gateway and relay between the body, limbic system, and cerebral cortex. Thalamic relay nuclei coordinate the projection of sensory information from the body and sensory organs, directing it to the appropriate somatosensory portions of the cerebral cortex—the most recent and "conscious" addition to the brain. The amount of the cortex reserved for any particular body area or function depends on its overall use, sensitivity, and relative importance for the animal's survival. Further, the area of the cerebral cortex allotted to any particular function corresponds proportionately to the relative size of the thalamic sensory nuclei relaying to it. Animals can be categorized into three basic types depending on which sensory function dominates: beholders, feelers, and listeners (Welker, 1973). Within this scenario, dogs probably fit into the listener-type category, indicating that a disproportionately large area of the canine cortex and thalamus is devoted to the representation and analysis of auditory information.

Besides relaying sensory and emotional input, the thalamus plays an important role in the expression of attentional behavior. In contrast to the general arousal functions served by the reticular formation, the thalamus mediates a more selective, "informed" attentional response toward sensory inputs. The thalamus enables a dog to selectively concentrate and focus on one thing at a time, whereas the reticular formation facilitates general alertness, causing all sensory inputs reaching an effective threshold to capture attention.

Unlike all other sensory inputs, which travel first to the thalamus before being relayed to other parts of the brain, olfactory sensory input moves directly from the olfactory bulb via the olfactory tract to the primary olfactory cortex (paleocortex). From the olfactory cortex, the olfactory input projects to the medial dorso nucleus of the thalamus, from where it is relayed to neocortical destinations (orbitofrontal cortex) for cognitive (associative) processing and the conscious perception of smell. A second major olfactory pathway originating in the primary olfactory cortex projects to the preoptic/lateral hypothalamus. Another important limbic destination of olfactory information is the amygdala. The corticomedial nucleus of the amygdala receives afferent input directly from the olfactory bulbs as well as forming connections with the olfactory cortex. Secondary olfactory projections terminate in various other related limbic areas, including the septum and hippocampus (Thompson, 1993). Clearly, many areas of the dog's brain receives olfactory information via parallel and interacting circuits. These various neural circuits serve such diverse functions as food and mate selection, kinship recognition, sexual behavior, memory, imprinting, motivation, emotion, and learning. Not surprisingly, a proportionately larger area of a dog's brain than the human brain is devoted to analyzing olfactory information.

Hypothalamus

The hypothalamus performs many regulatory functions over basic biological activities, including appetite, thirst, and various homeostatic functions like blood pressure, temperature regulation, and blood sugar levels. Besides controlling basic appetitive/homeostatic drives and regulating the expression of emotional behavior, hypothalamic nuclei also control sexual drive. Hypothalamic activity is intimately connected with the endocrine system and the regulation of the pituitary gland—the so-called master gland of the body. The hypothalamus exercises direct *chemical* regulatory control over the pituitary by the manufacture and secretion of releasing factors. Hypothalamic releasing factors circulate via the portal blood supply to the anterior pituitary, causing it to release various tropic hormones involved in growth, sexual behavior, maternal behavior, metabolism, and general biological stress reactions. The hypothalamus also controls the ANS, which is composed of two subsystems: the sympathetic nervous system and the parasympathetic nervous system. Together the sympathetic division and parasympathetic division perform numerous complementary functions designed to achieve biological homeostasis (Fig. 3.2). The sympathetic division provides immediate physiological preparation for emergency freeze-flight-fight reactions. Sympathetic arousal is regulated by the posterior hypothalamus, which when appropriately stimulated evokes a bodywide neuroendocrine preparation for vigorous action. Besides directly activating the biological systems needed for emergency action, sympathetic arousal stimulates the adrenal medulla to release the peripheral hormones epinephrine and NE into the bloodstream. Epinephrine reinforces and sustains ANS-triggered stimulation of such stress-related bodily changes as increased heart rate and respiration. This interaction between the hypothalamus and the adrenal medulla is known as the sympathetic-adrenomedullary system.

A neuroendocrine system associated with stressful arousal and homeostasis is formed by the hypothalamus, pituitary, and the adrenal cortex. Under conditions of stress, the hypothalamus secretes corticotropin-releasing factor (CRF), which signals the pituitary gland to secrete a tropic hormone—adrenocorticotropic hormone (ACTH)—into the bloodstream. ACTH stimulates the adrenal cortex

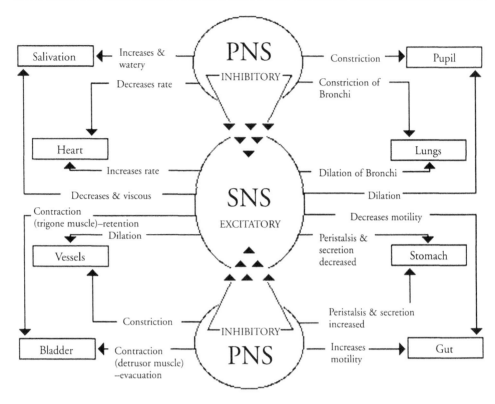

FIG. 3.2. Examples of complementary autonomic action produced by the interaction of the parasympathetic nervous system (PNS) and the sympathetic nervous system (SNS). The checks and balances between the PNS and SNS strive to achieve biological homeostasis.

to release various steroidal hormones, including cortisol (corticosterone). Cortisol serves many biological functions (regulation of blood pressure, control of glucose levels in the blood, and acceleration of the breakdown of protein into amino acids) to help an animal cope effectively with stress, injury, or defense. The release of cortisol into the bloodstream completes the circuit when it reaches the hypothalamus, where it restrains CRF production and thereby inhibits ACTH production by the pituitary. The reduction of circulating ACTH causes the adrenal cortex to decrease production and secretion of cortisol. This slower stress-activated system is known as the hypothalamic-pituitary-adrenocortical (HPA) system.

The parasympathetic branch of the ANS shadows the actions of the sympathetic system, but with an opposing calming influence more specifically targeted on the various organs and systems of the body activated by the sympathetic division. Although autonomic activity is aimed at achieving homeostatic balance of sympathetic and parasympathetic influences, some individuals appear to be genetically predisposed in one direction or the other (Kagan et al., 1987; Kagan and Snidman 1988). Some dogs are sympathetically dominant (prone to emotional reactivity and biological stress), whereas others, the parasympathetically dominant type, are inherently more calm and enjoy a more precise biological adaptation. The sympathetically dominant temperament type is more prone to develop behavior problems involving emotional reactivity and psychosomatic disorders than the parasympathetically dominant counterpart. Tests devised to evaluate relative sympathetic versus parasympathetic ANS reactivity in puppies could be potentially useful in conjunction with puppy temperament-testing procedures. Measures of heart rate, blood pressure, respiration, and cortisol levels under various conditions of stress could provide a reliable means to assess ANS dominance and temperament reactivity.

Gunnar (1994) reviewed several studies showing a correlation between cortisol levels and relative dominance-assertiveness in young children. This correlation is an interesting finding, since HPA activation is generally associated with emotional distress and fear. She reports an experiment performed by de Haan and colleagues (1993) demonstrating a direct relationship between dominance-aggressiveness and cortisol levels in 2-year-old children. In this experiment, salivary cortisol levels were measured during the first few days of nursery school. Subsequent interviews with the teacher and parents of the children tested revealed several positive correlations between high cortisol levels and a child's tendency to become a group leader, engage in aggressive behavior in school, and exhibit an "angry temperament" at home. On the other hand, more socially retiring children exhibiting shyness, with a tendency toward solitary play, and other signs of behavioral inhibition did not show significant cortisol indicators of HPA system arousal.

Studies with various animal species have shown a link between increased HPA system activity and stress. Sapolsky (1990) studied the dynamic interaction between social status, the stress response, and a variety of correlated hormonal changes exhibited differentially by dominant and subordinate free-ranging baboons. He found that resting cortisol levels are higher in subordinate males, but that, under acute stress, cortisol levels in dominant males overshoot that exhibited by subordinates under the same conditions:

> Cortisol is responsible for much of the double-edged quality of the stress response. In the short run it mobilizes energy, but its chronic overproduction contributes to muscle wastage, hypertension and impaired immunity and fertility. Clearly, then, cortisol should be secreted heavily in response to a truly threatening situation but should be kept in check at other

times. This is precisely what occurs in dominant males. Their resting levels of cortisol are lower than those of subordinate males yet will rise faster when a major stressor does come; exactly how this speedier rise is accomplished is not understood. (1990:120)

Similarly, Manogue and colleagues (1975) found that, among squirrel monkeys, individuals destined to play a dominant role in the group exhibited higher cortisol levels than subordinates during the early phases of the group's organization. Once the group became stable, the dominant monkey's cortisol level dropped below that of the subordinates. Under conditions of external distress, however, the dominant monkey exhibited emergency cortisol levels that quickly overshot that of subordinate group members. McLeod and coworkers (1995) have shown that urinary cortisol levels are increased under the influence of social stress among captive wolves. For example, they found that the lowest-ranking females exhibited the highest levels of cortisol in their urine. The presence of high levels of cortisol in the urine of subordinate females may help to account for the natural inhibition of estrus in such females via stress-mediated suppression of hypothalamic secretion of gonadotropin-releasing hormone. Haemisch (1990) investigated cortisol levels in guinea pigs undergoing social conflict in familiar and unfamiliar environments. Under conditions of social conflict occurring between an offensive individual and defensive individual, the defensive guinea pig exhibited significantly higher levels of plasma cortisol (about four times as much) under familiar environmental conditions than the offensive animal. When confrontations took place in an unfamiliar environment, the difference between the offensive and defensive individuals was not significant.

A study involving HPA activity in pointers found that genetically nervous dogs possessed significantly larger adrenal glands than normal controls (Pasley et al., 1978). Adrenal hypertrophy is commonly associated with chronic HPA-mediated stress. However, a subsequent experiment performed by Klein and colleagues (1990) failed to show a significant difference between nervous and normal pointers in terms of HPA system activity. The authors speculate that the lack of difference between the two strains of pointers may have resulted from the testing method employed (a static single-point baseline comparison), which may have missed significant differences in HPA activity occurring episodically at other times during the day. Another interesting finding relevant to hypothalamic-pituitary interaction involves differences in somatomedin/insulin-like growth factor (IGF-I) levels found in nervous and normal pointers (Uhde et al., 1992). Nervous dogs exhibit lower plasma levels of growth factor (GF) than normal controls. Nervous dogs appear to be smaller, perhaps a direct physical outcome of GF insufficiency. Further, nervous pointers are more prone to exhibit compulsive behaviors (especially oral ones like excessive licking, biting, and pulling) than normal pointers. Uhde and colleagues suggest that replacement GF might provide some therapeutic benefit for acral lick dermatitis (to date, an untested possibility).

Intense sympathetic arousal may precipitate pronounced parasympathetic rebound effects like diarrhea and urination resulting from increased alimentary and urinary motility. Another common outcome following intense sympathetic arousal is opponent-processed parasympathetic reduction of heart rate. Church and colleagues (1966) demonstrated that dogs stimulated with shock experience an initial sharp rise in heart rate (sympathetic arousal), but with the cessation of shock the subjects' heart rates fall far below their original quiet preshock levels. Konorski (1967) reported experiments in which a dog and several rabbits were caused to experience intense fear by being shot with noninjurious paper projectiles from a sham gun. Whereas the dog experienced an increase in blood pressure after being shot, the rabbits exhibited a sharp fall in blood pressure, with some experiencing an increase after the cessation of stimulation. A few of the stimulated rabbits died as the result of a precipitous and lethal fall in blood pressure. Another relevant study with respect to parasympathetic rebound effects on cardiac function was performed by Richter (1957), who immersed rats in water and observed their swimming behavior under various experimental conditions. One group

of swimmers had their whiskers (vibrissae) cut off before being placed in the swim tank. In rats, the whiskers are a very important sensory accessory for providing information about their immediate surroundings. According to Welker's nomenclature, previously discussed above, rats are *feelers* whose thalamo-cortical world is dominated by sensory information provided by the whiskers. The rats without whiskers panicked, apparently responding to the tank situation as though it were inescapable without the aid of whiskers; they swam frantically for a minute or so, before giving up and sinking to the bottom of the tank. Subsequent necropsies showed that the rats had not drowned but had suffered cardiac arrest. Ordinarily, rats can swim for long durations without stopping (up to 48 hours). The dewhiskered rats, however, were seized with intense sympathetic activation rapidly followed by an equal but opposed parasympathetic rebound, resulting in the loss of heart activity. In subsequent studies, Richter found that if he repeatedly immersed and rescued a rat before cutting off its whiskers, the animal did much better than controls not pretreated before exposure to immersion. Pretreated rats appeared to be partially immunized against an apparent "helplessness" effect generated by the removal of their whiskers.

LIMBIC SYSTEM

The limbic system is a complex loop of neural structures and circuits involved in the expression and experience of emotions. This pervasive and influential system also plays an important role in learning and memory. The primary structures composing the limbic system include the amygdaloid complex, the septohippocampal system (septal area and hippocampus), the diencephalon (hypothalamus and thalamus), and the limbic cortex. The limbic system has been investigated primarily by observing the effects of intracranial electrical or chemical stimulation or ablation of target areas (Table 3.1).

The limbic system appears to have evolved out of primitive structures involved in the analysis (intensity, quality, and direction) and interpretation of olfactory information. This

TABLE 3.1. Behavioral and emotional effects produced by stimulating or destroying various limbic areas

Limbic areas	Stimulation	Destruction
Cingulate gyrus	Tameness or aggression	Fearlessness (dog)
Thalamus		
Paramedian	Relaxation, sleep	—
Ventrolateral	—	Apathy
Midline	Affective aggression	—
Anterior	—	Docility
Dorsomedial	—	Rage
Hypothalamus		
Ventromedial nucleus	Hypophagia	Hyperphagia, rage (dog), affective aggression
Dorsomedial	Affective aggression	—
Posterior area	Alertness, excitement (dog)	Inactivity, sleep (dog)
Anterior area	Sleep (dog)	—
Lateral area	Quiet (predatory) attack; induces drinking and eating	Reduced affective aggression, adipsia, asphagia (dog)
Amygdala	Fear, wariness, affective aggression (dog)	Tameness, docility, passiveness (dog)
Septum	Defecation, urination, tameness, hypersexuality	Irritability, rage, reduced fearfulness (dog)

Source: From Swenson (1984) and Hoerlein (1971).

function of the limbic system is especially evident in reptilian species, in which the limbic system provides vital olfactory information regulating appetitive and sexual behavior, as well as various agonistic displays. In higher vertebrates like dogs, the limbic system has been diversified to serve a number of new and more complex emotional functions.

Among many other activities, interpretive olfactory functions are still performed by the amygdala. The amygdala is an almond-shaped complex of nuclei embedded in the white matter of the temporal lobe, just below the cortex and anterior to the hippocampus. The nuclei forming the amygdala are divided into three main groups: the basolateral nuclei (receive relayed sensory inputs from the thalamus as well as analyzed sensory inputs from the cortex), corticomedial nuclei (receive afferent inputs from the olfactory bulb and mediate higher cortical analysis of olfactory information), and the central nucleus (projects to the brain stem and hypothalamus and mediates the expression of fear). The amyg-

dala is interconnected with the hypothalamus by a bundle of fibers called the stria terminalis and a collection of fibers called the ventral amygdalofugal pathway.

In dogs and other mammals, the amygdala mediates the expression of fear and the modulation of aggression. Electrical stimulation of certain areas of the amygdala evokes intense vigilance together with generalized fear or rage reactions. On the other hand, surgical removal of the amygdala results in hyperactivity, marked hypersexual interest, compulsive orality, and a loss of fear and aggressiveness. Previously fearful or aggressive animals are "tamed" by amygdalectomy, allowing contact and petting without visible signs of nervousness or fear. Moyer reports a dramatic reduction in fear in an amygdalectomized rat:

> Normal albino rats freeze and remain immobile in the presence of a cat even though they have had no prior experience with that animal. However, if the rat is amygdalectomized, its behavior in the presence of the cat is not inhibited and it approaches the cat without reluc-

tance. In one case an amygdalectomized rat climbed onto the cat's back and head and began to nibble on the cat's ear. The resultant attack by the cat only momentarily inhibited the rat, which again crawled back on the cat's back as soon as it was released. (1976:257)

Many neurons found in the amygdala exhibit a low threshold of excitability and are prone to seizure, with collateral cortical irradiation and possible loss of conscious awareness. Dogs undergoing psychomotor seizure activity may exhibit a pronounced and unpredictable pattern of periodic explosive aggression followed by disorientation. Seizure activity in the amygdala has been associated with the development of psychomotor epilepsy. With the use of electroencephalograms (EEGs), abnormal electrical activity has been identified in the amygdala of aggressive persons. It does seem reasonable that some seizure activity in the amygdaloid complex could result in heightened aggressiveness, vigilance, intolerance, disorientation, and the periodic exhibition of inappropriate explosive rage. A study by Holliday and coworkers (1970) of epilepsy in dogs confirms that epileptic dogs frequently exhibit collateral abnormal behavior (sometimes as their most prominent symptom), including episodic rage, voracious appetites or inappetence, inappropriate vocalizations, aimless pacing and circling, viciousness toward inanimate objects, intense fearful reactions, persistent licking movements, restlessness, and "apparent blindness." Although psychomotor seizure activity may be associated with collateral aggressive behavior (Borchelt and Voith, 1985), aggressive behavior is infrequently diagnosed as a direct symptom of organic disease (Parker, 1990).

Moyer (1976) reports several studies indicating that the amygdala plays an important role in the modulation of predation and other forms of aggression in various animal species, probably through the modulation of fear. Electrical stimulation of different areas of the amygdala either inhibits or excites predatory behavior. Similarly, other amygdaloid locations modulate (differentially inhibit or excite) irritable or fear-induced aggressive displays. For instance, lesions in the central nucleus produce a lower threshold for irritable aggression in dogs. Once provoked, such aggression appears to escalate quickly without signs of fear or escape. In dogs, the spontaneous attack that is observed in cats with identical amygdala lesions (such cats attack conspecifics without any provocation from the target) does not occur. Instead, dogs exhibit increasing signs of irritability and frustrative arousal that quickly builds up and finally precipitates a full-blown and intense rage response—an *avalanche syndrome* (Fonberg, reported in Moyer, 1976). These behavioral changes suggest that the central nucleus may exercise a strong inhibitory influence (fear) over affective-irritable aggression, with disinhibition occurring when it is damaged.

The amygdala works in conjunction with other limbic structures, cortical association areas, thalamic nuclei, hippocampus (providing memories and context specificity to fear responses), and basal ganglia (giving the amygdala *effector* access to species-typical motor programs). As noted above, the amygdala also forms direct and diverse connections with the hypothalamus, including hypothalamic nuclei that control blood pressure, secretion of stress hormones, and the startle response (LeDoux, 1996). The majority of these projections are bidirectional with target structures projecting back to the amygdala, providing a switchboard of interchange between these various areas of the brain. The result is a system of checks and balances over amygdaloid functions, including the display of aggression and fearfulness. In addition to fear, the amygdala appears to play an important role in the mediation of social behavior and motivation. Fonberg and Kostarczyk (1960) observed various changes in the social motivation and behavior of dogs after lesioning the dorsomedial amygdala and/or the lateral hypothalamus. In addition to the expected loss of appetite, the dogs lost their ability to show normal social responsiveness to people, expressed no emotion, made no physical contact or effort to look at people, were unresponsive to petting and would often move away when being petted, lost their normal tail-wagging behavior, were easily distracted, were apathetic and slow moving, and, in general, were indifferent to the social environment. Apparently, the lesioned dogs lost their ability to derive pleasure from social interaction.

As is discussed in more detail later in this chapter, the amygdala appears to play a central role in emotional learning (LeDoux, 1994). This function is facilitated by a number of amygdala afferent inputs (basal and lateral nuclei) and efferent outputs (central nucleus) projecting to various somatomotor and autonomic areas controlling the expression of fear in the hypothalamus. The role of the amygdala in the classical conditioning of fear has been demonstrated in a variety of animals and situations (Davis, 1992). Most of these experiments have involved intracranial electrical stimulation or the lesioning of specific areas of the amygdala. Other studies have evaluated the effects of neurotransmitters, agonists, and antagonists on the learning of fear. For example, NE has been implicated in the learning of conditioned fear responses (Lavond et al., 1993). Injecting an NE antagonist (propranolol, a beta blocker) into the amygdala after avoidance training disrupts the subsequent performance of the previously learned avoidance task. Also, naloxone (an endogenous opioid antagonist) injected directly into the amygdala enhances the acquisition of avoidance behavior. The explanation for this improvement, however, does not rest on a direct effect of naloxone on amygdaloid activity but on an indirect causation involving the suppression of endogenous opioid activity. Apparently, endorphins interfere with the release of NE in the amygdala during avoidance training. Microinjections of an opioid agonist (levorphanol) also retard avoidance learning, providing additional support for the foregoing account. Ablation of the amygdala disrupts the acquisition and maintenance of avoidance learning. Previously learned avoidance responses are either quickly extinguished after amygdalectomy or may require greater aversive stimulation to be elicited (Thompson, 1967). On the other hand, stimulation of the central nucleus evokes many autonomic reactions correlated with fear: increased heart rate, respiration, and blood pressure. Such stimulation typically results in the inhibition of ongoing behavior and evokes various facial and motoric expressions associated with fear. The constellation of fearful responses evoked by amygdaloid stimulation is innately programmed and not dependent on learning for its full expression. What is acquired or learned is the range of stimuli and situations able to elicit them.

Conditioned emotional responses are learned when a neutral stimulus (e.g., a tone) is paired with an unconditioned fear-eliciting stimulus (e.g., shock). After a number of pairings in which the conditioned stimulus (CS) and unconditioned stimulus (US) are presented in a close temporal order, the CS will gradually acquire the ability to elicit the fear response without the presentation of the US. This connection between the CS and the US appears to be mediated by the amygdala in conjunction with the thalamus and other related brain sites. Lavond and colleagues (1993) reported a series of studies showing that the classical conditioning of foot-shock reactions (freezing reactions and increases in blood pressure) depends on the participation of various ancillary structures involved in the process of associating conditioned and unconditioned stimuli. Animals with lesions to auditory nuclei projecting from the thalamus (medial geniculate nucleus) to the amygdala fail to learn tone-foot-shock associations but readily learn a light-foot-shock association. Similarly, animals with hippocampal lesions fail to acquire context-foot-shock associations but still learn the tone-foot-shock association. Efferent projections from the amygdala to the hypothalamus also play an important role in classical conditioning of fear reactions. Lesions of the hypothalamus result in both the elimination of conditioned freezing and conditioned blood pressure responses.

In addition to amygdala-hypothalamus interactions, the expression and experience of emotion appear to require the collaboration of several limbic areas, collectively referred to as the Papez circuit (see below). This process begins with emotionally primitive inputs originating in the hypothalamus. These emotional inputs are projected to the anterior thalamus, where they undergo further elaboration and are in turn relayed via the thalamocortical pathway into the limbic cortex (e.g., the cingulate area). It has been speculated that the limbic cortex provides a kind of neural "screen" organized to receive and bring to awareness primitive emotional impulses originating in the diencephalon. An analogous relationship holds between a film projector and its receiving screen. Just as the image produced by the projector requires a screen to capture and focus its contents, the limbic cortex receives, transforms, and brings to awareness the emotional impulses generated by the hypothalamus. Prior to reaching the limbic cortical areas, emotional input lacks a hedonic quality and an *experienced* subjective content.

Besides its apparent role in the experience of emotion, the cingulate area appears to play a role in the regulation of motor activity. Stimulation of the anterior cingulate area excites motor activity, whereas stimulation of the posterior cingulate area inhibits it. The cingulate gyrus also appears to play an important role in the exhibition of sexual behavior. In males, cingulate lesions result in a reduction of sexual drive, whereas similar lesions in females have no effect on sexual drive but will disrupt maternal behavior, including patterns of nursing and audiovocal communication maintaining mother-progeny contact. Additionally, the cingulate appears to serve an important function in the facilitation of play (MacLean, 1986). The development of maternal behavior, distress vocalization, and play are limbic hallmarks differentiating the mammalian brain from that of the reptile. The reptile brain lacks a structure equivalent to the cingulate gyrus. An important implication of MacLean's work for dogs is the putative localization of separation-distress vocalization within the anterior cingulate gyrus.

Another limbic structure of interest is the septal area—a putative reward center. In humans, electrical stimulation of the septum results in the pleasurable sensation of building to, but never realizing, orgasm. Whereas the amygdala is largely involved with the expression and experience of emotions associated with self-preservation (e.g., escape-avoidance of aversive stimuli), the septal area mediates the experience of affects associated with sexual behavior (MacLean, 1986). Electrical stimulation of the septal area results in strong erotic feelings and increased libido. An im-

portant regulatory function performed by the septum is the inhibition of negatively motivated behaviors such as aggression. Self-stimulative electrodes implanted in the septum of human patients have been used to control impulsive aggression. In general, lesions of the septal area result in disinhibition of aggressive impulses together with exaggerated reactivity to startle—*septal rage syndrome.* Supporting this inhibitory function, the septum receives serotonergic projections from the raphe bodies in the brain stem. Apparently, the septal area performs an excitatory role over hedonically pleasurable affects (e.g., erotic sensations) while inhibiting aversive ones. Not surprisingly, it follows that septal damage adversely affects the animal's ability to play (Panksepp, 1998). Although cingulate lesions appear to negatively influence active avoidance learning (negative reinforcement), passive avoidance learning (positive and negative punishment) may be enhanced by such lesioning. In contrast, septal lesions interfere with passive avoidance learning (i.e., learning that requires strong inhibition) but do not appreciably interfere with active avoidance learning and, in some cases, may even improve it (Gray, 1971). Also, extinction and reversal learning in which a previously learned response must be abandoned or inhibited in order to learn a new one is disrupted by lesioning of the septal area.

Most investigations of subcortical and cortical limbic areas have been carried out with the aid of ablation techniques or electrical stimulation of target brain areas. This emphasis has naturally led some researchers to explore invasive procedures in the treatment of behavior disorders. Delgado (1969) has been particularly influential in this regard. In his famous demonstrations, a charging bull is halted in its tracks at the push of a button, showing in a very dramatic way that aggressive behavior can be controlled by remote electrical stimulation of the brain. His work offered hope that alternative treatment modalities for the control of intractable and otherwise untreatable behavior disorders might be on the horizon. Another area that has received some attention, including some rather horrifying applications in human patients, is neurosurgery. Although very little experimental work utilizing neurosurgery as a means to control abnormal behavior has been carried out in dogs, it would appear from basic research that neurosurgery could provide relief in some cases involving severe or intractable anxiety, phobia, and aggression (Beaumont, 1983), especially where euthanasia is the only alternative. Prefrontal lobotomies have been performed on dog-aggressive sled dogs (malamutes) and on family dogs with various aggression problems (Allen et al., 1974). The surgeries appeared to be most effective in the management of intraspecific aggression in the sled dogs but yielded only limited benefits for pet dogs exhibiting aggression toward people. Other targets for such surgery that have been mentioned in the literature include thalamocingulate projections (cingulectomy), the thalamocortical pathways, or various sites in the amygdala and hypothalamus. Since a considerable amount of surgical risk and cost is associated with such interventions, the procedure is rarely used. A major problem associated with neurosurgery is the brain's tendency to compensate for its losses, often resulting in short-lived benefits (for weeks to months) from limbic lesioning (Thompson, 1967).

In addition to neurosurgery, electroconvulsive therapy (ECT) has also been used to treat aggression problems in dogs (Redding and Walker, 1976). The authors reported a significant reduction in aggression exhibited by the treated dogs toward the owner, children, dogs, or other adults (both men and women) as the result of ECT. Redding (1978) also suggests that ECT may prove to be a useful therapeutic tool in the treatment of other behavior problems, including fear biting, neurodermatitis, destructive tendencies, flank sucking, tail biting, and excessive fear of loud noises. The effect of ECT in the treatment of these behavior problems has not been evaluated. Redding (1978) recommends a treatment program involving daily multiple convulsive exposures (under general anesthesia) carried out over a week. After day 3 or 4, marked changes are usually observed in aggressive dogs in the direction of increasing docility. He notes that repeated treatments and retreatments may be necessary to maintain the improved behavior. As is the case in human patients, ECT has a pronounced effect on memory:

> After ECT treatment an "aura" of confusion and apparent loss of memory is observed in all patients. Owners report that their dogs are confused at times for 2 to 4 weeks after the treatment, after which there is a gradual return of memory. Following treatment and release from the hospital, the dog may show no more interest in the owner than in any other person. The ability to recognize the owner returns relatively rapidly, however. (1978:695–696)

According to Redding, memory loss is associated with the therapeutic benefit of ECT. To my knowledge, little additional research has been carried out to evaluate the effectiveness and side effects of ECT. Like psychosurgery, ECT has an ethical stigma attached to its use, making it a last-resort option for the treatment of refractory aggression—if used at all.

LEARNING AND THE SEPTOHIPPOCAMPAL SYSTEM

The largest subcortical limbic structure is the hippocampal formation. The hippocampus appears to be involved in the processing of memory and, in collaboration with other limbic structures, various affective and cognitive functions. Damage to the hippocampus results in an animal's inability to store recent memory but does not interfere with memories already consolidated before damage occurred. The hippocampus in conjunction with the septum appears to play an important role in response inhibition and habituation. It also serves important sensory processing functions. One sensory function it performs is the detection of novelty and familiarity. This attentional feature of the hippocampus may represent a significant factor in the hippocampal-lesioned animal's inability to form certain memories. Some theories suggest that an attentional/contextualizing interference may cause the hippocampus to "attend" inaccurately to significant stimuli.

The hippocampus together with other prominent structures belonging to the Papez circuit (hypothalamic mammillary body, the anterior thalamic nuclei, and the cingulate gyrus) appears to play important interactive roles in the elaboration of emotional experience and expression (Steinmetz, 1994) (Fig. 3.3). According to the Papez circuit theory, emotional experience is generated when inputs from the hypothalamus are projected from the anterior thalamus into the cingulate cortex—the site where "environmental events are endowed with an emotional consciousness." Fibers from the cingulate cortex subsequently converge on the hippocampus, from where the loop is closed as the processed input is relayed back to the hypothalamus. Steinmetz summarizes the basic functions of this circuit:

> Each of these loops seems to serve a specific function that is associated with limbic system activity such as timing (septal loops), response processing (cingulate gyrus), processing of sensory stimuli (trisynaptic loop) and so on. The loop structure that is associated with the septo-hippocampal system provides sophisticated circuitry for information processing such as the processing that is necessary for generating emotional responses. Indeed, the neural processes that are involved in generating and regulating

emotional responses require the integration of much information such as assessing the organism's internal and external environments, matching present experiences with past experiences, and selecting responses (both autonomic and somatic) that are appropriate for the situation. A relatively complicated circuitry, such as the limbic system with its variety of structures and interconnections, is likely at the heart of generating and regulating emotional states. (1994:24)

An important correlation appears to exist between the hippocampus and the septal area in their joint inhibitory functions. Under conditions of arousal and septal-hippocampal inhibitory control over ongoing behavior, the hippocampus exhibits a steady theta brain wave in contrast to surrounding desynchronized activity occurring elsewhere in the brain. Theta waves are produced in the hippocampus by novelty, pain, and frustration. Lesions of various brain sites (medial nucleus of the septum and certain nuclei of the thalamus), as well as the effects of various drugs (especially barbiturates), abolish or disrupt

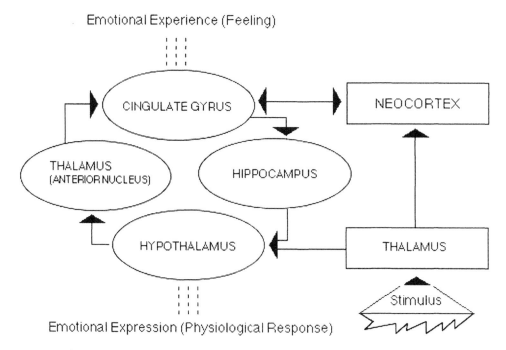

FIG. 3.3. The Papez circuit has been proposed as a primary pathway for the expression and experience of emotion.

these theta waves, which are believed to be associated with the normal inhibitory functioning of the septohippocampal system (SHS). Theta rhythms are generated by the hippocampus in an area called the dentate gyrus but are under the control of pacemaker cells in the medial septum (Gray, 1982).

In line with such a processing-modulatory function is Gray's speculation that the hippocampus, together with other limbic areas interacting with the SHS, serves to excite or inhibit behavior selectively (Gray, 1982). In conjunction with the ARAS, for example, the SHS appears to detect novelty in the environment and mediates the expression of surprise or startle. The SHS also mediates other forms of adaptation, including the most primitive form of stimulus learning—habituation. Orienting response studies performed by Sokolov and Vinogradova (reported in Gray, 1971) have shown that novelty and habituation are processed by a comparator mechanism located in the SHS. This mechanism compares ongoing stimulation with an animal's expectations of what should be occurring. If the results of this comparison between what is expected and what actually occurs are different, the effect produced is novelty (surprise/startle) and the evocation of an appropriate orienting response or intensified vigilance. If the stimulation is identical to what the animal expects, then habituation will occur—the dog gradually takes no notice of it. Habituation is highly specific, however. Sokolov's studies have shown that subtle changes of the stimulus complex (e.g., intensity, duration, quality, repetitive rate, and association with other stimulus events) may trigger a comparator "alarm" with a resultant recovery of the habituated orienting response. This subtle type of sensory sorting has led Gray to speculate that novelty reaches the SHS by a thalamocortical route rather than through the ARAS, which appears to be more dedicated to attentional functions arising from painful stimulation. An immediate outcome produced by novelty is the inhibition of ongoing behavior—a kind of "stop and think" hesitation occurs whenever a dog is faced with something significant and new. When the comparator finds a significant difference between what is expected and what actually happens, it signals and ac-

tivates the behavior inhibition system (BIS). The BIS inputs cause ongoing behavior to stop. The BIS is particularly associated with punishment or frustrative nonreward. Both punishment and frustration disrupt ongoing behavior and subsequently invigorate or potentiate instrumental responding.

Another general system outlined by Gray involves the display of unconditioned escape behavior and affective aggression in response to fear- or anger-evoking stimuli. The flight-fight system (FFS) is predominately under the regulation and control of the hypothalamus and the amygdala. As previously discussed, the hypothalamus controls both affective aggressive displays and quiet predatory attacks.

Finally, Gray has postulated a behavioral activation system (BAS) operating in dopaminergic reward centers (nucleus accumbens) associated with the basal ganglia, neocortical structures, and various regulatory activities provided by the SHS, including important comparator functions. The BAS is associated with both the acquisition of reward and the termination or avoidance of punishment. The determination of whether a particular response is followed by reward or punishment depends on a comparator function. Voluntary behavior is self-reflective, requiring that at each moment the SHS evaluates the convergence or divergence of expected outcomes with what actually occurs. These various functions are coordinated by the prefrontal cortex, resulting in organized learning based on positive-feedback loops involving a series of predictions and confirmations that culminate in general expectancies about behavioral outcomes. Three basic outcomes on voluntary behavior are possible as the result of such expectancies: acquisition, extinction, or maintenance. Behavior that is followed by positive consequences exceeding expected outcomes is strongly reinforced, whereas behavior attended by consequences that are overpredicted (receiving a reward smaller than expected) results in a weakening of the associated behavior. Finally, responses followed by outcomes that are well predicted lead to confirmation of previously established expectancies but result in no new learning.

The BAS and positive learning evolved to

maximize direct contact with rewarding events and to avoid their loss or omission. In contrast, the BIS is concerned with the recognition of signals anticipating punishment, nonreward, or startle/novelty. In the presence of such signals, the BIS prompts an animal to inhibit ongoing behavior and to become more vigilant. The FFS involves affective displays aimed at removing fear-eliciting or threat signals by flight or attack. Gray (1991) postulated a theory of temperament that involves a combined contribution of these three systems. The BIS encodes relevant pathways and individual difference in the area of anxiety and impulsivity with heightened sensitivity to learning involving punishment; the FFS encodes traits predisposing an individual to various degrees of aggressive and defensive behavior, and the BAS is relevant to an animal's willingness to learn or alter behavior for positive reinforcement.

According to Rogeness (1994), conduct disorder in children may be conceptualized within the general framework of Gray's model. A child who is predominately controlled by reward mechanisms belonging to the BAS may be unable to adequately control maladaptive impulses that lead to immediate satisfaction. Such individuals are unable to inhibit consummatory behavior when faced with the immediate prospects of reward acquisition or escape-avoidance opportunities. Also, children with an underactive BIS may not condition well to signals predicting loss of reward or other forms of punishment. Since the BAS is mediated by dopaminergic activity and the BIS governed by noradrenergic activity, one would expect in an impulse-biased child or dog greater dopamine activity and tone, as well as reduced noradrenergic function. An additional factor, especially relevant with regard to the expression of aggressive behavior in such cases, is serotonergic projections from the dorsal raphe bodies terminating in the amygdala—an important area for the inhibition of aggressive behavior. Serotonin plays an important role in the regulation and inhibition of aggressive behavior—decreased serotonergic activity in these systems is associated with an increased likelihood of aggressive impulsivity under conditions of threat or frustration.

A dog governed by a strong BAS (strong dopaminergic activity) tends to be one that gets into perpetual trouble, moving from one "jam" to another. Such dogs are swept up by the moment's opportunities and governed by the acquisition of immediate gratification and the calculation of escape-avoidance strategies with which to avoid punishment—all rewarding events. BIS (strong noradrenergic activity)-controlled dogs, on the other hand, are more circumspect and responsive to punitive events impinging on them; such dogs are more likely to inhibit their behavior in the future following punishment instead of perpetually making the same mistakes. Theoretically, dogs governed by strong BAS activity and regulated by a weak BIS together with reduced serotonergic modulation over amygdaloidal interconnections are more likely to behave impulsively, possibly with episodic aggression. Perhaps, a diagnostic test differentiated by two biochemical parameters would be useful for the evaluation of certain forms of aggression: (1) evidence of decreased noradrenergic/serotonergic activity and (2) evidence of increased dopaminergic activity. Clinical investigations of drugs that inhibit the reuptake of NE and serotonin (e.g., amitriptyline and clomipramine) in conjunction with appropriately selective dopamine antagonists might prove very useful for the management of canine impulsive behavior disorders, including some forms of hyperactivity and aggression.

CEREBRAL CORTEX

The cortex, which is the outermost and latest development in the evolution of the vertebrate brain, is believed to be the central site of consciousness and intelligence, performing the most complex associative and mnemonic functions. The gray matter (the fissured and convoluted outer surface) is largely composed of neuron cell bodies stacked approximately 3 mm thick. Underlying the cortex is a white medullary structure composed of myelinated axonal fibers that communicate with different parts of the cortex and other proximal and distal areas of the brain. Beneath the medullary white matter are the basal ganglia, a collection of subcortical nuclei involved in the mediation of complex movement, like walking and running. Removal of the cerebral cortex (but sparing the basal ganglia) results in the loss of sophisticated locomotor skills, but other motor activities, like running, walking, fighting, and sexual behavior, are not significantly affected. Besides motor functions, the cerebral cortex is intimately involved in the organization of somatosensory information and the elaboration of various cognitive functions, like learning and problem solving.

The cerebral cortex is divided into two large left and right hemispheres that are interconnected by the corpus callosum and other commissure fiber bundles, allowing the two sides of the brain to communicate with each other. An interesting feature of the cerebral cortex is that its two sides have a contralateral relationship with the body—for example, impulses originating on the right side of the cortex are responsible for motor activity on the left side of the body and vice versa. The cortex is functionally sectioned into several areas serving distinct roles: the frontal lobe (serving various unifying and associative functions), the temporal lobe or auditory cortex (responsible for receiving and processing auditory information), the precentral lobe or primary motor cortex (involved in fine motor activity), the parietal lobe (receiving somatic-tactual sensory input from the skin and body), and the occipital lobe (receiving and processing visual inputs).

The prefrontal cortex located in the frontal lobe receives input from many parts of the brain and assesses it in terms of a dog's changing needs, goals, and the current demands of the internal and external environment. In addition to the assessment of input, the prefrontal cortex decides on the course of action needed and directs the expression of programmed species-typical action patterns. The prefrontal cortex evaluates the effect of such behavior via reward-punishment outcomes (Suvorov et al., 1997). Consequently, pathways originating in the prefrontal cortex appear to play a very significant role in the coordination of goal-directed behavior, perhaps in conjunction with the behavioral activating system as previously described. Damage to the prefrontal cortex produces a

number of significant cognitive and emotional dysfunctions. Allen and colleagues (1974) found that dogs that had undergone prefrontal lobotomy exhibited a high degree of distractibility, but, paradoxically, once they managed to focus on something, they seemed to hold their attention on it for an unusual length of time. Emotionally, the dogs with prefrontal damage (especially involving the orbitofrontal area) appeared disorganized and uninhibited. For example, the authors mention one dog that "growled while experiencing seemingly pleasurable stimuli" (1974:207).

The frontal cortex is a unifying association structure, serving many cognitive, memory, emotional, and motor functions. The prefrontal lobes appear to play a prominent role in learning, especially learning that requires a mental representation of the world. Animals suffering lesions to this area of the brain can learn simple conditioned associations and perform appropriate instrumental responses as long as the necessary information required to learn the behavior and perform it are present and held constant (e.g., a discrimination task involving a positive and a negative stimulus). However, animals with prefrontal lesions do poorly when required to perform a delayed-response task. For example, if a prefrontally damaged dog is shown the location of a piece of food and then briefly removed from the room, the dog would display a much retarded ability to remember where the item was last seen a few moments before. Mastering a delayed-response task requires that dogs form a mental picture or representation of the context and the location of the item in that context. Such effects of lesioning suggest that the frontal cortex plays an important role (in conjunction with limbic structures like the hippocampus and amygdala) in the operation of working memory (Goldman-Rakic, 1992).

The temporal cortex, which is located laterally on the cortex toward the front, is primarily concerned with the organization of information derived from audition. Cortical functions originating in the temporal lobes also appear to play an important role in the formation of complex visual patterns. A dog's ability to recognize its owner's face from others probably involves the participation of the temporal lobe. This area is the only cortical structure to receive projections from all the sensory modalities. The temporal lobes play an important role in the higher elaboration and the conscious experience of emotion, receiving projections from the limbic system and more primitive input directly from the thalamus. Monkeys that have undergone extensive damage to the temporal lobes do not exhibit normal fears and anxieties, are unusually calm and placid while being handled, and tend to engage in compulsive oral behavior. For instance, unlike normal monkeys, lesioned animals may pick up snakes and lighted matches without exhibiting any apparent fear. These effects of temporal lobe lesioning and damage to underlying limbic structures located in the temporal lobes are collectively referred to as the Kluver-Bucy syndrome (Kluver and Bucy, 1937). The authors refer to these phenomena as examples of "psychic blindness," arguing that the absence of fear could not be fully explained by reduced emotional reactivity alone, suggesting that the lesioned animals may simply fail to "recognize" the items as innately feared objects.

Considering the important associative and regulatory functions that are performed by the frontal cortex, it would seem reasonable to conclude that the frontal cortex (especially localized in the prefrontal and orbitofrontal areas) probably plays a considerable role in the control of impulsive and episodic behavior, such as aggression and panic. In addition to exercising regulatory control over target subcortical trigger sites (e.g., the amygdala and hypothalamus) and motor programs in the basal ganglia, it is a central area for interpreting and integrating the hedonic arousal resulting from highly motivated behavior, thereby providing a means to enhance central control over such impulses through learning. Unfortunately, as noted by LeDoux (1996), the connections from the amygdala to the cortex are far stronger than the regulatory connections from the cortex to the amygdala—a functional asymmetry that may help explain the failure of some animals to gain full control over their fearful or aggressive impulses (Fig. 3.4). Also, some evidence suggests that the prefrontal cortex is affected by the dimorphizing influence of perinatal hormones (Kelly, 1991), perhaps affecting cortical regulatory control over fear and aggression, as well as influencing many other neural activities. This possibility is consistent with the general observation of trainers and behaviorists that male dogs present more frequently with aggression and other common behavior problems than female dogs. Although various mechanisms and neural sites are probably influenced by such hormonal activity, the prefrontal area may be particularly important because of the influence that it appears to exert on the perception of social signals and the

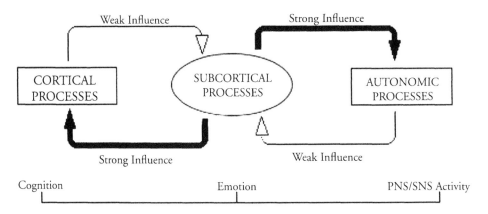

FIG. 3.4. Diagram of the asymmetrical interactions between cortical, subcortical, and autonomic neural processes. PNS, parasympathetic nervous system; SNS, sympathetic nervous system.

coordinated actions that it directs in response to that information. Brain and Haug describe the close relation between hormones and social communication:

> Hormones can be regarded as acting on situational factors by altering the perception of signalling between conspecifics. Evidence for hormonal involvement in perception has been obtained for all the major sensory systems. ... Hormones also may alter the probability of the production of signals that serve social functions. The most frequently modified signals are somatosensory, olfactory, visual, and auditory. For example, androgens and estrogens have major effects on olfactory social communications in both rodents and infra-human primates. (1992:543–544)

The parietal lobes, which are located on either side of the cortex toward the rear, make up a central cortical region mainly involved with processing somatosensory information from the body. This area is concerned with the senses of touch (pressure), warmth, cold, and pain. It is also responsive to proprioceptive sensory input from the muscles, tendons, and joints. The parietal area contains several mental representations of the body mapped out over its surface that correspond to various parts of the body. Depending on the amount of sensory input and the particular sensory modality's importance to the species involved, the size of any particular area represented in the cortex will vary. Rats (which depend on their whiskers to a great extent) have a disproportionately large area of their somatosensory cortex devoted to the mapping and representation of sensory input from their whiskers. Eichelman (1992) has noted that the mere clipping of a rat's whiskers has an equivalent suppressive effect on affective aggression as a bilateral amygdalectomy. The amount of the cortex mapped for any sensory modality is proportionately correlated with the relative size of the thalamic relay involved (Thompson, 1993). The occipital lobe is located at the rear of the brain and is primarily involved in the processing of visual information relayed to it by the thalamus. Extensive lesioning of the occipital lobe of the cerebral cortex results in blindness.

Even though a dog's behavior is strongly influenced by intrinsic neurobiological processes, it remains flexible and responsive to the adaptive influence of learning. An important function of behavioral intervention is to improve a dog's ability to focus attention, to exercise impulse control, and to develop a more adaptive repertoire of coping strategies. Most veterinary clinicians emphasize the importance of adjunctive behavior modification when administering psychotropic medications, such as fluoxetine. While the subcortical circuits mediating the expression of affective aggression can be modulated by such drugs, treatment is only lastingly effective if corresponding cortical regulatory control is enhanced at the same time through learning. In severe cases, medications may help dogs to obtain better self-control over their dysfunctional or problematic impulses, but such drugs can never take the place of sound training and behavioral intervention.

NEUROTRANSMITTERS AND BEHAVIOR

An important cellular function performed by neurons is the manufacture of chemical neurotransmitters. Neurotransmitters are produced in the cell body of specialized neurons by the endoplasmic reticulum, which is dispersed throughout most of the cytoplasm of the neuron. After manufacture, neurotransmitters are stored in vesicles produced by another cell structure called the Golgi apparatus. The vesicles containing the neurotransmitter are subsequently transported down the axon along microtubules and stored in the presynaptic terminal. This process is called axonal transport and includes both a slow and fast variety. Fast transport moves chemical transmitters quickly down the axon at a rate of 10 to 20 mm a day, whereas slow transport may move substances at a much slower rate of only about 1 mm per day. Axon transport takes place in both directions—both away from and back toward the cell body (Thompson, 1993).

Acetylcholine

As previously discussed, communication between neurons takes place at small gaps between neurons called synapses. Different chemical transmitters are involved, each possessing specific functions at different levels of neural organization. Peripheral neurons innervating skeletal muscle fibers act via the release of acetylcholine (ACh). The secretion of ACh into the synaptic cleft stimulates adjacent postsynaptic receptor sites to open ionic channels, resulting in the depolarization of the affected cell. The stimulative effects of ACh continue as long as it remains in the synapse. To open the synapse for additional transmissions, the receptor cell releases acetylcholinesterase (AChE), an enzyme that degrades ACh into acetate and choline. An interesting aspect of ACh in the body is that it exhibits an excitatory or an inhibitory effect depending on the muscle receptors involved. Skeletal muscles are excited by ACh, whereas the heart muscle is inhibited by it. Curare, a compound used experimentally to inhibit voluntary muscle activity, blocks the receptor sites for ACh in the skeletal muscles (resulting in paralysis) but has no effect on the heart muscle. Atropine, on the other hand, blocks the inhibitory effects of ACh on the heart muscle but has no discernible effect on skeletal muscles. Nicotine acts on skeletal muscle receptor cells in much the same ways as ACh. Sites sensitive to the excitatory effects of nicotine and ACh are referred to as *nicotinic* receptors. Muscarine (a poison derived from mushrooms) has an inhibitory effect much like that of ACh on the activity of the heart. As a result, ACh receptor sites that serve to slow the heart rate are called *muscarinic* receptors.

Glutamate and GABA

Synaptic transmission within the brain is also mediated by neurotransmitters synthesized from various amino acids derived from dietary protein. Excitatory transmissions are conducted by glutamate, whereas GABA is responsible for inhibitory transmission across neural synapses. Unlike ACh, glutamate and GABA are not broken down by enzymatic actions within the synaptic cleft but are reabsorbed by the presynaptic terminal through a reuptake process called pinocytosis. During the reuptake process, the presynaptic membrane enfolds around the transmitter molecule, drawing it back into the axon. Glutamate and GABA balance and check each other through a complex excitatory-inhibitory process of neural homeostasis. A complete loss of GABA in the brain would result in uncontrolled excitation and convulsions.

GABA has been implicated in the control of phobias and generalized anxiety disorders. Intense fear and anxiety problems in dogs are frequently treated with various benzodiazepine preparations. Such anxiolytics appear to affect benzodiazepine-GABA receptors concentrated along fear circuits communicating between the amygdala and hypothalamus. Benzodiazepine receptors are closely associated with GABA receptors. Medications such as diazepam (Valium) appear to work by modifying the binding of GABA to its receptor, thereby amplifying receptor activity and reducing fear and anxiety by inhibiting activity in fear circuits (Panksepp, 1998). Murphree (1974) tested the effects of several common psychotropic drugs on the extreme anxiety reactions of genetically fearful pointers. Of the various drugs tested, which included phenobarbital, chlorpromazine, amphetamine, and alcohol, Murphree determined that the benzodiazepines were "far superior." Nervous dogs treated with benzodiazepines learned a bar-pressing response more quickly and performed the response at a higher rate than dogs not treated. Since benzodiazepines have specific receptor sites mediating their effect on fear and anxiety, it has been speculated that the brain itself produces anxiolytic substances much like the analgesic opioids (endorphins) are produced in response to pain. Like morphine, benzodiazepines are potentially highly addictive.

Catecholamines: Dopamine and Norepinephrine

Another group of important neural transmitters are the catecholamines. Tyrosine (an amino acid) is converted through various chemical actions from L-dopa (L-3,4-dihydroxyphenylalanine) to dopamine, NE, and lastly epinephrine. Each of these chemical changes requires the action of a specific enzyme. Some neurons possess the necessary enzymes needed to produce dopamine, whereas others have an additional enzyme for the synthesis of NE (Fig. 3.5). Although epinephrine is not produced in the brain, its production is under hypothalamic influence via the adrenal medulla.

Most dopamine is produced and distributed through three brain systems: (1) The nigrostriatal system involves dopamine-producing neurons originating in the substantia nigra of the midbrain, with axons projecting into the basal ganglia (a forebrain area involved in coordinated movement). (2) The mesolimbic system originates in dopamine-producing cells within the ventral tegmental area (located adjacent to the substantia nigra). Mesolimbic axons project to various regions via the MFB, including the amygdala, lateral septum, hypothalamus, hippocampus, and nucleus accumbens. (3) The mesocortical system also originates in the medial tegmental area, with axons projecting to the limbic cortex (cingulate and entorhinal areas), prefrontal cortex, and hippocampus. In addition, a fourth dopamine system communicates between the hypothalamus and the pituitary gland. Both mesolimbic and mesocortical dopamine circuits have been implicated in the development of serious cognitive and behavioral disorders, such as schizophrenia (Kandel, 1991). It has been theorized that an affected person's brain contains either too much dopamine or too many receptor sites for dopamine activity. Phenothiazines are a class of major tranquilizers that bind with these receptor sites, thereby preventing dopamine from doing so. Chlorpromazine (Thorazine) is a commonly prescribed antipsychotic drug that functions specifically as a dopamine antagonist. On the other hand, depletion of dopamine can also result in serious problems, as observed in Parkinson's disease, which involves the second dopamine circuit (nigrostriatal) originating in the substantia nigra, with projections terminating in the basal ganglia. Parkinson's disease results from the depletion of dopamine and the destruction of dopamine-producing neurons. The disease is associated with several motor deficiencies, including repetitive movement, tremors, and loss of coordinated movement. Parkinson's disease is treated with the dopamine precursor L-dopa. Dopaminergic circuits have been implicated in the development of compulsive disorders in dogs. Finally, dopamine plays a central role in the mediation of classical and instrumental learning. Reward experiences occurring as the result of either negative or positive reinforcement appear to be dopamine dependent. The reinforcement effects derived from appetitive stimuli, as well as those occurring as the result of the successful avoidance of aversive stimulation, are both interfered with when dopamine activity is blocked (Carlson, 1994).

NE circuits in the brain originate in neurons belonging to the locus coeruleus located in the brain stem. Axonal fibers extending from these NE-producing neurons project into all major structures of the brain. These

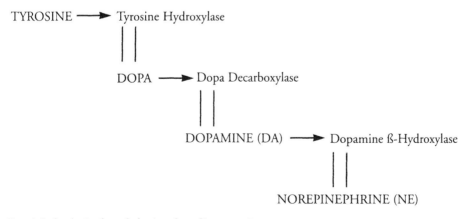

FIG. 3.5. Synthesis of catecholamines from dietary tyrosine.

diffuse projections contribute to the ARAS, providing a steady level of arousal or wakefulness within these divergent circuits and systems. NE axons often form synaptic terminals in a very different way than the basic pattern previously described. Instead of the conventional synapse, the NE axons form swollen protuberances along their surfaces. At each of these protuberances, NE is released as the action potential moving along the axon reaches these swellings. NE is reabsorbed through a reuptake mechanism. Among its many functions, NE is an excitatory transmitter of the ANS, stimulating increased heart rate and respiration during sympathetic arousal.

Serotonin (5-Hydroxytryptamine)

An important neurotransmitter in the neural economy of dogs is serotonin or 5-hydroxytryptamine (5-HT), which is especially important for the control of sleep cycles and has been implicated in the neurochemistry of stress, depression, and aggression. Specialized neurons manufacture serotonin from nutritional tryptophan (Fig. 3.6). Serotonin is stored in vesicles located in the presynaptic axon, and under appropriate stimulation, these serotonin-containing vesicles are released into the synaptic cleft. Serotonin molecules bind to specific serotonergic-receptor sites located on the postsynaptic neuron. Like other monoamines already discussed, serotonin is not broken down in the synapse like ACh but is recaptured through a reuptake mechanism. Excess amounts of serotonin are broken down by monoamine oxidase (MAO) within the presynaptic terminal. Serotonin-

producing neurons are located in the raphe nuclei located in the medulla, with projections into various parts of the brain. The raphe nuclei send serotonin-containing fibers to sleep-wake regulatory centers in the hypothalamus (suprachiasmatic nucleus), to the amygdala, hippocampus, septum, basal ganglia, and cerebral cortex. Besides controlling sleep-wake cycles, serotonin projections terminating in the limbic system play an important role in inhibiting anger and aggression. Further, serotonin directly attenuates the subjective experience of pain occurring during highly emotional displays involving anger or aggression, thereby mitigating against the effectiveness of physical punishment in the control of emotionally charged (affective) aggression.

Depression is often treated with drugs that either inhibit the reuptake of serotonin and NE or block the action of MAO—an enzyme that chemically breaks down the neurotransmitter. MAO inhibitors prevent the enzymatic breakdown of serotonin and other monoamines reabsorbed into the presynaptic terminal, thus making more of these substances available for use. Antidepressants like fluoxetine (Prozac) function to keep more serotonin in the synaptic cleft by selectively inhibiting its reuptake. Other antidepressants (tricyclics) like imipramine (Tofranil) and amitriptyline (Elavil) inhibit the reuptake of both serotonin and NE. The benefits of tricyclic medications on depression have led to theories implicating low levels of serotonin and NE in its development. Iorio and colleagues (1983) isolated a group of "depressed" beagles and tested various anxiolytic and psychotropic drugs on them. That re-

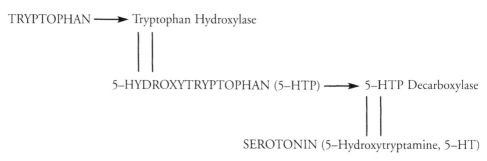

FIG. 3.6. Synthesis of serotonin from dietary tryptophan.

search group found a significant improvement in 50% of the dogs exposed to imipramine, amitriptyline, and isocarboxazid (an MAO inhibitor). Interestingly, the dogs tested all exhibited a 2-week (10- to 17-day) delay from the onset of treatment to the appearance of signs of improvement. None of the dogs showed immediate improvement under tricyclic treatment, and all (except one) returned to baseline levels of depression when medication was withdrawn after 28 days.

More recently, Rapoport and colleagues (1992) demonstrated a connection between serotonergic activity and acral lick dermatitis (ALD), a compulsive disorder in dogs. A total of 42 dogs exhibiting compulsive licking were exposed to controlled trials involving various drugs, including clomipramine (Anafranil) and fluoxetine (Prozac). The results of the study showed that clomipramine (a tricyclic antidepressant) and fluoxetine [a selective serotonin reuptake inhibitor (SSRI)] were both effective against ALD, whereas the other medications tested were not beneficial. The authors speculate from research carried out by Jacobs and coworkers (1990) in cats that a specific serotonin subsystem in the dorsal raphe may be inappropriately activated by chewing and licking, thus implicating it as a potential neural site for ALD.

Clomipramine has also been shown to be an effective medication for the treatment of fear and generalized anxiety in companion dogs not responsive to behavior therapy (desensitization and counterconditioning) or previous treatment with anxiolytics (diazepam) or other tricyclics lacking strong serotonin reuptake-blocking effects (Stein et al., 1994). The study involved five dogs of various ages and breeds presenting with symptoms of fear and generalized anxiety. All the dogs exhibited improvement (three of them much improved to very much improved) within 2 to 3 weeks under the influence of clomipramine. A previous study carried out by Tancer and colleagues (1990) evaluated the effects of imipramine (Tofranil, a related tricyclic drug) on 17 genetically nervous pointers but without much success. Imipramine is commonly prescribed for the control of panic disorder in humans. In the case of the nervous pointers, however, little

sustained improvement was observed in the dogs treated orally with 50 mg given twice daily.

Monoamines and the Control of Aggression

Several studies have implicated monoamines in the regulation of aggressive behavior (Siegel and Edinger, 1981). For example, quiet or predatory aggression is significantly reduced in animals by increasing the levels of NE in the hypothalamus and the medial nucleus of the amygdala. On the other hand, increased levels of NE stimulate affective hostility involving intruder-induced or pain-induced aggression. Eichelman and colleagues (1981) have reviewed the relevant literature regarding the biochemistry and pharmacology of aggression. Included was a series of studies by Reis (1972) demonstrating that electrically induced rage via the amygdala in cats results in the depletion of NE reserves in both forebrain and brain stem areas. Other studies of decerebrate cats have shown that electrical evocation of sham aggression results in a depletion of NE in the brain stem in proportion to the magnitude and duration of the rage evoked. This depletion is followed by a sharp increase of NE metabolism as evidenced by rising levels of tyrosine hydroxylase activity (Leventhal and Brodie, 1981). Tyrosine hydroxylase is the *rate-limiting factor* in the production of both dopamine and NE. The amount of this enzyme in the neuron determines how much NE it can produce. Sham rage is entirely suppressed in cases where catecholamine reserves are completely depleted and synthesis is chemically blocked. Lithium, a drug that reduces brain NE, attenuates shock-induced aggression, but this effect is confounded by a possible involvement of increased serotonin availability also caused by lithium.

Arons and Shoemaker (1992) studied the distribution of catecholamines (dopamine and NE) and beta-endorphin in different brain regions of three behaviorally distinct breeds: the Border collie, shar planinetz, and the Siberian husky. These breeds exhibit different predatory responses toward mice serving as prey, with the husky showing the most predatory and consummatory behavior and the shar showing the least predatory and consummatory behavior toward mice. They found significant differences in the relative concentrations of some of the neural transmitters measured, suggesting that breed-specific behavioral differences may be related to underlying neurochemical differences obtained through selective breeding. For example, in the lateral hypothalamus, a site associated with quiet attack, shars exhibited a significantly lower concentration of dopamine than found in collies or huskies. Despite the evident breed differences in catecholamine concentrations, the authors note that complex behavior patterns like predation are probably governed by a complex interaction of many neurotransmitter systems. One particular neurotransmitter differentiation between the breeds studied seemed especially suggestive. An important trait difference between collies, shars, and huskies is their general activity and exploratory levels. Collies and huskies tend to be more active and interactive with their immediate environment than are shars. NE is frequently associated with arousal and general activity levels. Consequently, it is not surprising to find that collies and huskies exhibit a 40% to 60% higher level of NE than shars in important NE areas of the brain (e.g., the locus coeruleus, brain stem, and diencephalic areas). NE levels may provide an important biological marker correlated with general activity and exploratory levels in different breeds of dogs.

Although cholinergic pathways in the brain are not as well studied as monoaminergic pathways, some studies have shown a linkage between ACh and aggressive behavior. Injections of ACh placed in the ventricular system (fluid-filled areas inside the brain) result in affective aggression and rage in cats. Further, direct cholinomimetic stimulation (carbachol) of the amygdala also results in aggressive behavior in cats. Cholinergic agonists injected into the lateral hypothalamus of nonkilling animals induces quiet attack behavior. This predatory response is blocked by the cholinergic antagonist atropine (Eichelman, 1987). Dopaminergic and beta-adrenergic blockers do not suppress cholinergic-induced aggression (Leventhal and Brodie,

1981).

Increasing evidence suggests that the indoleamine serotonin plays an inhibitory role over the exhibition of both predatory (quiet attack behavior) and affective aggression. Depletion of serotonin increases affective aggression in rats and quiet attack behavior in cats, whereas increased serotonin production reduces affective aggression in rats and reduces fighting behavior among isolated (usually more aggressive) mice. Recently, Reisner and colleagues (1996) demonstrated that the cerebrospinal fluid (CSF) of dogs exhibiting dominance-related aggression contains lower levels of serotonergic and dopaminergic metabolites than found in normal (nonaggressive) controls. Among the dominant-aggressive dogs studied, those that reportedly attacked without warning were found to have significantly lower concentrations of 5-hydroxyindoleacetic acid (5-HIAA) and homovanillic acid (HVA) in their CSF than those dogs that gave warning before biting. The investigators suggest that this difference between dogs that warn and those that do not may indicate an impairment of a serotonergic-mediated impulse control mechanism modulating such aggressive displays. Also, dogs studied that had a history of biting hard (puncturing or lacerating the skin) tended to have lower concentrations of 5-HIAA and HVA than did dogs not delivering damaging bites. Interestingly, Popova and colleagues (1991) found significant differences in the serotonergic activity of human friendly versus human aggressive/defensive silver foxes. Foxes selected for tame behavior have greater amounts of serotonin and related by-products in their brain tissue, suggesting increased serotonergic activity. Popova and coworkers speculated that increased serotonergic activity may play an instrumental role in the process of domestication, serving to reduce aggressive tendencies and replacing them with more prosocial and tame ones. They found a similar pattern of increased serotonergic activity in tame versus wild Norway rats.

The influence of serotonin on aggressive behavior appears to be linked to the strong inhibitory effect that the neurotransmitter has over emotional processes and impulsive behavior. Stein and coworkers reported findings indicating that a decrease in serotonergic activity results in "an inability to adopt passive or waiting attitudes, or to accept situations that necessitate or create strong inhibitory tendencies" (1993:10). Reducing the availability of serotonin by blocking its synthesis or available receptor sites negatively affects the suppressive effects of punishment, whereas the restoration of normal serotonin levels reverses this disinhibitory effect. Olivier and colleagues (1987) demonstrated strong inhibitory effects of serotonin-enhancing drugs on the frequency of various forms of aggression exhibited by mice and rats, including intermale aggression (mice), resident-intruder aggression (rats), isolation-induced aggression (mice), maternal aggression (rats), and mouse-killing behavior in rats. Especially strong inhibitory effects were observed in animals medicated with the serenics fluprazine and eltoprazine (serotonin agonists). Eltoprazine, in particular, exhibited very promising characteristics for the control of aggressive behavior. It not only inhibited a wide spectrum of aggressive behaviors, but seemed initially to be highly specific with few collateral side effects on other behavioral systems. Unfortunately, subsequent research seems to indicate that the aggression-reducing effects may be due to anxiogenic side effects. Dodman (1998) found that although eltoprazine did reduce aggression, it also appeared to elevate anxious behavior in the two dogs treated. Other research (Kemble et al., 1991) seems to support the conclusion that serenics elevate social anxiety, thus making their use highly questionable in the control of aggressive behavior.

The apparent connection between enhanced serotonin activity and the inhibition of aggressive behavior has led to the widespread use of SSRIs and tricyclic antidepressant medications for the control of canine aggression problems, especially dominance-related aggression (Dodman et al., 1996a). Another drug found to show some promise for the control of dominance aggression in dogs is lithium (Reisner, 1994). Physiologically, lithium decreases NE turnover and inhibits tyrosine hydroxylase activity, thus affecting dopamine production. In addition, lithium produces an increase in blood levels of tryptophan; increases serotonin production in the brain, while at the same time inhibiting its metabolism; and, in general, enhances the aggression-inhibiting functions of the serotonergic system (Leventhal and Brodie, 1981).

Diet and Enhancement of Serotonin Production

The brain's production of serotonin depends on nutritionally derived tryptophan. Tryptophan, like other precursor amino acids used in the manufacture of neurotransmitters, reaches the brain by passing through the blood-brain barrier. Research first carried out at the Massachusetts Institute of Technology under R. J. Wurtman has demonstrated that diets rich in protein tend to deplete brain tryptophan levels. This is a somewhat paradoxical finding, since tryptophan is a protein-forming amino acid and should be made more available to the brain as blood protein levels increase (Young, 1986). Even more paradoxical is a related finding that diets high in carbohydrates actually increase available tryptophan for serotonin synthesis, even if the food itself contains only modest amounts of tryptophan. The explanation for these apparent discrepancies involves two parts. (1) Naturally occurring tryptophan represents only a small proportion of the various amino acids making up protein (approximately 1% to 1.6%). The other larger and more prevalent amino acids all compete with tryptophan for a limited number of transport channels passing through the blood-brain barrier. The result of the foregoing biochemical scenario is that tryptophan is blocked out and the brain may be quickly depleted of available stores of the amino acid needed for the steady production of serotonin. (2) A more complicated metabolic process is needed to explain how a high-carbohydrate diet raises brain levels of tryptophan. Diets containing a proportionately higher level of carbohydrates than protein (at least 1 part protein to 5 to 6 parts carbohydrate) stimulates the secretion of insulin. An important effect of insulin production is its diversion of large neutral amino acids (other than tryptophan) into muscle tissue. Because of its unique molecular structure differentiating it from other amino acids, tryptophan is not similarly affected by the secretion of insulin. The outcome is that the proportion of plasma tryptophan is greatly increased, thus obtaining an advantage over other amino acids competing for transport through the blood-brain brain. As a result, the brain's production of serotonin is significantly increased.

For the increased movement of tryptophan to occur, the diet must be kept both low in protein and high in carbohydrates. In rats, a diet with protein levels exceeding 18% is sufficient to block the tryptophan effect (Spring, 1986). The exact percentages for dogs have not been determined but are assumed to be very similar (Dodman et al., 1996b). Unfortunately, these estimates have not been confirmed through appropriate physiological studies.

A common protein source in dog foods is corn. Corn, however, is unusually low in tryptophan and may represent some risk to animals sensitive to serotonergic underactivity. Lytle and colleagues (1975), who studied the effects of a restricted corn diet on pain thresholds in rats, found that a diet restricted to corn as the primary source of protein results in a significant reduction of plasma and brain levels of tryptophan, with a subsequent decrease in the production of brain serotonin. Serotonin has an important analgesic effect on pain. Animals fed a restricted corn diet exhibit a lower threshold for pain (measured by the magnitude of a flinch or jump response to electric shock) than controls on a balanced amino acid diet of casein. Test subjects fed a tryptophan-rich diet or receiving an injection of tryptophan soon recovered from the hyperalgesic effect induced by the corn diet.

The foregoing studies are suggestive for the management of pain and aggressive behavior in dogs. Ballarini (1990) proposed that dietary protein be routinely adjusted as part of a comprehensive treatment program involving aggression in dogs. A study carried out by Dodman and coworkers (1996b) showed a promising linkage between reduced dietary protein and some forms of aggressive behavior in dogs. Dogs exhibiting territorial

aggression with a strong component of fearfulness responded beneficially to a reduced protein diet (17%), while territorial aggressors of the dominant type showed no significant change. The study, however, is not without possible flaws, perhaps accounting for its failure to show a stronger response than reported. Three problematic areas stand out: (1) protein levels were not kept sufficiently low, (2) carbohydrate levels may not have been high enough to induce an increased passage of tryptophan across the blood-brain barrier, or (3) the dogs may not have been exposed to the diet for a sufficient time. Behavioral effects from the diet were measured only after a relatively short period (2 weeks), so perhaps added benefits might be expected from a longer-term exposure (6 to 8 weeks). Also, Aronson has noted that, in addition to the diet's beneficial effect on fear-related territorial aggression, it is "possible that a more radical reduction in dietary protein levels would produce a reduction of dominance aggression and hyperactivity as well" (1998:80).

An important area of basic research is obviously wanting: a determination of the relative protein/carbohydrate proportions and percentages needed to induce (or block) tryptophan influx in dogs. Before any conclusions can be drawn with regard to the effect of low-protein diets on impulsive agonistic behavior in dogs, such questions will need to be explored and answered in detail. Furthermore, no study to date has directly implicated dietary tryptophan depletion in the causation of canine aggression or hyperactivity, except by way of extrapolation from studies involving other animal species. Therefore, another important area of future research is determination of the effect of tryptophan depletion and supplementation on canine behavior. In a prototype study conducted by Chamberlain and colleagues (1987) in vervet monkeys, the monkeys were fed an identical diet except for the relative content of nutritional tryptophan. Three groups of monkeys were differentially fed diets containing normal tryptophan levels, high tryptophan levels, and low tryptophan levels. Although little benefit was seen with the provision of a higher percentage of tryptophan in the diet, a strong correlation was observed in terms of two parameters of aggression and the low-tryptophan diet. Monkeys fed a relatively low-tryptophan diet exhibited an increase of competitive aggression over food (dominance aggression) and spontaneous agonistic displays among themselves. The researchers also found a significant link between tryptophan depletion and an increase in general motor activity. Interestingly, in both cases, the observed behavioral effects of tryptophan depletion were restricted to male monkeys.

The level of tryptophan in the blood serum of assaultive alcoholics is at a lower than normal ratio to other amino acids, suggesting a possible connection between serotonin depletion in the brain and the exhibition of impulsive aggression among alcoholics. Morand and colleagues (1983) performed a pilot study with human patients to determine the effects of tryptophan on chronically aggressive schizophrenics. The study involved supplemental tryptophan at dosages of 4 to 8 grams a day. There was an approximately 30% reduction in the incidence of aggressive behavior while the patients received the tryptophan supplementation, but the response of patients was variable, with some becoming even more depressed and disorganized. Christensen (1996) wrote a critical review of the literature on the relationship between diet and behavior, providing a concise and objective summary of the current state of research in this important area.

Arginine Vasopressin and Aggression

Vasopressin has received considerable experimental attention, especially with respect to its influence over scent marking, dominance behavior, and affective aggression. Also known as antidiuretic hormone, vasopressin is a peptide hormone that controls water retention by the kidneys. In addition to this peripheral role, the hormone also appears to play a central neuromodulatory function over the expression of aggressive behavior. C. F. Ferris (University of Massachusetts Medical

School), who has studied the effects of arginine vasopressin (AVP) in golden hamsters for several years, found that the vasopressinergic system in the hypothalamus mediates the expression of several agonistic behavior patterns: flank marking (an AVP-dependent behavior), offensive aggression, and the formation of dominant-subordinate relationships (Ferris et al., 1986; Ferris and Potegal, 1988).

AVP receptors overlay androgen and estrogen receptors, suggesting that sex hormones and AVP may interact in the expression of aggressive behavior. In fact, the aggression-facilitating effect of AVP appears to *depend* on the presence of testosterone. Delville and coworkers (1996), for example, found that the hamster's behavioral response to microinjections of AVP varies depending on the presence or absence of testosterone. They showed that latency of attack is reduced by AVP microinjections into the ventrolateral hypothalamus (VLH), but only if the subjects are pretreated with testosterone prior to injection. Although AVP regulates the onset and latency of aggression via the VLH, it does so without concurrently affecting the behavior's strength or number of bites delivered—a dimension of attack behavior that appears to be controlled by the selective activation of AVP receptors in the anterior hypothalamus (AH). This work suggests that the VLH and AH play different functional roles in the expression of aggressive behavior.

The regulation of aggressive behavior is more complicated than the interactions of testosterone and AVP acting directly on the hypothalamic vasopressinergic system. Besides AVP and sex hormones, researchers have discovered a robust interaction between AVP and serotonin in the hypothalamus (Ferris and Delville, 1994). Both the ventrolateral hypothalamus and anterior hypothalamus exhibit a high concentration of serotonin-bearing axon terminals and binding sites. Interestingly, fluoxetine (Prozac) injected peripherally inhibits AVP-induced offensive aggression and retards the onset of resident-intruder attacks, with fewer bites occurring during the attacks (Ferris and Delville, 1994; Ferris et al., 1997). These studies suggest that serotonin directly modulates AVP neurons in the hypothalamus, thereby antagonizing AVP-system-facilitated aggression.

There are many potential implications of this work for dogs. Until recently, progestins were commonly used for the control of unwanted aggression and marking behavior. The most frequently mentioned target site of progestin action is the hypothalamus, perhaps including the targeting and disruption of AVP activity. An antivasopressinergic link would appear logical, since progestins produce a diminution of both urine marking and aggressive behavior in treated animals. More recently, the veterinary use of fluoxetine has become increasingly popular for the control of unwanted behavior, especially dominance-related aggression and various compulsive disorders. Fluoxetine is rarely prescribed for intraspecific or territory-related aggression; given the findings of Ferris, though, perhaps such a wider use might prove very beneficial, especially in cases of refractory dog fighting and territory-related aggression. Lastly, serotonin-enhancing drugs may play a beneficial role in the control of household urine marking by dogs.

NEURAL SUBSTRATES OF MOTIVATION (HYPOTHALAMUS)

Beginning with the pioneering work of Olds and Milner (1954), many studies have shown that direct stimulation of various parts of the brain produces pleasurable feelings. Although electrical stimulation of the anterior hypothalamus evokes intense sexual excitement, lesioning of the same site results in a loss of sexual drive and interest. In addition to the evocation of highly motivated and directed behavior, such intracranial stimulation of the anterior and lateral hypothalamus (especially the MFB) results in a pronounced experience of general pleasure and activation. Both areas of the hypothalamus function as brain reward sites. An interesting feature of hypothalamically stimulated pleasure is that it is not associated with actual consummatory satisfaction but instead results in the augmentation of appetitive need or desire for the reward object. Consequently, the pleasure areas of the hypothalamus appear to be more connected with

drive induction than drive reduction. Stimulation of sites associated with hunger, thirst, or sexual desire raises activity levels in the direction of those basic needs but does not appear to evoke a corresponding sense of satisfaction or satiety. It is interesting, also, that such stimulation does not appear to produce a sense of frustration or anger. On the contrary, the sensation of desire or appetite is immensely rewarding for many animals. The stimulation of neural sites associated with appetence for food may be rewarding because it simultaneously elicits cortical representations or imaginings of pleasurable affects previously associated with the satisfaction of hunger.

Observations from electrical self-stimulation experiments provide general neurological support for a deprivation theory of reinforcement (Premack, 1965; Timberlake and Allison, 1974). For any particular stimulus (or response) to be rewarding, an animal must feel a need or appetite for it. The hedonic direction of any behavioral consequence (i.e., its reward or punitive value) depends on the animal's relative deprivation or approach/attraction toward the item or opportunity in question. The drive or incentive to work for food may be experienced by hungry dogs as a conditionally rewarding state (drive induction), whereas the acquisition of the desired item (under the motivation of hunger) is an unconditionally rewarding event (drive reduction). Reinforcement, therefore, hinges on two distinct but interdependent functions: appetence and consummation. Without the presence of both factors, the reward may not be reinforcing. For example, food for a sated dog may actually be aversive, just as an opportunity to play could be punitive if the dog is overly tired or is sick. The hypothalamic activation of hunger sites both propels dogs into appropriate goal-directed behavior and provides conditional, positive reinforcement to the animals for doing so. Gray (1971, 1991) has postulated a behavioral activation system (BAS) facilitating these functions of brain-coordinated conditional reward or punishment. A feedback system appears to exist in which the animal is systematically guided toward stimuli promising satisfaction of a particular drive versus the avoidance of stimuli promising dissatisfaction or having been associated with previous punishment. Gray speaks about the role of hypothalamic reward sites in this regard:

> We suppose that stimuli which regularly precede the occurrence of a reward themselves acquire the capacity to activate the reward mechanism; and that, the closer in time to the innately rewarding stimulus they occur, the stronger is this capacity. The reward mechanism is so constructed that, via connections with the animal's "motor" system (i.e., those parts of the brain which issue commands to the limbs), it strives to maximize such conditioned or "secondary" rewarding stimulation. In this way, given a stable environment in which sequences of stimuli recur with a degree of regularity, it is able to guide the animal towards the innately rewarding stimulus. We could, in fact, liken the reward mechanism to a homing or "approach" device of the kind used by a guided missile to aim up a heat gradient at the hottest spot around. (1971:183)

Such a functional neural arrangement regulated by the hypothalamus makes sense, considering the many moment-to-moment homeostatic roles that it serves. Behavior directed toward the acquisition of some biologically needed item or experience receives endogenous conditional reinforcement from reward sites associated with the needed item until it is obtained and general homeostasis secured. In carnivores, such a system of conditional reinforcement is particularly appropriate, considering the often sustained effort and arduous work required to locate and kill prey. Without endogenous conditional reinforcement, the animal's effort may wane or be redirected toward easier or more immediately rewarding activities.

NEUROBIOLOGY OF AGGRESSION (HYPOTHALAMUS)

Many studies have demonstrated that the hypothalamus plays an important role in the expression of aggression. Two broad categories of aggressive behavior have been observed in the laboratory during intracranial stimulation: (1) quiet attack (predatory behavior) and (2) affective aggression (defensive and offensive displays) (Fig. 3.7). Electrical stimulation of the lateral hypothalamus results in the evocation of various predatory displays, including stalking, pouncing, and biting sequences. Quiet attack depends on the presence of a suitable prey object—that is, the evoked sequence is directed and dependent on a target. If an adequate target is not available, the stimulated animal may simply eat (if food is present) or become aroused and engage in searching or appetitive behavior involving sniffing and pacing. A differentiating feature of electrically stimulated predatory behavior is its emotionally *quiet* character. Quiet attack behavior occurs in the absence of visible agitation or sympathetic activation. Further, electrical stimulation of quiet attack behavior appears to be a hedonically pleasurable experience. Animals will self-stimulate

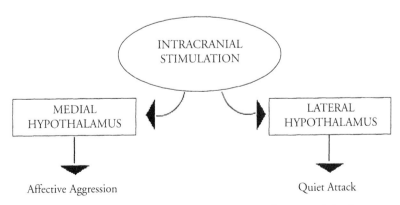

FIG. 3.7. Pathways mediating the expression of affective aggression and quiet attack (predatory aggression).

themselves through electrodes inserted into areas associated with quiet attack behavior (Panksepp, 1971). The reward experienced during stimulation of the lateral hypothalamus is similar to that seen during excitation of sites associated with drinking and eating. Essentially, quiet attack is an appetitive and consummatory response analogous to food or water seeking and ingestion.

Affective aggression is evoked by electrically stimulating the ventromedial hypothalamus. Unlike quiet predatory attack, affective aggression is a generalized response that may be targeted at any available object moving within the animal's reach. It is a highly emotional display associated with intense autonomic activation. In contrast to the pleasurable experience of quiet attack stimulation, intracranial stimulation of hypothalamic sites associated with affective aggression elicits a hedonically aversive experience that both cats and rats (and probably dogs) respond to as a punitive event. Research performed by Adams and Flynn (1966) appears to support this belief. They taught cats to jump on a stool to escape shock applied to their tails. After having obtained a vigorous escape response, they differentially stimulated sites in the lateral and medial hypothalamus and then compared the results on the previously trained escape response. Stimulation of the medial area resulted in strong escape responding in the cats, whereas stimulation of the lateral hypothalamus did not result in escape efforts. This different response to lateral versus medial stimulation supports the view that they are reward and punishment sites, respectively.

The Adams and Flynn experiment indicates that a linkage exists between affective aggression and escape behavior. Apparently, aggression is not only aversive to the animal, but it is also closely associated with painful stimulation and fear. Azrin and colleagues (1967) demonstrated that a definite relationship exists between aversive stimulation and the evocation of escape or attack behavior. Their findings show that escape is generally *prepotent* over attack; if attack ends the painful stimulation, however, it is easily conditioned as an avoidance response. Further-

more, during extinction (i.e., the phase of training where attack no longer served to postpone or terminate the aversive event) previously acquired attack behavior remained highly persistent and vigorous—even though it was consistently ineffective against the aversive event. The observations by Adams and Flynn are congruent with the prepotency theory of escape proposed by Azrin and coworkers. When sites typically associated with attack were stimulated, the cats tested readily emitted the learned escape response rather than attacking.

These laboratory observations are significant for understanding and controlling various forms of canine aggression. Tortora (1983) has developed a theory of aggressive behavior in dogs that incorporates a theoretical viewpoint that is consistent with the findings of Azrin and colleagues and the aforementioned research. He has argued convincingly that many common forms of canine aggression directed toward human targets are motivated by avoidance dynamics rather than an ethological causation like dominance-related competition. Many aggressive displays that are currently diagnosed as dominance aggression are, according to Tortora's analysis, aimed at avoiding some perceived aversive outcome rather than establishing or maintaining the offending dog's social status. Dominant dogs may be more prone to learn an active defensive coping strategy during social conflict in order to control (avoid or escape) aversive outcomes than a more submissive counterpart, but the underlying behavioral dynamics and motivations are not to enhance dominance status but simply to terminate a perceived threat. Within the framework of this model, subordinate or submissive dogs are more likely to react nonaggressively, that is, by freezing or fleeing—unless escape is prevented, whereupon they may attack as a last resort. Submissive dogs flee or freeze, not because of their lower relative status or some controlling deferential attitude, but rather because their primary mode of avoidance is flight or freezing. Both active and passive defensive modalities are aimed at avoiding an aversive or feared outcome.

Consistent with Tortora's viewpoint, Siegel and Edinger (1981) have argued that affective aggression appears to be neurally organized around the general purpose of self-preservation and survival. They have speculated that even such functionally disparate aggressive patterns as fighting, maternal aggression, and territorial defense may all be ultimately subsumed under the same general category of hypothalamically affective attack behavior. Evidently, stimulation of the same brain site evokes different forms of aggression, depending on the social and environmental conditions existing at the time.

NEUROBIOLOGY OF FEAR

The study of fear has made tremendous strides during the past decade. Several interacting and self-regulating circuits in the brain have been identified. The auditory-neural pathways involved in classical fear conditioning have been mapped by LeDoux and his coworkers at New York University (LeDoux, 1996). Since auditory fears (e.g., brontophobia and other loud noises) are common among dogs, it is appropriate to review these important findings in detail.

Primary Neural Pathways Mediating the Classical Conditioning of Fear

Although all sensory modalities are capable of forming conditioned links with central fear circuits, the pathways active during auditory conditioning are the most fully known (LeDoux, 1994). Auditory information reaches the brain via relay nuclei located in the brain stem and thalamus. Such information follows two primary pathways: a slow circuit visiting cortical destinations before projecting into the amygdala, and a fast circuit directly terminating in the lateral amygdala. Slow and fast circuits are both engaged during fear conditioning, and each circuit is capable of establishing conditioned fear independently of the other. In the fast circuit, auditory projections from the thalamus (medial geniculate body) are received by the lateral nucleus of the amygdala and relayed to the central nucleus and other amygdaloidal areas, chiefly the basal and accessory basal nuclei. The aversive US appears to form direct links to the lateral amygdala and indirect ones via thalamic relays (Carlson, 1994). It is within this general network that the auditory CS is associatively linked with the fear-eliciting US.

Outputs from the central amygdala are subsequently processed by other limbic and cortical regulatory circuits. Efferent projections from the central nucleus terminate in the hypothalamus, producing a variety of discrete emotional and physiological expressions of fear. The specific manifestation of fear exhibited by an animal depends on the location of arousal. Amygdala projections reaching the central periaqueductal gray matter produce freezing, outputs to the lateral hypothalamus increase blood pressure, and connections formed with the paraventricular hypothalamus stimulate the release of stress hormones.

In addition to direct thalamic input, the amygdala also receives regulatory inputs from limbic and cortical portions of the brain, especially the hippocampus. This additional information converges on the amygdala to produce rich emotional variety, meaning, and subtlety. The combination of these various neural influences on the amygdala modulates and refines the dog's ultimate emotional response to stimulation. The organization of emotional expressiveness and its adaptation depends on the harmonious interplay and the efficient regulatory functioning of these various neural networks. Innate or acquired dysfunctions occurring in any one of these interdependent pathways result in emotional and behavioral disorder.

Habituating and Consistently Responsive Neurons

Unlike conditioned stimuli that acquire their fearful properties by being associated with other startling or traumatic events, fears of loud noises are biologically *prepared*. The sound of fireworks or thunder, for example, requires no associative conditioning in order to elicit fear reactions in a sensitive and predisposed animal (Menzies and Clarke, 1995). Stimuli that evoke fearful reactions without conditioning appear to utilize *hardwired* neural pathways that are responsive only to a narrow range of stimulation and variability.

Recent research supports the hypothesis that a limbic substrate elaborates persisting unconditioned fear of loud noises. A series of experiments carried out by Fabio Bordi (see LeDoux, 1994) demonstrated that, within the lateral nucleus of the amygdala, two distinct neurons can be isolated: *habituating* and *consistently responsive.* By measuring activity in these cell groups, he found that the habituating cells eventually stop firing in response to repeated low-intensity acoustic stimulation. In contrast, however, consistently responsive cells are not subject to the effects of gradual habituation. Further, he found that only very loud noises activate consistently responsive cells. These cells invariably fire if sufficiently intense stimulation is produced by loud sounds.

It would seem reasonable to speculate that consistently responsive neurons in the amygdala mediate or play a significant role in the elaboration of loud-noise-phobic and thunder-phobic responses in dogs. These effects do not depend on learning but invariably result when a sufficiently intense unconditioned auditory stimulus is presented. A neural mechanism of this type may help to explain some of the difficulties associated with the treatment of thunder-phobic dogs. Because fearful responses to loud acoustic stimulation are unlearned and unresponsive to habituation, they would inherently resist behavioral training efforts.

It has been frequently observed that thunder phobia worsens with age. Although a dog may exhibit sensitivity to loud noises when young, the initial reactions are more or less under the animal's control. As the dog ages, and perhaps following a particularly intense exposure, its ability to cope with its fear of thunder may be compromised. This situation is particularly evident in dogs exhibiting chronic separation distress. These observations support the possibility that some neurological change may be occurring that compromises the dog's ability to cope with fear over time, although much more study in this area is needed before any firm conclusions can be drawn.

A possibility, though, of considerable interest involves the breakdown of regulatory control of the hippocampus. The hippocampus performs a regulatory function over the expression of fear. Under conditions of repeated or prolonged stress, the hippocampus may undergo degenerative changes that alter its ability to perform these functions. On the other hand, the amygdala appears to function more efficiently under stress. Over time with the impairment of hippocampal regulation, the strength of amygdaloidal outputs may be increased, with the appearance of excessive fear. Under conditions of fear, the hippocampus undergoes further degeneration, with increasing susceptibility to fear and the manifestation of increasingly exaggerated expressions of it. Besides the influence of possible hippocampal damage due to stress, strong evidence indicates that learning under fearful conditions is especially persistent and augmented by the facilitating presence of epinephrine. The potentiated response to thunder or anticipatory conditioned stimuli (atmospheric changes, lightning, etc.) exhibited by phobic dogs may be the combined accumulated effects of enhanced fear learning and stress. With these various effects in mind, it would make sense to consider pharmacological treatments that focus on the control or amelioration of negative stress effects and administering a medication capable of blocking epinephrine activity during thunderstorms.

Many thunder fears have a clear link with a specific event in a dog's past (Hothersall and Tuber, 1979), but many do not and instead follow a more gradual and progressively worsening course. Fears that have a specific link with an event in a dog's near past appear to be more responsive to simple counterconditioning efforts than fears developing over years of exposure.

Extinction of Conditioned Fear

Once conditioned fears are learned, they are encoded as relatively permanent emotional memories. These so-called *savings* are not subject to subsequent erasure through extinction (Kehoe and Macrae, 1997). Although extinction efforts (repeated presentations of the CS without the US) can temporarily attenuate the fearful CS, extinction is subject to a number of well-known recovery effects (Bouton and Swartzentruber, 1991). As noted above, fear conditioning does not require the activation of cortical circuits, but in order to extinguish fear a significant amount of cortical involvement is required (LeDoux, 1994). The importance of higher neural mechanisms for extinction is evident in the failure of extinction to occur in animals suffering cortical lesions. Although robust conditioned fear responses can be obtained in spite of extensive cortical damage, such lesions dampen or entirely eliminate the effects of extinction. Extinction is a higher learning regulatory process that attunes conditioned fears to changing environmental conditions and organismic needs.

Three significant aspects of fear conditioning and extinction have important implications for the treatment of behavior problems involving fear:

1. Once fear is learned, it is probably permanent.

2. Although extinction and counterconditioning efforts may ameliorate aversive affects and reduce fearful responding, such training efforts are subject to reversal and the reinstatement of unwanted behavior.

3. Since the extinction of fear is subject to recovery, behavioral training should include efforts to enhance voluntary impulse control over fear-related behavior.

Brain Areas Mediating Contextual Learning and Memory

Previous learning and contextual cues serve to modulate fearful behavior. A tiger safely confined behind bars and glass in a zoo represents a significantly different stimulus in terms of fear-eliciting potential than one roaming free in public. Contextual cues serve an occasion-setting function signaling those times and places when the feared event is likely to occur. For example, a dog that has been previously attacked by another dog will

become progressively more vigilant and defensive as it nears the place were the incident occurred. These various contextual cues associated with fear (and aggression) are organized by the hippocampus. Classical conditioning of specific fears (CS-US) are mediated by the amygdala, whereas fear associated with the context or configuration of stimuli present at the time of conditioning are mediated by the hippocampus. Contextual cues or configurations draw on information that is encoded and stored as nonsensory representations and relations.

Comparing the structural and functional differences between classical conditioning and contextual conditioning may help to explain how some fears are rapidly extinguished and others become persistent phobias. In the developing nervous system of mammals, the prominent systems of learning and memory mature at different rates and become functional at different times. Stimulus-specific fears mediated by the amygdala are operative early in the animal's life cycle, whereas contextually modulated fears are possible only after the hippocampus is functionally operative sometime around weaning (Jacobs and Nadel, 1985). This ontogenetic transition may play an important role in the appearance of the critical period for fear conditioning in 8- to 10-week-old puppies. Emotionally traumatic events occurring during this time can produce long-lasting fears. The period may be a vulnerable integrative phase articulating emotional and contextual learning. At the conclusion of this period, a puppy's contextual learning abilities and the various cortical regulatory influences mediated by hippocampus are ready for environmental exposure; in fact, this chain of events appears to follow the empirical evidence. As puppies near 10 or 12 weeks of age, they exhibit a more curious and confident attitude about exploring the environment extending beyond the immediate nesting site, making more and more ambitious excursions as they mature (Scott and Fuller, 1965). Besides exhibiting an increased interest in wider exploration of the environment, cortical articulation is evident in the observation by Nott that "puppies of this age gradually learn the relevance of their behaviours and are able to determine which behaviours are appropriate to specific situations" (1992:69).

The organization of learning and encoding of memories depends on the maturation of these different systems. The earliest fearful associations learned are encoded as unconscious or *implicit* memories. Although implicit memories are consciously inaccessible, they are not without widespread influence. Implicit unconscious memories activate physiological responses associated with fear. The conscious identification of the eliciting aversive stimulus and the context in which it occurred requires the participation of *explicit* memories formed by the hippocampus and related cortical systems. Explicit memories are the cold facts formed about the surrounding circumstances of fearful conditioning, whereas coordinated implicit memories provide the emotional content (Fig. 3.8).

Implicit and explicit memories are elaborated into conscious experiences through the integrative mediation of the working memory. The working memory system is a complex, short-term memory and neural organizing system of mental and sensory information that is intimately connected with conscious cognitive functions.

During fearful conditioning, both implicit and explicit memories are formed and are coupled together through the working memory so that they usually reach conscious attention together—but not always. This is especially the case involving memories formed

before the full maturation of the hippocampus (or in cases where hippocampal functioning is disrupted). Typically, such early memories remain unconscious and inaccessible but under appropriate environmental stimulation are capable of evoking strong autonomous emotional responses via the visceral brain and body. Fear conditioning that occurs independently of the contextualizing influence of the hippocampus produces a number of characteristics that correspond to symptoms observed in phobias, especially a tendency toward excessive generalization and context independence. Although infantile fears are forgotten, they may be reinstated under the influence of stress. According to Jacobs and Nadel (1985), stress-inducing environmental conditions disrupt hippocampal contextualization of memories while potentiating context-free associations formed by the amygdala. As is discussed below, stress plays a prominent role in the learning and unlearning of fear.

AUTONOMIC NERVOUS SYSTEM–MEDIATED CONCOMITANTS OF FEAR

Several physiological changes occur with the onset of fear. These reactions are mediated by the hypothalamus through the autonomic nervous system in conjunction with various hormonal mechanisms. The overall picture is one of emergency and preparedness to act in the face of danger. Common physiological concomitants of fear include pupillary dila-

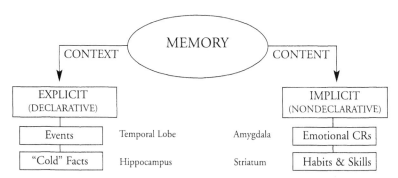

FIG. 3.8. Memory is functionally differentiated into explicit and implicit forms. Explicit and implicit memories depend on the operation of different areas of the brain. CR, conditioned response.

tion (mydriasis), retinal vasodilation (resulting in a reddish glow of the eyes), piloerection (hair standing on end), hypoalgesia (loss of sensitivity to pain), loss of appetite (both food and water), hyperpnea (rapid panting), alimentary irritability with diarrhea, increased perspiration (seen on the pads of the dog's feet), tachycardia (faster heart rate) with harder contractions, and reflex potentiation (stronger startle and withdrawal reflex actions). An important concomitant of sympathetic arousal is direct stimulation of the medulla and the secretion of epinephrine (adrenaline). Epinephrine stimulates and augments sympathetic processes and enhances an animal's ability to flee or fight. Under the influence of intense fear, a dog may urinate, release the anal glands, or defecate. Chronic anxiety may result in polyuria and irregular urination patterns. Lastly, appetitive behavior like eating and drinking is suppressed by fear.

Fear and Biological Stress

Fear is closely linked with biological stress. Stress occurs when any demand is placed upon a dog that requires the dog to change or adjust. Although stress is most commonly associated with hedonistically aversive demands, it is not necessary that the stressor be aversive. Any biological or psychological demand, regardless of its hedonistic valence, can result in stress (Selye, 1976). Whereas healthy stress is an everyday occurrence, pathological stress is associated with disease activity or psychological trauma. Chronic fear and anxiety may lead to stress-related disease, including atrophy of lymphatic glands, immunosuppression, and gastric ulcers. In addition, stress associated with chronic fear may undermine the brain's ability to cope adequately with fear by causing various degenerative effects, especially involving the hippocampus and its restraining influences over the hypothalamus.

The stress response is mediated by a complex loop of interconnected neural and hormonal mechanisms. During fearful stimulation, sensory information relayed by the thalamus prompts the amygdala to instruct the periventricular hypothalamus to secrete

CRF. Subsequently, CRF stimulates the anterior pituitary gland to release ACTH into the bloodstream. ACTH is a hormone that acts specifically on the cortex of the adrenal glands, triggering the release of a variety of adrenal steroids. Once in the bloodstream, these hormones excite the emergency activation of a dog's bodily defenses.

Among the steroidal hormones secreted by the adrenal glands is a group known as the corticoids, which include both inflammatory (aldosterones) and anti-inflammatory hormones (cortisol). In addition to its anti-inflammatory effects, cortisol also serves to calm fearful dogs while preparing them for action. Human subjects undergoing corticosteroid therapy report feeling an increased sense of well-being. It is likely that dogs experience a similar benefit. Urinary cortisol levels and other stress indicators (e.g., the presence of high levels of catecholamines) might well prove to be a valuable test for the detection of physiological changes associated with chronic anxiety. Beerda and coworkers (1996) compared urinary and salivary cortisol measures with the more invasive blood plasma measures. Both urinary and salivary samples provide equally valid measures of stress-induced cortisol activity in dogs. The researchers suggest that salivary cortisol measures may be particularly useful in quantifying acute stress reactions.

Neural Stress Management System and Fear Learning

The hypothalamic-pituitary-adrenal (HPA) axis is regulated by a biochemical negative-feedback loop controlled by cortisol levels dispersed in the bloodstream. High levels of circulating cortisol suppress ACTH via the suppression of hypothalamic CRF secretion. In addition, hypothalamic CRF production is modulated by the combined and opposing stimulatory influences of the hippocampus and amygdala. In the presence of a fear-eliciting stimulus/situation, the amygdala instructs the hypothalamus to secrete more CRF, whereas the hippocampus instructs the hypothalamus to slow down production of CRF. These excitatory and inhibitory control mechanisms provided by the amygdala and hippocampus serve to match and tune an animal's physiological response to the actual circumstances of relative danger/safety present in the environment (Fig. 3.9).

Under conditions of intense fearful arousal, strong associative memories are encoded, often causing lasting emotional disturbances that fail to dissipate over time. The hormone epinephrine appears to play a significant role in the formation of traumatic memories. The urine of humans suffering traumatic experiences (post-traumatic stress disorder) contains elevated amounts of catecholamines (epinephrine and NE), possibly providing a peripheral measure and diagnostic criterion of trauma-induced stress (Kosten

et al., 1987). In animals, retention of avoidance learning and aversive emotional memories is mediated by epinephrine and disrupted by epinephrine blockade (McGaugh, 1990). Rats, for example, given a post-training dose of epinephrine retain more about the training situation than untreated controls. McGaugh speculates that the mechanism mediating this facilitatory effect involves peripheral epinephrine (epinephrine is blocked at the blood-brain barrier) triggering opioid disinhibition of NE activity occurring in the amygdala. Interestingly, extinction occurring under response prevention contingencies is also facilitated by the administration of stress hormones (ACTH and epinephrine) shortly before carrying out response-blocked presen-

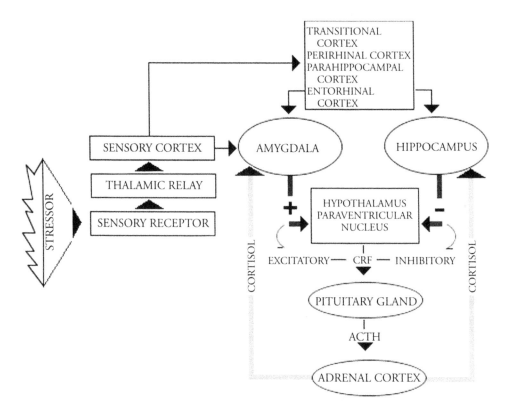

FIG. 3.9. Diagram showing the primary stress circuits. Note the bimodal modulatory effects of cortisol on the amygdala and hippocampus. In the amygdala, cortisol stimulates the transmission of signals to the hypothalamus that cause it to release corticotropin-releasing factor (CRF), whereas, in the hippocampus, cortisol exercises an inhibitory influence over the secretion of CRF. In sum, these influences regulate (augment or restrain) the activation of the physiological response to stress via CRF-mediated adrenocorticotrophic hormone (ACTH) release by the pituitary gland. After LeDoux, (1996).

tations of the aversive CS (Richardson et al., 1988). Riccio and Spear suggest that the hormonal enhancement of extinction is attributable to the reenactment of a more complete internal representation of the original fear occurring when the aversive CS is presented without the US:

> Further investigation is needed, but this finding is provocative in suggesting that, in addition to cognitive information about contingencies, elicitation of an affective response may contribute importantly to the elimination of fear-motivated behavior. (1991:232)

An opposite effect on learning appears to occur in the presence of endogenous opioids and narcotics (McGaugh, 1990). Opiates exert a strong inhibitory influence over noradrenergic neurons—an effect that is blocked by the administration of opioid antagonists (e.g., naloxone). NE-producing neurons projecting to the amygdala appear to play an important role in the retention of aversive associative learning. When narcotics are administered after aversive training, they interfere with the retention of fear conditioning. Also, increased opioid activity in the amygdala reverses the facilitatory effect of epinephrine on memory.

The memory-enhancing effect of epinephrine is dose dependent, with high doses stimulating the memory-blocking activity of the opioid system. These observations suggest that the brain may actually have a built-in memory modulating or "erasing" mechanism associated with particularly aversive traumatic events. During times of intense sympathetic arousal when large amounts of epinephrine are secreted, stressful memories may be disrupted or prevented from forming. These findings are highly suggestive with regard to the persistence of some conditioned stimuli to extinction. Fanselow (1991) notes that aversive conditioning results in conditioned stimuli capable of evoking endogenous opioid production. Consequently, the presentation of the aversive CS in the absence of the US may impede extinction of the CS by eliciting the simultaneous release of beta-endorphins, thereby physiologically obstructing the

reenactment or representation of the original fear-conditioning situation.

In general, though, emotionally significant events are better remembered than nonemotional ones. An interesting implication of these findings is the possible beneficial effects of blocking adrenergic activity shortly after the occurrence of traumatic events. LeDoux (1996) has suggested that the administration of an epinephrine-blocking agent may serve as a prophylaxis against the development of lasting fears, negative memories, and the elaboration of emotional disorders following a traumatic experience. Since, as already noted, the brain opioid system appears to interfere with memory formation and retention, it may not be such a bad idea after all to take a good stiff drink following a particularly traumatic event. A potential implication of these findings for dogs is that increased opioid activity might reduce learned social fears following agonistic encounters, perhaps facilitating subsequent reconciliation between combatants, as well. Evidence from rodent studies suggests that strong opioid activity does occur following defeat. Miczek (1983) found that mice confronted with inescapable defeat experience a "large, lasting pain suppression" that appears to be mediated by endogenous opioid activity. Endorphins have also been shown to reduce affective aggression. If a similar phenomenon is present in dogs, this may have potential value in understanding some important aspects of dog social behavior. The emotions associated with submission are clearly of a different origin and quality than those associated with fear and avoidance, the former of which may include some element of fear but, in addition, is well buffered with very strong affiliative overtones. Submissive dogs do not avoid dominant opponents but accept defeat and adopt a subordinate role without an appearance of lasting fear. The possible facilitatory social function of opioids following defeat is consistent with the proposed general role of endogenous opioids in the formation and maintenance of social attachment and bonding among dogs (Panksepp, 1988; Hoffman, 1996).

Stress-related Influences on Cortical Functions

The disruptive influences of stress extend beyond the limbic feedback loops and the HPA system. In addition to the impact of stress on subcortical and physiological mechanisms, acute and persistent stress can generate pronounced dysregulatory effects over higher cortical activities as well. As already discussed, the prefrontal area serves many vital integrative and executive functions, which include impulse control and the coordinated regulation of behavioral systems needed to meet the various internal and external demands placed on the animal to adjust. The provision of a flexible adaptational interface between the organism and the environment appears to be a prominent function of the prefrontal cortex. This prefrontal function is mediated by learning and the exertion of inhibitory and modulatory influences over subcortical processes. Under the adverse conditions of excessive stress, however, subcortical activities are amplified while, at the same time, corresponding cortical regulatory functions may be temporarily disrupted. In particular, acute stress has a robust excitatory effect on the amygdala, which, in turn, coordinates the expression of numerous preparatory systems that mobilize an organism for impending emergency action. During such stressful activation, increased levels of NE and dopamine are released in the prefrontal cortex. Although increased catecholamine activity appears to have a facilitatory effect on subcortical processes, the release of these neurotransmitters in the prefrontal area has an opposite effect, causing it temporarily to suspend its efficient functioning. Instead of enhancing prefrontal functions, as it does in the amygdala, increased dopamine (especially involving D_1 receptors) tends to suspend or disrupt cortical restraint over subcortical activity (Arnsten, 1998). As a result, the benefits of previous learning, impulse control, and social inhibition may be momentarily compromised or turned off, with control taken over by species-typical offensive and defensive action patterns. Under the influence of stress, the behavioral thresholds for these innate patterns are lowered while, simultaneously, their expression is amplified by limbic pathways enhanced by increased catecholamine and CRF activity.

These changes point to several significant effects of stress on the behavior of dogs. Foremost is the possibility that stress-mediated activation of the nervous system may disrupt normal cortical control over the expression of undesirable behavior associated with fear and anger. The foregoing findings underscore the importance of canine husbandry and management efforts that strive to reduce stressful influences in a dog's environment. Unfortunately, stress is a fairly ubiquitous phenomenon in the life of most dogs. Among the most common sources of adverse stress are excessive confinement, insufficient exercise and attention, sensory distress (e.g., exposure to loud noises), separation distress, poorly predicted and uncontrollable training events (especially excessive punishment), and frustration. The loss of predictability and control over significant aversive and appetitive events results in increased anxious arousal and frustrative persistence—both sources of stress associated with the development of many behavior problems. Although the connection between anxiety and the physiological mobilization of stress is well known and recognized, frustration is also an important source of stress (Coover et al., 1971). The combined influence of such behavioral sources of stress on the elaboration of behavioral dysfunction and disorganization are discussed at length in Chapter 9, which is dedicated to the influence of adverse learning conditions on behavior.

Exercise and the Neuroeconomy of Stress

Counteracting the effects of stress depends on a twofold process of altering the environment and providing training and socialization activities that are both highly predictable and controllable. Another common recommendation used to counteract the adverse effects of stress is exercise. The experimental study of exercise indicates that it exerts a considerable, and potentially therapeutic, influence on the physiology of dogs. For example, Radosevich and colleagues (1989) demonstrated that moderate exercise produces pervasive modulatory effects on both peripheral and central endocrine activity in dogs. In addition to the release of various HPA system hormones (beta-endorphins, ACTH, and cortisol), exercise also increases the production of NE. Surprisingly, under conditions of low-intensity exercise (running a treadmill at 4.2 miles/hour on a 6% incline for 90 minutes), a coordinated and commensurate increase of beta-endorphins and ACTH was observed; whereas, in the case of high-intensity exercise (4.2 miles/hour on a 20% incline for 90 minutes), the expected trajectory of increased production of these substances did not proceed linearly—that is, the release of beta-endorphins and ACTH is *dose dependent* on the amount of exercise received. Also, the cerebrospinal fluid (CSF) of exercised dogs contains greater amounts of NE.

Many studies with animals (especially rodents) have shown that neurotransmitter activity is influenced by exercise (Meeusen and DeMeirleir, 1995). Although acute and forced treadmill exercise appears to deplete NE stores in the brain (as observed in learned helplessness) and is physiologically stressful for animals, chronic exercise appears to enhance noradrenergic activity and increases the amount of NE stored in several parts of the brain. Besides enhancing noradrenergic activity, exercise was also found to increase serotonin levels in the central amygdala (Chaouloff, 1997). These combined influences are believed to be responsible for some of the beneficial mood effects associated with exercise.

The finding that exercise enhances serotonergic activity is of considerable importance with respect to the use of exercise for the management of stress-related behavior problems. Within the brain's neuroeconomy, serotonin plays an important modulatory role over stress and the control of undesirable impulsive behavior. Promising evidence in support of a functional link between serotonin production and exercise has been reported by Dey and his associates (1992), who demonstrated a significant alteration of central serotonergic activity in rats exposed to chronic exercise. Daily exercise was found to generate pronounced and sustained enhancement of serotonin metabolism in various areas of the brain, including the cerebral cortex. The authors suggest that the cortex is the most likely neural site mediating the beneficial effects of exercise over depression. They refer to other research with rodents that has shown that experimentally induced depression produces a decreased level of serotonin in the frontal area. Signs of depression in these animals were reversed by administering microinjections of serotonin into the frontal cortex, whereas similar microinjections of NE, dopamine, and gamma-aminobutyric acid failed to alleviate depression similarly. Interestingly, Dey (1994) found that long-term exercise (4 weeks) had a pronounced immunizing effect on rats exposed to stress-induced depression. Chronic exercise prevented the signs of behavioral depression and generated a "remarkable enhancement" of 5-HT_2 receptor subtype responsiveness. In general, the response of serotonin receptor subtypes to exercise was very similar to the effects produced by tricyclic antidepressants. A similar effect has been reported by Chaouloff (1997) with respect to NE. He found that exposure to chronic and free-choice wheel running has an immunizing effect against NE depletion resulting from uncontrollable and inescapable foot shock.

The aforementioned studies support the hypothesis that exercise, especially daily and long-term exercise, has potentially beneficial effects on the neuroeconomy of the dog. Many dog-behavior consultants and trainers have long recommended exercise for the amelioration of a wide variety of behavior problems. Although the research is far from conclusive, the beneficial influence of exercise in combination with appropriate behavioral (e.g., basic training and behavior modification) and environmental interventions is a sensible approach to the management of stress-related behavior problems.

NEUROBIOLOGY OF COMPULSIVE BEHAVIOR AND STEREOTYPIES

Emotional conflict and stress are considered to be significant etiological factors underlying the development of compulsive behavior disorders (CBDs). In addition, there is growing evidence linking CBDs with various neurological sources of causation. Wise and

Rapoport (1989) have argued that basal ganglia dysfunction underlies obsessive-compulsive disorder (OCD) in humans, reporting various historical and contemporary sources of evidence implicating its functional role. They evaluate two functions of the basal ganglia in support of their hypothesis: (1) the basal ganglia may be "repository for innate motor programs" (fixed action patterns), and (2) the basal ganglia performs a gating function over various sensory inputs (releasers). In addition, some sophisticated experimental work with OCD has identified a basal ganglia connection. For example, microinjections of amphetamine into the ventrolateral striatum results in compulsive forepaw licking in rats. The injection of a dopamine antagonist reverses the oral stereotypy (Stein et al., 1992). Luxenberg and colleagues (1988) discovered through x-ray computed tomography (CT) that the caudate nuclei of persons exhibiting OCD are bilaterally smaller than in persons not exhibiting the disorder. Another neuroimaging study implicating caudate involvement was performed by Baxter and coworkers (1987). Through positron emission tomography (PET), the researchers found that the caudate nuclei of OCD patients exhibits a higher glucose metabolic rate than that of controls. Lastly, horses challenged with apomorphine (a dopamine receptor stimulant) exhibit increased oral activity and compulsive licking and other oral stereotypies—symptoms that worsen with increasing apomorphine dosages (Fraser, 1985). Also, tight-circling behavior is induced in rats as the result of intracranial (striatal) microinjections of apomorphine (Koshikawa, 1994). These various studies suggest dopamine pathways play a mediational role in the elaboration of compulsive behavior and stereotypies.

In addition to the neural sites just discussed, an endogenous opioid mechanism has been suggested to play a role in the etiology and maintenance of certain CBDs. Both ALD in dogs (Dodman et al., 1988; White, 1990) and cribbing in horses (Dodman et al., 1987) are influenced by endogenous opioid activity. In these studies, a narcotic antagonist was dispensed to the affected animals. The drugs (naltrexone and nalmefene) effectively impede endogenous opioid activity by blockading opioid receptor sites. Evidently, some opioid mechanism underlies licking and cribbing, since both oral stereotypies were significantly reduced under the influence of the medication. Although significant benefits were observed in both dogs and horses, the decrement of compulsive behavior is drug dependent, with symptoms recurring soon after the narcotic antagonist was withdrawn.

As a word of caution, note that the endogenous opioid mechanisms involved in compulsive behavior are not fully understood. Although a connection has been established between compulsive behavior and opioid activity, it has not been determined how endorphins are related to compulsive behavior and vice versa—that is, it is not clear whether endorphin activity is causal or consequential to compulsive behavior. A couple of important questions need to be settled with regard to the role of endorphins in ALD and tail chasing: (1) does increased central endorphin activity precipitate (or facilitate) compulsive activity, or (2) is compulsive licking or tail chasing more primary in the chain of events—that is does self-stimulation in response to stress produce greater endorphin activity, thereby representing a kind of self-medication for a stressed or bored dog.

Additional support for a neurological causation is provided by the palliative effects of tricyclic antidepressants like clomipramine (Anafranil) and SSRIs, such as fluoxetine (Prozac), in its management. The efficacy of SSRIs implicates a serotonergic pathway, perhaps regulating a dopaminergic system at some level of organization. A report by Brown (1987) noted the reduction of fly-catching episodes and associated hyperactivity in a dog placed on a low-protein diet. The author concluded that the beneficial effect of diet change was due to a dietary allergy. However, another possibility underlying this improvement is a serotonergic connection via enhanced tryptophan transport through the blood-brain barrier (Ballarini, 1990). Evidence of direct serotonergic involvement has also been discussed in the literature. For instance, Jacobs and colleagues (1990) noted that a serotonergic subsystem within the dorsal raphe in cats is stimulated during licking and self-grooming. It is not known, however, whether the increment of neural activity is due to the action of oral movements or sensory feedback caused by such movement. Rapoport and colleagues (1992) extrapolated from these findings to the possibility that a dysfunction may exist in a similar system in some dogs suffering with licking disorders like ALD.

Other neural substrates have been implicated in the etiology and control of compulsive disorders. Uhde and coworkers (1992) reported, in passing, some alleged success in controlling ALD with growth hormone supplementation. Crowell-Davis and colleagues (1989) reported a case involving various compulsive symptoms, including hyperactivity, self-licking, and fly catching. The dog was observed to be especially symptomatic when in the presence of its owner. When isolated, most of the dog's compulsive behaviors abated, suggesting an attention-seeking or anxious-arousal mechanism of some sort at work. Despite such indications, the clinicians discovered that the dog exhibited EEG patterns that were consistent with epilepsy. Subsequent treatment with phenobarbital proved effective in controlling the dog's behavioral symptoms.

The HPA system has been implicated in the expression of compulsive behavior. Growing evidence suggests that a significant role is played by ACTH in the release and maintenance of compulsive ritualization (Swedo, 1989). ACTH is released under various circumstances of increased autonomic arousal and stress, including conflict and exposure to novelty. Rats injected intracranially with ACTH exhibit increased self-grooming behavior. Following intraventricular injection of ACTH (lateral ventricle), rats spent as much as 90% of their time over an hour engaged in self-grooming activity. ACTH-induced grooming is topographically similar to grooming exhibited by rats under conditions of novelty and conflict. It has been found that ACTH-induced grooming can be reduced with opioid antagonists (naloxone and naltrexone) and enhanced with low doses of morphine. Both ACTH and beta-endorphins are produced in the pituitary as part of a generalized response to stress. The subsequent release of peripheral cortisol by the adrenal cortex appears to play a regulatory role over the production of both beta-endorphins and ACTH, thus limiting the extent of their activation via a negative-feedback loop. Cortisol may also influence noradrenergic neurons, as well as provide a regulatory function over the blood-brain barrier. One can speculate on how this might impact on the transport of nutritional precursors like tryptophan and, indirectly, on how the serotonergic system may be secondarily affected by the cortisol-regulated mechanisms mobilized by stress.

NEUROBIOLOGY OF ATTACHMENT AND SEPARATION DISTRESS

MacLean (1985) has proposed that the neural substrates mediating separation distress, maternal care, and play belong to the same paleomammalian portion of the limbic system. According to his theory, these social behavior tendencies are all elaborated within the cingulate cortex and related neural structures. He has argued that the "separation call" or distress vocalization is the mammal's "earliest and most basic" vocalization pattern. More primitive forms of animal life (e.g., reptiles)—lacking a cingulate cortex—do not display evidence of maternal care, separation-distress vocalization, or play. Socially directed vocalization patterns may have originally evolved to maintain close contact between the mammalian mother and her immature offspring. In addition to maternal caregiving and separation distress, play between conspecifics also appeared with the evolution of mammals, perhaps serving to facilitate social harmony among litter mates.

Panksepp (1982) also views distress vocalization as stemming from a primal mammalian emotional system but more specifically originating in those areas of the brain that mediate panic and explosive behavior. In addition to the cingulate gyrus, other brain sites that contain dense concentrations of opioid receptors are implicated in the organization of attachment and separation distress. These areas include the amygdala, dorsomedial thalamus, hypothalamus, and the central gray area:

It is proposed that sites from which distress vocalizations and explosive agitated behavior can
be elicited represent the approximate trajecto-
ries of panic circuitry, the major adaptive function of which is to sustain social cohesion
among organisms whose survival depends on
reciprocity of care-soliciting and care-giving
behaviors. (Panksepp, 1982:414)

These various areas of the brain and interconnecting circuits are stimulated by the differential presence or absence of pertinent social
stimuli evoking or allaying social distress and
panic.

Limbic Opioid Circuitry and the Mediation of Social Comfort and Distress

Both MacLean and Panksepp have noted the
existence of a highly concentrated pattern of
opiate receptors in the neural circuits believed
to mediate social comfort, separation-distress
reactions, and various other relevant emotional responses. Panksepp's lab has performed numerous studies demonstrating a direct linkage between brain opioid activity and
the elaboration of separation distress, contact
comfort, and play (Panksepp et al., 1984).
After many years of study investigating imprinting and isolation-induced distress in
ducklings, Hoffman (1996) has concluded,
along with Panksepp, that social attachment
and bonding is probably mediated by opioid
receptors activated in the presence of adequate social stimuli. Social bonding and separation distress also appear to be closely related to opioid activity in monkeys. Keverne
and associates (1989) at Cambridge University measured significant elevations of beta-
endorphins in the cerebral spinal fluid of Ta-
lapoin monkeys upon being reunited with
conspecifics after a period of isolation. In addition, they have found that social grooming
among paired monkeys is probably mediated
by an endogenous opioid mechanism. Monkeys exposed to naloxone blockade engaged
in more grooming interactions, whereas low
doses of morphine reduced such affiliative exchanges. A similar differentiating effect is observed among rhesus monkeys, where *cooing*
(a primate separation-distress vocalization) is
decreased by the administration of morphine

and increased by naloxone (Kalin and Shelton, 1989).

Panksepp and colleagues (1980, 1988)
found that low doses of morphine significantly reduce separation-distress vocalizations
by puppies, guinea pigs, and chicks. In addition, the researchers demonstrated that socially deprived *kennel dogs* become more socially responsive and obedient after being
administered low doses of morphine and
more uncontrollable when given naloxone
(Panksepp et al., 1983). Knowles and
coworkers (1987) observed that well-socialized adolescent dogs (6 to 8 months old) exhibit increased care-seeking behavior (tail
wagging and social contact) under the influence of naloxone, whereas morphine reduces
such social behavior. It should be noted that
initial efforts to demonstrate a relationship
between naloxone and separation-distress vocalization in puppies failed. Although these
early efforts failed to show a relationship between naloxone blockade and separation-distress vocalization, the researchers did find a
significant relationship between naloxone and
other canine social behavior patterns, including separation distress, when an intermittent
operant element was involved:

> Recently we have measured other care-solicit-
> ing behaviors in the dog, and we find that
> naloxone can facilitate tail-wagging and face-
> licking. Also, we have recently observed that
> naloxone facilitates vocalizations in dogs when
> there is the possibility of a clear operant com-
> ponent. For instance, in several litters of pup-
> pies being tested for social motivation, we have
> observed naloxone-treated animals to vocalize
> more frequently when they are intermittently
> prevented from making social contacts. Ac-
> cordingly, our failure to see a clear facilitation
> of DVs [distress vocalizations] in puppies fol-
> lowing naloxone in a simple separation situa-
> tion does not constitute a negation of the hy-
> pothesis that opioid-blockade should increase
> care-soliciting behaviors. (Panksepp et al.,
> 1980:476)

Additional evidence for an opioid mechanism mediating social emotion and attachment has been reported in rodents by D'Amato and Pavone (1993), who measured
differences in pain thresholds between mice
paired with siblings versus controls paired

with unrelated mice of a similar age. Following 2 months of separation, reunited sibling mice exhibited a significantly higher pain threshold than controls. The full expression of the analgesic effect following the reunion of siblings took approximately 2 hours. The researchers found that the effect was blocked with the administration of naloxone, confirming the involvement of an opioid mechanism.

Not surprisingly, separation distress and panic manifest themselves behaviorally like symptoms of withdrawal from narcotics.

Hippocampal and Higher Cortical Influences

In addition to the aforementioned subcortical circuits, cortical systems are probably also involved in the regulation of separation distress, enabling dogs to cope with separation without experiencing excessive worry or panic. The amount of separation distress expressed by a dog appears to depend on the additive effects of social loss together with the relative novelty of the situation (time and place of separation) in which isolation occurs. For example, many adult dogs exhibit their first dramatic episodes of separation distress (excessive barking or howling, destructive chewing, or elimination problems) only after the family moves into a new home. Other dogs will remain relatively quiescent as long as they are confined in a familiar part of the house and the owner keeps a regular schedule. However, if they are confined in an unsocialized area (e.g., the basement or garage) or if the owner leaves early or returns late, they may become overly anxious and panic. The most intense separation-distress reactions appear to occur when a dog is left alone in an unfamiliar place. This general observation has been experimentally demonstrated with puppies by J. P. Scott and his associates (1973).

The central issue being raised here is whether two converging neural circuits (subcortical and cortical) might contribute modulatory influences over separation distress. Specifically, the hypothesis being advanced is whether two complementary circuits are in-

volved: a circuit that is responsive to the loss of socially significant stimuli, and a second one that is activated by contextual considerations like location (familiar/unfamiliar) and schedule (predictable/unpredictable). An analogous situation occurs in the classical conditioning of fear. During the conditioning of fear involving an acoustic CS, the auditory signal (e.g., tone) generated in the ear is directed via thalamic auditory relays to the amygdala, where it is associated with the fear-eliciting US (e.g., shock). The fearful association between the tone and shock is thereby learned and permanently stored as an emotional memory connecting the CS with the US. However, the animal must also learn in what contexts the fear-eliciting CS is really threatening. Such contextual learning depends on the additional involvement of a complex hippocampal-cortical circuit, which results in the production of consciously accessible memories defining the exact situations (time and place) in which the CS predicts an actual threat (LeDoux, 1994). Under conditions of chronic stress, these various contextualizing functions of the hippocampus may be disrupted. A great deal of evidence suggests that excessive and chronic stress produces degenerative effects on hippocampal regulatory functions (McEwen, 1992). On the other hand, as noted above, these same conditions of stress appear to augment amygdaloidal functions, potentiating emotional learning and responsivity associated with conditioned fear. In the case of separation-distressed dogs, it would seem reasonable to suppose that hippocampal functions may also undergo a similar progressive deterioration as the result of chronic stress associated with the disorder. The neural degenerative effects of stress may help to explain why separation-reactive dogs fail to adjust to the effects of chronic separation distress. It may also provide a possible clue for the higher incidence of other fears and phobias (especially fear of thunder) presenting with separation anxiety.

In the case of separation distress, traumatic experiences associated with the loss of significant social stimuli may be stored as inaccessible emotional memories (manifesting as a persistent and unmodifiable dread of being alone). Along similar lines of contextual learning in the case of fear, the context or situation in which separation occurs may also serve to modulate significantly the amount of anguish and distress expressed via consciously accessible memories of past experiences with separation and the participation of higher cortical coping mechanisms and control. Context may be defined here in terms of both spatial as well as temporal parameters, that is, referring to the place where the dog is confined, as well as the owner's schedule of departures and returns. In general, one might predict that as contextual familiarity and regularity (place and schedule) increase, the magnitude of separation distress should decrease. This seems to be precisely what occurs when dogs are successfully treated for separation-related problems. Whether such a regulatory coping circuit exists is not definitively known, but I would be surprised to discover that it did not.

Stress and Separation Anxiety

In addition to the HPA system readying the body for emergency action, another important CRF-mediated circuit within the brain itself modulates emotionally stressful states resulting from the distress and panic associated with social separation. Panksepp and colleagues (1988) describe an experiment in which CRF was intraventricularly injected into the brains of young chicks. The chicks exhibited pronounced distress vocalizations for 6 hours, even though they were in the presence of social stimuli that normally inhibited such reactivity. Within the CRF brain system, NE counterbalances and restrains CRF activity. Under conditions of prolonged stress, NE is depleted, resulting in the disruption of homeostatic balance between NE and CRF. Some CRF projections terminate in the area of the locus coeruleus and, perhaps, under conditions of chronic stress, CRF may exhaust the production of NE or, in conjunction with a parallel neuromodulatory system (e.g., the opioid system), impede efficient NE production. In addition to CRF-mediated activation of the locus coeruleus, CRF projections innervate the dorsal raphe.

It is known, for example, that endogenous opioids exercise a strong inhibitory restraint over NE-producing neurons (McGaugh, 1990). Under conditions of stressful regulatory imbalance, CRF-facilitated influences may prevail over the mood-enhancing influences of NE. Lowered levels of NE are associated with depression, and not unexpectedly many dogs suffering chronic separation distress also develop signs of depression. In addition to CRF circuits, other neuroendocrine (prolactin and oxytoxin) circuits may also play important roles in the modulation and expression of separation distress (Panksepp, 1992).

Strong evidence suggests that early stressful experiences produce lasting changes in the CRF stress-mediating systems of the brain. Relatively brief doses of separation distress produced by periodically removing rat pups from their mothers before they reach 21 days of age produce long-term changes in the rat's brain (Nemeroff, 1998). These early exposures to stress appear to alter permanently the CRF gene expression and, consequently, the rat's stress management system. These changes include the elevation of central CRF and proliferation of CRF receptor density, thereby intensifying the animal's response to CRF throughout its life. In addition to CRF system changes, early stress exposure elevates stress-induced ACTH secretion as well as plasma cortisol levels. Interestingly, the SSRI paroxetine (Paxil) appears to return CRF levels effectively to normal while adjusting the animal's increased receptor sensitivity to more normal levels, as well. In addition, the medication produces an overall reduction of undesirable fearful and anxious behavior. These palliative effects produced by paroxetine are apparently drug dependent. When treatment was discontinued, the earlier CRF levels, receptor sensitivity, and associated stress-mediated behavior returned to pretreatment levels. These findings suggest the possibility that early and repeated or traumatic exposure to separation may incline dogs to become overly responsive to stress-eliciting experiences, perhaps predisposing dogs to develop a variety of fear-related behavior problems and problematical separation anxiety as adults.

Finally, recent studies by Price and colleagues (1998) suggest that stress-related CRF system activation appears to exert a direct inhibitory influence over serotonin production in the dorsal raphe. This CRF-mediated restraint over serotonin production might obviously affect remote areas of the brain dependent on serotonin activity originating in the brain stem. The intimate link between CRF and serotonin output may help to explain the aforementioned stabilizing and serotonin-enhancing effects of paroxetine via CRF system regulation (or normalization). The evidence suggests that paroxetine might be a useful alternative for the management of stress-related behavior problems in dogs; however, currently it is not commonly employed by veterinary behaviorists (Overall, 1997; Dodman and Shuster, 1998). Considering the potential benefits, and the apparent lack of mitigating adverse side effects, perhaps some exploratory clinical trials with the drug should be carried out and evaluated.

Dexamethasone-Suppression Test

Clearly, a possibility exists that some functional dysregulation of the HPA system plays a role in the expression of adult separation-distress problems. Persons suffering depressive disorders frequently exhibit HPA dysregulation of cortisol production. To determine the presence of such dysregulation, depressed patients are administered an oral dose of dexamethasone (a synthetic cortisol), and plasma cortisol levels are measured at various times during the day. In persons exhibiting normal-functioning HPA system regulation, cortisol levels are suppressed; in persons exhibiting HPA system dysregulation, however, plasma cortisol levels are not suppressed. Some evidence indicates that children exhibiting severe separation anxiety show an abnormal response to the dexamethasone-suppression test (Livingston, 1991). Perhaps adult dogs exhibiting chronic or severe separation anxiety may suffer a similar dysfunction of HPA activity. The dexamethasone-suppression test might offer a diagnostic method for isolating such dogs from other dogs presenting with a more psychogenic etiology and symptomatology. Further, an abnormal dexamethasone-suppression test result appears to be moderately predictive of a positive response to antidepressant medications in human patients (Risch and Janowsky, 1986).

PSYCHOMOTOR EPILEPSY, CATALEPSY, AND NARCOLEPSY

Epilepsy

In cases of bizarre or unusual behavior occurring with little or no warning, one should suspect the possibility of a biological pathology involving the brain. Psychomotor seizure activity (limbic epilepsy) often presents with psychosomatic symptoms, like chronic vomiting or diarrhea (Reisner, 1991), and various behavioral signs. Although behavior problems associated with fear and aggression are typically viewed as learned patterns, some such patterns may be (in part or whole) the behavioral manifestation of seizure activity in the hypothalamus, limbic system, or temporal lobes (Aronson, 1998). The amygdala is particularly sensitive to seizure activity, perhaps an etiologically significant factor in the development of some forms of panic disorder and generalized anxiety. Holliday and coworkers (1970) studied 70 cases of canine motor epilepsy presenting with varying degrees of severity and duration. As the result of interviews taken with owners, they detected a number of behavioral sequelae occurring comorbidly with epilepsy in dogs, suggesting the possibility of a limbic system or temporal lobe involvement:

> Behavioral signs of varying duration and form were common before or after a generalized seizure or sometimes pre- and postictally. The behavioral abnormalities consisted of: wandering in circles, restlessness, somnolence, apparent blindness, viciousness, inappropriate barking, attacking inanimate objects, terror-stricken behavior, inappetence, voracious appetite, generalized trembling, champing of the jaws, licking movements, and behaviour as if one ear were painful. Such changes usually lasted a few hours at most, but were occasionally present for 3–4 days. In a few dogs the behavioral signs were the most prominent abnormality, appearing at times in the absence of generalized tonic-clonic seizures. (1970:283)

Unfortunately, such pathology is difficult to diagnose through conventional EEG tests done to verify somatomotor epilepsy. One way to determine whether a particular case is precipitated by underlying limbic seizure activity is to compare the differential effects of epileptogenic drugs and antiepileptic drugs on the expression of the behavior in question. Borchelt and Voith (1985) have described a case involving a male Lhasa apso that, when presented with food, would begin eating, lift his head, growl, and whirl about attacking the surrounding area. The bizarre, poorly directed, species-atypical character of the behavior prompted a pharmacological test. It was found that the dog's aggressive behavior could be kindled by injecting him intravenously with chlorpromazine regardless of the social context or ongoing environmental stimulation. On the other hand, if the dog was given an oral dose of diazepam before eating, he ate peacefully without exhibiting any aggressive behavior.

Dodman and colleagues (1992) have reported three cases of what they term *episodic dyscontrol syndrome* (aggression), all of which appear to be associated with limbic seizure activity. The dogs (a Chesapeake Bay retriever, cocker spaniel, and English springer spaniel) exhibited fairly well-directed, although inappropriate and exaggerated, species-typical aggressive behavior. The episodes of aggression were found to be associated with several features that suggested limbic seizure activity. It was noted that the dogs exhibited various premonitory mood changes in the directions of increased irritability and depression, several autonomic signs (excessive salivation, pupillary dilation and glazing of the eyes, and vomiting), and intense aggressive behavior at a high frequency under low or no apparent provocation. All of the dogs proved responsive to phenobarbital therapy—a confirmatory indicator of seizure activity.

Catalepsy

Catalepsy is a condition in which dogs lose muscular control over the body, with full or partial collapse. Under full cataleptic loss of voluntary control, dogs may fall into a trancelike condition during which the limbs exhibit a plastic rigidity remaining in the form they are placed (Fox, 1968). A common example of catalepsy is tonic immobility, a phenomenon that is widespread in the animal kingdom and that may have a biological self-preservative function when an animal is faced with environmental threat (Gallup and Maser, 1977). The behavior has been described as *feigning death* or *protective inhibition*. A very familiar example of the behavior is exhibited by the opossum, a marsupial that uses tonic immobility as a primary mode of defense against predation. Cataleptic tonic immobility can be induced in a variety of ways: "The conditions for induction have included eye contact, pressure on body parts, repetitive stimulation, inversion, and restraint" (Crawford, 1977:89). Dogs that are abruptly rolled on their sides, following a brief struggle, are often absorbed into a state of tonic immobility. Tonic immobility might be part of a parasympathetic rebound effect in response to intense sympathetic arousal. Another interpretation conceptualizes tonic immobility and catalepsy as a response to conflict provoked by incompatible motivations between active and passive defensive mechanisms; that is, when an animal is threatened with imminent physical danger during which escape is not possible and attack is equally ineffectual, the outcome may be cataleptic immobility. Grandin (1992) has argued that the induction of tonic immobility is an elemental part of some taming processes in animals (e.g., wild horses), claiming that the firm touch calms while the light touch excites. She has designed a *squeeze machine* for the treatment of autistic and hyperactive children, claiming that physical pressure promotes a lasting sense of calmness and well-being. This may be relevant to the beneficial effects of forced lateral recumbency on some dogs. Dogs exposed to such restraint for several minutes are often significantly calmer when finally released.

Narcolepsy

Narcolepsy is a sleep disorder that, in humans, is associated with catalepsy and the rapid onset of sleep. In dogs, it appears to be genetically determined, with breeds such as the Doberman pinscher, miniature poodle, and black Labrador retriever most often exhibiting the disorder (Voith, 1979). The condition is incurable. During episodes of narcolepsy, affected dogs move rapidly from an active state into a state of muscular weakness and collapse while apparently remaining in a trancelike conscious state. The onset of narcoleptic episodes is frequently associated with feeding times, during periods of general excitement, during or just after elimination, and sometimes during sexual activity. Regarding such attacks, Foutz and colleagues write,

> These attacks are frequently precipitated by the excitement of approaching desired goals, such as food, a play object or companion, or sexual activity. Some breeds such as Labradors often experience cataplexy more frequently when playing and exercising than when eating. Unpleasant experiences such as pain (caused by a hypodermic injection), fear, or parturition, do not appear to specifically elicit attacks. Cataplexy also appears to occur spontaneously. Very young puppies do not appear to be significantly responsive to food, but play activities are major precipitants for attacks. (1980:68–69)

Pavlov (1927/1960:319) appears to be describing narcolepsy when he writes concerning a highly inhibited dog that could not bear even a short delay of conditional reinforcement without becoming "drowsy and even fall[ing] asleep over its plate while taking the food."

Although the causes of narcolepsy are not definitively known, recent advances point to a dysfunction associated with the cholinergic innervation of the pontine reticular formation (PRF). Catalepsy associated with narcolepsy may result from the abnormal activation of these cholinergic mechanisms associated with the induction of REM (rapid eye movement) sleep. A colony of narcoleptic Doberman pinschers has been isolated and is currently being subjected to various experimental manipulations in an effort to determine the causal mechanisms involved. Reid and coworkers (1994) have directly measured ACh activity in the PRF via probes implanted into the pons of narcoleptic dogs. They have found a definite relationship between narcoleptic episodes and increased levels of extracellular ACh in the PRF of affected dogs. Interestingly, baseline levels of ACh in the PRF did not differ between controls and narcoleptic dogs.

The diagnosis of narcolepsy can be confirmed by EEG or by injecting narcoleptic dogs with imipramine. Reportedly, affected dogs quickly recover from the attack after being injected with the drug (Voith, 1979). In severe cases, CNS stimulants (*d*-amphetamine and methylphenidate) are sometimes prescribed to control the disorder (Foutz et al., 1980). Narcolepsy in dogs is often left untreated, since treatment is problematical (Hart, 1980). Medication with CNS stimulants may produce a variety of undesirable side effects and produce increasing tolerance over time.

REFERENCES

Adams D and Flynn JP (1966). Transfer of an escape response from tail shock to brain stimulated attack behavior. *J Exp Anal Behav*, 8:401–408.

Allen BD, Cummings JF, and DeLahunta A (1974). The effects of prefrontal lobotomy on aggressive behavior in dogs. *Cornell Vet*, 64:201–216.

Arnsten AF (1998). The biology of being frazzled. *Science*, 280:1711–1712.

Arons DC and Shoemaker WJ (1992). The distribution of catecholamines and beta-endorphin in the brains of three behavioral distinct breeds of dogs and their 2M hybrids. *Brain Res*, 594:31–39.

Aronson LP (1998). Systemic causes of aggression and their treatment. In N Dodman and L Shuster (Eds), *Psychopharmacology of Animal Behavior Disorders*. Malden, MA: Blackwell Science.

Azrin NH, Hutchinson RR, and Hake DF (1967). Attack, avoidance, and escape reactions to aversive shock. *J Exp Anal Behav*, 10:131–148.

Ballarini G (1990). Animal psychodietetics. *J Small Anim Pract*, 31:523–553.

Baxter LR, Phelps ME, Mazziotta JC, et al. (1987). Local cerebral glucose metabolic rates in obsessive-compulsive disorder: A comparison with rates in unipolar depression and normal controls. *Arch Gen Psychiatry*, 44:211–218.

Beaumont JG (1983). *Introduction to Neuropsy-*

chology. New York: Guilford.

Beerda B, Schilder MB, Janssen NS, and Mol JA (1996). The use of saliva cortisol, urinary cortisol, and catecholamine measurements for a noninvasive assessment of stress responses in dogs. *Horm Behav,* 30:272–279.

Borchelt PL and Voith VL (1985). Aggressive behavior in dogs and cats. *Comp Cont Educ Pract Vet,* 7:949–957.

Bouton ME and Swartzentruber D (1991). Sources of relapse after extinction in Pavlovian and instrumental learning. *Clin Psychol Rev,* 11:123–140.

Brain PF and Haug M (1992). Hormonal and neurochemical correlates of various forms of animal "aggression." *Psychoneuroendocrinology,* 17:537–551.

Brown PR (1987). Fly catching in the cavalier King Charles spaniel. *Vet Rec,* 120:95.

Carlson NR (1994). *Physiology of Behavior.* Boston: Allyn and Bacon.

Chamberlain B, Ervin FR, Pihl RO, and Young SN (1987). The effect of raising or lowering tryptophan levels on aggression in vervet monkeys. *Pharmacol Biochem Behav,* 28:503–510.

Chaouloff F (1997). Effects of acute physical exercise on central serotonergic systems. *Med Sci Sports Exerc,* 29:58–62.

Christensen L (1996). *Diet-Behavior Relationships: Focus on Depression.* Washington, DC: American Psychological Association.

Church RM, LoLordo V, Overmier JB, et al. (1966) Cardiac responses to shock in curarized dogs: Effects of shock intensity and duration, warning signal, and prior experience with shock. *J Comp Physiol Psychol,* 62:1–7.

Coover GD, Goldman L, and Levine S (1971). Plasma corticosterone increases produced by extinction of operant behaviour in rats. *Physiol Behav,* 6:261–263.

Crawford FT (1977). Induction and duration of tonic immobility. *Psychol Rec,* 1:89–107.

Crowell-Davis SL, Lappin M, and Oliver JE (1989). Stimulus-responsive psychomotor epilepsy in a Doberman pinscher. *J Am Anim Hosp Assoc,* 25:57–60.

D'Amato FR and Pavone F (1993). Endogenous opioids: A proximate reward mechanism for kin recognition? *Behav Neural Biol,* 60:79–83.

Davis M (1992). The role of the amygdala in fear and anxiety. *Annu Rev Neurosci,* 15:353–375.

de Haan M, Buss K, and Wegesin D (1993). Development of peer relations: Effects of prior experience, temperament, and stress reactivity on adjustment to preschool. Poster presented at the Society for Research in Child Development, New Orleans.

Delgado JMR (1969). *Physical Control of the Mind: Toward a Psychocivilized Society.* New York: Harper and Row.

Delville Y, Mansour KM, and Ferris CF (1996). Testosterone facilitates aggression by modulating vasopressin receptors in the hypothalamus. *Physiol Behav,* 60:25–29.

Dey S (1994). Physical exercise as a novel antidepressant agent: Possible role of serotonin receptor subtypes. *Physiol Behav,* 55:323–329.

Dey S, Singh RH, and Dey PK (1992). Exercise training: Significance of regional alterations in serotonin metabolism of rat brain in relation to antidepressant effect of exercise. *Physiol Behav,* 52:1095–1099.

Dodman N (1998). Pharmacologic treatment of aggression in veterinary patients. In N Dodman and L Shuster (Eds), *Psychopharmacology of Animal Behavior Disorders.* Malden, MA: Blackwell Science.

Dodman N and Shuster L (1998). *Psychopharmacology of Animal Behavior Disorders.* Malden, MA: Blackwell Science.

Dodman NH, Donnelly R, Shuster L, et al. (1996a). Use of fluoxetine to treat dominance aggression in dogs. *JAVMA,* 209:1585–1587.

Dodman NH, Miczek KA, Knowles K, et al. (1992). Phenobarbital-responsive episodic dyscontrol (rage) in dogs. *JAVMA,* 201:1580–1583.

Dodman NH, Reisner I, Shuster L, et al. (1996b). Effect of dietary protein content on behavior in dogs. *JAVMA,* 208:376–379.

Dodman NH, Shuster L, Court MH, et al. (1987). Investigation into the use of narcotic antagonists in the treatment of a stereotypic behavior pattern (crib-biting) in the horse. *Am J Vet Res,* 48:311–319.

Dodman NH, Shuster L, White SD, et al. (1988). Use of narcotic antagonists to modify stereotypic self-licking, self-chewing, and scratching behavior in dogs. *JAVMA,* 193:815–819.

Eichelman B (1987). Neurochemical bases of aggressive behavior. *Psychiatr Ann,* 17:371–374.

Eichelman B (1992). Aggressive behavior: From laboratory to clinic. *Arch Gen Psychiatr,* 49: 488–492.

Eichelman B, Elliot GR, and Barchas JD (1981). Biochemical, pharmacological, and genetic aspects of aggression. In DA Hamburg and MB Trudeau (Eds), *Biobehavior Aspects of Aggression.* New York: Alan R Liss.

Fanselow MS (1991). Analgesia as a response to aversive Pavlovian conditional stimuli: Cognitive and emotional mediators. In MR Denny

(Ed), *Fear, Avoidance, and Phobias: A Fundamental Analysis.* Hillsdale, NJ: Lawrence Erlbaum Associates.

Ferris CF and Delville Y (1994). Vasopressin and serotonin interactions in the control of agonistic behavior. *Psychoneuroendocrinology,* 19:593–601.

Ferris CF and Potegal M (1988). Vasopressin receptor blockade in the anterior hypothalamus suppresses aggression in hamsters. *Physiol Behav,* 44:235–239.

Ferris CF, Meenan DM, Axelson JF, et al. (1986). Vasopressin antagonist can reverse dominant/subordinate behavior in animals. *Physiol Behav,* 38:135–138.

Ferris CF, Melloni RH Jr, Koppel G, et al. (1997). Vasopressin/serotonin interactions in the anterior hypothalamus control of aggressive behavior in golden hamsters. *J Neurosci,* 17:4331–4340.

Fonberg E and Kostarczyk E (1960). Motivational role of social reinforcement in dog-man relations. *Acta Neurobiol Exp,* 40:117–136.

Foutz AS, Mitler MM, and Dement WC (1980). Narcolepsy. *Vet Clin North Am Adv Vet Neurol,* 10:65–80.

Fox MW (1966). Neuro-behavioral ontogeny: A synthesis of ethological and neurophysiological concepts. *Brain Res,* 2:3–20.

Fox MW (1968). *Abnormal Behavior in Animals,* 332–355. Philadelphia: WB Saunders.

Fraser AF (1985). Background to anomalous behaviour. *Appl Anim Behav,* 13:199–203.

Gallup GG and Maser JD (1977). Tonic immobility: Evolutionary underpinnings of human catalepsy and catatonia. In JD Maser and MEP Seligman (Eds), *Psychopathology: Experimental Models.* San Francisco: WH Freeman.

Goldman-Rakic PS (1992). Working memory and the mind. *Sci Am,* 267:111–117.

Grandin T (1992). Calming effects of deep touch pressure in patients with autistic disorder, college students, and animals. *J Child Adolesc Psychopharmacol,* 2:63–72.

Gray JA (1971). *The Psychology of Fear and Stress.* New York: McGraw-Hill.

Gray JA (1982). Precis of the neuropsychology of anxiety: An enquiry into the functions of the septo-hippocampal system. *Behav Brain Sci,* 3:469–483.

Gray JA (1991). The neuropsychology of temperament. In J Strelau and A Angleitner (Eds), *Explorations in Temperament.* New York: Plenum.

Gunnar M (1994) Psychoendocrine studies of temperament and stress in early childhood: Expanding current models. In JE Bates and TD Wachs (Eds), *Temperament: Individual Differences at the Interface of Biology and Behavior.* Washington, DC: American Psychological Association.

Haemisch A (1990). Coping with social conflict, and short-term changes of plasma cortisol titers in familiar and unfamiliar environments. *Physiol Behav,* 47:1265–1270.

Hart BL (1980). Behavioral aspects of canine narcolepsy. In BL Hart (Ed), *Canine Behavior (A Practitioner Monograph).* Santa Barbara, CA: Veterinary Practice.

Hoerlein BF (1971). *Canine Neurology: Diagnosis and Treatment.* Philadelphia: WB Saunders.

Hoffman HS (1996). *Amorous Turkeys and Addicted Ducklings: A Search for the Causes of Social Attachment.* Boston: Authors Cooperative.

Holliday TA, Cunningham JG, and Gutnick MJ (1970). Comparative clinical and electroencephalographic studies of canine epilepsy. *Epilepsia,* 11:281–292.

Hothersall D and Tuber DS (1979). Fears in companion dogs: Characteristics and treatment. In JD Keehn (Ed), *Psychopathology in Animals: Research and Clinical Implications.* New York: Academic.

Iorio LC, Eisenstein N, Brody PE, and Barnett A (1983). Effects of selected drugs on spontaneously occurring abnormal behavior in beagles. *Pharmacol Biochem Behav,* 18:379–382.

Jacobs BL, Wilkinson LO, and Fornal CA (1990). The role of brain serotonin: A neurophysiologic perspective. *Neuropsychopharmacology,* 3:473–479.

Jacobs WJ and Nadel L (1985). Stress-induced recovery of fears and phobias. *Psychol Rev,* 92:512–513.

Kagan J and Snidman N (1988). Biological bases of childhood shyness. *Science,* 240:167–171.

Kagan J, Reznick JS, and Snidman N (1987). The physiology and psychology of behavioral inhibition. *Child Dev,* 58:1459–1473.

Kalin NH and Shelton SE (1989). Defensive behaviors in infant rhesus monkeys: Environmental cues and neurochemical regulation. *Science,* 243:1718–1721.

Kandel ER (1991). Disorders of thought: Schizophrenia. In ER Kandel, JH Schwartz, and TM Jessell (Eds), *Principles of Neural Science.* Norwalk, CT: Appleton and Lange.

Kehoe EJ and Macrae M (1997). Savings in animal learning: Implications for relapse and maintenance after therapy. *Behav Ther,* 28:141–155.

Kelly DD (1991). Sexual differential of the nervous system. In ER Kandel, JH Schwartz, and

TM Jessell (Eds), *Principles of Neural Science.* Norwalk, CT: Appleton and Lange.

Kemble ED, Gibson BM, and Rawleigh JM (1991). Effects of eltoprazine hydrochloride on exploratory behavior and social attraction in mice. *Pharmacol Biochem Behav*, 38:759–762.

Keverne EB, Martensz ND, and Tuite B (1989). Beta-endorphin concentrations in cerebrospinal fluid of monkeys are influenced by grooming relationships. *Psychoneuroendocrinology*, 14:155–161.

Klein EH, Thomas T, and Uhde TW (1990). Hypothalamo-pituitary-adrenal axis activity in nervous and normal pointer dogs. *Biol Psychiatry*, 27:791–794.

Kluver H and Bucy P (1937). "Psychic blindness" and other symptoms following bilateral temporal lobotomy in rhesus monkeys. *Am J Physiol*, 119:352–353.

Knowles PA, Conner RL, and Panksepp J (1987). Opiate effects on social behavior of juvenile dogs as a function of social deprivation. *Pharmacol Biochem Behav*, 33:533–537.

Konorski J (1967). *Integrative Activity of the Brain: An Interdisciplinary Approach.* Chicago: University of Chicago Press.

Koshikawa N (1994). Role of the nucleus accumbens and the striatum in the production of turning behaviour in intact rats. *Rev Neurosci*, 5:331–346.

Kosten TR, Mason JW, Giller EL, et al. (1987). Sustained urinary norepinephrine and epinephrine elevation in post-traumatic stress disorder. *Psychoneuroendocrinology*, 12:13–20.

Lavond DG, Jeansok JK, and Thompson RF (1993). Mammalian brain substrates of aversive classical conditioning. *Annu Rev Psychol*, 44:317–342.

LeDoux JE (1994). Emotion, memory, and the brain. *Sci Am*, 270:50–57.

LeDoux J (1996). *The Emotional Brain: The Mysterious Underpinnings of Emotional Life.* New York: Simon and Schuster.

Leventhal BL and Brodie KH (1981). The pharmacology of violence. In DA Hamburg and MB Trudeau (Eds), *Biobehavioral Aspects of Aggression.* New York: Alan R Liss.

Livingston R (1991). Anxiety disorders. In M Lewis (Ed), *Child and Adolescent Psychiatry: A Comprehensive Textbook.* Baltimore: Williams and Wilkins.

Luxenberg JS, Swedo SE, Flament MF, et al. (1988). Neuroanatomical abnormalities in obsessive-compulsive disorder detected with quantitative x-ray computed tomography. *Am J Psychiatry*, 145:1089–1093.

Lytle LD, Messing RB, Fisher L, and Phebus L (1975). Effects of long-term corn consumption on brain serotonin and the response to electric shock. *Science*, 190:692–694.

MacLean PD (1985). Brain evolution relating to family, play, and the separation call. *Arch Gen Psychiatry*, 42:405–417.

MacLean PD (1986). Culminating developments in the evolution of the limbic system: The thalamocingulate division. In BK Doane and KE Livingston (Eds), *The Limbic System: Functional Organization and Clinical Disorders.* New York: Raven.

Manogue KR, Lesher AI, and Candland DK (1975). Dominance status and adrenocortical reactivity to stress in squirrel monkeys (*Saimiri sciureus*). *Primates*, 16:457–463.

McEwen BS (1992). Paradoxical effects of adrenal steroids on the brain: Protection versus degeneration. *Biol Psychiatry*, 31:177–199.

McGaugh JL (1990). Significance and remembrance: The role of neuromodulatory systems. *Psychol Sci*, 1:15–25.

McLeod PJ, Moger WH, Ryon J, et al. (1995). The relation between urinary cortisol levels and social behavior in captive timber wolves. *Can J Zool*, 74:209–216.

Meeusen R and DeMeirleir (1995). Exercise and brain neurotransmission. *Sports Med*, 20:160–188.

Menzies RG and Clarke CJ (1995). The etiology of phobias: A nonassociative account. *Clin Psychol Rev*, 15:23–48.

Miczek KA (1983). Ethopharmacology of aggression, defense, and defeat. In EC Simmel, ME Hahn, and JK Walters (Eds), *Aggressive Behavior: Genetic and Neural Approaches.* Hillsdale, NJ: Lawrence Erlbaum Associates.

Morand C, Young SN, and Ervin FR (1983). Clinical response of aggressive schizophrenics to oral tryptophan. *Biol Psychiatry*, 18:575–578.

Moyer KE (1976). *The Psychobiology of Aggression.* New York: Harper and Row.

Murphree OD (1974). Psychopharmacologic facilitation of operant conditioning of genetically nervous Catahoula and pointer dogs. *Pavlov J Biol Sci*, 9:17–24.

Nemeroff CB (1998). The neurobiology of depression. *Sci Am*, 278:42–49.

Nott HMR (1992). Behavioural development of the dog. In C Thorne (Ed), *The Waltham Book of Dog and Cat Behaviour.* Oxford: Butterworth-Heinemann.

Olds J and Milner P (1954). Positive reinforcement produced by electrical stimulation of septal area and other regions of rat brain. *J Comp Physiol Psychol*, 47:419–427.

Olivier B, Mos J, van der Heyden J, et al. (1987). Serotonergic modulation of agonistic behavior. In B Olivier, J Mos, and PF Brain (Eds), *Ethopharmacology of Agonistic Behavior in Animals and Humans.* Dordrecht, The Netherlands: Martinus Nijhoff.

Overall K (1997). *Clinical Behavioral Medicine for Small Animals.* St. Louis: CV Mosby.

Panksepp J (1971). Aggression elicited by electrical stimulation of the hypothalamus in albino rat. *Physiol Behav,* 6:321–329.

Panksepp J (1982). Towards a general psyschobiological theory of emotions. *Behav Brain Sci,* 5:407–467.

Panksepp J (1988). Brain opioids and social affect. In P Borchelt, P Plimpton, AH Kutscher, et al. (Eds), *Animal Behavior and Thanatology.* New York: Foundation of Thanatology.

Panksepp J (1992). Oxytocin effects on emotional processes: Separation distress, social bonding, and relationships to psychiatric disorders. *Ann NY Acad Sci,* 652:243–252.

Panksepp J (1998). *Affective Neuroscience: The Foundations of Human and Animal Emotions.* New York: Oxford University Press.

Panksepp J, Conner R, Forster PK, et al. (1983). Opioid effects on social behavior of kennel dogs. *Appl Anim Ethol,* 10:63–74.

Panksepp J, Herman BH, Vilberg T, et al. (1980). Endogenous opioids and social behavior. *Neurosci Biobehav Rev,* 4:473–487.

Panksepp J, Normansell L, Herman B, et al. (1988). Neural and neurochemical control of the separation distress call. In D Newman (Ed), *The Physiological Control of Mammalian Vocalization.* New York: Plenum.

Panksepp J, Siviy S, and Normansell L (1984). The psychobiology of play: Theoretical and methodological perspectives. *Neurosci Behav Rev,* 8:465–492.

Parker JP (1990). Behavioral changes of organic neurologic origin. *Prog Vet Neurol,* 1:123–131.

Pasley JN, Powell EW, and Angel CA (1978). Adrenal glands in nervous pointer dogs. *IRCS Med Sci,* 6:102.

Pavlov IP (1927/1960). *Conditioned Reflexes: An Investigation of the Physiological Activity of the Cerebral Cortex,* GV Anrep (Trans). New York: Dover (reprint).

Popova NK, Voitenko NN, Kulikov AV, and Avgustinovich DF (1991). Evidence for the involvement of central serotonin in the mechanism of domestication of silver foxes. *Pharmacol Biochem Behav,* 40:751–756.

Premack D (1965). Reinforcement theory. In D Levine (Ed), *Nebraska Symposium on Motivation.* New York: University of Nebraska Press.

Price ML, Curtis AL, Kirby LG, et al. (1998). Effects of corticotropin-releasing factor on brain serotonergic activity. *Neuropsychopharmacology,* 18:492–502.

Radosevich PM, Nash JA, Lacy B, et al. (1989). Effects of low- and high-intensity exercise on plasma and cerebrospinal fluid levels of ir-beta-endorphin, ACTH, cortisol, norepinephrine and glucose in the conscious dog. *Brain Res,* 498:89–98.

Ranson SW and Clark SL (1959). *The Anatomy of the Nervous System: Its Development and Function.* Philadelphia: WB Saunders.

Rapoport JL, Ryland DH, and Kriete M (1992). Drug treatment of canine acral lick: An animal model of obsessive-compulsive disorder. *Arch Gen Psychiatry,* 49:517–521.

Redding RW (1978). Electroconvulsive therapy. In BF Hoerlein (Ed), *Canine Neurology: Diagnosis and Treatment,* 694–696. Philadelphia: WB Saunders.

Redding RW and Walker TL (1976). Electroconvulsive therapy to control aggression in dogs. *Mod Vet Pract,* 57:595–597.

Reese WO (1991). *Physiology of Domestic Animals.* Philadelphia: Lea and Febiger.

Reid MS, Siegel JM, Dement WC, et al. (1994). Cholinergic mechanisms in canine narcolepsy: II. Acetylcholine release in the pontine reticular formation is enhanced during cataplexy. *Neuroscience,* 59:523–530.

Reis D (1972). The relationship between brain norepinephrine and aggressive behavior. *Res Publ Assoc Res Nerv Ment Dis,* 50:266–297.

Reisner I (1991). The pathophysiologic basis of behavior problems. *Vet Clin North Am Adv Comp Anim Behav,* 21:207–224.

Reisner I (1994). Use of lithium for treatment of canine dominance-related aggression: A case study [Abstract]. *Appl Anim Behav Sci,* 39:190.

Reisner IL, Mann JJ, Stanley M, et al. (1996). Comparison of cerebrospinal fluid monoamine metabolite levels in dominant-aggressive and non-aggressive dogs. *Brain Res,* 714:57–64.

Riccio DC and Spear NE (1991). Changes in memory for aversively motivated learning. In MR Denny (Ed), *Fear, Avoidance, and Phobias: A Fundamental Analysis.* Hillsdale, NJ: Lawrence Erlbaum Associates.

Richardson R, Riccio DC, and Ress J (1988). Extinction of avoidance through response prevention: Enhancement by administration of epinephrine or ACTH. *Behav Res Ther,* 26:23–32.

Richter CP (1957). On the phenomenon of sudden death in animals and man. *Psychosom Med,* 19:191–198.

Risch SC and Janowsky DS (1986). Limbic-hypothalamic-pituitary-adrenal axis dysregulation in melancholia. In LL Judd and PM Groves (Eds), *Psychobiological Foundations of Clinical Psychiatry*. Philadelphia: JB Lippincott.

Rogeness GA (1994). Biologic findings in conduct disorder. In M Lewis (Ed), *Child and Adolescent Psychiatric Clinics of North America: Disruptive Disorders*. Philadelphia: WB Saunders.

Sapolsky RM (1990). Stress in the wild. *Sci Am*, 262:116–123.

Scott JP and Fuller JL (1965). *Genetics and the Social Behavior of the Dog*. Chicago: University of Chicago Press.

Scott JP, Stewart JM, and DeGhett VJ (1973). Separation in infant dogs. In JP Scott and EC Senay (Eds), *Separation and Anxiety: Clinical and Research Aspects* (AAAS Symposium, Washington, DC).

Seligman MEP (1975). *Helplessness: On Depression, Development and Death*. San Francisco: Freeman.

Selye H (1976). *The Stress of Life*. New York: McGraw-Hill.

Shepherd GM (1983). *Neurobiology*. New York: Oxford University Press.

Siegel A and Edinger H (1981). Neural control of aggression and rage behavior. In PJ Morgane and J Panksepp (Eds), *Handbook of the Hypothalamus*, Vol 3, Part B: *Behavioral Studies of the Hypothalamus*. New York: Marcel Dekker.

Spring B (1986). Effects of foods and nutrients on the behavior of normal individuals. In RJ Wurtman and JJ Wurtman (Eds), *Nutrition and the Brain*, 7:1–47. New York: Raven.

Stein DJ, Borchelt P, and Hollander E (1994). Pharmacotherapy of naturally occurring anxiety symptoms in dogs. *Res Commun Psychol Psychiatry Behav*, 19:39–48.

Stein DJ, Hollander E, and Liebowits MR (1993). Neurobiology of impulsivity and the impulse control disorders. *J Neuropsychiatry*, 5:9–17.

Stein DJ, Shoulberg N, Helton K, and Hollander E (1992). The neuroethological approach to obsessive-compulsive disorder. *Compr Psychiatry*, 33:274–281.

Steinmetz JE (1994) Brain substrates of emotion and temperament. In JE Bates and TD Wachs (Eds), *Temperament: Individual Differences at the Interface of Biology and Behavior*. Washington, DC: American Psychological Association.

Suvorov NF, Shuvaev VT, Voilokova NL, et al. (1997). Corticostriatal mechanisms of behavior. *Neurosci Behav Physiol*, 27:653–662.

Swedo SE (1989). Rituals and releasers: An ethological model of obsessive-compulsive disorder. In J Rapoport (Ed), *Obsessive-Compulsive Disorder in Childhood and Adolescence*. Washington, DC: American Psychiatric Press.

Swenson MJ (1984) *Duke's Physiology of Animals*. Ithaca: Cornell University Press.

Tancer ME, Stein MB, Bessette BB, and Uhde TW (1990). Behavioral effects of chronic imipramine treatment in genetically nervous pointer dogs. *Physiol Behav*, 48:179–181.

Thompson RF (1967). *Foundations of Physiological Psychology*. New York: Harper and Row.

Thompson RF (1993). *The Brain: A Neuroscience Primer*. New York: WH Freeman.

Timberlake W and Allison J (1974). Response deprivation: An empirical approach to instrumental performance. *Psychol Rev*, 81:146–164.

Tortora DF (1983). Safety training: The elimination of avoidance-motivated aggression in dog. *J Exp Psychol Gen*, 112:176–214.

Uhde TW, Malloy LC, and Slate SO (1992). Fearful behavior, body size, and serum IGF-I levels in nervous and normal pointer dogs. *Pharmacol Biochem Behav*, 43:263–269.

Voith VL (1979). Behavioral problems. In EA Chandler, EA Evans, WB Singleton, et al. (Eds), *Canine Medicine and Therapeutics*. Oxford: Blackwell Scientific.

Welker WI (1973). Principles of organization of the ventrobasal complex in mammals. *Brain Behav Evol*, 7:253–336.

White NM and Milner PM (1992). The psychobiology of reinforcers. *Annu Rev Psychol*, 43:443–471.

White SD (1990). Naltrexone for treatment of acral lick dermatitis in dog. *JAVMA*, 196:1073–1076.

Wise SP and Rapoport JL (1989). Obsessive-compulsive disorder: Is it basal ganglia dysfunction? In JL Rapoport (Ed), *Obsessive-Compulsive Disorder in Children and Adolescents*. Washington, DC: American Psychiatric Press.

Young SN (1986) The clinical psychopharmacology of tryptophan. In RJ Wurtman and JJ Wurtman (Eds), *Nutrition and the Brain*, 7:49–88. New York: Raven.

4

Sensory Abilities

Each animal has its own Merkwelt (perceptual world) and this world differs from its environment as we perceive it, that is to say, from our own Merkwelt.

NIKO TINBERGEN, *The Study of Instinct* (1951/1969)

D OGS ARE equipped with a number of specialized sensory organs evolved to obtain biologically significant information from the environment. These various sensory systems gather and process chemical, mechanical, and physical inputs, transduce them into coded electrical impulses, and then conduct the raw sensory data to the brain. Once in the brain, the sensory data are further processed and encoded into meaningful representations about the surrounding environment. The animal is totally dependent on the reliability of this information processing for the procurement of vital biological needs and all forms of adaptive learning.

The sensory capacity of dogs can be divided into three broad categories:

1. *Exteroception*: Exteroceptors are sensitive to all stimulation acting on dogs from the external environment. These stimuli (including light, sound, chemical agents [taste and smell], heat, cold, and pressure) correspond to the special senses of sight, hearing, taste, smell, and touch.

2. *Interoception*: Interoceptors are responsive to stimulation arising from within the bodily organs, such as emotional reactions and some muscular sensations.

3. *Proprioception*: Proprioceptors coordinate kinesthetic sensations and reflexes of the body, including the sense of balance.

VISION

Much of the close social exchange that occurs between dogs and people depends on the visual recognition of subtle gestures and postural signals. This visual information provides a sensory foundation for socially significant communication and harmonious interaction. Another important function of sight is to scan the environment for biologically important changes in the dog's surroundings not detected by the other senses.

Retina

The dog's eye is structured so that reflected light energy can be efficiently gathered and focused upon the retina, which is composed of light-sensitive neural tissue located at the back of the eye. There are two types of photoreceptor cells located in the retina: the *rods* (sensitive to contrasts of light and dark) and the *cones* (sensitive to variations in color and detail). A dog's retina contains many more rods than cones, with the latter comprising only 3% of all the photoreceptor cells found in the canine eye (Peichl, 1991). The preponderance of rods makes the dog's vision better suited for discriminating light and dark and detecting movement than seeing color and detail.

An important structural difference between the dog and human retina is the absence of a fovea. The fovea is a tightly concentrated area of cone and ganglion cells located at the center of the field of vision in the human eye. Nearly half of the human visual cortex is involved in representing information originating in the fovea (Thompson, 1993). Although not possessing a fovea, the central portion of the dog's retina does exhibit a higher concentration of cone cells than found in other retinal areas, with cones making up approximately 20% of all the receptors found there (Parry, 1953). Instead of possessing a fovea, the dog's retina contains a *visual streak* and a concentration of ganglion cells called the *central area*. The visual streak is an elongated oval concentration of light-sensitive receptors and ganglion cells situated along the central portion of the retina. The visual streak and central area are believed to play important roles in enhancing visual acuity, binocular vision, and horizontal scanning. Peichl (1992), who compared the visual streaks of dogs and wolves, found that wolf retinas consistently possessed a pronounced visual streak, whereas the visual streak in dog retinas varied considerably (moderate to pronounced) among the different breeds studied. He attributed these differences to the effects of domestication and breeding, thus providing additional physiological support for what Hemmer (1990) has termed the decline of "environment appreciation" in dogs and other domestic animals due to sensory and neurological degeneration resulting from domestic breeding (see Chapter 1).

Clarity of vision requires that an optical image is precisely focused on the retina. This function is achieved by the cornea, lens, and the aqueous media within the eye. Like humans, many dogs are either farsighted (hyperopia) or nearsighted (myopia). In the case of farsightedness the image is focused behind the retina, whereas in nearsightedness the image is focused in front of the retina. Myopia is not a general characteristic of canine vision (as has been sometimes suggested), but its incidence is relatively more common among certain breeds. For example, Murphy and colleagues (1992) found that 64% of the Rottweilers they tested were myopic. They also determined that 53% of the German shepherds tested (clinical population) were myopic, but, interestingly, of the German shepherds participating in a guide-dog program, only 15% were affected by the condition. This finding suggests that dogs with poor focusing abilities had been excluded from the guide-dog population as the result of other behavioral shortcomings arising during their training. Certainly, dogs like the German shepherd and Rottweiler should be tested for myopia before being trained for various utilitarian tasks requiring good eyesight.

Color Vision

Until recently, many dog authorities believed that dogs lacked color vision or, at best, it was considered a very weak aspect of canine vision. This opinion was based on early color-vision studies carried out by Smith (1912) and by Orbelli (1909, cited in Windholz, 1989) before him. Smith performed a series of color-brightness discrimination experiments (primitive by contemporary standards) with dogs and concluded that, although dogs appeared to exhibit a rudimentary ability to discriminate color, this ability was "highly unstable and cannot be supposed to play any part in the animal's normal existence" (Smith, 1912:190). Pavlov (1927) also reported disappointing results following a number of color-vision experiments performed by his laboratory associate Orbelli, whose early findings were consistent with Smith's results. During a series of color discrimination studies, Orbelli was not able to demonstrate a differential response to color, although he was able to achieve some apparent color recognition in one dog—a feat that was accomplished only after great effort and difficulty. Pavlov reported,

> The results obtained by other investigators, both Russian and foreign, lead to the conclusion that colour vision in dogs, if present, is only of a very rudimentary form, and that in most dogs it cannot be detected at all. (1927:132–133)

After several frustrated experimental efforts, Orbelli concluded that dogs did not differentiate between colors but rather responded to changes of brightness in the samples presented to them. However, other researchers during this same period—ostensibly implementing controls for brightness—reported conflicting results regarding color vision in dogs. A significant procedural difference between these experiments and the ones performed by Orbelli was the use of Pavlov's salivary method versus instrumental methods in which a dog is required to make a voluntary response indicating a choice between color samples. Experimenters using instrumental discrimination methods involving a voluntary response found that dogs did, in fact, possess some significant color vision. Stone (1921) criticized these early efforts to establish the existence of color vision in dogs, arguing that they had failed to control adequately for differences of brightness associated with the color samples presented. He suggested that positive studies indicating the presence of color vision in dogs were confounded by uncontrolled brightness factors, and concluded along with Smith and Orbelli that "the dog possesses only very rudimentary

sensitivity to colors and depends very little, or not at all, on color distinctions in daily life" (1921:415).

The question of color vision in dogs has remained controversial ever since. However, highly controlled vision studies carried out by Neitz and colleagues (1989) and Jacobs and coworkers (1993) have demonstrated that dogs do possess significant abilities to perceive and use color. Neitz and coworkers, for example, determined through a series of color discrimination experiments (e.g., sample-matching discriminations) that dogs can differentiate dichromatic colors having spectral absorption peaks at 429 nm (blue-violet range) and 555 nm (yellow-green range). Spectral neutrality (colorlessness) was found to occur at 480 nm (i.e., the greenish blue range). The dog's dichromatic color vision enables a dog to discriminate bluish objects from yellow ones, but dogs are unable to differentiate between many other colors that are vivid to humans, for example, red, orange, and green—colors that dogs probably perceive as tints and shades of yellow or blue. The various colors that dogs see are affected by a composite of perceptual inputs other than saturated hue, for example, value (lightness/darkness) and intensity (brightness/dullness). Miller and Murphy (1995) noted that dogs are unable to differentiate between greenish blue and gray. This observation is based on findings by Neitz and colleagues (1989) that the range between 475 and 485 nm (greenish blue to humans) is spectrally neutral (i.e., colorless) to dogs. The dog's inability to discriminate between greenish blue and gray occurs, on the one hand, because a dog's dichromatic vision cannot perceive the greenish blue hue but, also, because the normal value of greenish blue is in the gray range. These current findings conflict with an earlier study performed by Rosengren (1969), in which dogs (three female cocker spaniels) were ostensibly trained to discriminate between red, blue, green, and yellow hues. In addition, she found that the dogs could distinguish these various colors from gray samples of different values.

In contrast to earlier reports indicating the existence of only minimal (if any) color vision in dogs, Neitz and colleagues (1989) found that dichromatic color discriminations were rapidly mastered by the dogs they studied (two Italian greyhounds and a toy poodle), noting that color discrimination was evident after only a single day of training. They concluded that "color vision for the dog is not simply a laboratory curiosity, but rather may provide a useful source of environmental information" (1989:124).

Jacobs and colleagues (1993) confirmed the findings of Neitz et al. by means of sophisticated optometric instruments for measuring relative absorption rates of the photopigments contained in the dog's cone receptor cells (electroretinogram flicker photometry). They found that dogs, like the foxes, possess two different photopigmented cones that reach spectral absorption peaks at 430 to 435 nm and 555 nm, respectively. In the case of trichromatic vision, blue-sensitive cones reach absorption peaks at 420 nm, green-sensitive ones at 534 nm, and red-sensitive pigments at 563 nm. In general, mammalian photosensitivity is limited to a narrow electromagnetic wavelength range between ultraviolet and infrared, that is, approximately 380 to 760 nm (Schmidt-Nielsen, 1989).

Vision in Subdued Light

Although the dog's ability to recognize detail and color is limited, dogs possess significant abilities to see under conditions of subdued light or in darkness. Unlike humans, who are phylogenetically adapted to diurnal (daytime) activities, dogs are biologically adapted to a crepuscular rhythm of activity—that is, they are most active around dawn and again at dusk. Selective pressures have resulted in the evolution of structures and mechanisms facilitating vision under subdued light conditions. Night vision is made possible by a photosensitive chemical called rhodopsin contained in the rod receptors. When light energy falls on the rods, the rhodopsin is chemically altered or "bleached" out, transducing a neural signal that is relayed via bipolar cells to the retinal ganglion and, finally, to the optic nerve and brain. When the light source is removed, the photochemical gradually recovers to its original state. Unlike cones, which are linked to

individual fibers in the optic nerve, numerous rods are synaptically connected in the retina to the same neural fiber. This "wiring" is a structural feature of canine vision that yields a loss of visual detail but an increase in light and movement sensitivity.

The dog's vision under subdued light is enhanced by a special reflecting surface, called the tapetum lucidum, located behind the retina. Under conditions of low lighting, the pupil dilates, allowing as much light as possible to enter the eye. Unabsorbed light passing over the retina is concentrated on the tapetum and reflected back over the light-sensitive rod receptors, thus causing added bleaching of rhodopsin and a greater sensation of light. The reflective glow of a dog's eyes when exposed to bright light in darkness is caused by the mirrorlike tapetum. Located below the tapetum lucidum in the lower part of the eye is a heavily pigmented tapetal structure called the tapetum nigrum, which is believed to absorb excessive light entering the eye and thereby reduce glare and scatter effects. Whereas the tapetum lucidum is adapted to accommodate light reflected from the darker earth, the tapetum nigrum is adapted to handle brighter light coming from the sky. These two tapetal structures work together to optimize the amount of illumination reaching the retina.

Binocular Vision and Depth Perception

In general, the eyes of predators are set toward the front of the head, giving them a much sharper and wider field of binocular vision than experienced by prey animals. The eyes of prey animals are usually located more toward the side of the head, giving them an ability to scan the surrounding environment widely for approaching danger. Binocular vision depends on a field of ocular overlap between left and right eyes and a network of complex retinal projections involving both sides of the visual cortex. Such visual abilities enable predators to precisely locate, focus, and track a prey's movement. As the result of the placement of the eyes and the presence of a prominent muzzle blocking a full frontal view, the average dog exhibits only approximately 40 to 60 degrees of overlap between the right and left eyes. This gives dogs binocular capabilities that are good but inferior to human abilities. Such anatomical limitations, however, are a gain in terms of peripheral vision. Whereas human peripheral vision extends to about 180 degrees, the average dog's peripheral range is approximately 250 degrees. Of course, the amount of binocular and peripheral vision varies considerably from breed to breed depending on how the eyes are set in the skull and various neural substrates mediating visual perception.

An important aspect of binocular vision is depth perception. Although a dog's binocular vision is good, a dog's ability to perceive depth is somewhat mitigated by a lack of full binocular vision. Since a dog's binocular vision is limited to a more or less narrow frontal range, a dog's ability to perceive depth is also restricted to a narrow field of vision located directly in front of it. Miller and Murphy (1995) have pointed out, however, that depth perception does not rely on binocular vision alone. Monocular depth perception is also possible as the result of head movements that produce an appearance that objects are moving at different speeds relative to one another, thus providing information about relative distances and depth between them. Other sources of important information concerning depth include foreground/background contrast, atmospheric or aerial perspective (clarity of contour), relative size/scale of objects, linear perspective, overlapping, and vertical location in the field of vision.

Shape and Form Discrimination

Humphrey and Warner (1934) reported an interesting study suggesting that a dog's ability to form clear object images is limited both under close-up conditions and at distances, indicating that dogs may have a very narrow range of effective vision. They reported a study by Karn (1931; Karn and Munn, 1932) in which dogs were trained to discriminate between two triangles, one with its apex pointing up and the other pointing down. These triangles had 9-inch sides, and the dogs were permitted to approach as closely as they liked before choosing between them. Karn found that the dogs usually made

choices only after they were within 20 inches of the triangles. By progressively making the triangles smaller, he was able to obtain reliable discrimination between triangles with 3-inch sides but no smaller. Humphrey and Warner note that a parallel deficiency in human vision would result in our not being able to read a book unless it had "letters three inches high."

Karn and Munn's results conflict somewhat with earlier findings by Pavlov's associate, Shenger-Krestovnikova, who experimented with very subtle shape discriminations in dogs (Pavlov, 1927). In one of her experiments, dogs were required to discriminate between a circle and an ellipse. Over the course of several trials, the shape of the ellipse was gradually expanded in the direction of a circular shape. This was accomplished by altering the ratios of the semiaxes of the circle to the ellipse from 3:2, 4:3, 5:4 ... 9:8. She found that dogs could master discriminations as fine as 9:8 but only with great difficulty. A few of the dogs studied developed striking neurotic sequelae as a result of the perceptual and emotional distress caused by the difficult visual discrimination (see Chapter 9). I once participated in a feasibility study involving military scout dogs that required them to perform a number of sophisticated remote tasks. These tasks were shaped through progressive preliminary training that began with a simple pattern discrimination in a Y maze. The cards (checker patterned and blank) were approximately 12 inches square and placed about 15 feet away from the decision point. The dogs showed great difficulty in mastering this simple discrimination task. After several days of frustrated effort, a flashing light stimulus was added to augment the positive card and to facilitate the discrimination required. The difficulty exhibited by the dogs (German shepherds bred at Biosensor Research for trainability and intelligence) may have been related to a perceptual factor similar to the one discovered by Karn—that is, perhaps the choice point was too far away for them to differentiate accurately between the discriminative stimuli being presented.

Despite the dog's apparent difficulty in discriminating stationary shapes and patterns, most dogs unquestionably possess excellent abilities to discriminate between individuals at distances and in groups—a common and readily demonstrable observation. This ability may be due to an acute sensitivity to movement and subtleties of gesture. Whitney (1961) reported that dogs that had been previously addicted to morphine would copiously salivate whenever they saw him coming toward their kennel. When approached by strangers, the salivation effect was never evident unless he happened to be part of the group. Whitney claims to have observed, through field glasses, addicted dogs salivating as he approached their kennel at variable distances up to 120 feet away. Miller and Murphy (1995) reported a study performed in 1936 with 14 police dogs. In this study, dogs that could identify moving objects at 810 to 900 meters (m) could only recognize these same objects when stationary at much closer distances (585 m or less).

Blindness

Occasionally, dogs lose their sight. Some common causes of blindness or loss of visual acuity include cataracts, progressive retinal atrophy, and glaucoma. Although sight is an extremely important sensory ability for dogs, blindness need not be a cause for euthanasia. Dogs appear to adjust well through compensatory reliance on other senses like hearing and smell and probably with the help of kinesthetic learning of the environment. Chester and Clark (1988) carried out a survey of 50 dog owners with blind dogs. Only 22% of those surveyed noticed a change in their dog's temperament. The most common temperament changes reported were an increase of dependency and attention-seeking behavior. Other changes included increased fearfulness toward family members or other dogs. Of the owners, 74% reported that there was no change in their dog's response to strangers; 12% reported that their dog failed to compensate adequately within familiar surroundings. Only two dogs were reported to experience an increase in aggressiveness—one of which was explained as the result of painful glaucoma and "resentment" about being medicated. This is a somewhat surpris-

ing finding, since many behavioral specialists regard blind and deaf dogs as being more prone to develop aggression problems.

To facilitate a blind or vision-impaired dog's adjustment, appropriate training and management efforts must be carried out. Much of what such dogs performed effortlessly in the past may need to be laboriously relearned. Managing to climb up and down stairs, for example, often proves to be a particularly difficult challenge for blind dogs, but, with patient and gentle encouragement, most blind dogs can learn to climb steps without assistance. Blind dogs appear to form a mental map of the house and quickly learn to avoid bumping into things, provided that the owner is careful not to rearrange furniture or leave objects in the dog's path (e.g., kitchen chairs left out from under the table). Such dogs should be fed in the same place and, for added safety, crated when the owner is absent. Also, the owner might wear a bell as an auditory means to communicate his or her whereabouts to the dog (Campbell, 1992). Olfactory cues (e.g., citronella oil) can be dabbed lightly on the corners of doorways, furniture, and other objects that may be bumped into as the dog moves through the house. The strategic placement of gates and other barriers is also useful. As in the case of deaf dogs, training blind dogs is based on the utilization of sensory modalities other than the disabled one, especially hearing and touch. Van der Westhuizen (1990) has recommended teaching dogs to respond to directional cues such as "left" and "right" to help guide their movements. He suggests that heeling lessons are facilitated by allowing the dog to make contact or lean into the handler's leg, thus providing additional means to orient the dog's movement while walking in close quarters. In addition to the use of gentle physical prompts, training blind dogs depends on the use of expressive verbalization, using tonal variations and inflections to promote effective communication. Both blind and, as will be seen in a moment, deaf dogs are at considerable risk of being injured by pedestrians (e.g., bicyclists and skaters) or by vehicular traffic and should be leashed whenever away from home.

AUDITION

The dog's ear is composed of an outer ear (pinna), auditory canal, and various structures designed to convert sound waves into auditory information. The pinna gathers and directs sound into the auditory canal, where it is carried to the tympanic membrane or eardrum. The eardrum is an extremely sensitive and elastic membrane reacting to the slightest vibrations on its surface: movement of less than one-tenth the diameter of a hydrogen atom can produce an audible sensation (Thompson, 1993). The vibrations caused by the pressure of sound waves on the eardrum are mechanically conducted to the cochlea through the mediation of three tiny bones or ossicles: the malleus, the incus, and the stapes. The cochlea is a snail-like tubular structure that is innervated by the auditory nerve. Sound vibrations are passed into the cochlea at the oval window. These vibrations cause a fluid wave in the cochlear fluid, which causes a rippling effect against the surrounding basilar membrane. The vibratory displacement of the basilar membrane stimulates auditory receptors (called hair cells) to bend rhythmically, thereby evoking a nerve potential that is carried by individual fibers into the auditory nerve. Different sounds are distinguished by the specific pattern of wave motion that they generate. The vibratory wave movements in the cochlear fluid selectively activate certain groups of receptor cells while passing over others as they flow against the surrounding basilar membrane. Audibly different sensations are produced by the distinctive pattern and topography of the wave involved. Auditory sensations are conducted by the auditory nerve to the cochlea nuclei located in the medulla oblongata before being relayed to the thalamus.

Frequency Range of Hearing

The dog's range of hearing has been shown to be superior to human audition in many respects. Dogs can easily hear sounds outside the human range of audibility [20,000 cycles per second (cps)]. Estimates vary from 26,000 cps (Fuller and DuBuis, 1962),

41,000 to 47,000 (Heffner, 1983), 30,000 to 40,000 (Schmidt-Nielsen, 1989), and 60,000 to 65,000 cps (Houpt, 1991); whatever the case may be, dogs do hear ultrasound—sound that is imperceptible to normal human ears. Dogs can also hear sounds of very low frequencies at 15 cps. The general range of hearing estimated by Fox and Bekoff (1975) is 15 to 60,000 cps. To place these numbers into perspective, 28 cps is the frequency of the lowest key on the piano and 4180 cps is the frequency of sound produced by the highest key. Apparently, dogs hear best at around 4000 cps, compared with humans at 1000 to 2000 cps. Lipman and Grassi (1942) compared human hearing with that of dogs and found that under comparable sound intensities (decibels) dogs and humans did about equally well with regard to the perception of low frequencies (125 to 250 cps). They observed, however, that dogs do progressively better as the frequencies increase with "markedly superior" abilities between 4000 and 8000 cps, and concluded that "the dog lives in a broader and deeper acoustic world, thus gaining direct contact with natural events which are imperceptible to man" (1942:88).

Auditory Localization

Another way that the dog's sense of hearing is better than ours is its ability to locate the origin of sounds coming from a distance. A variable ability to localize the origin of sounds is evident in puppies as early as 16 days of age (Ashmead et al., 1986). Adult dogs are able to pinpoint the origin of sound with a great accuracy with the aid of their movable earflaps (pinnas). Locating the origin of sound, however, involves much more than facile movement of the ears. Sound location depends on complex brain calculations that rely on the dog's ability to register narrow time differences between the sound reaching each of its opposing ears. The ear closest to the source of sound is struck slightly sooner than the opposite ear. Determining the direction of the sound's origin depends on a cooperative mediation of information between the cochlear nuclei and time-sensitive neurons located on either side of the brain stem in a structure known as the superior olive. These neurons can detect delays of stimulation between one ear and the other on the level of microseconds (a millionth of a second). The slightest movement of the head toward the source of stimulation provides additional information about distance. A change in the dog's head position relative to the sound provides spatial information that can then be used by the brain to triangulate and compute the sound's distance (Thompson, 1993). The common tendency for a dog to cock its head to one side when listening carefully to an unusual sound is probably a reflexive effort to pinpoint a more exact location, perhaps involving a dimension of height relative to the ears when positioned parallel to the ground.

Ultrasound and Training

A potential application utilizing the dog's ability to hear in the ultrasonic range is to use high-frequency sounds in dog training. Of course, the Galton or "silent" whistle has been used for many years as a signaling device, especially for recall. Recently, however, many battery-powered ultrasonic devices have come onto the market for use in behavioral training as "humane" forms of punishment for nuisance barking and other behavior problems (Landsberg, 1994). An assumption underlying the use of such devices is that the ultrasound stimulation produced by them is aversive to dogs—that is, that it hurts their ears. This assumption, however, has not been borne out by personal experience or experimental testing. For example, Blackshaw and coworkers (1990) tested the auditory reaction of several dogs, ranging widely in size and breed type, to variable frequencies of ultrasound under controlled conditions. They found that ultrasonic devices producing high-frequency sounds between 14 to 36 kHz resulted in remarkably little apparent aversion in the dogs, mostly yielding a "no effect" response or minimum signs of interest as indicated by brief pricking of the subjects' ears. A few dogs reacted aversively to the sound by turning away from it. Small dogs appeared to be slightly more sensitive to ultrasound than

are medium or large dogs. This latter finding is consistent with Galton's early observation that small dogs responded to his silent whistle while large dogs did not. However, this apparent difference between small and large dogs does not appear to depend on the size of the dog's head or auditory apparatus. Heffner (1983) found that the upper limits for high-frequency hearing are remarkably similar from breed to breed, regardless of their size and ear shape: Chihuahua, 47 kHz; dachshund, 41 kHz; poodle, 46 kHz; pointer, 45 kHz; and St. Bernard, 47 kHz. Perhaps smaller dogs are simply more behaviorally reactive to ultrasound than are large breeds.

These devices have not proven to be very reliable, effective, or aversive to most dogs. I have been disappointed by my own experiences with the products, finding them unreliable or ineffective beyond an initial "What's that?" or a mild annoying effect that dogs readily habituate to after a few trials. One popular bark-activated model that I tested actually jammed on a continuous mode and would have continued producing the ultrasound until it "fried" or the batteries ran down. Fortunately, it was not on a dog; unfortunately, the product is still on the market and widely used.

A possible explanation for the relative ineffectiveness of ultrasonic devices may be the result of insufficient power to drive the ultrasonic pulse. In other words, the small battery-powered models may not be strong enough to produce an aversive auditory effect. Ultrasound requires relatively more energy and amplitude than sound generated at lower frequencies. Frequencies above a dog's optimal range of hearing require progressively more amplitude boosting to be heard. For instance, to obtain an orienting response to the sound of a silent whistle, the effort needed to blow the whistle adjusted at a high frequency is much more forceful than required when it is adjusted to a lower one.

Ultrasound has two other distinct characteristics limiting its usefulness: narrow field of directionality and limited effective range. Unless the device is pointed directly at a dog's head at a close range, its effectiveness is drastically diminished. In the case of bark-activated collars, the ultrasonic burst may be blocked by the dog's neck and jaw, requiring that the sound stimulus reach the dog's ears by way of echoes from surrounding objects rather than from the collar itself. This further mitigates its usefulness in situations where nearby objects are not present, such as outdoors. Lastly, dogs may not be biologically prepared to readily associate ultrasound stimuli (even at high levels of stimulation) with threat without additional aversive conditioning. Ultrasound may possess some innate significance as a directional indicator for detecting and locating small prey animals, whose distress vocalizations are expressed at ultrasonic frequencies.

No adequate learning studies (that I am familiar with) have been carried out that demonstrate the effectiveness of ultrasound as a punisher or negative reinforcer in dogs. Considering the cost of the devices, and the ready availability of consistently more effective alternatives, one should resort to their use only in rare cases of special need, for example, with especially sensitive dogs or where auditory-mediated punishment needs to be silent. Although the use of ultrasound as an auditory punisher is not recommended, low-intensity ultrasound can be usefully employed in dog training as a means for signaling and controlling learned behavior (e.g., the silent whistle). Pairing unobtrusive ultrasonic cues with trained behaviors proves very effective in place of verbal commands in certain situations where silent control is desirable. Unfortunately, ultrasound is currently most often applied as a punitive device rather than a potentially valuable training tool for the delivery of discriminative signals and secondary reinforcement.

An additional problem raised by the dog's sensitivity to ultrasound is the advisability of ultrasonic flea deterrents. Ultrasonic collars are frequently used by pet owners to control flea infestation. This is unfortunate, both because they do not work (Dryden et al., 1989) and because the sounds produced by such devices are audible to dogs and cats exposed to them (Roe and Sales, 1992). Obviously, the possibility exists that ultrasonic flea collars may produce significant annoyance to dogs with sensitive hearing abilities. Ultrasonic flea

collars produce frequencies well within the range of a dog's hearing capability, at approximately 40,000 cps (92 dB amplitude at a distance of 10 cm). A serious question must be raised regarding the impact of daily exposure to pulsing ultrasound stimulation at these levels to a dog's quality of life. This is especially pressing since ultrasonic collars have been proven uniformly ineffective against flea infestation. While the directionality of ultrasound at the aforementioned frequencies probably prevents it from directly reaching the dog's ears while wearing the device, it does not prevent echoes from reaching the dog's ears indirectly or prevent the ultrasound from reaching resident dogs or cats exposed to its unobstructed output.

Deafness

Deafness occurs in dogs as a congenital disorder or may be acquired as the result of disease or physical damage to the auditory mechanism. Congenital deafness appears to be linked to pigmentation, with the likelihood of deafness increasing with the amount of white pigmentation present in the dog, especially in dogs that exhibit an absence of normal iris pigmentation. The merle gene (e.g., the Australian shepherd, Harlequin Great Dane, Old English sheepdog, and others) and piebald gene (e.g., bullterrier, Dalmatian, Great Pyrenees, and others) have been associated with an increased incidence of deafness (Strain, 1996). Dalmatians commonly exhibit congenital deafness, with as many as 30% of the puppies born exhibiting the disorder in one or both ears. Temporary hearing loss (elevated thresholds) may result from exposure to intense auditory stimulation exceeding 100 dB. For example, hunting dogs exposed to repeated close-range gunfire may experience significant noise-related hearing loss.

Determining whether a dog is deaf is best accomplished by the brain stem auditory evoked response (BAER) test, which detects electrical activity in the cochlea and other auditory nervous pathways in the brain. The test is conducted by directing a brief auditory stimulus (a click) into both ears and measuring the evoked electrical patterns produced by the stimulation. Deaf dogs will present a flat-line appearance. A major advantage of the BAER test is that it can isolate deafness in one ear (unilateral) or both (bilateral) ears (Strain, 1996). Bilateral deafness can also be detected by the absence of an appropriate response to loud startling noises or a failure to acquire various conditioned associations that depend on hearing to learn (e.g., the dog's name and other verbal/auditory cues used in training).

According to the reports of many deaf dog owners (Becker, 1997), deaf dogs can make a good adjustment to domestic life. Success with such dogs depends on careful training and other management efforts needed to protect the hearing-impaired dogs from injuries that might be sustained as the result of their inability to hear, especially the threat of vehicular injury. Like blind dogs, deaf dogs learn to rely on other sensory modalities to obtain environmental information, including vision, touch, and olfaction. Consequently, deaf dogs can be taught to respond to a wide variety of visual cues and hand signals, as well as various common forms of tactile stimulation used routinely in dog training. Obviously, training a deaf dog poses many unique problems, such as securing and maintaining the dog's attention, especially when the handler is out of the dog's field of vision. Campbell (1992) recommends the use of beanbags to condition dogs to keep their attention on the handler. When a dog's attention wavers, the beanbag is tossed at the dog's legs. The handler then turns and walks in an opposite direction while encouraging the dog to follow along. As the dog approaches, the handler crouches down and reinforces the following behavior with petting. Other ways to hold a deaf dog's attention include consistently reinforcing attention with treats, tossing toys into the dog's field of vision, stomping on the floor, and using flashlights and lasers (Becker, 1997). Remote-activated electronic collars are sometimes used for the control of undesirable behavior and to train dogs to come. A rather unique application of such devices set at a very low level is to pair the mild stimulation produced by the collar with food and other rewards. As a consequence, the stimulation can then be used to reinforce desirable behaviors conditionally in much the same manner

as applying other common conditioned reinforcers (e.g., "Good"). Remote-activated vibratory devices are also used for such purposes. Finally, even though dogs cannot hear, Tanner has emphasized that trainers should still speak to dogs as though the dogs can hear, since "we transmit our feelings and desires to our dogs through facial expressions as well as oral commands" (1970:23).

Deaf puppies are routinely euthanized, in part, as the result of the widespread belief that congenital bilateral deafness represents a significant risk factor for the development of a variety of behavior problems, including aggression—presumably developing as the result of repeated and unpredictable startle. The linkage between deafness and aggression is a highly controversial topic, with little current evidence available other than anecdotal reports and clinical impressions supporting the assumption that deaf dogs are more prone to bite. What most authorities do agree on is that deaf dogs require considerably more focused care and training than hearing dogs—a factor that the prospective owner of a deaf dog should realistically assess before making the decision to adopt.

OLFACTION

The dog's sense of smell has attracted a great deal of enthusiastic attention from both applied and scientific quarters but has only slowly received appropriate experimental study. Historically, almost supernatural capabilities were attributed to a dog's nose, often resulting in the promulgation of some rather fantastic and insupportable claims about canine olfactory abilities. In addition, many equally incredible theories have been posited regarding the way in which a dog's olfactory apparatus works (McCartney, 1968). These theories have ranged from the absurd to the occult. For example, one fanciful account hypothesized that irradiated energy emanating from living cells was absorbed by various materials stepped upon, and then re-emitted and detected by the dog's nose. Other discarded theories posited the notion that electrical waves or vibrations were responsible for the extraordinary feats of canine olfaction. One speculative adherent of the wave theory actually proposed that a pendulum be employed as an instrument for measuring the dog's olfactory acuity. Over the years, many important advances have been made in the study of olfaction, largely supplanting theories like the foregoing with more scientifically grounded alternatives. Currently, the science of smell is making important strides toward a more complete understanding of the intricate biochemical and neurological substrates of olfaction.

Mechanics of Smell

The sense of smell enables dogs to analyze the environment for significant chemical signs or disturbances. During the process of smelling, a sample of air containing the odor is sniffed and directed deep into the posterior portion of the left and right nasal cavities. Once in the nasal cavity, the odor accumulates on a mucous layer containing millions of odor-sensitive cilia. The cilia are hairlike dendritic elaborations of the olfactory receptor neuron. Each olfactory receptor has 10 or more immotile cilia that collect odorant molecules. The convoluted epithelial membrane containing these olfactory receptors is supported by a complex structure of turbinate bones. This arrangement allows for maximal contact between the collected odor and the olfactory mucosa. In addition, the cilia themselves add considerably to the overall membrane surface area exposed to odorant molecules. A dog's olfactory neuroepithelium contains as many as 250 million receptor cells. When stretched out, the surface area of the olfactory epithelium has been estimated to range (depending on the breed) from 20 to 200 square centimeters. In comparison, the human olfactory neuroepithelium covers a mere 2 to 4 square centimeters and contains only about 5 million receptor cells per nasal cavity (Cain, 1988).

Olfactory Transduction

Sensory data from these millions of receptor cells is conducted through the cribriform plate into the nearby olfactory bulbs within the cranium. Once in the olfactory bulbs, the axons converge upon the glomeruli. The glomeruli are spherical structures that integrate and organize olfactory input. There are far fewer glomeruli than olfactory receptor axons, requiring that many thousands of axons share individual glomeruli. Within each glomerulus, olfactory axons form synapses with second-order olfactory neurons called mitral cells. From the glomeruli, the information is passed onto other parts of the brain for higher processing, associative identification, and interpretation (see Chapter 3). As one might expect, the olfactory bulbs in dogs are considerably larger than those in humans.

The manner in which olfaction occurs is not fully understood, but important advances in the study of olfactory reception have been made by Axel and his associates at Columbia University (Axel, 1995). By using molecular genetics and sophisticated biochemical procedures, they have been able to isolate a large gene family dedicated to the synthesis of olfactory receptor proteins (Buck and Axel, 1991). The researchers have found that the olfactory neuroepithelium contains neurons possessing about 1000 different receptors, coded by an incredible 1% of the mammalian genome. In rats, one in every 100 genes is involved in the reception of odors, making olfactory receptor genes the largest family of genes currently known to exist. Each receptor protein is highly selective and will bind only to a select group of odorants. In combination, these diverse receptors yield an extraordinary diversity of smells. Whereas humans are believed to discriminate around 10,000 separate odors, dogs are probably able to detect a far larger number. These findings are extraordinary when one considers a comparison with all of the rich diversity of human color vision that is provided by only three kinds of photoreceptors differentially sensitive to three overlapping bands of visible light. Given that 1000 different olfactory receptors appear to exist, the potential number of smells available to the mammalian nose is staggering.

Each olfactory neuron expresses a receptor specialized for the detection of a specific type of odor molecule. All of these many receptor proteins are coupled to G proteins concentrated on the distal portion of the cilia. The receptor protein in conjunction with the G protein activates a cascade of biochemical events mediated by a second messenger within the cell, resulting in the depolarization of the olfactory neuron and the production of an action potential or signal. These olfactory receptor neurons are distributed randomly in several specialized zones on the olfactory epithelium (Ressler et al., 1993). The axons of olfactory neurons with the same receptor converge on the same glomeruli in the olfactory bulb (Axel, 1995). This is an extraordinary finding, since these receptor neurons are destroyed and shed after a functional life of 6 to 8 weeks. Olfactory neurons are being constantly replaced by underlying stem cells that subsequently send axons to the same locality in the olfactory bulb. How this is accomplished is not known.

Olfactory Acuity

Numerous studies have demonstrated that a dog's sense of smell is extremely sensitive. W. Neuhaus (McCartney, 1968; Passe and Walker, 1985) employed an olfactometer for mixing and delivering odorant samples at very low concentrations. His method involved evaporating the sample into a controlled airstream and directing it out through three separate ports, two of which contained air without any odorant. The dog was trained to choose between the three by pressing its nose against a box located behind the port associated with the sample. The concentration of the odorant sample was progressively lowered until the dog could no longer select the correct port. Surprisingly, he found that some substances were not detected by dogs at concentrations much lower than that detectable by humans. In most instances, however, the dog's ability was much superior. For example, he estimated that a dog's ability to detect butyric acid (a component in sweat that smells like dirty socks) is from 1 million to 100 million times better than a human's ability. These results (if true) mean that dogs may be able to detect 1 milligram of butyric acid in 100 million cubic meters of air. Pearsall and Verbruggen illustrate the extent of these incredible findings with a striking analogy:

Comparison with our own nose is difficult, but an example may help: One of the substances released by human perspiration is butyric acid. If one gram of this chemical (a small drop in the bottom of a teaspoon) were to be spread throughout a ten-story building, a person could smell it at the window only at the moment of release. If this same amount were spread over the entire city of Philadelphia, a dog could smell it anywhere, even up to altitude of 300 feet. (1982:5)

Butyric acid is a prominent feature of the scent picture utilized by dogs while tracking. Wright makes a number of probing observations and calculations based on assumptions drawn from Neuhaus's findings and the abilities of tracker dogs:

There are several sources of skin secretions: sweat glands, "odour glands", fat glands, and various others. The sole of the foot has only sweat glands, but they are present in large numbers: up to 1000 per square centimetre. Therefore the sweat glands are likely to be the most important. Over a period of 24 hours, the human body secretes about 800 c.c. of sweat, and from the two million or so sweat glands on the sole of each foot, about 2 per cent of the daily production, or about 16 c.c., would be released. Human sweat has about 0.156 per cent acid of which about one-quarter is aliphatic. If only 1/1000 of this penetrates steadily through the sole and the seams of the shoe, it can be calculated that of an acid such as butyric acid, at least 2.5×10^{11} molecules would be left behind in each footprint. This is well over a million times the threshold amount for the dog, and could still give a detectable smell when dispersed in 28 cubic meters of air. (1964:76)

These numbers are staggering, especially if one considers that some bloodhounds can follow trails several days old over rough terrain and then pick out the tracked person from a lineup of 10 people (Sommerville and Green, 1989).

Ashton and colleagues (1957) also found that a dog's ability to detect various odorants was not equally proficient for all sample substances. An apparent factor is related to the size of the molecule involved. Fatty acids differing by only a single atom of carbon resulted in significantly different olfactory thresholds. The more carbon atoms the molecule possessed, the lower was the dog's olfactory threshold for its detection. A possible explanation for this finding is that organic molecules with long carbon chains possibly trigger action potentials in a correspondingly greater number of olfactory receptor neurons than do molecules composed of fewer carbon atoms. The lower thresholds may be obtained because more receptor neurons are fired by molecules possessing a greater number of carbon atoms than those possessing only a few.

More recent and carefully controlled studies have compared the dog's olfactory ability with that of humans. These experiments have found somewhat less dramatic differences between humans and dogs—at least with respect to the substances investigated. Krestel and colleagues (1984) compared the dog's ability to detect amyl acetate with that of human subjects. Using a conditioned suppression technique, they determined that dogs can detect the substance at a concentration 2.6 log units lower (i.e., about 400 times better) than human test subjects. Marshall and Moulton (1981) determined that dogs could detect alpha-ionone at concentrations 3 to 4 log units lower than that detectable by humans (i.e., approximately 1000 to 10,000 times better).

Certainly not all dogs possess such incredible olfactory sensitivity. To obtain a general indication of the dog's olfactory sensitivity, Myers (1991) developed a home test for evaluating a dog's sense of smell. Eugenol, a pure olfactory stimulant, is used in a series of progressively dilute solutions and is systematically presented to a dog. The dog's reaction to each sample is noted. The odorant evokes a range of unconditioned reactions in dogs, including moving the head, licking the nose, or sniffing. This method of evaluating olfactory function has at least two potential shortcomings. First, the dog's reaction to the substance must be interpreted by the owner, who may or may not evaluate its reaction correctly. Secondly, the owner may inadvertently (unconsciously) provide the dog with cues to help it perform better. These problems suggest that the method is best suited for determining gross functions rather than subtle olfactory thresholds.

Biological and Social Functions of Smell

Besides the obvious usefulness of an acute sense of smell for the detection of prey animals, many social functions are coordinated by olfaction. Most dogs engage in scent marking and scent-mark investigation. Dunbar and Carmichael (1981) studied the urinary elimination patterns of laboratory beagles, finding that male dogs spend significantly more time investigating and marking samples of urine belonging to strange males than samples belonging to themselves or other males with whom they are familiar. Their study suggests that dogs are not responding to the smell of urine per se but to some specific pheromonal identifier within the context of urine that excites interest and triggers a marking response. Supporting the view that an olfactory signal triggers the marking response, Shafik (1994) has demonstrated in dogs an olfactory micturition reflex between the nasal mucosa and the urethral sphincters. Electrostimulation of the nasal mucosa appears to relax urethral sphincter muscles in dogs. The author speculates that this reflex induces elimination in the absence of a full bladder, thus contributing to the tendency of dogs to eliminate repeatedly in response to specific odorants rather than in response to signals from pressure receptors in the bladder wall. Other studies have shown that the frequency of sniffing and urinary marking is significantly reduced in animals that have been castrated or rendered anosmic. Among rats, testosterone has been proven to play a significant role as a hormonal enhancer of olfactory acuity (Pietras and Moulton, 1974). Perhaps the decline of sniffing and marking in castrated males is due to relevant pheromones failing to reach thresholds detectable by altered dogs.

Defecation may also serve some olfactory-signaling purpose, although few dogs examine the fecal droppings of conspecifics with the same degree of interest that they exhibit toward urinary scent marks. Some co-prophagic dogs may be very interested in the feces of other dogs, but not apparently for the signaling value of the excrement, but rather for its potential nutritional content. The anal glands secrete a strong-smelling substance into the fecal bolus just before it is excreted. The function of these anal secretions is not known, although dogs will copiously and violently express them when aroused with intense fear. Perhaps anal fluids contain chemical signals that dogs use alone or in conjunction with other chemosensory and physical cues to express or communicate some, as yet unknown, psychosocial intention or meaning. Among wolves, the alphas are most likely to deposit anal gland secretions into their feces and to concentrate their depositions in one area (Asa et al., 1985). Houpt (1991) has speculated that dogs scratch the ground after defecating in order to spread the fecal scent around, but this is an unlikely explanation for such behavior. Most dogs rarely (if ever) disturb their excrement (or urine marks) as the result of such scratching activity. Peters and Mech (1975) observed that wolves actually step away from deposited scats and urine marks before scratching. Some species do scatter their feces around after elimination (e.g., the hippopotamus), ostensibly to mark or maintain territory, but dogs do not engage in this sort of ritual. Two potentially significant outcomes of scratching after eliminating is the deposition of identifying pheromonal scents from the paws, augmented by impressive (perhaps, even provocative) visual signs of general size, weight, and vigor impressed into the earth with claws like a signature. This latter observation is consistent with the finding that only high-ranking wolves scratch after eliminating.

The sense of smell aids dogs in identifying the sexual status and receptivity of potential mates (Beach et al., 1983). Females begin depositing pheromonal clues about their pending status long before they are actually prepared to accept the males' advances. Such advanced invitation is widely advertised through increased urine marking on the female's part. Upon detecting this evidence of incipient estrus on their excursions, male dogs may become highly aroused and motivated by the female's sexual status but will be roundly rejected if they locate her. Desmond Morris speculates that the reason for these mixed signals is simple—the female secretes these early olfactory signals (pheromones) to maximize the probability of finding a mate:

> This may seem like a pointless period of teasing the male. If she will not accept him, why send out all those appealing scent signals? The answer is that it is important for her to ensure that all potential mates are well aware of her condition, so that when the crucial moment comes she will not find herself mateless. Ovulation occurs spontaneously on the second day of the estrus period proper. A day or two after that the bitch is ready to be fertilized. If males are absent then she will have to wait another six months for her next chance. (1986:92–93)

The dog is highly attracted to the vaginal secretions of the estrous female, which he persistently licks, hounding her until at last she consents to his courtship efforts.

Another important function of olfaction is kinship recognition. Hepper observed that puppies recognize littermates and prefer contact with them over nonlittermates, and he speculated that some combination of olfactory and visual information mediates such kin recognition and contact preference: "Pups oriented to the cage by visual cues and then used olfactory cues for 'close-up' recognition" (1986:289). Mekosh-Rosenbaum and coworkers (1994) demonstrated that puppies do use olfactory cues to identify littermates. Puppies at various ages were exposed to the bedding of both kin and nonkin conspecifics. Young puppies (20 to 24 days old) spent significantly more time investigating and making contact with kin bedding than with nonkin bedding. After 31 days of age, however, puppies began spending approximately equal time investigating kin and nonkin bedding. Interestingly, between days 52 and 56, male puppies were significantly more attracted to nonkin bedding. They speculate that this shift coincides with a "weakening of the mother-litter bond, leading toward the pups' ultimate independence" (1994:498).

This change coincides with the optimum time for placing a puppy in its permanent human home at around 7 weeks of age.

The canid habit of rubbing on strong-smelling substances is as common as it is intriguing. The habit appears in puppies as young as 3 months of age. Dogs scented in such a manner are immensely interesting to other dogs, attracting the active attention of conspecifics with whom they happen to come into contact. To the chagrin of the owner, the behavior is often exhibited immediately following a bath. The most commonly posited theory for the habit is olfactory camouflage. By rubbing in the strongest ambient smell, a predator might enjoy some slight advantage while stalking its prey. Although this theory seems plausible enough, it has been rejected by some authorities, based on the hunting techniques of the wolf. A second theory suggests that the habit provides a kind of scent identity shared by the pack—with any strong odor being a sufficient stimulus to excite socially infectious and ecstatic rubbing—regardless of the source. Captive wolves have been observed rubbing in the same scented spot until the whole pack is scented with the odor (E. Klinghammer, personal communication). While the object of such behavior is typically carrion or dung, any strongly odiferous substance will attract the response from wolves—even expensive perfume! (Mech, 1970). Fox has suggested that dogs may be motivated by "an aesthetic appreciation of odors" (1972:222) or, perhaps, such behavior may serve to enhance social recognition and contact (1971a). Kleiman (1966) suggested that the typical physical movement associated with the pattern is intended to impart the animal's scent to the object rubbed upon—not necessarily to receive odor from it. Morris (1986) rejected this suggestion, arguing that if the canid's intention was to mask the odor it would deposit an equally intense smell (feces or urine)—not simply rub on it. He speculated that a possible purpose for the habit is to obtain and share information about the surrounding environment with other pack members via various scents the scouting wolf has rolled upon. Although pack members show great interest in the returning scout and appear to delight in the smells that he has collected, whether this exchange ever results in the initiation of a hunting sortie has not been determined. To my knowledge, there has not been a controlled scientific investigation of this interesting phenomenon.

Ability to Detect and Discriminate Human Odors

Besides playing an important role in the social identification of conspecifics, the sense of smell is also used by dogs to identify people. Furthermore, the manner in which dogs smell and where they smell may be significant. Millot and colleagues (1987) reported that during spontaneous interaction between dogs and children, dogs more commonly sniffed the face during appeasing and friendly interaction, directed smelling to arms and legs during competitive encounters, and directed olfactory interest to the child's chest and legs when he or she was not behaving in any special way toward the dog. Smell may give observant dogs many clues about the emotional status of their owner or guest. Dogs appear to react differentially to the smells of people according to their emotional states and health. Owners have frequently commented on such abilities being exhibited by their dogs. Reportedly, Montaguer (LeGuerer, 1994) has found that dogs exhibit a repulsion toward the odor of psychotic children. According to LeGuerer, Montaguer performed a series of experiments with child-like dummies, with one dummy wearing undergarments saturated with the smell of a psychotic child while the other one wore undergarments imbued with the odor of a normal child. The dog actively avoided coming into contact with the dummy wearing underwear having the odor of the psychotic child.

Edney, who has studied a group of dogs believed to possess the ability to anticipate epileptic seizures in their owners, has speculated that affected dogs may be responding to "distinctive odors generated in the aura phase of epilepsy" (1993:337). Strong and associates (1999) have recently confirmed that *seizure-alert* dogs can be specifically trained to detect signs of impending seizure. The dogs included in the study were able to warn their owners of impending seizure from 15 to 45 minutes prior to the seizure's onset. An apparent beneficial by-product of such dogs was a significant reduction of seizure activity in their owners. Another interesting area involves dogs belonging to diabetics. Lim and colleagues (1992) found 15 cases in which some dogs appear to detect and react to hypoglycemic episodes in their owners. In another study, Smith and Sines (1960) found that rats could be trained to discriminate reliably between sweat samples taken from schizophrenics and sweat samples taken from nonschizophrenic controls. Perhaps, in the future, dogs will serve chemosensory diagnostic functions as yet not fully exposed—for example, the early detection of various mental and physical disease conditions. In addition, a dog's nose might be usefully employed for the detection of environmental pollutants at concentrations below the threshold of currently available mechanical means.

The dog's ability to detect and identify human scent is extraordinary. For example, King and coworkers (1964) found that dogs could detect the presence of a single fingerprint placed on a glass slide that was up to 6 weeks old (indoor samples). In their experiment, each discrimination trial involved four blank slides and one fingerprinted slide. Correct choices required that the dog sit in front of the fingerprinted slide. They compared the dogs' accuracy of detection along two separate dimensions of scent viability: age of scent and the effect of outdoor weathering. Toward this end, some of the slides were carefully preserved indoors while others were exposed to outdoor conditions for varying lengths of time before testing began. The dogs could easily detect indoor fingerprint samples after 3 weeks but were successful only 50% of the time after 6 weeks. They failed to detect outdoor samples reliably after 2 to 3 weeks. Fingerprints on slides covered by a film of water could not be detected.

Kalmus (1955) evaluated the dog's ability to discriminate between the scent of different people, including family members and twins. He demonstrated that dogs could easily and reliably make such discriminations, even be-

tween family members—unless they happened to be identical twins. He used freshly laundered handkerchiefs that had been scented from the armpits by the test subjects. The dogs were trained to sniff the hand of the subject and then to select the handkerchief that had been handled by that person. In the case of identical twins, the dogs appeared to treat the handkerchiefs scented by them as identical. This outcome suggests that the *preferred* scent cues were not incidental olfactory stimuli like clothing, diet, or emotional states. The really interesting result of Kalmus's study, however, occurred during tracking tests. On the whole, dogs that were given the scent of one twin would readily follow the other, *unless* both twins laid the track side by side and then split off in opposite directions. Under such conditions, one of the dogs studied consistently tracked the twin who had actually provided the sample scent, suggesting that under certain conditions dogs might rely on other *secondary* olfactory markers (perhaps incidental and transient) to differentiate the human scent.

A more recent study by Hepper (1988) found that both genetic and environmental factors affect a dog's ability to discriminate between twins. The experiments used a matching-to-sample method. Twins were instructed to wear two T-shirts over a 48-hour period. The dog was presented with one of the T-shirts to sample for several seconds. Meanwhile, the matching T-shirt along with the other twin's T-shirt had been crumpled and placed into a small plastic trough standing 10 feet away from the dog and handler. The dog was sent to retrieve one of the two T-shirts. Hepper found that dogs could accurately discriminate between twins so long as they differed in one of two directions: genetic relatedness or environment factors (e.g., diet). The dogs were unable to discriminate between infant identical twins if they had been fed the same diet.

A few years ago, Brisbin and Austad (1991, 1993) evoked a controversy by suggesting that dogs could not reliably match scents collected from different parts of the body to the correct human donor, thus contradicting Kalmus's previous finding that scent samples taken from the armpit could be accurately matched with scents taken from the hand. Their study aimed at determining the extent to which dogs could generalize scent discrimination training and matching abilities to scents collected from different parts of the body. The study was limited to three dogs—all previously trained to discriminate scent articles (AKC Utility Test) from scent collected from the hands only. None of the dogs had any previous experience involving the discrimination of scent from other parts of the body or law-enforcement experience. The researchers found that when the dogs were prompted to discriminate the scent sample taken from their owner's elbow from the scent samples collected from the hands of a stranger, they were only successful 57.9% of the time (results not rising above statistical chance).

In reply to Brisbin and Austad, Sommerville and colleagues (1993) criticized their study, arguing that the resulting findings suffered from an inherent ambiguity stemming from the way in which the dogs were trained and tested. For one thing, the dogs involved were trained to discriminate only scent collected from the hands and were naive with regard to the discrimination of scents obtained from other parts of the body. Ostensibly, the dogs had learned the scent signature of hands but not a reliable specifying signature of a person's identity per se. According to Sommerville and associates, the results reported by Brisbin and Austad were inconclusive, measuring an artifact resulting from inadequate preparatory training rather than a lack of ability to generalize or match scent accurately. The researchers subsequently carried out a much more extensive study of their own to test this general hypothesis (Settle et al., 1994). In contrast to the negative findings of Brisbin and Austad, they demonstrated that, if properly selected and trained, dogs can reliably discriminate and match body scents collected from different parts of the body to the correct donor:

> Our results show that dogs can efficiently match objects bearing the scents of individual humans whom they do not know even when the scented objects have been in contact with different parts of the body and collected with no particular precautions to avoid environmen-

tal contamination. … Our results suggest that if dogs are selected well, sympathetically trained and entirely dedicated to scent discrimination in a well-managed unit they are likely to maintain a dependably high performance over long periods. (1994:1446–1448)

The significance of the Brisbin-Sommerville controversy is to underscore the importance of careful selection, extensive training, and testing/certification of dogs used by law enforcement for tracking and identifying suspects.

Localizing the Origin and Direction of Odors

The primary function of olfaction in dogs is to detect and locate odors emanating from the surrounding environment. Von Bekesy (1964) performed a series of experiments to determine whether olfactory localization occurred in a manner analogous to directional hearing. He discovered that in the process of sniffing there exists a small time delay between the odorant entering one nostril before reaching the other, unless the source of the odorant is located directly in front. A difference of as little as 0.3 millisecond between nostrils was found sufficient to calculate the odorant's general direction of origin. He also found that differential olfactory analysis of the relative concentration of the left sample as compared with the right one provided additional information about the odorant's location. From this information, a gradient is formed from which a dog can calculate the approximate direction of the origin of the odorant by the differences of concentration entering the respective nostrils.

Schwenk (1994), who has studied the chemosensory locating abilities of snakes, has shown that a snake's tongue serves a similar direction-finding function as that performed by the separated nostrils of mammals. Scent gathered by one fork of a snake's flicking tongue is slightly more or less concentrated than scent gathered by the other. By comparing these differences via the vomeronasal organ (VNO), a snake is able to trail and locate prey animals wounded with venom. If the forked portion of the tongue is severed, a snake is unable to trail. Further, if one side of the VNO is blocked, a snake tends to trail in the direction of the unblocked side, consequently moving about in a wide circular path.

Few trails in nature are found at their source but are crossed and detected at some arbitrary point along their length. Determining which way to go once a trail is located is a challenge to the olfactory abilities of predators. This is also a problem of considerable importance for dogs trained to track people. McCartney (1968) discussed early directional tracking experiments carried out by Belleville, a Berlin police officer, who found that trained tracker dogs, when led to the midpoint of a track and started at right angles to it, chose the correct direction in only 47% of the trials. He concluded that the correct determination of track direction by the dogs was probably based on little more than chance. Other disappointing reports confirmed that the directional choice appeared to be based on statistical chance (Morrison, 1980; Schwartz, 1980). Similar results were found by MacKenzie and Schultz (1987), who tested 22 dogs trained to track but not trained to determine the direction of the track. Although six of the dogs exhibited perfect scores, the overall statistical picture for the group of dogs as a whole was not much better than random chance.

In contrast to these earlier difficulties with directional tracking, Steen and Wilsson (1990) found that professional tracker dogs can reliably choose the right direction on the basis of olfactory information alone. The researchers laid 50-m tracks on grass and on an asphalt airstrip. After 20 to 30 minutes, the dogs were brought to the track, faced in a perpendicular direction relative to the track, and unleashed. The dogs reliably determined the correct direction of the track.

Thessen and colleagues (1993) have confirmed the earlier findings of Steen and Wilsson with dogs previously trained for directional tracking. They tested German shepherd tracking dogs on fresh tracks 20 minutes old on grass and 3 minutes old on concrete (10 trials per dog on each surface). The dogs were equipped with a remote microphone and transmitter that recorded sniffing sounds. Other movements were recorded by a video recorder. The researchers found that directional tracking involves three distinct phases. (1) A searching phase during which the dogs moved and sniffed rapidly. The dogs sniffed at a rate of approximately 6 times per second during all phases. (2) A deciding phase characterized by slower movements and longer sniffing periods and with the dog's nose placed closer to the ground. The deciding phase lasted 3 to 5 seconds and involved the dogs sniffing at two to five footprints before choosing a direction. (3) A tracking phase involved more active movement and sniffing, similar to those observed during the searching phase.

Steen and Wilsson (1990) have hypothesized that a dog's ability to determine the direction of the track depends on a comparison of olfactory concentrations emanating from consecutive steps, thereby forming an olfactory intensity gradient. If this is true, it empirically confirms the incredible power of the dog's nose:

> If we assume that each footprint smelled the same at the moment it was set, and that the scent evaporated at a constant rate, we can get an idea of the dogs' sense of smell. We walked at a rate of one step per second and tracks were 30 min (1800 s) old when the dogs were tested. The smell from one print should therefore theoretically be 1/1800 stronger than that of the foregoing. This indicates that the dogs were highly sensitive to an odour difference of this magnitude. (Steen and Wilsson, 1990:534)

As extraordinary as these numbers seem at first glance, most trails in nature are far older and demand even greater sensitivity for determining their directionality than required by the experimental arrangements producing the above estimates.

William Carr and associates (Blade et al., 1996; Miller et al., 1996) at Beaver College (Glenside, PA) have studied various factors believed to influence the acquisition of directional tracking. Of particular interest is testing the intensity-gradient hypothesis proposed by Steen and Wilsson. The intensity-gradient hypothesis presumes that dogs can detect a difference of polarity/intensity existing between successive steps made by a track layer, possibly because the scent associated with the preceding step has undergone perceptible diminishment relative to the scent adhering to the succeeding step. To test this hypothesis, they have performed a number of directional tracking experiments comparing the dog's performance on normal and polarity-enhanced tracks.

In one experiment, two previously trained dogs were tested (Blade et al., 1996). One of them was tested on a normal track laid at a rate of 1 step per second. The second dog received identical testing but on a polarity-enhanced track laid at a rate of 1 step per 10 seconds. This was accomplished by the track layer resting upon a walker and holding the trailing step up for 10 seconds before stepping down again. The operative assumption here is that an increased delay between successive steps would make it easier for dogs to detect differences between them, perhaps as the result of scent dissipation or some unknown qualitative change in the scent picture. As expected from previous experiments, the first dog responded correctly on 14 of 20 trials, whereas the second dog, working on the polarity-enhanced track, responded correctly in 17 of 20 trials—a 21% improvement over this dog's previous score on a normal 1 step/second track. In another experiment (Miller et al., 1996), the interval between critical steps at the choice point was increased to 80 seconds between steps. This arrangement resulted in correct directional choices in 80% to 90% of trials. These experiments appear to confirm the earlier findings of Steen and Wilsson regarding a trained dog's ability to determine the direction of track above chance levels of significance, as well as provide significant evidence supporting the intensity-gradient theory of directional tracking.

VOMERONASAL ORGAN

The vomeronasal organ (VNO) is a specialized sensory apparatus located in the anterior portion of the palate, with ducts opening into the mouth just behind the front teeth. The organ is an elongated pouchlike structure that is lined with olfactory receptor cells. These cells are similar to those found in the olfactory mucosa except that they use microvilli instead of cilia. Scent information received by these receptor cells is projected via the accessory olfactory bulb (AOB) directly into the limbic system (amygdala and medial hypothalamus). Although there is some overlap between the olfactory system and the VNO, the latter is particularly well suited for the detection of pheromone molecules of a higher weight than reliably detected by olfaction (Cain, 1988). This difference makes the VNO more sensitive for the detection of nonvolatile chemical messages deposited in the urine and other bodily secretions. An important function of the VNO is the detection and subcortical analysis of these sexual pheromones. Destruction of the VNO results in the loss of normal sexual activities and several other vital functions (e.g., maternal care, aggressiveness, and secretion of sex hormones) in many mammals.

Although dogs do not exhibit the "lip curl" flehmen response observed in other mammals, many dogs do exhibit an analogous response called *tonguing*. When tonguing, the dog's tongue is pushed rapidly against the roof of the mouth, with the teeth sometimes chattering and expressing profuse foam sometimes collecting on the upper lip. Tonguing is frequently observed after a dog licks a urine spot or "tastes the air," following the exchange of mutual threat displays between two rival males. As the antagonists separate, one or the other may project his nose upward and initiate rhythmic sniffing and tonguing movements. The tonguing dog may actually extrude his tongue slightly in an effort to collect a sample. There is often a wide retraction of the lips together with a slight elevation of the muzzle. This action is accompanied by several brief sniffs and wide searching side-to-side movements of the head.

Eccles (1982) showed that the VNO in cats is regulated by the autonomic nervous system. He studied the flehmen response in cats, discovering that the vomeronasal pouch or lumen suctions or expels depending on current sympathetic or parasympathetic stimulation. Under parasympathetic tone, the organ is constantly flushing and developing droplets around vomeronasal ducts. These droplets absorb airborne odorant or tastant samples that are then conducted via a sympathetic-induced pumping action into the lumen of the organ. After the odorant/tastant is sampled, it is expelled with a vigorous flushing action, thus clearing the organ and preparing it for another sample.

Whether dogs exhibit a true flehmen response remains controversial, with many authorities believing that dogs do not display the pattern (Bradshaw and Nott, 1995), although some canid species (e.g., the coyote, side-striped jackal, and bushdog) do appear to exhibit a flehmen response (Ewer, 1973). Overall (1997) suggested that the vomeronasal complex lacks functionality altogether, noting that the vomeronasal sacs are without chemoreceptors. This is clearly not the case, though, according to Adams and Wiekamp, who identified several types of receptors in the vomeronasal epithelium and concluded that the canine VNO is "highly developed and unique amongst that of adult mammals" (1984:781). In addition, Salazar and coworkers (1992, 1994) described vomeronasal nerves and traced their destination to glomeruli in the accessory olfactory bulb. Although the VNO system may be less well developed in dogs than in some other animals (e.g., rats and cats), it is a functional organ of some importance to dogs. Unfortunately, the significance of VNO information for dogs is not known, but it likely serves some functional role in the exchange of pheromone information about social status and the animal's reproductive state.

Some preliminary evidence supporting a sexual function for the VNO system has been found in the study of the wolf's response to methyl p-hydroxybenzoate, a sexual pheromone. Klinghammer (unpublished data, personal communication) has discovered an intriguing phenomenon involving this pheromone among wolves. During the breeding season, captive wolf subordinates may court and mount an estrous female without interference from the alpha male, that is, until he detects the presence of this important sexual releasing hormone, at which point he actively defends his rights of exclusivity. The appearance of methyl p-hydroxybenzoate in a female wolf's uterine secretions apparently coincides with ovulation and

standing heat. The compound has also been found in the estrous secretions of female dogs and has been shown to elicit sexual arousal and mounting behavior in males when applied to the vulvas of spayed females (Goodwin et al., 1979).

GUSTATION

The ability to taste depends on the activation of gustatory receptor cells concentrated in the taste buds. The taste buds are found in various papillae (foliate, fungiform, and circumvallate to name the most common) that are distributed over the surface of the dog's tongue. Taste buds contained in the fungiform papillae are located on the anterior two-thirds of the tongue and transmit gustatory information via the chorda tympani, a branch of the facial nerve (seventh cranial nerve). The posterior third of the tongue is associated primarily with the circumvallate papillae, which are innervated by the lingual branch of the glossopharyngeal nerve (ninth cranial nerve). Both the seventh and ninth cranial nerves form central synapses in the nucleus of the solitary tract located in the medulla. Ascending pathways are relayed from the solitary tract via the pontine nucleus to the ventral posteromedial (VPM) nucleus of the thalamus and then to higher somatosensory cortical areas associated with the conscious experience of taste. Another pathway from the pontine nucleus carries taste information via the lateral hypothalamus, amygdala, and basal forebrain areas. These subcortical pathways may be involved in the production of affective qualities associated with taste and the memory processes underlying taste aversions. In addition, some investigators have theorized that taste input to the lateral hypothalamus mediates the reinforcing effects of food (Shepherd, 1983; Carlson, 1994).

Taste buds are normally washed in a coating of saliva stimulating a baseline or zero firing rate. When stimulated with a chemical tastant, the taste receptor is either excited or inhibited. In both cases, a taste sensation is generated. In dogs, the most common receptors are those excited by sugar and various sweet-tasting amino acids. Substances like citric acid also act on these same sweet taste receptors by inhibiting their rate of firing and thereby producing a sensation similar to what humans experience as sourness.

Similar papillae and taste buds in humans are specialized for the preferential detection of sugar (tip of the tongue), salt (to the front and side), sour (along the sides), and bitter (toward the back). Several taste studies reviewed by Kitchell (1976) indicated a similar localization pattern of taste receptors on the dog's tongue. The available evidence indicates that salty, sugary, and sour tastes are localized toward the front two-thirds of the tongue, while gustatory responses to bitter tastes are located toward the rear third of the tongue. Although the various taste qualities are most strongly responded to in these specific areas, taste sensations are not site exclusive but may be detected in various degrees and qualities over the surface of the tongue (Shepherd, 1983). There exists some disagreement in the literature regarding a dog's ability to taste salt. For example, according to Kitchell, several studies have demonstrated that dogs have a clear gustatory response to salt. In opposition to this view, Boudreau (1989) found that dogs totally lack salt-specific taste receptors. He noted that the ability to taste salt is common among mammals, especially herbivores, who need to find it in order to supplement a salt-deficient vegetarian diet. Since the carnivorous diet is already salt balanced, dogs (and cats) presumably have no need to seek salt in the environment and therefore do not possess the necessary taste capabilities for its detection. Interestingly, dogs are unique among many mammals studied in that dogs can taste furaneol, a sweet flavor found in fruits. Boudreau has speculated about the evolutionary function of the dog's ability to taste furaneol in terms of its omnivorous eating habits:

> Besides being intensely sweet, this compound also has a fragrant odor and is a character impact compound for many fruits. It is believed that this furaneol taste system is specific for fruit and is linked with the seed dispersing function of the dog. The presence of this taste system and its absence is readily detectable in the natural eating behavior of canines and felids. In a natural environment canines will supplement their small animal diet with fruit of the season, unlike felids. (1989:136)

The differentiation of tastes is biologically significant in terms of the animal's search for nutrients and the avoidance of poisons. Sour tastes may be used to estimate the relative acid/alkaline content of a food item, perhaps determining thereby its state of decay and available nutritive value. Dogs are especially sensitive to bitter substances, a biologically prepared tendency that may have survival value, since poisonous items are frequently bitter (Thompson, 1993). Like olfactory receptor cells, the taste buds are frequently replaced with new ones approximately every 10 days (Shepherd, 1983). Also, taste shares olfaction's sensitivity to the effects of habituation and adaptation, perhaps accounting for the dog's preference for novel food items over more familiar ones.

Taste has been much less studied than olfaction. It is known, however, that gustation is a precocious sense, being present in neonatal puppies at the time of birth and probably before. This has been confirmed by both conditioned-response testing (Stanley et al., 1963) as well as by direct measurement of nerve activity caused by gustatory stimulation (Ferrell, 1984a). Ferrell recorded the gustatory response of several puppies by inserting electrodes into the chorda tympani nerve bundle and then exposing them to various kinds of sugar. She found that puppies exhibited a stronger gustatory response to fructose than to other sugar flavors sampled (xylose, lactose, maltose, sucrose, and glucose). Interestingly, she found an almost equal spike occurring in the record when the pups' were exposed to distilled water. The gustatory response to fructose in neonatal puppies was found to be comparable to that of adult dogs.

The experience of flavor and taste preference depends on a composite of olfactory and gustatory factors, as well as past experience and learning. Garcia and colleagues (1966) found that intense and lasting taste aversions can be readily established toward a novel food item if its ingestion is followed by the induction of nausea. Such *taste aversions* occur even if nausea is induced after a delay of an hour or more. Pavlov (1927) reported an experiment performed by Zitovich that suggested that learning may play an important role in the development of food preferences. The subjects were puppies that had been taken away from their mother and hand reared. They were fed only milk for a "considerable" period of time. A fistula was implanted in the pups' salivary ducts to measure salivation output. When the puppies were finally shown food (meat or bread), they failed to exhibit a salivary response to the sight or smell of it. It was only after the puppies were encouraged to eat solid food that they began salivating in response to the sight or smell of such food.

Food preference is a somewhat complicated matter, involving four broad factors: genetic preparedness to recognize the sample as a potential food item, past experience with the food item, palatability of the food item, and its novelty. Kuo (1967) reported a study in which he removed chow puppies from their mothers at birth and divided them into three feeding groups: Group 1 was reared exclusively on a soy diet. Group 2 was fed a fruit and vegetable diet. Group 3 was sustained on a diet containing a variety of plant and animal ingredients. The various diets were supplemented with vitamins, minerals, and salt. Very young puppies were fed a liquid diet by hand and progressively moved to solid food as they matured. Kuo found that each group developed a specific preference for the food toward which it was accustomed. For instance, group 2 pups were familiar only with fruit and vegetable foods and refused to eat meat when offered it at 6 months of age. Group 1 pups were equally selective, refusing all food other than that made of soy. A puppy belonging to group 3 would readily eat almost any food offered to him. Kuo concluded that dogs exposed to limited novelty tend to develop exclusive preferences for familiar foods. Mugford (1977) reported conflicting results involving basenji and terrier puppies. He introduced puppies to assigned foods at weaning, maintaining them on those same food items for 16 weeks before testing. He found that two primary factors influenced food preferences: (1) preference was highly

influenced by the relative palatability of the food (e.g., moistness), and (2) a lack of previous exposure to the food item (novelty) increased a puppy's preference for it. More specifically, he determined that novelty without palatability produced a short-term preference, whereas novelty plus a high degree of palatability produced a more long-term shift in preference. These results appear to contradict those of Kuo. Contrary to Kuo, Mugford found that puppies fed a restricted diet *preferred* novel foods over familiar ones. It should be noted, however, that an important independent variable differed between these two experiments: Kuo removed the puppies from their mother at birth, whereas Mugford waited until after weaning to do so. Apparently, prior to weaning, young dogs may be especially prone to develop lasting preferences for familiar food items, whereas such preferences may be more flexible after weaning.

A potential factor influencing taste preference overlooked by both of these studies is the possible role of fetal taste experiences. Some evidence suggests that the fetus may taste or swallow amniotic fluids, and Cain (1988) noted that these prenatal gustatory experiences may have an important effect on the development of taste preferences. For example, Smotherman (1982) found that an increased preference for apple juice by adult rats could be produced by exposing fetal rats to a solution of apple juice injected into the amniotic fluids shortly before birth (day 20 of gestation). As adults, the rats were tested and compared with regard to their relative appetites for apple juice, maple syrup, or tap water. Rats exposed to in utero apple juice solution exhibited a distinct preference for apple juice as adults. Interestingly, Smotherman also found that the treated rats were significantly less reactive (i.e., exhibited less pituitary-adrenal activity) to stressful stimulation as adults than were fetal controls injected with saline water. Also, Pedersen and Blass (1982) obtained additional evidence for the development of such prenatal preferences by exposing rat fetuses to citral (a tasteless lemon scent). Pups that had been exposed to citral in utero and again immediately after birth were attracted to nipples coated with the scent. However, control pups that had been (1) exposed in utero only, (2) immediately after birth only, or (3) not exposed at all were not attracted to the nipples washed with citral. This study suggests that both prenatal and postnatal influences interact in combination to affect certain preferences.

Galef and Henderson (1972), who studied the food preferences of weanling rats, were particularly interested in determining the extent to which the mother's dietary intake influenced her young's preferences in food. They found that cues associated with food eaten by the lactating female are passed along (probably) through milk. Weanling rats tended to preferentially seek out food that the mother had eaten during lactation, even though it was less palatable than other food made available at the same time. The researchers pointed out that many substances—including antibiotics, sulfonamides, alkaloids, salicylates, bromides, quinine, alcohol, nicotine, DDT, and amphetamines (to name just some)—pass directly from the mother's milk into her suckling puppies. Additionally, they referred to a study by Ling and colleagues (1961) in support of the notion that complex taste and smell molecules associated with the mother's food may be passed into her milk. Ling and his associates found that the flavor of cow's milk is influenced by the sort of food eaten by her. Galef and Henderson concluded that it is reasonable to assume that taste preferences for specific foods are acquired (to some extent) through taste cues provided in the mother's milk prior to an animal's first experience with solid food.

Weanling puppies (2 to 4 months of age) are able to display a pronounced appetitive preference between foods containing as little as a 2% to 4% difference in fructose versus sucrose content. Moistened food containing 17% fructose is much more attractive than the same food containing 15% sucrose sweetening (Ferrell, 1984b). Other studies have shown that dogs exhibit a preference for cooked meat over raw (preferring beef over pork, lamb, chicken, and horsemeat—in that order) and sweetened foods. Dogs rendered anosmic still prefer sweetened foods and meat over dry food but do not exhibit the same range of preference for individual meats that smelling dogs do (Houpt, 1991). Dogs are especially fond of dairy products like cheese and butter. In addition to identifying preferred food items, taste mobilizes the gastrointestinal system to secret appropriate digestive juices. Both gastric acid and pancreatic enzyme secretions are differentially increased by direct taste stimulation of the dog's tongue (Powers et al., 1990).

Although dogs may have a preference for highly palatable and novel food, they can be persuaded to tolerate and thrive on a monotonous daily ration of dry food and fresh water. Acquiescing to a dog's novelty demands usually results in a finicky eater and what Fogle (1987) has aptly termed *starvation games*. One dog that I recall was so manipulative that he successfully trained his owner to feed him nothing but cheese steaks (less the rolls), a diet that may have played a significant physiological role in the dog's development of heightened irritability and aggressive behavioral problems (Mugford, 1987; Dodman et al., 1994). Dogs exposed to diets filled with daily novelty become progressively finicky and harder to please. Flavor-enhanced feeding and between-meal snacks, though highly desirable from a dog's viewpoint, may cause a dog to overeat and develop a weight problem. A recent survey performed by Kienzle and colleagues found that obese dogs often belong to obese owners who tend to "interpret their dog's every need as a request for food" (1998:2780S). Also, such dogs may become dangerously possessive over the desired food item when it is presented. Most finicky dogs will come around and eat what is presented to them after a day or two of hunger. A dog that has lost interest in food as the result of congestion or other olfactory dysfunction can be encouraged by putting food in the dog's mouth, thereby directly stimulating the taste buds and possibly eliciting appetitive interest (Hart and Hart, 1985).

SOMATOSENSORY SYSTEM

The dog's body is equipped with a variety of receptors sensitive to stimuli impinging on the skin or arising from within the body itself. Specific receptors have evolved for the detection and measurement of pressure, vibration, heat and cold, chemicals, and various noxious stimuli. In addition, internal receptors sensitive to joint location, muscle stretch, and tendon tension provide kinesthetic information about the relative location, direction, and action of the body. In combination, these highly specific sensory organs provide a tremendous amount of information about the external and internal environment and a dog's moment-to-moment orientation within it.

Dogs exhibit significant differences with respect to their individual responses to somatosensory stimulation. Some dogs are much more sensitive to touch than are others. Thresholds for stimulation are profoundly affected by an individual dog's emotional state, general physical condition, and past experience (learning). For example, fearful or hypervigilant dogs will likely respond to nociceptive stimulation at a much lower level of intensity than dogs that are relaxed and confident. Fearful dogs are also more likely to exhibit emotionally reactive behavior when stimulated. Similarly, dogs suffering from disease or deprivation may show significant changes in their relative responsiveness to certain kinds of stimulation. Hypothyroidism, for example, may cause affected dogs to seek warmth and avoid cold areas. Likewise, hungry dogs are more alert to stimuli associated with the acquisition of food. Somatosensory responsiveness is also significantly influenced by experience. A dog's response to stimulation may be decreased or increased depending on the presence or absence of previous habituating or sensitizing exposure to the evoking stimulus. The amount of past socialization received by a dog will also influence how that dog interprets and responds to tactile stimulation. Well-socialized dogs, for example, will more likely accept and respond in a friendly way to petting and hugs, whereas undersocialized dogs may only begrudgingly tolerate such tactile contact—if at all. Although the way in which dogs ultimately interpret and respond to sensory input is highly variable and dependent on many factors, the manner in which sensory input is obtained from the impinging external and internal environment follows a regular pattern of processing.

Mechanoreceptors

The largest sensory organ in the body is the skin, which contains numerous receptors adapted and specialized for the reception of specific sensory input. There are five basic categories of somatosensory receptors in the skin: nociceptors (associated with noxious or painful stimulation), proprioceptors (sensitive to body movement and position), thermoreceptors (responsive to heat and cold), chemoreceptors (sensitive to chemical stimulation), and mechanoreceptors (sensitive to physical changes, twisting, stretching, and pressure). Mechanoreceptors are the most numerous receptors in skin. At the base of each hair follicle, for example, is a group of pressure-sensitive hair-follicle receptors that are activated whenever the hair is disturbed by external movements that cause the surrounding tissue to stretch or bend. Follicle receptors of special importance to dogs are those associated with the vibrissae or whiskers located at various points on the face. The vibrissae provide dogs with information about nearby objects, coordinate the movement of the muzzle and mouth toward nearby objects, and may serve an important protective function against ocular injury by avoiding accidental collisions. In addition to direct mechanical stimulation, the vibrissae are responsive to vibrations and the subtle movement of air currents. The sensory information from the vibrissae is especially important for rats and cats. As noted in Chapter 3, Welker (1973) categorized rats as *feelers*, stemming from their extraordinary reliance on their whiskers for survival. In addition to indicating the presence of a nearby object to rats while in darkness, the vibrissae also appear to provide supplemental information about its shape, texture, and distance (Bear et al., 1996). An interesting possible cause of reflexive aggressive behavior occasionally exhibited by some dogs to a puff of air blown into their face may be related to a species-typical defensive reaction mediated by vibrissae. During combat between dogs, vibrissae may provide information about the opponent's close location and movements, perhaps mediating some measure of defense through the reflexive organization of combative behavior. Motile vibrissae on the muzzle quickly flare and reorient in a forward direction when a dog is aggressively aroused, suggesting that they play some functional role. Sensory information originating in the face, including receptors associated with the vibrissae, is conducted by the trigeminal nerve. In addition to providing mechanoceptive and proprioceptive information about the face and jaw, the trigeminal nerve is an important conduit for the transmission of chemoceptive information resulting from the chemical stimulation of the nasal and oral mucosa (e.g., the nonolfactory sensation of alcohol vapor to the nose or the burning sensation it produces if placed on the tongue).

A number of other mechanoreceptors have been identified in the skin of mammals (Martin and Jessell, 1991). The skin is composed of two layers: the dermis and the epidermis. In the epidermal layer, a pressure-sensitive and slowly adapting receptor known as Merkel's receptor is found. Merkel's receptors respond to indentations produced near the surface of the skin. In humans, specialized pressure and vibration receptors are located in the elevated ridges of the epidermis, forming fingerprints. These Meissner's corpuscles are responsive to both touch and low-frequency vibrations (50 Hz). Meissner's corpuscles exhibit an extremely small receptive field and are employed to form fine tactile discriminations. Unlike Merkel's receptors, Meissner's corpuscles are rapidly adapting.

Deeper within the dermis are other pressure receptors called pacinian corpuscles. These onionlike structures are composed of several concentric layers of connective tissue that variably respond according to the amount of pressure applied to them. Pacinian corpuscles are responsive to a large receptive field involving both pressure and vibration but in a higher frequency range than observed in Meissner's corpuscles, approximately 200 to 300 Hz. They respond quickly and rapidly adapt to continuous stimulation. Other mechanoreceptors located in the dermis are Ruffini's corpuscles. Like pacinian corpuscles, Ruffini's corpuscles exhibit a relatively large receptive field. Unlike pacinian corpuscles, however, Ruffini's corpuscles are much slower to adapt to long periods of continuous stimulation.

Nociceptors

Nociceptors are free, unmyelinated (bare) nerve endings in the skin and body that respond to noxious stimulation that either damages or threatens to damage body tissue. The subjective experience of nociception is pain. Painful stimulation elicits species-typical escape reactions that serve to separate the organism from the source of noxious stimulation. Nociceptors are divided into four types, depending on the source of stimulation: mechanical (responds to sharp pressure), thermal (extremes of burning heat or freezing cold), chemical (stinging sensation of ammonia or pepper), and polymodal (nociceptors that combine sensitivity to a combination of mechanical, thermal, and chemical stimuli).

Pain results from the stimulation of nociceptive nerve endings terminating on the skin's surface and enervating most of the body's major organ systems. In addition to the direct stimulation of these specialized receptors, traumatic stimulation may also cause local tissue damage and the rapid release of pain-enhancing hormones, such as prostaglandin. The secretion of prostaglandin sensitizes nociceptive nerve endings to histamine—an inflammatory by-product of cell damage (Carlson, 1994). Aspirin and other anti-inflammatory medications produce their analgesic effects by disrupting the production of prostaglandins. Pain information is relayed along two pathways: a fast pain system and a slow pain system (Thompson, 1993). The fast pain system informs the brain immediately of the traumatic event ("Yelp!") followed by the slow pain system (throbbing, aching, and burning sensations), which maintains the feeling of constant painful sensation—even though the original stimulus has been removed. The fast pain system terminates in two thalamic nuclei: the ventrobasal complex (also associated with touch and pressure) and the posterior nucleus. From these thalamic nuclei, the impulse is relayed to the cerebral cortex. The slow pain system passes through the reticular formation and projects to the hypothalamus and the limbic system (amygdala)—areas involved in the emotional interpretation of pain and the motivation of flight-freeze-fight reactions. The fast pain system is limited to surface nociception (the skin and mucosa) and is a more recent evolutionary development than the slow pain system, which services all bodily tissue except the brain, which is not sensitive to pain.

One effect of the slow pain system is the production of endorphins (a contraction of endogenous morphine). Endorphins are peptides (short protein molecules) produced by the brain in response to slow pain, pressure, and touch. Endorphins are also produced by the pituitary gland (beta-endorphins), which are released into the bloodstream together with other hormones such as adrenocorticotropic hormone (ACTH) as part of the general adaptation stress response. Endorphins circulate throughout the brain to various opioid receptor sites, including the hypothalamus, amygdala, and intralaminar thalamic nuclei. Interestingly, the fast pain system bypasses the emotional and motivational centers associated with avoidance learning and aggression. The fast pain system is a pure pain/startle reaction relayed directly to the cerebral cortex. It is not affected by endorphin activity or the effect of morphine. Naloxone, a molecule resembling morphine in many details, is an active antagonist of morphine and endorphins. Naloxone has little obvious effect on an animal, but it binds with opioid receptors in the brain. Consequently, the complementary pain-reducing and pleasure-enhancing effects of increased opioid activity are impeded. Naloxone is commonly used as a medication for the temporary management of some compulsive behavior disorders (Brown et al., 1987; Dodman et al., 1988), presumably based on the assumption that such disorders are, at least partially, mediated by the endogenous opioid system.

Proprioceptors

Proprioceptive sensitivity is essential for the smooth locomotor functioning of the body. The perception of the body's orientation in

space and its coordinated movements are under the control of various brain centers, including the sensory motor cortex and cerebellum. Sensory information mediating this process is produced by proprioceptors located in the muscles and joints. These receptors provide fast moment-to-moment information about the body's movements and its orientation relative to the location of its different parts. There are two common proprioceptors: muscle spindles and Golgi tendon organs. Muscle spindles respond to the rate and amount of stretching that the working muscle undergoes. (Incidentally, stretch-sensitive receptors in the detrusor muscle of the bladder send signals indicating that the bladder is full and needful of evacuation.) Golgi tendon organs measure the amount of force being exerted by the muscle on the tendon. In addition, many other mechanoreceptors located in the surrounding connective tissue provide information about physical changes in the joint, including angle and velocity of movement. Besides providing information about the body's orientation and movement, proprioceptors also provide sensory information about the external world resulting from the physical manipulation of objects.

Balance

In addition to proprioceptive information, the ability to coordinate bodily movement and balance is made possible by sensory information provided by two vestibular structures in the inner ear: the semicircular canals and the vestibular sacs. The semicircular canals are composed of three tubular structures extending from the cochlea and set at 90 degree angles to one another. The canals are filled with a fluid substance called endolymph that shifts in a direction opposite to the body's movement. The displacement of cochlear fluid during rotational movement causes hairlike receptors to bend, thereby generating a nerve impulse. During linear movement or while standing still, balance is controlled by information from the vestibular sacs (the utricle and saccule). These sacs contain a jellylike substance in which otoliths or tiny stones are suspended. Gravity pulls the otoliths against receptor hair cells that, in turn, produce signals about the relative position of the head to the line of gravity. Information from the semicircular canals and vestibular sacs is gathered in the vestibular nerve and relayed to the cerebellum and sensory motor cortex, where balance is finely coordinated.

Effects of Touch

Many studies have confirmed the enormous importance of touch for the ontogeny of normal emotional and social behavior. Harlow and Zimmerman (1959), for example, studied the comfort-seeking behavior of rhesus monkeys: Infant monkeys who had been separated from their biological mothers shortly after birth were offered two surrogate mother alternatives, one made of carpet and the other made of wire. The researchers found that the infant monkeys preferred surrogate mothers made of soft carpeting material and shunned artificial mothers made of wire, despite the fact that the wire surrogate provided milk whereas the carpet one did not. When Igel and Calvin (1960) replicated this experiment with puppies, they discovered that puppies also preferred a cloth nonlactating surrogate mother over a wire one that provided milk. In a series of experiments studying separation distress in puppies, Pettijohn and coworkers (1977) compared the effect of various stimulus conditions on the amount of distress vocalization exhibited by puppies that were briefly isolated from their mother and littermates (see Chapter 2). They found that separation distress vocalization was reduced by soft comfort objects (e.g., a piece of cloth), but food (novel and familiar) or hard play toys had no discernible effect on separation-related behavior. Curiously, the researchers also observed a decrease in distress when a mirror was put inside of the holding pen. Ostensibly, the puppies were comforted by viewing the image of themselves, and some even rubbed up against the mirror, apparently in a futile effort to make physical contact with the image.

The first systematic effort to quantify the calming effect of touch on dogs was performed by Gantt and coworkers (1966). Gantt observed that dogs in distress are calmed by social contact, exhibiting a significant decrease in both heart and respiratory rates while being petted. He referred to this phenomenon as the *effect of person.* Lynch and McCarthy (1969) reported that shock-elicited aversive arousal (as indicated by heart and respiratory rates) was reduced by petting. Also, they found that during classical conditioning, if the dogs were continuously petted during the preshock and postshock periods, heart rates were strongly dampened immediately before (anticipatory arousal) and after the shock was delivered (Lynch and McCarthy, 1967). Tuber (1986) noted the usefulness of massage, or what he calls the "soft exercise," for promoting calmness in dogs. He advised that training dogs to relax should be just as important as other training activities. Recently, Hennessy and colleagues (1998) reported evidence suggesting that it is not only petting but the way in which petting is done that yields the best effect on objective measures (e.g., cortisol levels) associated with reduced stress. The best results were obtained by utilizing deep muscle massage or long firm strokes of petting from the head to hindquarters. These findings underscore the value of massage for reducing stress in dogs. Massage and relaxation training have many applications in the management of dog behavior, especially in situations involving aversive emotional arousal.

Since Gantt's discovery, subsequent studies have shown that the effect of person is reciprocal, with humans also experiencing pronounced cardiovascular benefits from tactile contact with dogs (Katcher, 1981; Friedmann et al., 1983). Vormbrock and Grossberg (1988) confirmed previous studies indicating that petting causes a reduction of blood pressure in humans. In addition, they found that these physiological effects are not due to cognitive or conditioned associations but depend on direct tactile interaction between a person and a dog. The mere physical presence of a dog is insufficient; the dog must also be the object of petting to lower blood pressure (see Chapter 10).

Animals handled early in life exhibit many lasting benefits as the result of such exposure. Experiments with rats show that a minimum amount of preweaning handling results in increased vitality and activity levels, more confidence, and greater resistance to disease; handled subjects are larger and more socially dominant; and, finally, handling has a significant positive impact on learning and problem-solving abilities, as well as reducing reactive emotionality (Morton, 1968; Fox, 1971a). Puppies handled early in life appear to obtain many similar benefits (Fox, 1978).

Touch mediates a great deal of social communication between a dog and others with whom the dog comes into contact (Lynch, 1970). Most training efforts exploit hedonically pleasurable or aversive responses mediated by touch receptors. Dogs learn to value gentle petting as a reward and rough handling as a punishment. Touch is also an important modality of canine emotional expressiveness, whether it be a gentle lick on the chin, a casual pawing movement for attention, or a hard bite on the leg—the dog, too, understands the power of touch. Consequently, touch provides a basic medium for direct communication and intimate exchange based on analogous experiences of pleasure and pain shared by the human and the dog. Through the agency of touch, we develop an intuitive appreciation of dogs as emotional beings. Dogs react to our handling (whether positive or negative) in ways that are comparable to our own reactions undergoing similar stimulation. Humans and dogs appear to share an empathetic appreciation of one another through the modality of touch and tactile communication. Dogs cannot speak about how they feel, but they are, perhaps, more direct and transparent than virtually any human can be when communicating how they feel through the agency of physical posture, gesture, and various subtle movements and expressions of touch.

REFLEXIVE ORGANIZATION

Much of a dog's behavior is under the reflexive control of involuntary mechanisms. As discussed in Chapter 2, neonatal puppies exhibit a great variety of reflexes that are predominately geared to maintaining contact with the mother to secure basic survival needs. These early neonatal reflexes gradually disappear and are replaced by more centrally

controlled behaviors as puppies mature. Neonatal reflexive behavior has been carefully studied and cataloged (Fox, 1964). Understanding how the body's reflexes work was the primary emphasis of Sherrington's (1906) experimental work. He discovered that many of the dog's apparently voluntary behaviors were to some extent under the control of involuntary reflexive mechanisms. A dog's scratch reflex, for example, could be elicited by applying an electrical "itch" to its skin. Although mechanical and stereotypic, the scratch response was organized and well directed toward the source of the itch. What makes this noteworthy is that the dogs involved were decerebrate, having undergone previous surgeries to cut nervous pathways going to (afferent) or leaving (efferent) the brain. Other surprising abilities of decerebrate dogs included unsteady treadmill walking, withdrawal and crossed extensor reflexes to pain (the stimulated leg flexes while the opposing leg extends in order to push away from the noxious stimulus), and differential gustatory responses (a swallow reflex was elicited by milk whereas noxious substances were expelled).

The Russian physiologist Ivan Sechenov, the father of reflexology, made several discoveries about reflexive behavior that anticipated the findings of Sherrington. The following is a description of one of his famous experiments with frogs:

> Cut off the head of a frog and place the decapitated animal on the table. For a few seconds it seems to be completely paralyzed; but before a minute has passed you see that it has recovered and assumed the posture peculiar to the frog when in a state of rest on dry land: its hind legs are tucked under it and it supports itself on the front legs like a dog. If you leave it alone, or to be more precise, if you do not touch its skin, it will remain motionless for a very long time. But the moment you touch its skin, it starts and then resumes its quiet posture. Pinch it somewhat stronger and it will, in all likelihood, jump as if trying to escape from pain. (1863/1965:6–7)

The above reflex actions (and many others) do not require voluntary effort but result from the wiring of nervous connections between sensory receptors, motor neurons, and *interneurons* (a simple neural relay system) located in the brain stem and spinal cord.

Sherrington divided reflexive behavior into two broad categories: phasic and tonic. Phasic reflexes are those that occur quickly with a brief response, such as the patellar reflex (knee jerk). Tonic reflexes are those that involve sustained adjustments and equilibrating efforts over flexor/extensor dominance. An interesting example of tonic reflex action is thigmotaxis. Two instances of thigmotaxis can be readily observed in dogs. Fearful dogs tend to lean against their owner's body or may lay down on the ground as though pushing into it. This reaction is called positive thigmotaxis and is a common tonic reflex in fearful animals. Another example involves a dog's reaction to opposing pressure or force. Whenever a dog's body is pushed or pulled, the dog tends to react reflexively by responding in an opposing direction to the direction of the force applied to its body. Oppositional reflexes enable dogs to maintain physical equilibrium or to sustain a course of action when exposed to opposition. An especially common instance of this effect is seen when a dog pulls during walks, a tendency that is evoked by the owner's habit of pulling against the dog's forward movement. Such reflexive oppositional reactions explain why most trainers recommend that the leash be held in a slack manner and that the dog be corrected with a snapping action rather than a slow continuous pull.

Sherrington described several factors influencing the elicitation of reflexive action:

Threshold refers to the minimum stimulus intensity sufficient to elicit the reflex. A *high threshold* means that a relatively strong stimulus is needed to elicit a response, whereas a *low threshold* suggests that a relatively weak stimulus is needed to elicit a response. Altering response thresholds is an important part of effective behavior modification, especially involving emotional systems under the regulation of reflexive mechanisms.

Latency refers to the duration from the moment of stimulation to the onset of the reflexive action. Latency depends on the intensity of the stimulus involved and on the readiness of the animal to respond.

Irradiation refers to the tendency of an especially strong stimulus to elicit a generalized reaction extending to surrounding or associated neural systems.

Reciprocal inhibition neural systems refers to the tendency of elicited muscle actions to inhibit the actions of an opposite type. The elicitation of muscle reflexes involves three possible actions: flexion, extension, or a tonic combination of the two. Stimulating a group of muscles to flex causes the simultaneous inhibition of opposing extensor muscles. The concept of reciprocal inhibition was later adopted by Wolpe (1958) to describe the effect of counterconditioning and the process of systematic desensitization. Wolpe argued that relaxation/appetite and anxiety/fear are mutually exclusive affects that regulate each other through a mechanism of reciprocal inhibition—that is dogs cannot simultaneously feel anxious while relaxed or fearful while eating. The third characteristic of reciprocal inhibition (flexor/extensor tonic equilibrium) is analogous to situations in which opposing emotional alternatives are held in a stasis of conflict between the available options.

Fatigue occurs when repeated elicitation of a reflex action causes it to weaken or habituate. Habituation is the most basic form of learning observed in all animals from humans to sea snails.

Many basic biological functions are under the control of reflexive mechanisms. Although some reflexes can be influenced by voluntary efforts, most reflexes occur automatically, given the presence of a sufficiently salient stimulus. For instance, one can resist and possibly inhibit or slow the blink reflex elicited by touching the eyelashes, but it is much more difficult (if not impossible) to control pupillary constriction in the presence of bright light, stop salivation in the presence of food, or inhibit heart rate acceleration while in a fear-eliciting situation. Pavlov (1927) discovered that these sorts of behavioral and physiological events could be brought under the control of normally neutral stimuli through a conditioning process. The basic procedure was carried out by pairing the sound of a bell with the presentation of food. After a number of such contiguous pairings between the neutral stimulus (bell) and the unconditioned stimulus (food), the previously neutral bell becomes a conditioned stimulus that is able to elicit a conditioned response—that is, a response that is similar to the original or unconditioned response. As is discussed in Chapter 6, classical conditioning is an important tool in a trainer's armamentarium for managing and controlling dog behavior.

EXTRASENSORY PERCEPTION

Do dogs possess a sixth sense? Many authors writing to a popular audience, among them trainers, veterinarians, and behavioral consultants, have suggested that dogs may use information derived from sources other than the normal senses (Fox, 1972, 1981; Woodhouse, 1982; Vine, 1983; Campbell, 1986). These beliefs have been reinforced in the public's mind by animal psychics claiming to communicate with dogs telepathically and to perform extraordinary feats, ranging from locating lost pets (both dead and alive) to diagnosing behavioral and medical problems by psychically "talking" with the distressed animals. Such extraordinary abilities have not been successfully demonstrated under controlled laboratory conditions; nonetheless, they are widely held to be real abilities and supported by the testimonies of many satisfied customers. Some dog trainers, most notably Woodhouse (1982), claim that a very active telepathic linkage exists between trainer and dog:

> It is extraordinary how dogs pick up praise straight from your brain almost before you have time to put it into words. A dog's mind is so quick in picking up your thoughts that, as you think them, they enter the dog's mind simultaneously. I have great difficulty in this matter in giving the owners commands in class, for the dog obeys my thoughts before my mouth has had a chance to give the owner the command. (1982:72)

What makes such statements so difficult to accept without a high degree of skepticism is that such abilities would be so easy to confirm or disprove through a series of simple experiments. If confirmed, a whole new vista of human-animal communication would be opened up, but to the best of my knowledge such confirmation has not been obtained. Although impressive anecdotal evidence has been collected over the years, together with some inconclusive scientific evidence (especially by J. B. Rhine and colleagues at Duke University), overall the picture provides little in the way of confident support for the existence of extrasensory activity. Nothing seems very authoritative or conclusive about this literature, although defenders believe that it is enough to "prove" the existence of such phenomena (Bardens, 1987). Undoubtedly, subtle links of communication exist between humans and animals that are not fully understood, but these links are most probably examples of extraordinary senses and empathetic exchange rather than extrasensory mediation and arcane abilities.

Clever Hans

To study extrasensory perception (ESP) from a scientific viewpoint, one must approach it with the same methods and attitude used to investigate natural phenomena. In essence, this means that adequate experiments must be devised to test the claims of persons attributing events and experiences to paranormal causation. Without such investigation, no conclusions regarding such phenomena can be legitimately drawn.

The story of Clever Hans (Pfungst, 1911/1965) provides an edifying backdrop for appreciating the need for safeguards and a scientific method when studying such phenomena. Hans, a Russian trotting horse, belonged to Wilhelm von Osten, a retired German schoolteacher and amateur horse trainer. Von Osten appears to have honestly believed that he had discovered a training method for instructing animals to communicate on a more sophisticated level with humans. He was able to convince many critical observers of the legitimacy of his horse's extraordinary ability to tap out answers with his hoof to mathematical problems, and to respond to other questions posed to him. This latter feat was accomplished by von Osten assigning numerical values to letters, with which Hans could spell words by tapping out their numerical equivalence.

Hans's fantastic abilities were received with far-reaching international astonishment and interest. Various explanations were proposed to explain the horse's amazing abilities. Taken together, these accounts form a virtual monument to Ockham's razor (*Entia non sunt multiplicanda praeter necessitatem*: Entities are not to be multiplied beyond necessity) and the law of parsimony. These accounts ranged from trickery on the owner's part to telepathy. One of the scientific investigators of the Clever Hans phenomenon was O. Pfungst (1911/1965), who reported his observations in a book devoted to the subject. He described several of these theories, including one posited by a researcher (he refers to as a "natural philosopher") who wrote, "On the basis of most careful control, I have come to the conclusion, that the brain of the horse receives the thought waves which radiate from the brain of his master; for mental work is, according to the judgment of science, physical work" (1911/1965:28–29). This rather absurd concatenation of pseudoscience and mysticism echoes some of the current ways unexplained phenomena are explained in paranormal terms. The mystery of Clever Hans was finally solved when Pfungst demonstrated that the horse was actually responding to subtle cues emanating from his owner that told him when to stop tapping. The cues involved were slight and subtle upward head movements, barely perceptible upward movements of the eyebrows, and the flaring of the owner's nostrils. The size of the movements were estimated to be on the order of less than a millimeter and, in some instances, a mere deflection of one-fifth of a millimeter was accurately responded to by the horse.

Nora, Roger, and Fellow: Extraordinary Dogs

As Hans's fame spread through Europe, two dogs—Nora and Roger—also appeared on the scene, exhibiting fantastic abilities similar to those of Hans. Nora, a spaniel type, belonged to Emilio Rendich (an artist). After observing von Osten and Hans in action, the observant painter noted that von Osten constantly watched Hans's hoof tapping, while Hans, for his part, constantly observed his trainer. He surmised, like Pfungst, that Hans was responding to subtle cues emanating from his trainer: in particular, forward-leaning and backward-leaning movements. Also, Rendich believed that Hans had learned, more importantly, when to stop tapping rather than when to start. To test these hypotheses, using subtle forward and backward body movements as signals, he set out to train Nora (sometime before 1905) to paw and to stop pawing on cue. Reportedly, Nora could perform many of the same feats that Clever Hans exhibited (Candland, 1993).

In 1907, *Century Magazine* published an article titled "A Record of a Remarkable Dog," which was written about a dog named Roger under the pseudonym of B.B.E. Roger, a 3- to 4-year-old spaniel mix, came into B.B.E.'s possession with a history of trouble and problems. Before being adopted by B.B.E., Roger had been rejected from two previous homes as an "impossible" puppy. Withdrawn and depressed, Roger had apparently received some abusive treatment, but after 3 months of gentle handling, he gradually emerged and slowly began to exhibit an increased interest, attentiveness, and trust toward his new owner and surroundings. As his confidence improved, B.B.E. commenced efforts to educate him, starting with simple parlor tricks and progressing to more elaborate objectives as the dog's ability permitted. Roger proved to be a very intelligent and willing learner. For example, B.B.E. was able teach Roger to pick up individual playing cards from a pile of eight cards laid out in front of him. His method was crude but effective. He simply grasped Roger's paw and placed it over the selected card and then repeated its type and suit—for example, "That is the ace of clubs, Roger—ace of clubs." This was repeated four or five times. Roger was then given a cookie as a reward for his cooperation. Gradually, Roger learned to voluntarily place his paw on the selected card for which he would receive a treat.

B.B.E. carried out these training activities daily for 10-minute periods over 2 months. In the beginning, the correct card was kept in the same position, but as Roger's skills improved, it was placed in random locations relative to the other eight cards. After an additional month of training, Roger was taught to locate another card—this time, the ace of hearts. However, to B.B.E.'s amazement, Roger learned this new card trick after only a single trial of training. Subsequently, Roger learned to locate all eight cards in rapid succession, apparently having acquired a "learning set" that made variations of the task progressively more easy to learn. The next training goal was to teach Roger how to spell his name. This task was accomplished by placing Roger's paw sequentially on the various cards spelling out his name. Each trial was followed by the appropriate command "Where is the first letter?" and then "Where is the second?" and so on. Amazingly, Roger learned to spell his name within five or six sessions. B.B.E. also taught Roger how to add every combination of 2 up to 12. For example, B.B.E. would command "Show me 2 + 6" and would then place Roger's foot on the correct card containing the number 8. B.B.E. commented that Roger at this point in his education seemed never to forget, even after a single exposure. Finally, B.B.E. discovered to his great astonishment that Roger could spell "dog" and could even translate it into German (*hund*) and French (*chien*)—tasks that he had learned with no previous training!

B.B.E. performed a series of experiments to determine how Roger was performing these incredible feats of learning. In one of these experiments, he instructed Roger to add 2 + 3; however, instead of looking at the correct card, he looked at another card with the number 8 drawn on it. As he expected, Roger placed his foot on the card marked 8 instead of the one marked with the number 5. B.B.E. erroneously inferred from the evidence that Roger was responding to a visual image produced in his mind. He conjectured that this visual image was somehow unconsciously transmitted to the telepathically re-

ceptive dog: "All the time when he seemed to be learning rapidly, he had been simply getting the cards of which I thought" (B.B.E., 1907/1908:601). B.B.E. adopted the now familiar ESP explanation for his dog's remarkable abilities, speculating that he had tapped some previously unappreciated channel of interspecies communication with Roger:

> May it not be possible that between our minds and the minds of the lower animals there is a deep and quite subtle connection which may yet be explained in the future, but only by the use of the utmost sympathy and love? (1907/1908:602)

Century Magazine asked R. M. Yerkes of Harvard University to investigate. During Yerkes's initial observations of B.B.E. and Roger, he was unable to detect any obvious signals coming from B.B.E. that might explain the dog's extraordinary abilities. On a later occasion, however, following a 6-week separation between B.B.E. and Roger, Yerkes observed that B.B.E. did, in fact, provide Roger with subtle guidance. These movements were made more evident since Roger had been out of practice and apparently needed extra help. However, Yerkes (1907/1908) noted that "these movements were not readily seen by the observer when Roger is in practice and does his best. It is highly probable that the dog's visual sensitiveness to movement is greater than ours."

Another dog that attracted considerable fame and notoriety as the result of his remarkable learning abilities was a German shepherd named Fellow (Warden and Warner, 1928). The dog was owned and trained by J. Herbert, an avid fancier and breeder. Fellow appeared in a number of movies, playing the typical roles assigned to dogs during the 1920s. What made Fellow special among dogs was his reputed ability to understand over 400 different words, forming definite associations between them and specific objects, places, and actions. According to Warden and Warner, Herbert made no extraordinary claims about the possible operation of higher reasoning powers or extrasensory abilities underlying Fellow's proficiency at understanding commands. In fact, it was Herbert who contacted Warden and

Warner—both psychologists at Columbia University—to evaluate the extent of Fellow's accomplishments. The researchers conducted a number of tests with Fellow, concluding that he did possess most of the abilities attributed to him by his owner. In one series of tests, the experimenters and Herbert concealed themselves behind a screen from where commands were issued to Fellow. Even under such difficult conditions, the dog was still able to respond accurately to over 50 verbal commands of the type "Sit," "Down," "Take a walk," and "Step back." Although these so-called type I responses were readily performed by Fellow, other commands that required him to move toward some specific place or object—type II responses—were performed much more poorly and hesitatingly under such conditions. They observed that Fellow made few mistakes performing type II tasks (e.g., "Jump on the table," "Go and look out the window," and "Put your head on the chair") as long as he remained in full view of Herbert. However, when signaled to perform these same tasks from behind the screen, he made many more errors. Consequently, Warden and Warner performed an additional experiment to isolate the pertinent visual cues influencing Fellow's performance:

> It was now decided to make a deliberate attempt to confuse the dog, by having Mr. Herbert come from behind the screen and issue the commands, at the same time looking away from the place or object which the dog was supposed to approach in performing, with the following result:
>
> 1. "Go put your head on the chair"—dog jumps up on table at which Herbert is looking.
> 2. "Jump over the chair, good dog"—dog goes over to window at which Herbert is looking.
> 3. "Go over to the door"—approaches table at which Herbert is looking.
> 4. "Go over to the door, now I say"—goes to window slowly, toward which Herbert has turned.
> 5. "Go take a walk around the room"—dog goes to door at which Herbert is looking.
>
> Mr. Herbert was then blindfolded and the test repeated to see whether Fellow got his cue

from watching his master's eyes or from the general orientation of head and body. Similar results were now obtained showing that the latter factor is most likely the important one. (Warden and Warner, 1928:22–23)

These various tests and experiments confirmed that Fellow had attained an extraordinary ability to understand and respond to a variety of verbal and gestural cues. However, the most important question remains unanswered—How? According to Herbert, Fellow's successful training resulted from a regular practice of speaking to him "constantly almost from birth" onward in the manner of a parent to a child. Herbert claimed to have refrained from the use of corporal punishment, and only occasionally scolded Fellow when discipline was necessary. Unfortunately, little more was written about Herbert's accomplishment as a trainer and the finer details of his methodology.

Although the foregoing examples may lack the mystery and excitement of ESP, such extraordinary perceptual and learning abilities are of tremendous significance in themselves for an appreciation of the dog's perceptual abilities and the dog's relationship with humans. In all of the aforementioned cases involving extraordinary abilities, one factor seems to stand out above all others—the importance of close familiarity between the performing animal and human trainer. Hediger (1981), for example, argued persuasively in this regard that the crucial factor in Clever Hans's success was the high degree of familiarity existing between him and his trainer von Osten. Without the medium of intimate familiarity, unconscious gestures of such refinement as those employed by von Osten would never have been observed by the horse. Clearly, Hans's ability to read the unintentional cues of his trainer was an inadvertent outcome of the close relationship resulting from the training process itself and not dependent on extraordinary abilities or telepathy. Likewise, in the cases of Nora and Roger, a high degree of familiarity and affection was also evident, with B.B.E.'s revealing attribution of "sympathy and love" serving as a testimonial to the relevance of such factors in the development of remarkable animals. Finally, Herbert's method for instructing Fellow depended on close interaction and intimate communication between himself and the dog. These observations emphasize the relevance of enhanced affection, communication, and trust in the training process. Without such familiarity and affection-informing training activities, both dogs and trainers suffer a great loss. The dogs, on the one hand, will likely never reach their full potential and, on the other, the trainers are cheated of the full range of benefits and joy derived from affectionate companionship with dogs.

Extrasensory or Extrasensitive?

Although not all psychic phenomena can be explained by appealing to familiarity, intimacy, and affection; undoubtedly such factors do play a role in some forms of "telepathic" communication between intimate friends or human-animal companions in which the parties appear to know what each other is privately thinking or feeling without actually needing to communicate it directly. However, such connectedness may not depend so much on *extrasensory* abilities as it does on *extrasensitive* abilities. Many examples of animal ESP (e.g., amazing tales of psi trailing, anticipating important events like earthquakes before they occur, and experiencing the distress of a loved one suffering at a remote location) have been noted and discussed in various contexts, but to my knowledge none have fared very well under scientific scrutiny. Even though some experts in the field have expressed affirmative opinions concerning the possible existence of psychic phenomena, it remains a highly speculative area needful of much more research. Obviously, the many questions regarding ESP and animals are not going to be answered without such study. In the meanwhile, perhaps, the best one can do is maintain an open but critical mind with regard to such claims and phenomena.

Finally, it should be noted that at least some "paranormal" phenomena may be the result of sensory abilities not yet identified. For example, bats use echolocation to navigate around objects in their flight path and to locate prey insects, but before Griffin's discoveries concerning how this process actually worked, it remained unknown and liable to unprofitable speculation. The echolocating apparatus is incredibly sensitive. Even under conditions of pitch darkness, bats can recognize prey insects from similar nonprey insects on the basis of shape differences derived from echo information alone. Humans, too, can derive significant information from echoed sounds:

> Blind people, and blindfolded volunteers who have had considerable practice, can detect and classify objects in their vicinity by emitting audible sounds and hearing subtle differences depending on the presence of the object. But, curiously enough, many of the most proficient do not consciously recognize that they are accomplishing this by the sense of hearing. Instead they report that they simply feel that something is out there, and a common term for this ability is "facial vision." ... Nevertheless the feeling and the alleged "vision" cease almost totally if they can make no sounds or if their hearing is blocked. (Griffin, 1992:238)

It is not hard to see how these abilities could be wrongly interpreted as being the result of paranormal causation by persons wishing to interpret them as such. In addition to echolocation, many similar examples can be cited that testify to the phenomenal and varied sensory abilities of animals, including the fascinating dances of bees described by von Frisch, the remarkable migratory journeys of animals navigated by electromagnetic information, the infrared-radiation-sensing abilities of snakes, the electricity-sensing ability of some fishes, and the olfactory sensitivity of moths—many of these abilities might have been (and were) considered extrasensory 50 years ago and accounted for by various supernatural explanations instead of being recognized as belonging to the animal's special sensory accoutrements (Rhine and Pratt, 1957).

Perhaps dogs do possess some not fully understood extrasensory ability, but only scientific research will answer the question definitively one way or the other. Actually, all of the canine senses are capable of extraordinary sensitivity and incredible feats without resorting to extrasensory help. Besides the quality of the dog's inherited sensory abilities, ultimately the most influential factor in the actualization (or degeneration) of the dog's sensory and mental capacities is experience. Sensory abilities are both dynamic and conservative. Although they appear to remain the same from day to day, they actually change under the demands made upon them. These various changes are often slow and imperceptible, but changes do occur, educating the dog to see, hear, smell, taste, touch, and to move about with precise coordinated movements. The mind of the dog obtains a clear awareness of the environment through the effortful exercise and training of the senses. The refinement of sensory acuity and intelligence depends on these actualizing influences and the organizing functions provided by daily training and practice. Some experiences reported by scientific observers, though, simply cannot be so neatly explained, so I offer the following anecdote provided by Worden to remind the reader that the book is not yet closed on the issue of extrasensory perception in dogs:

> Belief in the popularly termed "sixth sense" of the dog is widespread, and one is always coming across almost incredible stories—told usually in an attempt to demonstrate the dog's "intelligence". It must be conceded that we have not as yet adequate explanations of homing behaviour or of many other surprising canine feats. I can add one bonafide case, in a Scottish terrier, Sheila, who was devoted to me and who remained with my parents at East Barnet from 1940 onwards, when she was seven years old, while I was working at Cambridge. As often as I could—but sometimes at intervals of some weeks—I would return home, or call in on my way to London, but my visits were usually unannounced, at different times of the day, and by any of a considerable number of local trains with which I had connected at Hatfield. Yet almost invariably Sheila would rise in pleasurable anticipation when the particular train bearing me was heard, some half a mile away, approaching the local station, and thereby inform my mother of my coming. There were over thirty stopping trains a day traveling in that direction. (1959:973)

REFERENCES

Adams DR and Wiekamp MD (1984). The canine vomeronasal organ. *J Anat*, 138:771–787.

Asa C, Mech LD, and Seal US (1985). The use of urine, faeces, and anal-gland secretions in scent-marking by a captive wolf (*Canis lupus*) pack. *Anim Behav*, 33:1034–1036.

Ashmead DH, Clifton RK, and Reese EP (1986). Development of auditory localization in dogs: Single source and precedence effect sound. *Dev Psychobiol*, 19:91–103.

Ashton EH, Eayrs JT, and Moulton DG (1957). Olfactory acuity in the dog. *Nature*, 179:1069–1070.

Axel R (1995). The molecular logic of smell. *Sci Am*, 273:154–159.

Bardens D (1987). *Psychic Animals*. New York: Henry Holt.

B.B.E. (1907–1908). Roger: A record of the performances of a remarkable dog. *Century Mag*, 59:599–602.

Beach FA, Beuhler MG, and Dunbar I (1983). Development of attraction to estrous females in male dogs. *Physiol Behav*, 31:293–297.

Bear MF, Connors BW, and Paradiso MA (1996). *Neuroscience: Exploring the Brain*. Baltimore: Williams and Wilkins.

Becker SC (1997). *Living with a Deaf Dog*. Cincinnati, OH: Susan Cope Becker.

Blackshaw JK, Cook GE, Harding P, et al. (1990). Aversive responses of dogs to ultrasonic, sonic and flashing light units. *Appl Anim Behav Sci*, 25:1–8.

Blade D, Miller EJ, Hamilton J, and Carr WJ (1996). Chemosensory directional tracking in companion dogs. Paper presented at the Eastern Psychological Association, Philadelphia, 30 March 1996.

Boudreau JC (1989). Neurophysiology and chemistry of mammalian taste systems. In R Teranishi, RG Buttery, and F Shahidi (Eds), *Flavor Chemistry: Trends and Developments*. Washington, DC: American Chemical Society.

Bradshaw JWS and Nott HMR (1995). Social communication behaviour of companion dogs. In J Serpell (Ed), *The Domestic Dog: Its Evolution, Behaviour, and Interactions with People*. New York: Cambridge University Press.

Brisbin IL and Austad SN (1991). Testing the individual odour theory of canine olfaction. *Anim Behav*, 42:63–69.

Brisbin IL and Austad SN (1993). The use of trained dogs to discriminate human scent: A reply. *Anim Behav*, 46:191–192.

Brown SA, Crowell-Davis S, Malcolm T, and Edwards P (1987). Naloxone-responsive compulsive tail chasing in a dog. *JAVMA*, 190:884–886.

Buck L and Axel R (1991). A novel multigene family may encode odorant receptors: A molecular basis for odor recognition. *Cell,* 65:175–187.

Cain WS (1988). Olfaction. In RC Atkinson, RJ Hernstein, G Lindsey, and RD Luce (Eds), *Stevens' Handbook of Experimental Psychology,* Vol 1: *Perception and Motivation.* New York: John Wiley and Sons.

Campbell WE (1986). *Owner's Guide to Better Behavior in Dogs and Cats.* Goleta, CA: American Veterinary Publications.

Campbell WE (1992). *Behavior Problems in Dogs.* Goleta, CA: American Veterinary Publications.

Candland DK (1993). *Feral Children and Clever Animals: Reflections on Human Nature.* New York: Oxford University Press.

Carlson NR (1994). *Physiology of Behavior.* Boston: Allyn and Bacon.

Chester Z and Clark WT(1988). Coping with blindness: A survey of 50 blind dogs. *Vet Rec,* 123:668–671.

Dodman NH, Reisner I, Shuster L, et al. (1994). The effect of dietary protein content on aggression and hyperactivity in dogs [Abstract]. *Appl Anim Behav Sci,* 39:185–186.

Dodman NH, Shuster L, White SD, et al. (1988). Use of narcotic antagonists to modify stereotypic self-licking, self-chewing, and scratching behavior in dogs. *JAVMA,* 193:815–819.

Dryden MW, Long GR, and Gaafar SM (1989). Effects of ultrasonic flea collars on *Ctenocephalides felis* on cats. *JAVMA,* 195:1717–1718.

Dunbar I and Carmichael M (1981). The response of male dogs to urine from other males. *Behav Neural Biol,* 31:465–470.

Eccles R (1982). Autonomic innervation of the vomeronasal organ of the cat. *Physiol Behav,* 28:1011–1015.

Edney ATB (1993). Dogs and human epilepsy. *Vet Rec,* 132:337–338.

Ewer RF (1973). *The Carnivores.* London: Weidenfeld and Nicolson.

Ferrell F (1984a). Gustatory nerve response to sugars in neonatal puppies. *Neurosci Biobehav Rev,* 8:185–190.

Ferrell F (1984b). Preference for sugars and non-nutritive sweeteners in young beagles. *Neurosci Biobehav Rev,* 8:199–203.

Fogle B (1987). *Games Pets Play.* New York: Viking.

Fox MW (1964). The ontogeny of behavior and neurologic responses in the dog. *Anim Behav,* 12:301–311.

Fox MW (1971a). *Behaviour of Wolves, Dogs and Related Canids.* New York: Harper and Row.

Fox MW (1971b). *Integrative Development of Brain and Behavior in the Dog.* Chicago: University of Chicago Press.

Fox MW (1972). *Understanding Your Dog.* New York: Coward, McCann and Geoghegan.

Fox MW (1978). *The Dog: Its Domestication and Behavior.* Malabar, FL: Krieger.

Fox MW (1981). *How to Be Your Pet's Best Friend.* New York: Coward, McCann and Geoghegan.

Fox MW and Bekoff M (1975). The behaviour of dogs. In ESE Hafez (Ed), *The Behaviour of Domestic Animals,* 3rd Ed, 370–409. Baltimore: Williams and Wilkins.

Friedmann E, Katcher AH, Thomas SA, et al. (1983). Social interaction and blood pressure: Influence of animal companions. *J Nerv Ment Dis,* 171:461–465.

Fuller JL and DuBuis EM (1962). The Behavior of Dogs. In ESE Hafez (Ed), *The Behaviour of Domestic Animals.* Baltimore: Williams and Wilkins.

Galef BG and Henderson PW (1972). Mother's milk: A determinant of the feeding preferences of weaning rat pups. *J Comp Physiol Psychol,* 78:213–219.

Gantt WH, Newton JE, Royer FL, and Stephens JH (1966). Effect of person. *Cond Reflex,* 1:146–160.

Garcia J, Ervin F, and Koelling RA (1966). Learning with prolonged delay of reinforcement. *Psychon Sci,* 5:121–122.

Goodwin M, Gooding KM, and Regnier F (1979). Sex pheromone in the dog. *Science,* 203:559–561.

Griffin DR (1992). *Animal Minds.* Chicago: University of Chicago Press.

Harlow HF and Zimmerman RS (1959). Affectional responses in the infant monkey. *Science,* 130:421–432.

Hart BL and Hart LA (1985). *Canine and Feline Behavioral Therapy.* Philadelphia: Lea and Febiger.

Hediger H (1981). The Clever Hans phenomenon from an animal psychologist's point of view. *Ann NY Acad Sci,* 364:1–17.

Heffner HE (1983). Hearing in large and small dogs: Absolute thresholds and size of the tympanic membrane. *Behav Neurosci,* 97:310–318.

Hemmer H (1990). *Domestication: The Decline of Environmental Appreciation.* Cambridge: Cambridge University Press.

Hennessy MB, Williams MT, Miller DD, et al. (1998). Influence of male and female petters on plasma cortisol and behaviour: Can human interaction reduce the stress of dogs in a public animal shelter? *Appl Anim Behav Sci,* 61:63–77.

Hepper PG (1986). Sibling recognition in the domestic dog. *Anim Behav,* 34:288–289.

Hepper PG (1988). The discrimination of human odor by the dog. *Perception,* 17:549–554.

Houpt KA (1991). *Domestic Animal Behavior.* Ames: Iowa State University Press.

Humphrey E and Warner L (1934). *Working Dogs.* Baltimore: Johns Hopkins Press.

Igel GJ and Calvin AD (1960). The development of affectional responses in infant dogs. *J Comp Physiol Psychol,* 53:302–305.

Jacobs GH, Deegan JF, Crognale MA, and Fenwick JA (1993). Photopigments of dogs and foxes and their implications for canid vision. *Vis Neurosci,* 10:173–180.

Kalmus H (1955). The discrimination by the nose of the dog of individual human odours and in particular of the odours of twins. *Brit J Anim Behav,* 3:25–31.

Karn HW (1931). Visual pattern discrimination in dogs [Master's thesis]. Pittsburgh: University of Pittsburgh Press [reported in Humphrey and Warner (1934)].

Karn HW and Munn NL (1932). Visual pattern discrimination in the dog. *J Genet Psychol,* 40:363–374.

Katcher HA (1981). Interactions between people and their pets: Form and function. In B Fogle (Ed), *Interrelations Between People and Pets.* Springfield, IL: Charles C Thomas.

Kienzle E, Bergler R, and Mandernach A (1998). A comparison of the feeding behavior and the human-animal relationship in owners of normal and obese dogs. *J Nutr,* 128:2779S–2782S.

King JE, Becker RF, and Markee JE (1964). Studies on olfactory discrimination in dogs: 3. Ability to detect human odour trace. *Anim Behav,* 7:311–315.

Kitchell RL (1976). Taste perception and discrimination by the dog. *Adv Vet Sci Comp Med,* 22:287–314.

Kleiman D (1966). Scent marking in Canidae. *Symp Zool Soc,* 18:167–177 [reported in Mech (1970)].

Krestel D, Passe D, Smith JC, and Jonsson L (1984). Behavioral determination of olfactory thresholds to amyl acetate in dogs. *Neurosci Biobehav Rev,* 8:169–174.

Kuo ZY (1967). *The Dynamics of Behavior Development: An Epigenetic View.* New York: Random House.

Landsberg G (1994). Products for preventing or controlling undesirable behavior. *Vet Med,* 89:970–983.

LeGuerer A (1994). *Scent: The Mysterious and Essential Powers of Smell.* New York: Kodansha International.

Lim K, Wilcox A, Fisher M, and Burns-Cox CJ (1992). Type 1 diabetics and their pets. *Diabetes Med,* 9(Suppl 2):S2–S4.

Ling ER, Kon SK, and Porter JWG (1961). The composition of milk and the nutritive value of its components. In SK Kon and AT Cowie (Eds), *Milk: The Mammary Gland and Its Secretion,* Vol 2. New York: Academic.

Lipman EA and Grassi JR (1942). Comparative auditory sensitivity of man and dog. *Am J Psychol,* 55:84–89.

Lynch JJ (1970). Psychophysiology and development of social attachment. *J Nerv Ment Dis,* 151:231–244.

Lynch JJ and McCarthy JF (1967). The effect of petting on a classically conditioned emotional response. *Behav Res Ther,* 5:55–62.

Lynch JJ and McCarthy JF (1969). Social responding in dogs: Heart rate changes to a person. *Psychophysiology,* 5:389–393.

Mackenzie SA and Schultz JA (1987). Frequency of back-tracking in the tracking dog. *Appl Anim Behav Sci,* 17:353–359.

Marshall DA and Moulton DG (1981). Olfactory sensitivity to alpha-ionone in humans and dogs. *Chem Senses,* 6:53–61.

Martin JH and Jessell TM (1991). Anatomy of the somatic sensory system. In JC Kandel, JH Schwartz, and TM Jessell (Eds), *Principles of Neural Science.* Norwalk, CT: Appleton and Lange.

McCartney W (1968). *Olfaction and Odours.* Berlin: Springer-Verlag.

Mech LD (1970). *The Wolf: The Ecology and Behavior of an Endangered Species.* Minneapolis: University of Minnesota Press.

Mekosh-Rosenbaum V, Carr WJ, Goodwin JL, et al. (1994). Age-dependent responses to chemosensory cues mediating kin recognition in dogs (*Canis familiaris*). *Physiol Behav,* 55:495–499.

Miller E, Houghton R, and Carr WJ (1996). Chemosensory tracking in dogs: Enhancing the track's polarity. *Chem Senses,* 20:743–744.

Miller PE and Murphy CJ (1995). Vision in dogs. *JAVMA,* 207:1623–1634.

Millot JL, Filiatre JC, Eckerlin A, et al. (1987). Olfactory cues in the relations between children and their pets. *Appl Anim Behav Sci,* 19:189–195.

Morris D (1986). *Dogwatching.* New York: Crown.

Morrison H (1980). He went that-a-way. *Off-Lead,* 9(6):10–11.

Morton JRC (1968). Effects of early experience "handling and gentling" in laboratory animals. In MW Fox (Ed), *Abnormal Behavior in Animals.* Philadelphia: WB Saunders.

Mugford RA (1977). External influences on the feeding of carnivores. In MK Kare and O Maller (Eds), *The Chemical Senses and Nutrition*, 25–50. New York: Academic.

Mugford RA (1987). The influence of nutrition on canine behavior. *J Small Anim Pract* 28:1046–1085.

Murphy CJ, Zadnik K, and Mannis MJ (1992). Myopia and refractive error in dogs. *Invest Ophthalmol Vis Sci*, 33:2459–2463.

Myers LJ (1991). Use of innate behaviors to evaluate sensory function in the dog. *Vet Clin North Am Adv Comp Anim Behav*, 21:281–298.

Neitz J, Geist T, and Jacobs GH (1989). Color vision in the dog. *Vis Neurosci*, 3:119–125.

Overall K (1997). *Clinical Behavioral Medicine for Small Animals*. St. Louis: CV Mosby.

Parry HB (1953). Degeneration of the dog retina: I. Structure and development of the retina of the normal dog. *Br J Ophthalmol*, 37:385–401.

Passe DH and Walker JC (1985). Odor psychophysics in vertebrates. *Neurosci Biobehav Rev*, 9:431–467.

Pavlov IP (1927/1960). *Conditioned Reflexes: An Investigation of the Physiological Activity of the Cerebral Cortex*, GV Anrep (Trans). New York: Dover (reprint).

Pearsall MD and Verbruggen H (1982). *Scent: Training to Track, Search, and Rescue*. Loveland, CO: Alpine.

Pedersen PE and Blass EM (1982). Prenatal and postnatal determinants of the 1st suckling episode in albino rats. *Dev Psychobiol*, 15:349–55.

Peichl L (1991). Catecholaminergic amacrine cells in the dog and wolf retina. *Vis Neurosci*, 7:575–587.

Peichl L (1992). Morphological types of ganglion cells in the dog and wolf retina. *J Comp Neurol*, 324:590–602.

Peters RP and Mech DL (1975). Scent-marking in wolves. *Am Sci*, 63:628–637.

Pettijohn TF, Wong TW, Ebert PD, and Scott JP (1977). Alleviation of separation distress in 3 breeds of young dogs. *Dev Psychobiol*, 10:373–381.

Pfungst O (1911/1965). *Clever Hans: The Horse of Mr. von Osten*. New York: Holt, Rinehart and Winston (reprint).

Pietras RL and Moulton DG (1974). Hormonal influences on odor detection in rats: Changes associated with the estrous cycle, pseudopregnancy, ovariectomy, and administration of testosterone propionate. *Physiol Behav*, 12:475–491.

Powers MA, Schiffman SS, Lawson DC, et al. (1990). The effect of taste on gastric and pan-

creatic responses in dogs. *Physiol Behav*, 47:1295–1297.

Ressler KJ, Sullivan SL, and Buck LB (1993). A zonal organization of odorant receptor gene expression in the olfactory epithelium. *Cell*, 73:597–609.

Rhine JB and Pratt JG (1957). *Parapsychology: Frontier Science of the Mind*. Springfield, IL: Charles C Thomas.

Roe DJ and Sales GD (1992). Welfare implications of ultrasonic flea collars. *Vet Rec*, 130:142–143.

Rosengren A (1969). Experiments in colour discrimination in dogs. *Acta Zool Fenn*, 121:1–19.

Salazar I, Barber PC, and Cifuentes JM (1992). Anatomical and immunohistological demonstration of the primary neural connections of the vomeronasal organ in the dog. *Anat Rec*, 233:309–313.

Salazar I, Cifuentes JM, Quintero S, and Garcia-Caballero T (1994). Structural, morphometric, and immunohistological study of the accessory olfactory bulb in the dog. *Anat Rec*, 240:277–285.

Schmidt-Nielsen K (1989). *Animal Physiology: Adaptation and Environment*. Cambridge: Cambridge University Press.

Schwartz C (1980). Project: Which way? *Off-Lead*, 9(7):22–24.

Schwenk K (1994). Why snakes have forked tongues. *Science*, 263:1573–1577.

Sechenov IM (1863/1965). *Reflexes of the Brain: An Attempt to Establish the Physiological Basis Of Psychological Processes*, E Belsky (Trans). Cambridge: MIT Press (reprint).

Settle RH, Sommerville BA, McCormick J, and Broom DM (1994). Human scent matching using specially trained dogs. *Anim Behav*, 48:1443–1448.

Shafik A (1994). Olfactory micturition reflex: Experimental study in dogs. *Biol Signals*, 3:307–311.

Shepherd GM (1983). *Neurobiology*. New York: Oxford University Press.

Sherrington CS (1906). *The Integrative Action of the Nervous System*. New Haven: Yale University Press.

Smith EM (1912). Some observations concerning color vision in dogs. *Br J Psychol*, 5:119–203.

Smith K and Sines JO (1960). Demonstration of a peculiar odor in the sweat of schizophrenic patients. *Arch Gen Psychiatry*, 2:184–188.

Smotherman WP (1982) In utero chemosensory experience alters taste preferences and corticosterone responsiveness. *Behav Neural Biol*, 36:61–68.

Sommerville B and Green M (1989). The sniffing detective. *New Sci*, May:54–57.

Sommerville BA, Darling FM, and Broom DM (1993). The use of trained dogs to discriminate human scent. *Anim Behav*, 46:189–190.

Stanley WC, Cornwell AC, Poggiani C, and Trattner A (1963). Conditioning in the neonatal puppy. *J Comp Physiol Psychol*, 56:211–214.

Steen JB and Wilsson E (1990). How do dogs determine the direction of tracks? *Acta Physiol Scand*, 139:531–534.

Stone CP (1921). Notes on light discrimination in the dog. *J Comp Psychol*, 1:413–431.

Strain GM (1996). Aetiology, prevalence, and diagnosis of deafness in dogs and cats. *Br Vet J*, 152:17–36.

Strong V, Brown SW, and Walker R (1999). Seizure-alert dogs: Fact or fiction? *Seizure*, 8:62–65.

Tanner JS (1970). Training a deaf dog. *Dog World*, (Sept):23, 74.

Thessen A, Steen JB, and Doving KB (1993). Behaviour of dogs during olfactory tracking. *J Exp Biol*, 180:247–251.

Thompson RF (1993). *The Brain: A Neuroscience Primer.* New York: WH Freeman.

Tinbergen N (1951/1969). *The Study of Instinct.* Oxford: Oxford University Press (reprint).

Tuber DS (1986). Teaching rover to relax: The soft exercise. *Anim Behav Consult Newsl*, 3(1).

Van der Westhuizen C (1990). Training a blind dog. *Off-Lead*, 21:22–23.

Vine LL (1983). *Your Neurotic Dog: Advice from a Leading Veterinarian on How to Remedy Canine Behavior Problems.* New York: Dial.

Von Bekesy G (1964). Olfactory analogue to directional hearing. *Appl Physiol*, 19:369–373.

Vormbrock JK and Grossberg JM (1988). Cardiovascular effects of human-pet dog interactions. *J Behav Med*, 11:509–517.

Warden CJ and Warner LH (1928). The sensory capacity and intelligence of dogs, with a report on the ability of the noted dog "Fellow" to respond to verbal stimuli. *Q Rev Biol*, 3:1–28.

Welker WI (1973). Principles of organization of the ventrobasal complex in mammals. *Brain Behav Evol*, 7:253–336.

Whitney LF (1961). *Dog Psychology.* New York: Howell Book House.

Windholz G (1989). Orbelli's experimental work on color discrimination in dogs. *Pavlov J Biol Sci*, 24:133–137.

Wolpe J (1958). *Psychotherapy by Reciprocal Inhibition.* Stanford: Stanford University Press.

Woodhouse (1982). *No Bad Dogs the Woodhouse Way.* New York: Summit.

Worden AN (1959). Abnormal behaviour in the dog and cat. *Vet Rec*, 71:966–978.

Wright RH (1964). *The Science of Smell.* New York: Basic.

Yerkes RM (1907/1908). The behavior of 'Roger,' being a comment on the foregoing article based on personal investigation of the dog. *Century Mag*, 59:602–606.

5

Biological and Dispositional Constraints on Learning

At every moment an animal's sense organs are being bombarded by physical energy in many forms. To this chiaroscuro it responds selectively. The selectivity in its responsiveness must influence what it can learn.

R. A. HINDE AND J. STEVENSON-HINDE *Constraints on Learning* (1973)

THE EPIGENESIS of behavior is guided by a complex mix of innate and experiential factors. The evolved sensory and neurobiological organization exhibited by dogs predispose them to behave in unique species-typical ways. Although biology contributes a great deal to the way dogs behave and how they adapt to the environment, without the nurturing influence of experience and learning, this innate potential would remain dormant and unactualized.

NATURE VERSUS NURTURE

The relative importance of biology (nature) versus experience (nurture) for the organization of behavior is the central issue fueling the nature-nurture controversy. This circular (and somewhat self-serving) dispute is maintained, on the one hand, by proponents of nature (often ethologists), who emphasize the importance of evolution and phylogenesis. On the other hand, proponents of nurture (usually behaviorists) underscore the ultimate importance of experience and learning. Obviously, both sides of the debate are partly right, with both genes and experience contributing to the development of behavior. However, to compare the relative importance of the two factors separately is analogous to asking whether hydrogen or oxygen is more important in the makeup of water. In the words of Lorenz, "any attempt to separate phylogenetically and individually adapted characters and properties of behavior, either conceptually or in the course of practical experiments, must necessarily be considered as hopeless and devoid of sense, as any trait of behavior, however minute, is automatically regarded, on principle, as being influenced by both factors achieving adaptation" (1965:5). The fact is that it takes both hydrogen and oxygen to make water. Without hydrogen there is no water and, likewise, without oxygen there is no water. A similar interdependent relationship holds between the influence of nature and nurture in the ontogeny of behavior. The important issue at stake here is not the relative dominance of one factor over the other but the dynamic interplay of the two in developing animals. Genes per se do not impact directly on behavior, just as behavior per se does not impact on genes. Genes exercise an indirect influence on behavior by regulating the operation of biochemical mechanisms underlying the expression of behavior. Conversely, although genes cannot be directly affected by experience, the expression of genes and the biochemical substrates that they regulate can be influenced by behavior and experience.

A dog's behavior is the outcome of a de-velopmental process (epigenesis) in which inherited genotypic characteristics interface with and adapt to the surrounding environment, thereby expressing the dog's behavioral phenotype (Fig. 5.1). Behavioral and biological development take place within a context of inherited constraints, sufficiently variable to allow for change according to the necessity dictated by an animal's unique experience and interaction with the environment. This adjustment to the demands of the physical and social environment depends on learning, but learning is possible only to the extent that an animal is genetically prepared to learn. Further, the organization of behavior itself is genetically programmed to be flexible and variable but only within definite limits. Survival depends on an animal learning from past experiences, adjusting its behavior appropriately to current circumstances, and forming reliable predictions about similar situations in the future. In essence, biology and genetics define the limits of how and what an animal learns, whereas experience dictates the moment-to-moment direction of these behavioral changes.

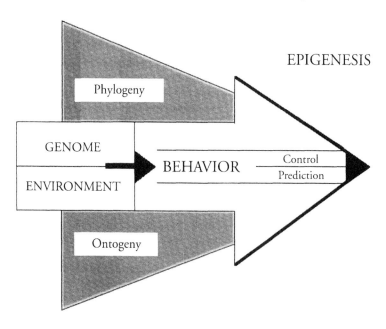

FIG. 5.1. The dog's development occurs under the influence of a complex set of biological and experiential factors.

INSTINCTS, "FIXED" ACTION PATTERNS, AND FUNCTIONAL SYSTEMS

The experimental study of animal behavior has produced great strides in our understanding of how animals learn. Unfortunately, however, the majority of this research has been confined to a narrow range of animal species (especially pigeons and rats) and limited to an arbitrary set of behaviors (e.g., maze learning, key pecking, lever pressing, and various other simple behaviors). Although the scientific productivity of such concentration is undeniable, over the years it has become increasingly evident that such investigation has failed in many important respects. Early on, Beach (1950/1971) criticized several aspects of this situation. He expressed strong reservations about the excessive reliance on rats as experimental animals and the rather exclusive experimental focus on learning and conditioning phenomena. He argued that the scientific study of animal behavior was at risk of becoming dangerously narrow and specialized—a psychology of pigeons and rats "which may or may not apply to other species and other situations" (1950/1971:12). He observed that such studies far outnumbered and overshadowed the investigation of other important areas of animal behavior research. According to Beach, an area of research that has suffered the most from this overconcentration is *instinct*:

> Another very important disadvantage of the present method in animal studies is that because of their preoccupation with a few species and a few types of behavior, psychologists are led to neglect many complex patterns of response that stand in urgent need of systematic analysis. The best example of this tendency is seen in the current attitude toward so-called "instinctive" behavior. ... The growing emphasis upon learning has produced a complementary reduction in the amount of study devoted to what is generally referred to as "unlearned behavior." ... Data relevant to all but a few "unlearned" reactions are too scanty to permit any definite conclusion concerning the role of experience in the shaping of the response. And those few cases in which an exhaustive analysis has been attempted show that the development of the behavior under scrutiny is usually more

complicated than a superficial examination could possibly indicate (1950/1971:12).

Although pigeons and rodents remain the most common animals studied in laboratories, since Beach's admonitory address the learning ability of many other species has been investigated (Bitterman, 1988; Krasne and Glanzman, 1995).

The importance of instinctual mechanisms and species-typical action patterns should not be overlooked in the analysis of behavior and understanding its motivation. Among other things, instincts preserve genetic information about an animal's biobehavioral past. Nature is conservative and under natural circumstances many biological constraints and pressures are maintained from generation to generation in the interaction between animals and the environment. These constants have resulted in the gradual genetic codification of vital biological information produced by the interaction of an animal species with the surrounding environment over the course of its evolution. Although behavior itself is not directly encoded in an animal's genome, various genetic instructions are orchestrated by the genome that provide the biological substrate for the expression of species-typical behavior.

An instinctive mechanism that has drawn a tremendous amount of attention is the fixed action pattern (FAP). Complex and regular patterns of stereotypic behavior, not dependent on learning for their expression, are referred to as fixed action patterns. Although some disagreement exists regarding just how "fixed" such motor patterns are, the concept is a useful one for understanding many more or less unlearned features of dog behavior. Although FAPs are instinctive, instincts are not identical with FAPs. For example, maternal care in dogs is not an FAP, yet certain components of maternal care are innately programmed FAPs. Thus, immediately after birth, the mother removes the allantoic sac and severs the umbilical cord with her carnassial teeth—this behavior is highly stereotypic from puppy to puppy. The puppy is licked dry and the umbilical cord cut shorter if necessary. Such licking and stimulation elicits various muscular reflexes and breathing. Another maternal FAP is the mother's stimulation of elimination. Newborn puppies are unable to eliminate voluntarily for about the first 2 weeks of life, thus requiring that the mother elicit elimination by licking the anogenital area and ingesting the neonate's excreta. The exact signs or releasing stimuli controlling these two epimeletic (care-giving) patterns are not known. Likewise, not all of the components involved in the dog's sexual behavior can be characterized as FAPs, but some sequences are FAPs. For instance, the female's practice of averting her tail to one side before intromission or the male's action of clasping and thrusting are FAPs. These actions are stereotypic and *hardwired* motor programs mediated by specific innate releasing mechanisms (IRMs).

FAPs depend on an inner readiness (appetitive, emotional, and hormonal) for action, a releasing or sign stimulus of sufficient strength to trigger the IRM, and the excitation of an appropriate motor program. Although experience and learning modify to some extent most instinctive behavior patterns, the general form and expression of an FAP is innately programmed and not subject to learning. It is useful to divide FAPs into two distinct components: appetitive and consummatory. Among animals of the same species, appetitive patterns of behavior may vary greatly, but the manner in which they consummate drive-directed behavior is uniform and stereotypic from individual to individual. However, an FAP's evocation is subject to change depending on an animal's accumulating readiness to act or, what Lorenz has termed, the ever-changing action-specific potential (ASP). Animals under a high motivational influence tend to respond to a minimum sign or releaser stimulus, whereas animals under a low ASP may require a correspondingly stronger releaser to evoke the appropriate FAP. Animals under a high level of "drive energy" may spontaneously discharge an FAP without appropriate stimulation. These spontaneous FAP discharges are referred to as vacuum activities. Lorenz views the canine custom of urinary scent marking as a good example illustrating these various motivational features underlying the FAP:

The motor patterns of urination performed by a male dog show all the phenomena here under discussion. A very strong releasing stimulus situation, such as the smell of a rival's mark in the dog's own territory, will cause him to lift his leg even when the amount of urine at his disposal is, at the moment, negligible. Even under the pressure of a much higher urinating potential, the dog will still look for releasing stimulus situations, such as upright objects, preferably on exposed corners, at which to lift his leg. Under extreme internal pressure he will forgo every external stimulation and even forget the conditioned inhibition of house training and urinate on the carpet—in this pitiable situation usually without even lifting his leg. (1982:186)

In addition to elimination, urinary behavior patterns serve many important social and reproductive functions—imperatives belonging specifically to the species. Given the presence of an appropriate releasing stimulus (a scent post overmarked by a strange dog), an intact adult male dog will readily mark with a distinctive leg-lifting movement. This movement does not depend on learning to occur but is mediated by a genetically encoded IRM, hormonal influences, and specific releasing stimuli (perhaps a pheromone) impinging on the dog from the environment. The autonomous character of this behavior makes its initial expression almost comical in effect. Many young dogs when first discovering this new ability may hop along with head cocked around curiously observing the perplexing action *happening* to them. The leg-lifting movement does not appear to be an action that they voluntary choose to express, but rather one that comes over them under the right set of circumstances. As is characteristic of many fixed action sequences, it is very hard to train a dog to lift its leg on command, even though the dog may perform the action many times a day. The resistance of leg lifting to voluntary control supports the view that it is an instinctive response controlled at a primitive level of neural organization. This points to an important criterion of the FAP: that its occurrence is spontaneous and not subject to learning (or much learning) for its display. Although the FAP is not dependent on learning for its appearance, it is not entirely independent of the actualizing influence of experience either. Without an experiential context or field of action the FAP will remain in a dormant and potential state.

INSTINCTUAL LEARNING

The historical antagonism between ethology and behaviorism was based to a large extent on the relative importance each discipline placed on the role of learning in the development of behavior. This opposition was embodied in the careers and theoretical orientations of B. F. Skinner (1974) and Konrad Lorenz (1982). Skinner emphasized the importance of experimental analysis and learning as they occur under controlled laboratory conditions. Lorenz, on the other hand, downplayed the importance of experimentation and stressed instead direct observation of animal behavior occurring within its natural setting. Whereas behaviorists believed that behavior could be best explained in terms of learning, ethologists objected to this narrow focus and emphasized the significance of phylogenetic or biological contributions governing behavior. Both of these positions have turned out to be excessively exclusionary and doctrinaire. Certainly, the behavior of many animals is guided by instinctual mechanisms and various programmed motor patterns, but these innate contributions are not necessarily rigid nor entirely outside of the influence of learning. Further, in conjunction with an animal's biological endowment, learning itself is an evolutionary adaptation that determines (in terms of general potential) what animals will learn and how they will learn it. Some adaptations are learned readily, some slowly, and some not at all.

William James defined instinct "as the faculty of acting in such a way as to produce certain ends, without foresight of the ends, and without previous education in the performance" (1890/1950:383). According to James, instinctive behavior consists of reflexes and impulses linked together to form complicated behavior patterns and tendencies. Although many behavioral adjustments to the environment are biologically encoded as predispositions or even imperatives to action, such instinctive impulses are not entirely immune to the influence of experience. For ex-

ample, in the case of animals possessing a well-developed memory, the first expression of an instinctive behavior may be a spontaneous response occurring without much purpose, but subsequent displays will be progressively influenced by experience and the effect of learning. The behavior is still instinctive but is now expressed under the additional influence of some expectation of producing a result (Thorpe, 1956/1966).

Unlike many of his contemporaries, James did not believe that instincts were regulated by rational self-control—at least directly: "Reason, per se, can inhibit no impulses; the only thing that can neutralize an impulse is an impulse the other way" (1890/1950:393). In other words, instincts are regulated by the operations of other instincts. However, through inferences derived from experience, an animal may learn how to control impulsive behavior indirectly by evoking opposing impulses to block its expression. For example, the impulse to act aggressively is not inhibited by a dog's exercise of better judgment, but through the simultaneous evocation of opposing instincts like fear of reprisal or affection for the object of anger. Fear is not overcome by telling oneself that there is nothing to fear, but by evoking opposing impulses to fear like relaxation or appetitive arousal.

Seligman and Hager described the relationship between learning and instinct in terms of a continuity in which "'learning' is continuous with 'instinct'" (1972:5), whereas Kuo employed a much more colorful terminology when referring to this functional relationship: "like one of a pair of inseparable, monstrous Siamese twins with one side of the body in common from head to toe, the term learning cannot by redefinition be detached from the concept of instinct" (1967:140). Long ago, David Hume eloquently characterized the close relationship between learning and instinct, while emphasizing the similarities existing between humans and animals with regard to the way each benefits from experience and observation:

> When we have lived any time, and have been accustomed to the uniformity of nature, we acquire a general habit, by which we always transfer the known to the unknown, and con-

ceive the latter to resemble the former. By means of this general habitual principle, we regard even one experiment as the foundation of reasoning, and expect a similar event with some degree of certainty, where the experiment has been made accurately and free from all foreign circumstances. It is therefore considered as a matter of great importance to observe the consequences of things. ... But though animals learn many parts of their knowledge from observation, there are also many parts of it, which they derive from the original hand of nature; which much exceed the share of capacity they possess on ordinary occasions; and in which they improve, little or nothing, by the longest practice and experience. These we denominate instincts, and are so apt to admire as something very extraordinary, and inexplicable by all the disquisitions of human understanding. But our wonder will, perhaps, cease or diminish, when we consider, that the experimental reasoning itself, which we possess in common with beasts, and on which the whole conduct of life depends, is nothing but a species of instinct or mechanical power, that acts in us unknown to ourselves; and in its chief operations, is not directed by any such relations or comparisons of ideas, as are the proper objects of our intellectual faculties. Though the instinct be different, yet still it is an instinct, which teaches a man to avoid the fire; as much as that, which teaches a bird, with such exactness, the art of incubation, and the whole economy and order of its nursery. (1748/1988:99)

Dancing Bees

Even among insects, learning serves many adaptive functions. Von Frisch (1953) demonstrated the importance of learning for the bee's adaptation and success as a species. He observed, for example, that individual bees are typically flower constant, that is, they tend to forage on a single kind of flower rather than sampling many different types. This aspect of bee foraging is of great benefit to flowers, which depend on bees for pollination. If bees moved haphazardly from one flower species to another, they would not be a very efficient vehicle for the distribution of pollen between flowers of the same species. Von Frisch found that such constancy also provided bees with an important advantage.

Each flower species poses special problems for bees with regard to the harvesting of nectar. It may take as many as five or six visits before a bee can easily find and harvest the nectar. The harvesting of nectar is an acquired skill that is mastered by practice. By specializing on one flower, a bee learns how to procure the hidden nectar inside most effectively without wasting time.

Next, von Frisch asked, how do bees discriminate the right flowers from all the rest competing for their attention? According to his experiments, bees acquire the ability to recognize the right flower through associative learning processes mediated by the senses of smell and sight. In one experiment, bees were fed sugar water while being exposed to the odor of bitter orange. After a number of visits, the bees showed a strong preference for the odor. Von Frisch next performed an experiment in which the odor was placed inside a box with a hole drilled into it so that the bees could freely enter. The box with the preferred scent was lined up with several other boxes, so that the bees had to choose the correct one containing bitter orange and sugar water from many other scents vying for attention. He found that the bees were able to discriminate the scent of bitter orange from over a dozen odors placed inside the other boxes.

To test the role of sight in this flower selection process, he performed another series of experiments. First, the bees were fed sugar water in a blue box scented with the oil of jasmine. The bees quickly learn to go to the blue box in search of sugar. Subsequently, he removed the sugar water and jasmine scent and placed it into an uncolored box located some distance from the blue one. The bees, again, oriented toward the blue box while in flight. However, upon discovering that the scent of jasmine was not present, they did not enter but searched the other boxes for the preferred scent of jasmine. When they finally found the scented box, they entered without hesitation. From these experiments, he concluded that bees use sight to locate a prospective flower from a distance but use smell to confirm that it is the correct one before alighting on it to forage. Other studies have shown that bees also estimate the availability of food according to a time reference (Gallistel, 1990). An interesting example of how bee learning forms coherent sets or learning units was discovered while studying the bee's ability to time access to food. In one experiment, bees were fed unscented food, except for a brief half-hour period each day. Subsequent tests showed that bees chose unscented food over scented food, except during that same half-hour period. Not only are color, scent, and time learned as a set but add also shape, landmarks, and locality—if one element is changed, the entire set must be relearned. Even more extraordinary feats of learning and communication are found in the bee's dances. Such dances give other foraging hive members specific information about the location (direction and distance) of food resources. Excellent secondary information concerning this behavior can be found in Gould (1982) and Griffin (1981).

The way that bees learn is rigidly programmed. As just noted, bees can quickly learn to associate a specific color and odor with food, but how they learn this sort of discrimination is strictly defined. Gould (1979) reviewed bee research that showed that bees associate color with food for *only* a brief 2-second moment just before landing and learn landmarks associated with the food's location *only* as they fly away. Further, finding its way back to the hive depends on highly programmed learning. The bee appears to learn significant landmarks associated with the hive on the first departure each day. If the hive is moved a few feet from its original location, returning bees exhibit great confusion and disorientation. However, if the hive is moved several miles overnight, the bees have no problem in learning the new location and finding their way home, so long as it remains in the same place after the first departure of the day:

> Learning, for the bee, has thus become specialized to the extent that specific cues are learned only at specific times—and then only in specific contexts. In fact, the learning programs of bees are even more specialized than that: although the insects acquire each bit of knowledge separately and at a different rate, once acquired, their knowledge forms a part of a coherent and holistic set, that is, a unit that

cannot be reduced to discrete component elements. (Gould, 1979:71)

Digging Wasps

The digger wasp also exhibits some rather extraordinary *instinctive* learning abilities. This particular wasp carefully prepares a burrow into which she deposits an insect or caterpillar that has been paralyzed by her sting. The wasp then deposits an egg on the host. When the egg hatches, the new larva feeds on the bee or caterpillar. One species of the digger wasp, *Ammophia pubescent*, exhibits incredible programmed learning and memory abilities. This particular wasp species provides provisions for as many as a dozen burrows containing young at various stages of development and nutritional needs. The wasp inspects each burrow and makes an inventory of what is needed for each larva. She then goes about the business of finding the required provisions. The Dutch ethologist G. P. Baerends (cited in Gould, 1982) found that the female wasp only retrieves the amount of food needed by each larva. Burrows containing an egg receive no caterpillars and small larva receive one to three caterpillars, whereas large larva receive more and pupating larva receive no food at all. By altering the contents of the various burrows while the wasp was out foraging, Baerends made a series of fascinating discoveries. If a burrow, for example, containing a large larva was excavated and replaced with a small larva or an egg, the wasp would provide it with the correct amount of food only if the alteration took place before the morning inspection. If the change was made after the morning inspection, the wasp would place an amount of food calculated from those morning observations, regardless of the actual needs of the larva placed into the burrow by the experimenter in her absence:

> During the morning inspection, Baerends reasoned, the wasps must make some sort of "shopping list," in which the detailed needs of each burrow are inscribed in association with its location and relevant landmark information. Working from her original shopping list the wasp, having learned more in a few minutes than many humans could—perhaps as many as

forty-five items in sets of three—proceeds to organize the rest of her day as mindlessly as a machine. This sort of learning, then, phenomenal as it is, is as stereotyped as any other piece of insect behavior. (Gould, 1982:262)

The digger wasp is specialized to obtain and act upon specific information derived from the environment at certain times of the day. However, the nature of this information and the manner in which it is obtained is subject to encoded rules and rigid mechanisms of acquisition. Tinbergen (1951/1969) described an experiment in which 20 pine cones were arranged around a digger wasp's (*Philanthus triangulum*) burrow while she was still inside. As the wasp left her burrow, she took a 6-second aerial reckoning of the immediate surroundings before flying away. While she was gone, the experimenter rearranged the pine cones, placing them several feet away from the burrow. On her return, the wasp went directly to the pine-cone circle in search of her burrow. This experiment was repeated several times with the same disorienting result. The wasp was unable to find the location of her burrow until the pine cones were finally returned to the original place around the burrow.

Of course, the dog's style of learning is very different from that exhibited by the honeybee and wasp, yet it may be profitable to study such learning as a means of gaining insight into aspects of the learning process not made explicit by laboratory investigations. Although finding parallel examples of fixed program learning in dogs is not easy, the dog is clearly programmed to learn some things at certain times more rapidly than at other times. Fox (1966), for example, found that avoidance learning was most rapidly obtained during a short sensitive period between 8 and 10 weeks of age. Scott and Fuller (1965) found that social identity and many social behavior patterns are learned during a brief period running between 3 and 12 weeks of age. Tinbergen observed that some Greenland Eskimo dogs had their first copulatory experience, defended home territory, and avoided neighboring territories all within the course of 1 week. Prior to this time, the dogs ran roughshod over the terri-

tories of other packs, a behavior that resulted in severe and repeated reprisal. According to Tinbergen, it was as though the dogs simply could not get the idea: "They do not learn the territories' topography and for the observer their stupidity in this respect is amazing" (1951/1969:150). Thus, habits, appetites, and aversions are optimally acquired at specific times in a dog's ontogenesis, suggesting that efficient training and socialization is a process dependent on proper timing as much as proper training.

PREPAREDNESS AND SELECTIVE ASSOCIATION

Learning is a basic adaptive mechanism exhibited by the vast majority of animals. It plays a profound role in a dog's success or failure in adjusting to its social and physical surroundings. As noted above, learning takes place within a biobehavioral context formed of many unlearned, innate mechanisms that supply a dog from birth (and before) with a varied repertoire of reflexive and instinctive adjustments to the environment. All animals come into the world preadapted to sense and attend to a limited set of stimuli; predisposed to feel and respond to a select group of unconditioned stimuli with emotionally significant arousal; programmed to act within a fixed range of ways (albeit variably within that range); and prepared to learn certain things and select associations, but not all things are learned or associated with an equal ease (Seligman, 1970). For example, although puppies can easily master the house-training routine, another animal like the chimpanzee, although considered by ethologists to be much more intelligent than the dog, may require laborious efforts to achieve voluntary control over alimentary functions—if at all. The chimp's evolutionary niche has placed little selective pressure on such variability in its elimination habits. The preparedness hypothesis suggests that certain conditioned stimuli and unconditioned stimuli are more readily associated than others, and, in the case of instrumental learning, the connection between a particular response and its consequences is more rapidly learned than others.

Preparedness affects dogs in both beneficial and adverse directions. Many phobic and emotional reactions are innately programmed and readied for potentiating experience (Seligman, 1971; LoLordo and Droungas, 1989). Dogs are prepared to enjoy close social contact with conspecifics and human companions but are unprepared to cope with loneliness and extended periods of separation. They are prepared to adjust socially within a highly structured and regimented social order but may become socially confused and overly competitive within an environment lacking the presence of a dominant figure modulating such competitive tendencies. The dog's sensory capabilities, like other animals, are attuned to a narrow field of species-typical activity. Not only must dogs be able to differentiate relevant from irrelevant information impinging on their senses, they must also be able to isolate it from competing background stimulation, attend to the specifics over time, and organize the information into meaningful associations from which to assess its significance and to decide on a course of effective action. Many of these functions occur more or less automatically by virtue of the way information is obtained and processed in the animal's brain.

Sensory Preparedness

Organisms are biologically prepared to selectively attend and respond to stimuli, depending on an apparent innate recognition of their significance. For example, Tinbergen (1951/1969) observed that young ducks and geese selectively respond to a cardboard silhouette depending on its orientation and direction of movement. When the model was moved to the right, it had the appearance of a short neck and long tail or hawklike attributes that evoked strong escape reactions. On the other hand, when the model was moved toward the left, it had the appearance of a long neck and short tail, i.e., the attributes of a goose in flight. This latter presentation evoked no response in the birds tested. Tinbergen also theorized that predators develop a *search image formation* in order to locate difficult-to-find prey animals equipped with *antipredator* adaptations (Fantino and Logan, 1979). Through experience involving successful hunts, the animal learns what to look for that is specific to the camouflaged or hidden prey animal. Gradually, the predator learns to attend to these specific attributes when searching for food.

Although not experimentally demonstrated in the laboratory, dogs appear to be more alert and attentive to the presence of accelerating (slow to fast) movements as opposed to decelerating (fast to slow) ones. Accelerating movements may be innate *sign stimuli* for escape/withdrawal behavior. Under natural conditions, slow-to-fast movements are more often associated with danger (e.g., a falling rock, swooping hawk, or stalk-and-chase movements of predators), certainly more so than movements exhibiting a fast-to-slow pattern (e.g., retreat). These opposing patterns of motion may be recognized by the distinctive patterns of retinal stimulation they produce. Command cues spoken with a clipped slow-to-fast inflection are typically much more effective than commands spoken in a drawn-out fast-to-slow manner. Similarly, strange and loud noises attract more attention than familiar and quiet sounds.

Dog trainers and owners alike have long recognized the value of altering the tone and amplitude of the voice to influence a dog's behavior. Repeated "kiss" sounds and whistles are familiar ways to stimulate a dog's attention and to arouse action. Similarly, soft and drawn-out word tones are commonly used to calm an agitated dog, whereas abrupt and repeated verbal prompts may be used to alert and put a dog on guard. Although dogs may not be able to understand the precise conceptual meaning and intent of the words used to communicate with them, they are very keen and responsive to the manner in which the words are spoken. For example, saying "No" in a high-pitched and upbeat tone of voice will likely evoke in a dog a preparatory response in anticipation of a rewarding outcome rather than worrying the dog about the possibility of impending punishment. Of course, in this example, classical conditioning probably plays an important role in the elaboration of the dog's response. However, it does appear that high and gentle tones of voice are more easily associated with rewarding outcomes, whereas low and forceful tones are more rapidly connected with punitive ones. Clearly, the tone and other characteristics of auditory stimulation appear to influence how dogs interpret information conveyed by verbal communication. Tone of voice conveys information to dogs about a trainer's emotional state and his or her immediate intentions, much like whining and growling convey very specific and different intentions among dogs. In other words, the meaning of the word signal appears to be most dependent on the *way* it is asserted rather than any abstract meanings conveyed by the word itself.

These observations suggest that dogs exhibit some degree of innate responsiveness to auditory stimulation based on the qualitative or quantitative characteristics of the acoustic signal presented. Clearly, socially significant auditory signals utilize various means to shape and infuse intentional meaning into the signals used to communicate needs. Patricia McConnell has explored the possibility that various physical alterations of acoustic stimuli may elicit differential changes in a dog's general activity level. Her investigation into this phenomenon began by interviewing over 100 trainers from all over the world (McConnell, 1990b). She found that the general style of auditory signaling used by animal trainers shared a fairly universal and definite pattern. The vast majority of trainers used rapidly repeated auditory signals to excite activity, whereas they used long and drawn-out signals to inhibit activity. Besides vocal sounds and whistles, she found that most trainers used repeated hand claps, finger snaps, tongue clucks and clicks, leg slaps, or "lip smooches" to increase activity in dogs. According to her interview records, no trainer ever mentioned using such signals to inhibit behavior. She observed that animal trainers would often give one sort of signal (e.g., two brief whistle blasts) to direct a dog into some action and then rapidly repeat the same sound to speed up the desired response. In one study comparing the effects of various signals on the approach behavior of puppies,

McConnell found that the strongest approach response toward a hidden person was evoked by repeated hand claps.

As a result of these interviews and related observations, she hypothesized that short and repeated ascending tones tend to stimulate behavioral excitation, whereas long and descending tones tend to exert an inhibitory effect over behavior. To test this hypothesis, she raised a mixed group of 20 Border collie and beagle puppies, carefully avoiding the use of expressive tones of voice, finger snaps, whistles, and claps (McConnell, 1990a, 1992). Only quiet and monotonic speech was permitted around the puppies, with most control being exercised by employing visual signals. At 4 months of age, 14 of the puppies were divided into two groups that received training to come or sit-stay on signal. Group 1 was trained to come in response to four brief ascending tones (150 milliseconds at 1500 Hz ascending to 3500 Hz) and to stay in response to one continuous descending tone (750 milliseconds at 3500 Hz descending to 1500 Hz). Conversely, group 2 was trained to come or stay in response to the same signals used to train group 1, but in reverse—that is, the continuous descending tone was associated with coming, whereas the repeated ascending tone was used to signal puppies to stay. After 10 days of training, the signals presented to the two groups were reversed. Although an apparent trend toward more efficient acquisition and increased activity was evident in group 1 (i.e., when "come" training was carried out in the presence of the repeated ascending tone), the overall effects of the training arrangement reached statistical significance only after the two groups were retrained to respond to the opposite set of signals. Even so, the significance detected by the study was not based on acquisition measures per se but rather stemmed from the elicitation of increased activity levels (viz., forepaw steps) occurring as the result of the presentation of the repeated ascending tone. Unfortunately, the study failed to show a significant differentiation between the two signals with respect to stay training and the acoustic inhibition of behavior. Overall, the results are somewhat disappointing and inconclusive with regard to the existence of an innate acoustic mechanism differentially sensitive to repeated and continuous signals—at least in the form used in the study. In the case of puppies, the differential effects of the signals presented show a definite trend consistent with McConnell's hypothesis; however, the results fail to demonstrate a very robust effect. Further, some effort should have been made to isolate potentially confounding influences differentially exerted by ascending versus descending tones on the behavioral effects attributed to repeated versus continuous signals. This would have required the incorporation of additional compound stimulus test arrangements such as repeated-descending versus continuous-ascending groups, with which to compare any additive or subtractive influences of tonal direction on activity in the presence of continuous or repeated signals.

From these findings, it appears that dogs are biologically prepared to increase nonspecific activity in response to brief and repeated acoustic signals. Although McConnell's study does not show a corresponding behavioral inhibition resulting from the presentation of long and continuous signals, it is clear from common experience that long and continuous signals do exert a calming and inhibitory effect on a dog's behavior. Many situations in nature attest to the activational effect of repeated tones, ranging from distress vocalizations in puppies to mating calls in birds. McConnell speculates that the dog's responsiveness to ascending repetitious sounds may be related to species-typical distress vocalizations, including whining, yelping, other repetitive sounds associated with intense arousal and care-seeking activity. Agonistic behavior may also provide an innate basis for the differential elicitation of increased activity versus decreased activity in response to acoustic stimulation of differing duration and tonal direction. A comparison of rapid alarm barking versus slow and continuous growling reveals distinctive innate features and effects. Rapid alarm barking serves to attract the attention and excitement of nearby conspecifics, alerting them and, perhaps, mobilizing them to join in and participate—that is, it has an excitatory effect on the group.

On the other hand, growling (a long, continuous social signal) may certainly attract the attention of the recipient, but it is more likely to elicit an inhibitory effect or result in the slow withdrawal or immobilization of the recipient target.

Cognitive Preparedness

The influence of behavioral preparedness should be given careful consideration when designing programs for modifying canine behavior. Dogs learn to perform some actions more rapidly or slowly, depending on the biobehavioral compatibility of the signal used and the behavior required to occur in the presence of that signal. Some signals and responses are more easily associated than others. For example, Lawicka (1964; Dobrzecka et al., 1966) found that dogs prefer spatially lateralized discriminative signals when learning a directional discrimination (go left/go right), while go/no go discriminations are more easily acquired when the discriminative cues are presented from the same location but varied in terms of tonal quality (Fig. 5.2). For example, in a simple go left/go right discrimination experiment, he found that dogs could learn the directional discrimination only if the discriminative tonal cues (high and low pitch) were presented from different locations relative to dogs. Although directional discriminations depend on spatially separated signals, such learning does not depend on the lateralization of the signals on a left-right axis. In fact, he demonstrated that dogs could learn to discriminate the correct left or right direction even if the signals were presented along a vertical axis, that is, by placing one sound source above the other. However, if the two signals were presented from the same location (a single speaker), then the go left/go right discrimination was frustrated and learned only with much difficulty, if at all. In another experiment, he found that dogs learned a go/no go discrimination much more easily if the discriminative cues came from the same source but varied in terms of tone. If the tonal signals were lateralized relative to the dogs, then the go/no go discrimination was impeded. Lawicka's exper-

STIMULUS

	Low Tone	Above
	High Tone	Below
	Speaker facing front	Speaker placed above or below dog
	QUALITY	LOCATION
GO/NO GO	Rapid Acquisition	Slow Acquisition
GO LEFT/ GO RIGHT	Slow Acquisition	Rapid Acquisition

RESPONSE

FIG. 5.2. Matrix shows the various relations tested in the Lawicka experiment. Note that acquisition rates differ depending on the sort of response being learned and the type of stimulus presented. After Miller and Bowe (1982).

iments clearly show that dogs are prepared to learn directional discriminations with spatially separated signals and go/no go discriminations from signals varied in tone but coming from the same location.

Prepared Connections: Taste Aversion

Another interesting study often discussed in the context of preparedness was performed by Garcia and Koelling (1966). Two groups of rats were given either water having a sweet taste (saccharine flavor) or water presented together with a compound audiovisual (light and noise) stimulus. These two groups were divided and differentially exposed to radiation or shock while they drank the water. The investigators found that radiation was selectively associated with the sweet water but

not with the bright-noisy audiovisual stimulus. After exposure, radiated rats avoided sweet water but continued to drink bright-noisy water. In the case of rats exposed to shock while drinking, the bright-noisy stimulus was selectively associated with shock, but shock was not associated with the sweet water. After exposure to shock, the rats would avoid bright-noisy water but continued to drink sweet water (Fig. 5.3). These experiments suggest that rats are biologically prepared to associate taste with nausea and, likewise, to associate light-noise with shock, but unprepared to make the converse associations, that is, to associate taste with shock or light-noise with nausea.

Additional evidence for biological preparedness in taste aversion was provided by a study performed by Wilcoxin and colleagues

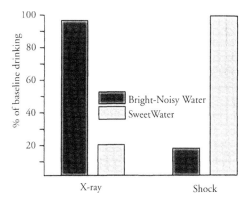

FIG. 5.3. This Garcia and Koelling (1966) study demonstrates the principle of selective association. The animals studied selectively associated nausea with sweetness and shock with auditory and visual stimuli, but not vice versa.

(1971), who compared the differential acquisition of taste aversion in rats and quail. The subjects were variously presented with water having a sour taste, water colored dark blue, or water that was both sour and dark blue. Rats experiencing nausea after drinking these combinations of color and flavor responded to flavor cues but not visual cues. Quail, on the other hand, were able to associate either the color or the taste of the water with nausea, provided the cues were presented separately; however, if both taste and color were presented together, the color cue overshadowed the flavor cue. When later offered sour or colored water, the quail drank sour water but not colored water. An obvious conclusion to be drawn from this experiment is that quail are prepared to make the taste-aversion association more effectively through the modality of sight than taste, whereas rats are better prepared to acquire a taste aversion through the modality of gustation only.

Many animal species are programmed to wait for some fixed period after ingesting a new food item in order to determine whether it is toxic to them (Gould, 1982). A blue jay, for example, hunts and eats butterflies, but if it happens to eat a monarch butterfly, it will soon become ill and vomit. Illness is induced by cardiac glycosides stored in various parts of the butterfly's body. These substances are obtained by the butterfly larva feeding on the

milkweed. After a single exposure to the nausea-producing monarch butterfly, a blue jay will avoid hunting them in the future (Brower, 1969). The most significant avoidance cue for blue jays is the butterfly's colorful wing pattern. Interestingly, the monarch butterfly's wing color and pattern has been mimicked by other butterflies (most notably, the viceroy butterfly), ostensibly providing them with safety from previously "trained" blue jays. Gould (1982) contends that taste aversion or "rapid food-avoidance conditioning" is a widely distributed form of programmed learning in the animal world. Each species is responsive to a specific set of cues that identify the most salient feature or sign stimulus associated with the evocation of illness. Tinbergen describes other cases involving learned food avoidance and mimicry. Songbirds exhibit a learned avoidance toward wasps due to illness induced by eating them:

> When a songbird such as a Redstart meets with a wasp for the first time in its life, it captures it. Sometimes, but that is relatively rare, the wasp will manage to sting the bird. The bird then lets go, and may show in various ways that the sting affected it rather unpleasantly; it may shake its head, and wipe its bill. Anyway it shows no further interest in the wasp. Usually however the wasp does not sting, it is killed before it can do so. Then it becomes evident that a wasp is distasteful: the bird does not finish it, and if it is eaten, it is often brought up again afterwards. Mostler has shown that most songbirds learn from one or a few such experiences to leave wasps alone. That they recognize such unpalatable insects by their colours is evident from the fact that from then on such a bird avoids not only wasps, but all similarly coloured insects. (1953/1975:95–96)

Many birds exhibit a similar avoidance toward the caterpillar of the cinnabar moth. After a single ingestion, birds learn to refuse all larvae with the caterpillar's distinctive black-and-yellow pattern of marking.

Studies with wild canids have demonstrated that taste aversion can be effectively employed to deter appetitive interest toward highly desirable prey animals. Coyotes have been conditioned to avoid sheep after being exposed to mutton and wool tainted with lithium chloride (LiCl) (Gustavson et al., 1974). Presumably, these treated coyotes had some previous safe exposure to the prey in the past. Besides coyotes, many other animals have shown a similar response to the taste-aversion procedure (Garcia et al., 1977; Gustavson, 1977). Mugford (1977) demonstrated that a strong taste aversion toward a highly palatable food item could be produced in cats if ingestion of the food was followed by treatment with LiCl. Gustavson and Gustavson (1982) compared the suppressive effects of peripheral versus internal aversive stimuli (nausea) presented at different points during the feeding sequence—that is, while rats approached or after they had consumed a highly desirable food item (an Oreo cookie). The peripheral stimuli included shock and repellents (ammonia, mustard, and quinine). Nausea produced by LiCl injections provided the internal aversive stimulation (taste aversion). They examined the suppressive effects of these aversives across three contexts: treatment cage, home cage, and novel cage (Table 5.1). Only taste aversion was shown to in-crease the latency of approach in all three training situations but only if the rats had consumed some of the cookie prior to the induction of nausea. Rats shocked as they approached the cookie exhibited significant hesitation when later tested in the treatment cage, but showed little evidence of transfer of suppression when tested in the home-cage and novel-cage situations. Interestingly, consumption measures indicated that rats exposed to quinine and mustard ate more of the cookie when it was presented in the home cage. Rats exposed to ammonia while they were eating exhibited significantly more hesitation when given a cookie in the novel test situation. A similar suppressive effect in the novel situation was not produced by quinine or mustard. In general, these findings suggest that aversion training using peripheral stimulation tends to be more context specific, whereas flavor-associated aversive internal stimulation (nausea) has cross-contextual implications: the suppression of appetitive and consummatory behavior. The authors illustrate the effect:

TABLE 5.1. Comparison of peripheral versus internal aversive conditioning

Training phase

APPROACH GROUP—Aversive stimulation presented as the animal approached the cookie

Testing phase		No stimulus	Shock	Ammonia	Mustard	Quinine	LiCl
Testing Contexts	Treatment	+	hes +	+	+	+	+
	Home	+	+	+	+	+	+
	Novel	+	+	+	+	+	+

Training Phase

CONSUMPTION GROUP—Aversive stimulation presented as the animal ate the cookie

Testing phase		No stimulus	Shock	Ammonia	Mustard	Quinine	LiCl
Testing Contexts	Treatment	+	hes +	+	+	+	000
	Home	+	+	+	++	++	000
	Novel	+	+	hes +	+	+	000
Key	+ Ate		++ Ate more		hes + Hesitated before eating		000 Did not eat

Note: The conditioned effects of peripheral and internal aversive stimulation occurring in different contexts. Note that only LiCl-induced nausea produced appetitive avoidance in all three testing situations. Source: After Gustavson (1996).

Conditioned taste aversions alter the palatability of the food, and make the flavor unacceptable whenever or wherever it is encountered. ... Anecdotally, if one wants to prevent a dog from eating biscuits in the parlor, but allow the dog to eat them in the yard, a peripheral aversive stimulus should be repeatedly applied to the animal when it approaches the biscuits in the parlor, but it should never be applied in the yard. However, if the desired impact is to prevent the eating of biscuits under any circumstances, then the dog should be made ill following consumption of biscuits on one or two occasions. (Gustavson and Gustavson, 1982:339)

While I cannot imagine anyone being so annoyed by a dog's interest in biscuits that they would want to apply a taste-aversion procedure to discourage it, the foregoing technique might be useful for the control of appetitive excesses of a more serious nature, such as intractable pica or coprophagia (Gustavson, 1996).

Efforts to test the suitability of taste aversion for the control of predatory behavior in dogs have not met with the success that might be expected from the aforementioned studies with wild canids and rodents. Hansen and colleagues (1997) treated two Alaskan huskies that exhibited a strong drive to chase and attack sheep; however, (apparently) neither of the dogs had actually killed or eaten sheep as prey in the past. The study consisted of feeding the dogs mutton mixed with wool and fat that had been tainted with LiCl. Although the dogs developed an aversion toward sheep meat, it was neither permanent (within 6 months, the dogs readily ate mutton) nor was it effective as a means to reduce the dogs' predatory behavior. In fact, the authors found that the procedure actually decreased the latency of predatory chase/attack behavior rather than increasing it as they had anticipated. They also noted several side effects, including an increase in intraspecific aggression, stiffness, trembling, and coordination deficits resulting from the ingestion of LiCl. A possible explanation for the study's failure to demonstrate a positive effect resulting from taste aversion may be due to the absence of a history of predatory behavior toward sheep that had resulted in the ingestion of sheep meat. The dogs apparently did not

associate the chase routine and the target prey with the meat they had developed an aversion toward. Further, since the authors were unclear about the predatory history of the dogs tested, one cannot be certain that the behavior of "chasing and attacking" was strictly motivated by predatory interests and the obtainment of food. For example, the dogs may have been engaging in predatory play, having no interest in eating their victims. Perhaps, better results with the taste-aversion method for controlling predatory behavior in domestic dogs would be obtained in cases that involve dogs who do exhibit a strong appetite for killing and eating the target prey animal.

Phylogenetic Differences: Habit Reversal and Matching

Bitterman (1965) compared the performance of various species learning the same tasks, that is, two discrimination procedures: habit reversal and matching. Habit reversal is a two-choice discrimination procedure where a previously conditioned positive stimulus S^D is made negative and a previously conditioned negative stimulus S^Δ is made positive. Bitterman found that some species (e.g., monkeys, rats, pigeons, and turtles) learn this sort of discrimination quickly, whereas others (e.g., fish, cockroaches, and earthworms) acquire the habit reversal poorly—if at all. The other task studied examined probability learning and matching behavior. The matching procedure involves presenting two discriminative stimuli in a choice situation. In an ordinary two-choice discrimination situation, reinforcement is associated 100% of the time with the positive stimulus and 0% of the time with the negative stimulus for a probability ratio holding between the two stimuli and reinforcement of 100:0. When reinforcement is presented so that, for example, 70% of the available reinforcement occurs in the presence of one stimulus (S^D1) and the remaining 30% occurs under the signalization of another (S^D2), some animals will tend to maximize by exclusively choosing only the stimulus with the highest likelihood of producing food (S^D1-70:S^D2-0), whereas other animals will tend to match their behavior—

that is, they tend to divide their time proportionately between the two stimuli (S^D1-70:S^D2-30). Surprisingly, Bitterman found that rats tend to maximize, whereas fish tend to match. This is a rather counterintuitive finding, since one would expect the "brainier" rats to "figure out" the probabilities of reinforcement more accurately than fish would and then to proportion their responses according to these probabilities. In fact, however, he discovered that decorticated rats performed the visual matching task better than normal controls, suggesting that the substrate locus of such matching behavior is at a subcortical level. Bitterman speculated that these differences in learning are phylogenetically significant and pertain to an animal's specific needs and adaptations within its respective evolutionary niche and ecological environment.

INSTINCTIVE DRIFT AND APPETITIVE LEARNING

Just as innate defensive reactions often obstruct efficient avoidance learning, interfering appetitive and exploratory tendencies sometimes surface during reward training that can significantly impede positive learning (Bolles, 1972). Animals trained to perform simple chains of behavior for food reinforcement often spontaneously exhibit adjunctive behavior patterns that distract them from completing the trained sequence. This interference occurs in spite of intensive and lengthy training efforts. In fact, it appears as though such interference worsens as conditioning proceeds. Animal trainers (Breland and Breland, 1961) using operant conditioning to train a variety of species to perform for entertainment and commercial purposes found that a number of the tasks were interfered with by species-specific appetitive and exploratory behaviors that spontaneously appear during the course of training. These interference effects resulting from food reinforcement are collectively referred to as *instinctive drift*. For example, in one case, a pig was trained to pick up wooden coins with its mouth and to deposit them in a piggy bank. The pig readily learned the task but over time began to play with the

coins by repeatedly picking them up and dropping them down again, throwing them into the air, or rooting them about with its snout—all behaviors associated with normal pig exploratory and appetitive behavior. Similarly, raccoons that had been taught a similar task would persistently fondle the coins before dropping them into the bank or, perhaps, periodically dip the coin into the bank as though washing it. When provided with more than one coin at a time, the raccoons would tend to rub them together instead of dropping them into the box as they had been trained to do. The Brelands formulated the following conclusion regarding instinctive drift:

> The general principle seems to be that wherever an animal has strong instinctive behaviors in the area of the conditioned response, after continued running the organism will drift toward the instinctive behavior to the detriment of the conditioned behavior and even to the delay or preclusion of the reinforcement. In a very boiled-down, simplified form, it might be stated as "learned behavior drifts toward instinctive behavior." (1961:684)

It is interesting to note that the sensory-motor modalities involved in this phenomenon are consistent with an interpretation involving corticothalamic dominance previously discussed (see Chapter 3). Under Welker's (1973) model of thalamocortical dominance, pigs are *rooters*, raccoons are *feelers*, and pigeons are *beholders*. Furthermore, some self-reinforcement stemming from hypothalamic-limbic feedback occurring during the emission of appetitive behavior may help to explain instinctive drift while at the same time preserving reinforcement theory. The locus of reinforcement supporting instinctive drift is internally articulated on brain reward sites associated with drive induction and preparatory appetitive responding. The arbitrary operant, on the other hand, may be more adequately conceptualized as belonging to or conditionally associated with the consummatory action and subsequent drive reduction. Although both are reinforcing, the action of preparing to eat may be intrinsically more rewarding than eating itself. Motivationally, this makes a lot of sense, since it requires a lot more effort (therefore, a lot more incentive and conditional reinforcement prior to consumption) to find food than to eat it.

Many other problems with the traditional conceptualization of appetitive operant learning have emerged in the laboratory. Brown and Jenkins (1968) discovered that pigeons could learn the key-peck response without being trained to do so by the experimenter. They found that pigeons readily acquired the habit of key pecking by simply exposing the birds to an active key that was programmed to light for 8 seconds and then shut off just before the presentation of food. The process, known as *autoshaping*, has drawn a great deal of attention, since it implies that the key-peck response may not be, strictly speaking, an operant at all but rather an elicited response acquired without depending on contingent positive reinforcement. It should be noted that while the initial key-peck response was not shaped or prompted, subsequent pecks at the lighted key were linked with the lighted key (conditioned reinforcement) and the presentation of food (i.e., positive reinforcement). The explanation for autoshaping may simply rest on the pigeon's high operant level for pecking and the occurrence of incidental reinforcement (i.e., superstitious learning). Seligman (1970) speculated that the autoshaping phenomenon depends on a high degree of preparedness in pigeons to associate pecking with the acquisition of food.

Subsequent experiments have yielded results that are even more difficult to explain by resorting to reinforcement theory. Williams and Williams (1969) designed an experiment in which key pecking never resulted in the acquisition of food but actually postponed it, that is, the bird was punished for pecking. Despite the negative punishment contingency, the pigeons maintained the key-peck response at a low rate (responding in one-third of the trials) and persisted in performing the response over the course of several hundred trials without stopping—even though the effort resulted in the omission of reinforcement. This finding is consistent with the observations of Breland and Breland. In effect, animals that are learning a response

closely linked with an innate appetitive-consummatory action tend to *drift* into its performance despite apparent reinforcement contingencies. The appetitive-consummatory action itself overshadows the arbitrary operant being rewarded. Jenkins and Moore (1973) observed that pigeons autoshaped to peck at a key for water or grain exhibited distinctively different response topographies. Pigeons trained to peck for grain exhibited a response resembling that used during eating, whereas those trained to peck for water did so in a manner topographically similar to drinking. This has led to some speculation that what is being learned is not an operant at all but rather a classically conditioned consummatory response.

While key pecking is rapidly acquired during appetitive training, not all responses are equally easy to shape. For instance, teaching dogs to scratch, yawn, or lift the rear leg in the typical urination posture is very difficult. Thorndike (1911/1965) found that cats worked much harder to escape problem boxes than did dogs. Many dogs would simply accept confinement in the box and not make the requisite effort to escape and obtain the proffered food reward. Thorndike noted that dogs tended to remain in the front of the box, fixed attentively on the food that remained out of reach. Unlike the cat, the dog "wants to get to the food, not out of the box" (1911/1965:59). Even among general obedience exercises, some behaviors are learned more easily than others. While the average dog readily learns to sit in exchange for a treat, many dogs "resent" being prompted to lay down and may actively resist such training efforts, even when it is carried out with food rewards alone.

CONTRAFREELOADING

Another troubling exception to the predictions of classical reinforcement theory is a phenomenon known as *contrafreeloading* (CFL). Neuringer (1969), for example, seriously questioned the importance of deprivation in animal studies, suggesting from his investigation of CFL that animals will work regardless of their motivational state (e.g., presence of threat or deprivation), even in the presence of free food. Several other studies have shown that animals will work under certain conditions for food doled out on a contingency basis, even though identical food is readily available in abundant quantities for free [Jensen (1963); also, see Osborne's review (1977)]. Many researchers studying CFL have suggested that the phenomenon reflects a preference for reinforcement with stimulus change or conditioned reinforcement over food presented ad libitum without stimulus change.

Inglis and coworkers (1997) offered another possible interpretation of this odd behavior, suggesting that CFL might serve an adaptation-enhancing function by providing information about a less than optimal food source. According to this theory, rather than exploit the immediately present, but possibly temporary, source of food, the animal works for food on a contingency basis to learn more about how to best manage and control (optimize) a potentially more reliable food source. Studies involving response-produced stimulus change seem to support such an informational purpose or imperative driving CFL (Wallace et al., 1973; Osborne and Shelby, 1975). CFL is especially interesting since it suggests that learning does not depend exclusively on consummatory events, but rather appetitive learning (at least) includes informational incentives that occur before the presentation of food.

Another possibility underlying CFL is the potentiating effects of conditioned reinforcement on learned behavior. For example, Marx and Murphy (1961) trained two groups of rats to nose poke for reinforcement. One group was exposed to classical conditioning where a buzzer was presented just before the presentation of reinforcement. Afterward, the two groups of rats were trained to run an alleyway. After a bit of practice, the two groups were exposed to the buzzer in the start box. The researchers found that the rats previously conditioned to the buzzer ran much faster than the controls. Stimulus change in this situation may be interpreted as an expectancy effect that augments general arousal and speed of performance. Expectancy as an in-

formation incentive makes sense here and in the case of CFL as well.

In several respects, CFL mirrors instinctive drift, except in one very important way—that is, CFL does not depend on a food-producing response for its maintenance. In fact, if stimulus change is discontinued and the target food-producing response is followed by the reinforcer only, the animals studied almost immediately neglect the food-producing response and turn instead to the free food now presented with antecedent stimulus change (Wallace et al., 1973). In the case of instinctive drift, the object cue associated with reward becomes the target of excessive behavior—for example, the raccoon's habit of repeatedly handling or "pretending" to wash the wooden coins and, consequently, failing to deposit them in the toy bank as required for reinforcement. Tomie (1996) reviewed a large body of literature showing that the manipulandum takes on special properties when it serves both as a reward cue and a mechanism for instrumental manipulation. According to this analysis, instinctive drift (a topic that he discusses at some length) is the result of a maladaptive repetition of preparatory responses that preclude actual completion of the sequence to obtain and consume primary reinforcement. Excessive manipulation of the cue/manipulandum may be a model for understanding some forms of compulsive behavior and drug abuse. Tomie, for example, argues that addictive behavior is driven to a considerable extent by the coincidence of the reward cue and the manipulandum (e.g., handling the syringe or holding and puffing the cigarette) occurring immediately prior to the pleasurable effects of the drug's action. The syringe or cigarette itself is implicated as playing an important role in the maintenance of the addiction.

GENETIC PREDISPOSITION AND TEMPERAMENT

Each individual—human or animal—is born with a definite tendency toward varying degrees of emotional reactivity in the direction of behavioral inhibition or excitability (Gray, 1991; Kagan and Snidman, 1991). The dog's general emotional reactivity or threshold to emotionally evocative stimulation is definitely a predisposing factor in the development of many common behavior problems. To a large extent, differences in emotional thresholds are affected by a limbic/autonomic inheritance present at birth. Some individuals are genetically disposed to being more calm and emotionally balanced under the influence of limbic modulation and parasympathetic tone (parasympathetic dominant), whereas others (sympathetic dominant) are much more sensitive and reactive to fright-freeze-fight stimulation, are hyperemotional, tend to perseverate in negative emotional states, are subject to neurotic elaborations and disequilibrium, and are prone to develop psychosomatic disease.

Schneirla (1965) has proposed that approach-withdrawal patterns are the fundamental organizing components regulating animal behavior and emotional development. These opposed tendencies are integrated at the level of the autonomic nervous system. Approach behavior is evoked by low-intensity stimulation and is closely paralleled by parasympathetic activity, that is, steady-state biological functions like resting heart rate and respiration. On the other hand, withdrawal is evoked by high-intensity stimulation, paralleling the activation the sympathetic system and the elicitation of various states of biological readiness, like increased heart rate and respiration. Thresholds for approach behavior and withdrawal behavior are ontogenetically defined, with approach behavior being dominate during neonatal developmental stages and withdrawal tendencies like fear and defensive reactions becoming progressively more dominant as a dog develops (see Chapter 2).

With maturation, these various autonomic adjustments move toward homeostatic balance and set the dog's relative emotional reactivity as an adult. As a result, some individuals are more emotionally labile, whereas others tend toward emotional stability and calmness. Approach-withdrawal dynamics are regulated according to various threshold differences—differences that are influenced by a dog's genetic constitution and early experiences. As development progresses, primitive

approach behavior becomes transformed into "seeking" or appetitive behavior (modified through the incentives of positive reinforcement), while withdrawal is elaborated into various learned patterns of escape and avoidance behavior (modified through the incentives of negative reinforcement). In domestic dogs, approach behavior is perpetuated so that competing withdrawal tendencies (flight, freeze, or fight) are kept in check. In some dogs, as the result of genetic disorders or adverse experiences, withdrawal thresholds are lowered and flight-fight reactions amplified, thus making the dogs more fearful or aggressively reactive to social contact.

As previously discussed (see Chapter 3), an important neural locus of emotional behavior is the hypothalamus, a brain structure orchestrating parasympathetic and sympathetic nervous activity. Besides regulating the expression of emotion, the hypothalamus has direct neural and hormonal connections with the pituitary gland, a structure responsible for the release of various tropic hormones, including adrenocorticotropic hormone (ACTH). The hypothalamic-pituitary-adrenal (HPA) system is a complex loop of biochemical feedback mechanisms regulating the body's reaction to stress and threat. ACTH stimulates the adrenal cortex to secrete various steroidal hormones, including cortisol, a hormone serving many general emergency functions as well as instructing the pituitary to stop producing ACTH. Additionally, the hypothalamus innervates the adrenal medulla, which, under sympathetic arousal, releases epinephrine directly into the bloodstream to support sustained emergency action.

The hypothalamus also appears to play a role in the regulation of androgen secretions. A negative-feedback mechanism exists between the level of testosterone in the blood and the hypothalamus (Hart, 1985). If the level of testosterone declines, the hypothalamus is stimulated to secrete gonadotropin-releasing factor, thereby causing the anterior pituitary to release luteinizing hormone into the bloodstream. Luteinizing hormone in male dogs stimulates the testes to produce increased amounts of testosterone. As testosterone reaches optimal plasma levels, the hypothalamus ceases the production of the releasing factor, which causes the pituitary to stop producing luteinizing hormone. Gonadal hormones appear to play a significant, although variable, role in determining a dog's general temperament by modulating thresholds for the expression of various sexually dimorphic and species-typical behavior patterns. Perinatal and pubescent androgens may predispose male dogs to exhibit a wider variety and greater frequency of behavior problems than exhibited by females as adults (Hart and Hart, 1985). In general, the effect of androgens on behavior is twofold: (1) the androgenization of testosterone-sensitive neural substrates mediating sexual and aggressive behavior (perinatal), and (2) modulating activities in these substrates once they are elaborated and functioning (pubescent).

Because of the apparent role of testosterone in the expression of certain forms of aggression, neutering is often recommended as a method for controlling such behavior. However, a great deal of controversy surrounds the effects of castration on aggressive behavior in dogs. Although castration appears to reduce intermale aggressive behavior in many mammalian species, the effect of castration is not so dramatic or clear-cut among dogs. Le Boeuf, for example, compared the adult behavior of dogs castrated at 40 days of age with the behavior of intact littermates. He found that prepubertal castration "seems to have little effect on sexual responsiveness, sexual attractiveness, or aggressivity" (1970:134). Similarly, Salmeri and colleagues (1991) found that prepubertal neutering (7 weeks of age) produced little difference in comparison with conspecifics neutered at 7 months. Surprisingly, the only dimensions of significant behavioral change resulting from prepubertal neutering were excitability and general activity levels but moving in an opposite direction than expected. They found that castrated dogs tended to become *more* active and excitable than intact controls. Even intermale aggression was only modestly decreased. Other studies have shown more dramatic effects resulting from neutering (Hopkins et al., 1976; Neilson et al., 1997). These studies involved populations of dogs exhibiting various behavior problems at the time of castration. The results indicate that the behaviors most likely to be affected by neutering are those associated with sexual maturation—that is, those depending on the presence of circulating testosterone for their full expression or maintenance.

A possible cause for the variable effect of castration on sexual behavior and aggression may be due, in part, to the influence of perinatal androgenization. The puppy's nervous system is androgenized just before birth and after birth by a surge of testosterone, thus predisposing the dog to exhibit many sexually dimorphic physical and behavioral characteristics as an adult male. Another surge of testosterone occurs at the time of puberty beginning around 6 months of age, reinforcing and sensitizing the earlier androgen effects on neural tissue. Evidence from studies with mice and rats suggests that prenatal secretion of testosterone may also affect the development of female fetuses that happen to be situated between males in the uterus. Such androgenized female rodents tend to exhibit more malelike behavior and aggressive tendencies as adults (Knol and Egberink-Alink, 1989). These effects have been demonstrated in other species (e.g., ungulates) and, at least theoretically, are possible in dogs (Overall, 1997). In fact, Coppola (1986, reported in Borchelt and Voith, 1996) has found that female dogs born in litters predominantly composed of male puppies are more likely to exhibit dominance aggression and various masculine tendencies as adults. Another potential source of prenatal influence on the emotional reactivity of offspring is the effect of anxious stress on the mother. Thompson (1957) performed a carefully controlled study in which rat mothers were differentially exposed to stressful stimulation versus normal laboratory conditions over the period of gestation. Subsequent tests revealed that the young of stressed mothers were significantly more "emotional" than controls born to unstressed mothers.

Obviously, many contributing factors affect the emotional reactivity of dogs. Scott notes that while susceptibility to emotionally provocative stimulation is undoubtedly subject to genetic variation, emotion per se does not exist on a genetic level:

> Emotions do not exist in genetic systems but are created as a result of the organizing activity of genetic systems interacting with other systems in the processes of development. There is no "gene for" an emotion or emotionality; these are phenomena that exist only on higher levels of organization. (1988:22)

He goes on to propose that the general function of emotion is to prolong momentary stimulation. The prolongation of emotional arousal motivates purposeful behavior in the direction of satisfying the emotional demand. The various emotions experienced by an animal are the motivational forces facilitating both adaptive and maladaptive behavior. In the case of maladaptive behavior, highly charged emotional reactions contribute to the development of dysfunctional behavior when the evoking situation does not provide outlets for adequate coping responses or, alternatively, a viable means of escape from the source of stimulation when other means of adaptation are not possible.

A common source of such excessive emotional stimulation in dogs is separation distress. Separation-distressed dogs are highly motivated to reestablish social contact denied to them by isolation or confinement. Under such conditions, dogs may engage in various distressed behaviors like barking and howling, destructiveness, and loss of eliminatory control. Some dogs simply fall into a state of depression. The evoking emotions and situation conform to Scott's conditions of maladaptive behavior: a high degree of emotional arousal, absence of adequate coping alternatives, and no means of escape. The degree of separation reactivity exhibited by a dog is influenced by both genetic variations (some breeds appear more reactive to separation) and experience, with both factors contributing to the determining threshold and magnitude of separation distress.

Although many genetic and other biological factors play a significant part in the expression of emotional traits, the majority of behavior problems presented for training are acquired as the result of adverse learning experiences and, therefore, can be more or less remedied through behavior therapy and training. While the behavioral traits exhibited by the various dog breeds differ considerably in detail, the broad preparedness for learning is very similar among dogs regardless of their breed affiliation. Consequently, the dog's genetic and biological endowment is often treated as a virtual constant. One result of such biological similarity is the ease with which the various breeds undergo formal obedience training in a group setting without much in the way of special consideration for breed-specific needs. The most significant variable in analyzing and modifying adjustment problems is the learned component; however, inherited emotional factors cannot be ignored, especially in cases involving severe emotional disorders and aggression. Statistical evidence suggests that some breeds are more prone to develop behavior problems than others (Landsberg, 1991). These breed variations with respect to the incidence of behavior problems may be the result of selective breeding for potentially problematic traits (e.g., increased aggression or activity levels). In other cases, abnormal tendencies may have been inadvertently transmitted without intentional selective pressure (e.g., shyness and various common dysfunctional behavior patterns like fear biting and low-threshold dominance aggression).

BREED VARIATIONS

Among the various dog breeds, great variability can be seen regarding the ease with which they learn different tasks. The Border collie possesses a superb propensity for herding sheep—an ability not available to nonherding breeds. No amount of training will turn a black-and-tan coonhound into an able sheep-herding dog, nor a Border collie into a steady trailing hound. Willis (1989) noted that the Border collie's ability to herd sheep not only depends on a genetic endowment (e.g., traits like crouching and *showing eye*) and intensive training but also on the selective breeding of sheep willing to be herded. Some breeds of sheep (notably African and Latin American varieties) do not respond by grouping tightly together and fleeing when challenged by a Border collie but instead may attack the dog when provoked.

Even highly specific behavioral traits involve an apparent heredity factor. For example, Dalmatians were often kept as coach dogs in the past. These dogs were expected to run under the carriage and to maintain an ideal position just behind the horses. Keeler and Trimble (1940) found that the dog's position preference (trailing behind the carriage, lingering to the rear of the carriage, or running under the front axle) was to some extent determined by heredity. They bred several dogs together ranked in terms of their respective position preferences. At 6 months of age, the resulting puppies were yoked to an experienced coach dog to train them to perform the activity. After a brief period of training, the pups were released from the control of the experienced dog and observed. It was found that the trainees exhibited position preferences consistent with their parents' preferences. Although not conclusive, it appears that coach position is to some extent an inherited trait.

Clearly, genetic factors predispose dogs to exhibit certain inevitable behavioral strengths or weaknesses (Mackenzie et al., 1986). Sometimes these genetically wired behavioral predispositions are antagonistic with specific training goals, requiring extra effort to overcome or incorporate. Most of what a dog does can be interpreted in terms of innate behavioral predispositions manifested under the actualizing influence of learning. The important issue at stake here is not whether a dog exhibits innately prepared or instinctive behavior, but that such behavior exhibits sufficient variability and flexibility to be modified through training. Dogs are extremely adaptable animals both in terms of their range of biological diversification and their modes of behavioral expression. One need only bring to mind the delicate Italian greyhound standing in the shadow of a monumental Neapolitan mastiff in order to appreciate the incredible genetic variability of dogs. The morphological contrast between the two breeds is so striking that it is understandably hard for some people to believe that they derive their appearances and behavior from the same ancestral gene pool.

Hall (1941) referred to the animal's temperament endowment as the "raw stuff of individuality." This is especially true in the case of tendencies in the opposing directions of inhibition-introversion or excitability-extroversion. Some dogs are innately more inhibited and introverted, whereas others are more excitable and extroverted. Inherited temperament traits influence the way dogs learn and how they are most effectively trained. Measuring or objectively representing this "raw stuff" in dogs has prompted factor analyses (Royce, 1955; Cattell and Korth, 1973; Draper, 1995; Goodloe and Borchelt, 1998), efforts to quantify and describe breed attributes (Scott and Fuller, 1965; Hart and Hart, 1985), and predictive temperament tests (Pfaffenberger, 1963; Campbell, 1972; Vollmer, 1977, 1978). Various behavioral profiles have been devised to help potential dog owners to make rational decisions about their chosen breed's compatibility with their lifestyle and expectations of dog companionship (Tortora, 1980; Hart and Hart, 1988). The Waltham Centre for Pet Nutrition has organized a counseling service called Selecta-dog for assisting dog owners in search of the ideal canine companion. The service counsels around 4500 inquirers a year (Edney, 1987). All of these scientific and applied activities are based on the assumption that a considerable portion of a dog's behavior is affected by inherited tendencies and traits.

Temperament Testing

Various tests have been devised to assess the temperament of puppies, presumably to assist in the placement of puppies into appropriate homes. However, some skepticism about the reliability of early temperament testing has accumulated over the years, especially with regard to predicting dominance tendencies and dominance aggression—a behavior problem believed to depend on social learning and maturation, as well as genetic predisposition. Margaret Young (reported in Fogle, 1990) has questioned the effectiveness of early aptitude and temperament testing for predicting specific traits in adult dogs. She found that many dogs that later proved to be difficult or aggressive were not detected by her battery of tests performed between 6 and 8 weeks of age:

> Social attraction, following and acceptance of stroking, did not reliably distinguish puppies that were later aloof and independent from those that were attracted toward people, readily trainable and handleable. Nor did tendencies identified by the test at seven weeks as dominant or submissive reliably predict later tendencies toward dominance or submissiveness. (1990:94)

However, she found that all puppies that displayed overt aggressive behavior (growling and barking) during testing were most likely to exhibit aggressive tendencies as adults. A study performed by Beaudet and colleagues (1994) questioned the reliability of puppy temperament testing for the detection of a predictive dominance factor in the temperament of young dogs. The researchers evaluated 39 puppies at 7 weeks of age according to the procedures recommended by Campbell (1972) and then once again at 16 weeks of age. The results were surprisingly negative. The study indicates that temperament-test results of 7-week-old puppies were not predictive of relative dominance exhibited by the same puppies when they were retested again at 16 weeks of age. According to the authors, "the test has no predictive value regarding future social tendencies. In fact, the total value of the behavioral scores for social tendencies between the two age groups showed a trend toward regression from dominance to submission" (Beaudet et al., 1994:273). These findings are consistent with the fluctuating dominance values found between these age groups by Scott and Fuller (1965). They early on discovered that relative dominance is a rather fluid social process that becomes progressively more stable and permanent as puppies mature.

Wright (1980) has also noted a great deal of individual variation with respect to competitive behavior and social dominance in puppies at the ages of 5.5, 8.5, and 11.5 weeks. One factor that was consistently correlated with competitive success was a willingness to explore a strange-complex situation

actively: "Those puppies that were the least neophobic were also the ones that were able to control a desirable object in a competitive situation" (1980:23). Mahut (1958) also reported a significant correlation between a dog's willingness to explore novel and fear-eliciting objects and its relative fearlessness and aggressivity. Of the 10 breeds she studied, the ones most willing to explore and "tease" the fear-eliciting objects presented to them were also the ones known as "fighters, killers, and ratters." Pawlowski and Scott (1956) found clear evidence of hereditary influence on the expression of relative competitive dominance among various breeds of dogs (basenji, beagle, cocker spaniel, and wirehaired fox terrier), speculating that the more dominant breeds (basenji and terrier) possess a lower threshold for external stimulation and the arousal of fighting behavior. Another study supporting the general supposition that relative dominance is inherited was performed by James (1951), who cross-fostered two mixed litters of terrier and beagle pups, so that the litters were comprised of half beagles and half terriers. He observed that the social organization that developed between the puppies was a linear dominance hierarchy with terriers on top. Beagles and terriers tended to congregate in separate groups. Evidence of territorial expansion based on dominance was also found in the study. Terriers not only took the food presented, they also tended to defend the area against the trespass of beagles.

Among other predictive trait correlations that have been found between puppy and adult behavior, especially significant are early measures of general activity and excitability. Martinek and Hartl (1975), for example, reported a stable correlation between excitability and habituation rates in dogs at 4 months of age and their subsequent performance as guard dogs at 14 months. These early measures of excitability/habituation were highly predictive of an adult dog's trainability. Dogs situated on either extreme of the excitability continuum performed poorly during training as adult dogs. Those dogs exhibiting moderate excitability levels as puppies proved to be most trainable as adult guard dogs. Humphrey and Warner (1934) also found a positive correlation between high energy (excitability) and adult aggressiveness. Additional support for this general hypothesis comes from studies by Goddard and Beilharz (1986), who determined that low activity levels in 12-week-old puppies were positively correlated with fearfulness in adult dogs. From 8 weeks onward, consistent individual differences in the expression of fear were observed—an observation consistent with findings reported previously by Fox (1966). The retrieving test was particularly reliable with regard to predicting *confidence* in adult dogs—fearful or emotionally inhibited puppies refused to fetch a ball.

Jackson Laboratory Studies

Scott and Fuller (1965) performed numerous experiments in an effort to quantify the relative contribution of heredity versus environment on the ontogenesis of the dog's behavior. They studied several generations of five breeds of dogs (basenji, beagle, cocker spaniel, wirehaired fox terrier, and Shetland sheepdog) and various crosses between them. The dogs were reared under similar conditions and then tested to compare and evaluate the inheritance of breed differences, including relative emotional reactivity, trainability, and problem-solving behavior. Clear differences were observed between the breeds studied. For example, wirehaired terriers, basenjis, and beagles were found to be much more emotionally reactive than cocker spaniels and Shetland sheepdogs, with the cocker spaniel being rated the most emotionally stable of the breeds studied. In terms of trainability, cocker spaniels also proved to be more responsive (both while being weighed and during leash training) than the other breeds tested. Somewhat surprisingly, the shelties were rated below the other breeds in terms of leash training, receiving most of their demerits as the result of jumping up or winding the leash around the handler's legs. The basenjis received high scores in terms of fighting the leash, whereas beagles exhibited the most reactive vocalizations during training. Cockers also performed better during an obedience test in which the dogs were trained

to stay on a table for 30 seconds and then to jump off on command. Again, the basenjis proved the least cooperative of the five breeds. In terms of problem-solving behavior, the hunting breeds (basenjis, beagles, cockers, and terriers) outperformed the shelties. Scott and Fuller speculated that selective breeding may have had a direct bearing on these differences:

> This is probably because most of the tests were deliberately designed to test independent capacities motivated by food rewards; and it is noteworthy that the beagle, which is normally used for hunting without direction, shows the best over-all performance in terms of number of first ranks. By contrast, the Shetland sheep dogs, whose ancestors have been selected for their ability to perform complex tasks under close direction from their human masters, performed badly. Indeed, in many of the tests, the shelties gave the subjective impression of waiting around for someone to tell them what to do. Furthermore, while all the hunting breeds are strongly motivated by food, sheep dogs in general have been selected away from this trait. (1965:257)

An important factor influencing the outcome of many of the trainability and problem-solving tests was a dog's relative emotionality and degree of confidence or fear.

INHERITANCE OF FEAR

Krushinskii

Many studies have shown that emotional extremes involving fearfulness are inherited. Thorne (1944), for example, found that a "fear biting" basset hound named Paula had a tremendous genetic influence on a large group of her descendants in terms of their relative fearfulness. Of 59 dogs related to this highly reproductive female, 43 (73%) were shy and unfriendly. Thorne concluded that shyness was the result of a dominant trait and, therefore, not responsive to modification through learning and training. Krushinskii (1960) took exception to Thorne's conclusion that the shyness trait was unalterable through the influence of learning. He tracked the inheritance and expression of active defensive reactions (ADRs) and passive defensive reactions (PDRs) in dogs. In the case of PDRs, if both parents exhibited the trait, the majority of the offspring would also show fearful tendencies. However, the expression of PDRs is highly dependent on environmental factors, especially socialization effects and environmental exposure. In opposition to Thorne, Krushinskii argued that the expression of shyness depended on both genotype and training conditions. The absence of active socialization together with environmental isolation tends to augment PDRs (shyness), whereas active socialization and the provision of environmental exposure tends to increase the exhibition of ADRs (aggressiveness). Krushinskii concluded that, although heredity plays a vital role in the expression of PDRs and ADRs, various environmental factors are also important in determining the final character of a dog's temperament.

Although experiential factors play an actualizing role in the expression of temperament excesses and deficits, breed differences clearly do exist. Thus, some breeds (and individuals) are more predisposed to become shy, while others are more prone to become aggressive. To quantify and compare these breed differences, Krushinskii studied the PDRs of German shepherds, Airedale terriers, and Doberman pinschers under conditions of home rearing and kennel isolation. He determined that decisive genetic differences exist between these different breeds, predisposing each to develop distinctive and varying degrees of passive defensive behavior. For example, the German shepherds were more prone to exhibit fearful behavior, regardless of the conditions of rearing. Further, while both German shepherds and Airedale terriers exhibited increased levels of passive defensive behavior following exposure to conditions of isolation, the shepherds exhibited more fearfulness than the terriers exposed to the same amount of isolation. Interestingly, Doberman pinschers were much less prone to exhibit increased PDRs as the result of isolation. Even when reared under extreme conditions of isolation, the expression of fearfulness in the Doberman pinschers studied was approximately the same as that exhibited by German shepherds that had been raised in a home environment.

Nervous Pointers

Murphree (1973) and his associates at the VA Hospital in Little Rock, Arkansas, found that a dog's tendency to develop fearful behavior toward humans is inherited. They have been systematically breeding a normal strain and a nervous strain of pointers for many years. The normal pointers, or A-dogs, are described as being active, socially outgoing, and very compliant to experimental tasks. They are able learners and resistant to the induction of experimental neurosis. The nervous pointers, or E-dogs, are prone to fearful extremes in behavior, exhibiting an intense aversion toward human contact. In the presence of humans, the E-dogs retreat and become tense (catatonic rigidity) and wide-eyed; in general, a stark contrast to the normal pointers. E-dogs are further distinguished by being smaller and more prone to develop severe mange, a condition that may be related to stress-induced immunosuppression.

Several physiological differences have been observed between normal and nervous pointers. The HPA system is directly affected by chronic fear and stress. However, as noted in Chapter 3, Klein and coworkers (1990) were unable to demonstrate significant differences between normal and nervous dogs with regard to HPA system activity (e.g., increased ACTH and cortisol levels). This finding conflicts with an earlier study performed by Pasley and colleagues (1978) that found that E-dogs had larger adrenal glands than A-dogs. Klein and colleagues attributed this apparent conflict of findings to the influence of episodic stress taking place only in the presence of humans and, therefore, not detectable by their baseline measurements. It should be noted in this regard, that E-dogs appear normal and relaxed while interacting with other pointers; it is only when they come in contact with humans that they show signs of fear. Uhde and coworkers (1992) found clear differences in the body weights of normal versus nervous dogs, with the most fearful patterns of behavior being exhibited by female dogs weighing the least. Additionally, they found that an inverse relationship existed between a dog's degree of fearfulness, her body weight, and plasma levels of insulin-like growth factor I (IGF-I). Fearful dogs exhibited significantly lower levels of IGF-I, suggesting that chronic fear may adversely affect the hypothalamic-growth hormone axis. With respect to brain substrate differences, Lucas and colleagues (1974) found distinct differences in hippocampal theta-wave activity between normal dogs and nervous dogs. Spontaneous hippocampal theta-wave activity is associated with arousal occurring in the presence of familiar stimuli or following habituation to novelty. On the other hand, desynchronization of theta-wave activity is evoked during the elicitation of the orienting response, during escape from aversive stimulation, and following intracranial stimulation of the reticular formation. A decrease in theta-wave activity indicates momentary neural inhibition and increased vigilance, whereas increased rhythmic theta-wave activity is associated with a relaxed, alert state. Nervous pointers exhibit less hippocampal theta-wave activity than normal counterparts. This evidence seems to implicate the hippocampus as important neural substrate mediating lower fear thresholds and prolonged states of generalized anxious arousal in such dogs:

> These data indicated to us that nervous pointer dogs do not exhibit a normal response in their hippocampogram to environmental stimuli. We believe that these animals remain in the initial phase of the orienting response (desynchronization of the hippocampogram) and that habituation fails to occur. (Lucas et al., 1974:612)

Lastly, while in the presence of humans, the heart-rate patterns of normal and nervous dogs differ significantly (Newton and Lucas, 1982). Nervous dogs exhibit reduced heart rates both when a person is in the room (without petting) and also when petted. In contrast, normal dogs exhibit an *increase* in heart rates only when a person enters the room, but a slower rate (returning to baseline) while being petted.

A striking sensory difference between nervous and normal pointers is the existence of a much higher incidence of deafness in nervous dogs. Klein and colleagues (1988) found that most of the nervous dogs that they tested were deaf. Despite this finding, the researchers emphasize that nervous behavior occurs independently of a dog's hearing ability, with hearing and deaf nervous dogs exhibiting similarly abnormal behavior. In another study, involving a colony of pointers studied at the National Institute of Mental Health (Bethesda, MD), 21 of 28 nervous dogs were found to be deaf. In contrast, among the 16 normal pointers tested, 15 had normal hearing, with one exhibiting loss of hearing in one ear (Steinberg et al., 1994).

Although nervous dogs are more prone to exhibit fearful behavior toward humans than are normal pointers, the former do respond variably (with some benefit) to rehabilitative efforts, including supplemental socialization and graduated desensitization. For example, Reese (1978) reported an experiment in which a litter of six nervous-strain puppies were divided so that three of them were home reared while the other three were raised under ordinary laboratory conditions. The home-reared and laboratory-reared puppies were then tested and compared. The results indicated that the home-reared puppies exhibited some improvement in terms of social responsiveness to humans that was not evident in lab-reared siblings. However, the benefit of home rearing was short-lived. By 12 months of age, little difference between the two groups was observed in terms of their response to human contact. In another rehabilitative experiment, an effort was made to train nervous pointers to hunt (McBryde and Murphree, 1974). Surprisingly, the researchers discovered that after patient training, involving gradual desensitization and social facilitation, the pointers not only became successful hunters (practically indistinguishable from normal pointers), they also learned to tolerate close working contact with humans while in the field. This apparent benefit did not, however, generalize back to the laboratory setting—test scores within that context remained essentially constant.

Murphree and Newton (1971) found that avoidance responding could be attenuated somewhat by providing lab-reared puppies with intensive supplemental socialization and exposure to positive human contact. This additional socialization included daily 30-minute sessions of affectionate holding and play. While nervous puppies showed limited benefit from such additional social contact, normal puppies exhibited a much more pronounced benefit as a result of such treatment. Experiments like the foregoing led Reese (1978) to speculate that the basic difference between nervous E-dogs and normal A-dogs was their variable responsiveness with respect to negative and positive reinforcement. He contended that E-dogs were more sensitive to negative reinforcement, whereas normal A-dogs were more sensitive to the effects of positive reinforcement. The outcome of this selective sensitivity was that nervous dogs were more negatively influenced by the aversive effects of routine handling and testing. On the other hand, A-dogs responded more readily to the positive events occurring during the same routine handling, thus accounting for their increased benefit from supplemental socialization efforts. Reese concluded, "The fact that a high percentage of A's remain friendly and cooperative seems just as remarkable as the fact that a high percentage of E's do not" (1978:172).

HEREDITY AND INTELLIGENCE

Intelligence is a complex and largely indeterminate aspect of a dog's cognitive endowment. Serious attempts to quantify it as an independent factor have been frustrated by both conceptual and experimental inadequacies. Even finding agreement on what is signified by the word *intelligence* is not easily obtained from one authority to the next. Intelligence is embedded in a web of interactive factors, including sensory abilities, motor skills, emotional reactivity, general motivation, and previous learning experiences. To my knowledge, no controlled experiments with dogs have been performed to measure intelligence while at the same time properly excluding the influence of these extraneous factors. The results of most animal intelligence studies to date are confounded by experimental shortcomings that measure more than intelligence per se. Instead of measuring intellectual ability, IQ tests measure a cluster

of factors among which intelligence may or may not play a prominent role.

Measuring Intelligence

To rectify this problem, a reasonable starting point for the study of dog intelligence might begin with the design of an adequate series of controlled experiments. One *hypothetical* possibility is to compare multiple subjects in terms of their differential rate of learning and problem solving in a situation where all other variables are controlled for except *rate of learning* or *insight*. The next step would be to isolate and group these animals into slow and fast learners. To ensure that this apparent difference is of an innate origin, genetic studies would have to be undertaken to breed selectively for slower and faster learners from the segregated groups. By genetically augmenting their respective strengths and weaknesses, two strains of efficient and deficient learners would theoretically be produced. Additionally, the hypothetical study could be extended to include a comparison of genetically slow and fast learners with regard to their acquisition of other diverse skills, thereby determining the extent to which the proposed intelligence factor generalizes to other problem-solving situations. However, even if such careful studies were actually carried out, they would probably prove to be a waste of time and effort.

In fact, many behavioral studies like the above have been performed on rats. Early on, Tolman (1924) and Tryon (1929, 1934) found that maze-learning ability in rats was inherited. Both researchers selectively bred maze-dull and maze-bright rats, thereby developing two distinct strains of rats based on maze-learning ability. Speculation that such enhanced learning ability resulted from a general intelligence factor was not supported by subsequent experimentation, however. The deciding factor in maze learning was not intelligence but rather differences of emotional reactivity exhibited by the two strains. Searle (1949) tested the two strains of rats under various maze conditions and concluded that maze-dull rats were simply more fearful and timid of the maze situation—not less intelligent. Further, additional studies involving maze-bright and maze-dull rats demonstrated that maze-bright rats are not necessarily better learners than maze-dull rats when tested on tasks other than maze learning (Wahlsten, 1972). Intelligence appears to be an epiphenomenon compounded of many underlying predisposing factors and experiential contributions, including emotional reactivity, locomotor ability, sensory acuity, and sensitivity to hedonically significant outcomes (positive and negative training events).

E. G. Sarris (University of Hamburg) performed a series of experiments and observations to assess intelligent behavior in dogs, especially in terms of trial-and-error learning and "insight." He posed a number of problems for a variety of dogs at various ages, involving varying degrees of difficulty. Besides evaluating maze performance, he recorded learning styles and strategies used by dogs to solve problems requiring the physical manipulation of ropes, boxes, doors, stairs, and wagons as aids. What makes Sarris's study so intriguing and valuable is the care he took to describe the behavior he patiently observed. The report, published as a four-part series in the *American Kennel Gazette* (Sarris, 1938–1939), contains a diary of notes and photographs illustrating his findings. Sarris emphasized the need for appreciating the dog's special "umwelt" or subjective schema with which it organizes its experience of the environment. He argued that temperament and intelligence are mutually interdependent influences that inform a dog's umwelt and problem-solving behavior. Problems are conceived of as unaccustomed umwelt conditions that require a dog to vary customary patterns of behavior in novel ways to arrive at a solution: "Everything originating in the human 'Umwelt' has to be transformed in to 'dog things,' in order that the brain of the dog can grasp and co-ordinate it" (Feb 1939:24). In this regard, a dog's ability to play provides a decisive factor. Sarris notes that play is an "infallible" individualizing indicator of a dog's temperament and relative intelligence. Play appears to mediate intelligent adaptations by allowing a dog to discover and to explore options fearlessly outside of the usual pattern. The quality of a dog's intelligence and temperament are expressed through its ability to play. Although Sarris accomplishes his goal of demonstrating the existence of individual differences in dogs, more importantly his patient observations captured unique glimpses into the range and potential sagacity of canine intelligence that are often overlooked under less natural conditions of study.

Measuring Differences in Intelligence

Clearly, the measurement of dog intelligence and its relative distribution among dog breeds will not be advanced by pop psychology, simplistic IQ tests, and contrived intelligence rankings à la Coren (1994). Scott and Fuller, after reviewing the results of 13 years of highly controlled testing and evaluation of dog problem solving and learning ability in various breeds, concluded with respect to dog intelligence that all dogs exhibit a similar profile when other factors like emotional reactivity and motivation are held constant or factored out:

> On the basis of the information we now have, we can conclude that all breeds show about the same average level of performance in problem solving, provided they can be adequately motivated, provided physical differences and handicaps do not affect the tests, and provided interfering emotional reactions such as fear can be eliminated. In short, all the breeds appear quite similar in pure intelligence. (1965:258)

Scott and Fuller concluded that all dogs do about equally well so long as they can be comparably motivated and relaxed during training and testing. Further, they note that a dog's relative ability to solve problems and to learn is not due to a genetically transmitted intelligence factor per se, but, more significantly, such ability depends on the presence of emotional attributes that are compatible with the tasks required.

There is a tendency among dog owners to equate intelligence with trainability. But does a dog's trainability and obedience depend on its intelligence? The available scientific evidence indicates that a willingness to accept training and to perform obediently are not necessarily correlated with intelligence. Fox succinctly denies a relationship between intelligence and obedience: "Obedience, however, like trainability, is not a sign of intelligence, and obedience training to stay, sit, retrieve, and so on are not measures of intelligence per se" (1972:112).

Many ethologists studying wild canids have expressed the belief that wolves are more intelligent than domestic dogs, yet even hand-reared wolves are very difficult to train and often refuse to perform the most rudimentary obedience tasks; they are simply not prepared to learn such things—at least under conventional methods of training. Dogs, on the other hand, readily learn to exchange obedience for reassuring affection and are easily subordinated by threats and compulsion. When wolves are exposed to formal obedience training, they may attempt to flee and, if escape is blocked, may struggle or attack. The wolf's responses to forceful handling are biologically programmed species-typical defensive reactions. While an intelligence factor is undoubtedly present, the average dog's trainability is more influenced by the way the dog reacts to rewards or emotionally provocative coercion. Although intelligence may be an important factor in training, other traits and predispositions prepare some dogs to learn more efficiently—for example, a high degree of emotional dependency, ease of subordination to handler control, and low reactivity to physical aversive stimulation. These traits and others conducive to obedience training are selected for, especially in the herding and retriever-type dogs.

There can be little doubt that some dog breeds accept obedience training better than others. However, this does not necessarily imply that breeds performing well in obedience competition are more or less intelligent than counterparts not performing as well in the ring. Preparedness to learn a task is often confused with intelligence, and contrapreparedness to learn is considered something akin to stupidity. Dogs are specialists, so it is extremely misleading to compare the rate that different breeds learn an arbitrary skill (like obedience) for which they are not equally prepared through selective breeding to learn. The intelligence of dogs is remarkably similar from breed to breed. In fact, as

Scott and Fuller (1965) have noted, the greatest differences in intelligence exist between individuals belonging to the same breed rather than between the various breeds. However, many of these intrabreed differences (where they exist) are probably more the result of early training and rearing practices than the workings of an innate intelligence factor.

The dog's versatility as a domestic species is reflected in the ease with which it is trained and adapted to so many varied roles and environments. As the result of many thousands of years of conscious and unconscious selective breeding, dogs have accrued many adaptive behavioral changes, including an aptitude for training and a desire for close social contact with humans. While a dog's behavior is informed by an ancient phylogenetic heritage, its success as "man's best friend" is not governed by genes alone but by the dog's ability to learn. As will be repeatedly emphasized throughout the remainder of this book, our dogs' ability to learn from the consequences of their actions, and thereby to adjust their behavior to fit more precisely the demands of the surrounding environment, is central to the dog's success as humankind's closest animal ally and companion.

References

Beach FA (1950/1971). The snark was a boojum. *Am Psychol*, 5:115–124 (reprint).

Beaudet R, Chalifoux A, and Dallaire A (1994). Predictive value of activity level and behavioral evaluation on future dominance in puppies. *Appl Anim Behav Sci*, 40:273–284.

Bitterman ME (1965). Phyletic differences in learning. *Am Psychol*, 20:396–410.

Bitterman ME (1988). Vertebrate-invertebrate comparisons. In HJ Jerison and I Jerison (Eds), *Intelligence and Evolutionary Biology*. Berlin: Springer-Verlag.

Bolles RC (1972). Reinforcement, expectancy, and learning. *Psychol Rev*, 79:394–409.

Borchelt PL and Voith VL (1996). Dominance aggression in dogs (Update). In VL Voith and PL Borchelt (Eds), *Readings in Companion Animal Behavior*. Trenton, NJ: Veterinary Learning Systems.

Breland K and Breland M (1961). The misbehavior of organisms. *Am Psychol*, 16:681–684.

Brower LP (1969). Ecological chemistry. *Sci Am*, 220:22–29.

Brown PL and Jenkins HM (1968). Autoshaping of the pigeon's key-peck. *J Exp Anal Behav*, 1:1–8.

Campbell WE (1972). A behavior test for puppy selection. *Mod Vet Pract*, 12:29–33.

Cattell RB and Korth B (1973). The isolation of temperament dimensions in dogs. *Behav Biol*, 9:15–30.

Coppola MC(1986). Dominance aggression in dogs. Master's thesis. Department of Psychology, Hunter College, New York, NY.

Coren S (1994). *The Intelligence of Dogs: Canine Consciousness and Capabilities*. New York: Free Press.

Dobrzecka C, Szwejkowska G, and Konorski J (1966). Qualitative versus directional cues in two forms of differentiation. *Science*, 153:87–89.

Draper TW (1995). Canine analogs of human personality factors. *J Gen Psychol*, 122:241–252.

Edney ATB (1987). Matching dogs to owners: 10 years of "Selectadog." *J Small Anim Pract*, 28:1004–1008.

Fantino E and Logan CA (1979). *The Experimental Analysis of Behavior: A Biological Perspective*. San Francisco: WH Freeman.

Fogle B (1990). *The Dog's Mind: Understanding Your Dog's Behavior*. New York: Howell Book House.

Fox MW (1966). The development of learning and conditioned responses in the dog: Theoretical and practical implications. *Can J Comp Vet Sci*, 30:282–286.

Fox MW (1972). *Understanding Your Dog*. New York: Coward, McCann and Geoghegan.

Gallistel CR (1990). *The Organization of Learning*. Cambridge: MIT Press.

Garcia J and Koelling RA (1966). Relation of cue to consequence in avoidance learning. *Psychol Sci*, 4:123–124.

Garcia J, Rusiniak KW, and Brett LP (1977). Conditioning food-illness aversions in wild animals: *Caveant canonici*. In H Davis and HMB Hurwitz (Eds), *Operant-Pavlovian Interactions*. Hillsdale, NJ: Lawrence Erlbaum Associates.

Goddard ME and Beilharz RG (1986). Early prediction of adult behaviour in potential guide dogs. *Appl Anim Behav Sci*, 15:247–260.

Goodloe LP and Borchelt PL (1998). Companion dog temperament traits. *J Appl Anim Welfare Sci*, 1:303–338.

Gould JL (1979). Do Honeybees Know What They Are Doing? *Nat Hist*, 88:66–75.

Gould JL (1982). *Ethology: The Mechanisms and Evolution of Behavior*. New York: WW Norton.

Gray JA (1991). The neuropsychology of temperament. In J Strelau and A Angleitner (Eds), *Explorations in Temperament*. New York: Plenum.

Griffin DR (1981) *The Question of Animal Awareness: Evolutionary Continuity of Mental Experience*. New York: Rockefeller University Press.

Gustavson CR (1977). Comparative aspects of learned food aversions. In LM Barker, MR Best, and M Domjan (Eds), *Learning Mechanisms in Food Selection*. Waco, TX: Baylor University Press.

Gustavson CR (1996). Taste aversion conditioning versus conditioning using aversive peripheral stimuli. In VL Voith and PL Borchelt (Eds), *Readings in Companion Animal Behavior*. Philadelphia: Veterinary Learning Systems.

Gustavson CR and Gustavson JC (1982). Food avoidance in rats: The differential effects of shock, illness and repellents. *Appetite J Int Res*, 3:335–340.

Gustavson CR, Garcia J, Hankins WG, and Rusiniak KW (1974). Coyote predation control by aversive conditioning. *Science*, 184:581–583.

Hall CS (1941). Temperament: A survey of animal studies. *Psychol Bull*, 38:909–943.

Hansen I, Bakken M, and Braastad BO (1997). Failure of LiCl-conditioned taste aversion to prevent dogs from attacking sheep. *Appl Anim Behav Sci*, 54:251–256.

Hart BL (1985). *The Behavior of Domestic Animals*. New York: WH Freeman.

Hart BL and Hart LA (1985). Selecting pet dogs on the basis of cluster analysis of breed behavior profiles and gender. *JAVMA*, 186:1181–1185

Hart BL and Hart LA (1988). *The Perfect Puppy*. New York: WH Freeman.

Hinde RA and Stevenson-Hinde J (1973). *Constraints on Learning: Limitations and Predispositions*. New York: Academic.

Hopkins SG, Schubert TA, and Hart BL (1976). Castration of adult male dogs: Effects on roaming, aggression, urine marking, and mounting. *JAVMA*, 168:1108–1110.

Hume D (1748/1988). *An Enquiry Concerning Human Understanding*. Buffalo, NY: Prometheus (reprint).

Humphrey E and Warner L (1934). *Working Dogs*. Baltimore: Johns Hopkins Press.

Inglis IR, Forkman B, and Lazarus J (1997). Free food or earned food? A review and fuzzy model of contrafreeloading. *Anim Behav*, 53:1171–1191.

James W (1890/1950). *The Principles of Psychology,* Vol 2. New York: Dover (reprint).

James WT (1951). Social organization among dogs of different temperaments, terriers and beagles, reared together. *J Comp Physiol Psychol,* 44:71–77.

Jenkins HM and Moore BR (1973). The form of the autoshaped response with food or water reinforcers. *J Exp Anal Behav,* 20:163–181.

Jensen GD (1963). Preference for bar pressing over "free-loading" as a function of rewarded presses. *J Exp Psychol,* 65:451–454.

Kagan J and Snidman N (1991). Infant predictors of inhibited and uninhibited profiles. *Psychol Sci,* 2:40–44.

Keeler CE and Trimble HC (1940). Inheritance of position preference in coach dogs. *J Hered,* 31:51–54.

Klein E, Steinberg SA, Weiss SRB, et al.(1988). The relationship between genetic deafness and fear-related behaviors in nervous pointer dogs. *Physiol Behav,* 43:307–312.

Klein EH, Thomas T, and Uhde TW (1990). Hypothalamo-pituitary-adrenal axis activity in nervous and normal pointer dogs. *Biol Psychiatry,* 27:791–794.

Knol BW and Egberink-Alink ST (1989). Androgens, progestagens and agonistic behaviour: A review. *Vet Q,* 11:94–101.

Krasne FB and Glanzman DL (1995). What we can learn from invertebrate learning. *Annu Rev Psychol,* 46:585–624.

Krushinskii LV (1960). *Animal Behavior: Its Normal and Abnormal Development.* New York: Consultants Bureau.

Kuo ZY (1967). *The Dynamics of Behavior Development: An Epigenetic View.* New York: Random House.

Landsberg GM (1991). The distribution of canine behavior cases at three behavior referral practices. *Vet Med,* 86:1011–1018.

Lawicka W (1964). The role of stimuli modality in successive discrimination and differentiation learning. *Bull Pol Acad Sci,* 12:35–38 [reported in Mazur (1986)].

Le Boeuf BJ (1970). Copulatory and aggressive behavior in the prepubertally castrated dog. *Horm Behav,* 1:127–136.

LoLordo VM and Droungas A (1989). Selective associations and adaptive specializations: Taste aversions and phobias. In SB Klein and RR Mowrer (Eds), *Contemporary Learning Theories: Instrumental Theory and the Impact of Biological Constraints on Learning,* 145–179. Hillsdale, NJ: Lawrence Erlbaum Associates.

Lorenz K (1965). *Evolution and Modification of Behavior.* Chicago: University of Chicago Press.

Lorenz K (1982). *The Foundations of Ethology: The Principal Ideas and Discoveries in Animal Behavior.* New York: Simon and Schuster.

Lucas EA, Powell EW, and Murphree OD (1974). Hippocampal theta in nervous pointer dogs. *Physiol Behav,* 12:608–613.

Mackenzie SA, Oltenacu EAB, and Houpt KA (1986). Canine behavioral genetics: A review. *Appl Anim Behav Sci,* 15:365–393.

Mahut H (1958). Breed differences in the dog's emotional behaviour. *Can J Psychol,* 12:35–44.

Martinek Z and Hartl K (1975). About the possibility of predicting the performance of adult guard dogs from early behavior: II. *Activ Nerv Supl (Praha)* 17:76–77.

Marx MH and Murphy WW (1961). Resistance to extinction as a function of the presentation of a motivating cue in the start box. *J Comp Physiol Psychol,* 54:207–210.

Mazur JE (1986). *Learning and Behavior.* Englewood Cliffs, NJ: Prentice-Hall.

McBryde WC and Murphree OD (1974). The rehabilitation of genetically nervous dogs. *Pavlov J Biol Sci* 9:76–84.

McConnell PB (1990a). Acoustic structure and receiver response in domestic dogs, *Canis familiaris. Anim Behav,* 39:897–904.

McConnell PB (1990b). Lessons from animal trainers: The effect of acoustic structure on an animal's response. In Bateson P and Kloffer P (Eds), *Perspectives in Ethology.* New York: Plenum.

McConnell PB (1992). Louder than words. *Pure-Bred Dogs Am Kennel Gaz,* May.

Miller JD and Bowe CA (1982). Roles of the qualities and locations of stimuli and responses in simple associative learning: The quality-location hypothesis. *Pavlov J Biol Sci,* 17:129–139.

Mugford RA (1977). External influences on the feeding of carnivores. In MK Kare and O Maller (Eds), *The Chemical Senses and Nutrition,* 25–50. New York: Academic.

Murphree OD (1973). Inheritance of human aversion and inactivity in two strains of pointer dogs. *Biol Psychiatry,* 7:23–29.

Murphree OD and Newton JEO (1971). Crossbreeding and special handling of genetically nervous dogs. *Cond Reflex,* 6:129–136.

Neilson JC, Eckstein RA, and Hart BL (1997). Effects of castration on problem behaviors in male dogs with reference to age and duration of behavior. *JAVMA,* 211:180–182.

Neuringer AJ (1969). Animals respond for food in the presence of free food. *Science,* 166:399–401.

Newton JEO and Lucas LA (1982). Differential heart-rate responses to person in nervous and normal pointer dogs. *Behav Genet,* 12:379–393.

Osborne SR (1977). The free food (contrafree-loading) phenomenon: A review and analysis. *Anim Learn Behav,* 5:221–235.

Osborne SR and Shelby M (1975). Stimulus change as a factor in response maintenance with free food available. *J Exp Anal Behav,* 24:17–21.

Overall K (1997). *Clinical Behavioral Medicine for Small Animals.* St. Louis: CV Mosby.

Pasley JN, Powell EW, and Angel CA (1978). Adrenal glands in nervous pointer dogs. *IRCS Med Sci,* 6:102.

Pawlowski AA and Scott JP (1956). Hereditary differences in the development of dominance in litters of puppies. *J Comp Physiol Psychol,* 49:353–358.

Pfaffenberger CJ (1963). *The New Knowledge of Dog Behavior.* New York: Howell Book House.

Reese WG (1978). Familial vulnerability for experimental neurosis. *Pavlov J Biol Sci,* 13:169–173.

Royce JR (1955). A factorial study of emotionality in the dog. *Psychol Monogr Gen Appl,* 69:1–27.

Salmeri KR, Bloomber MS, Scruggs SL, and Shille V (1991). Gonadectomy in immature dogs: Effects on skeletal, physical, and behavioral development. *JAVMA,* 198:1193–1203.

Sarris EG (1938–1939). Individual difference in dogs [four parts]. *Am Kennel Gaz,* Nov 1938, Dec 1938, Jan 1939, Feb 1939.

Schneirla TC (1965) Aspects of stimulation and organization in approach-withdrawal process underlying vertebrate behavioral development. In DS Lehrman, RA Hinde, and E Shaw (Eds), *Advances in the Study of Animal Behavior,* 7:1–74. New York: Academic.

Scott JP (1988). Genetics, emotions and psychopathology. In M Clynes and J Panksepp (Eds), *Emotions and Psychopathology.* New York: Plenum.

Scott JP and Fuller JL (1965). *Genetics and the Social Behavior of the Dog.* Chicago: University of Chicago Press.

Searle LV (1949). The organization of hereditary maze-brightness and maze-dullness. *Genet Psychol Monogr,* 39:279–325.

Seligman MEP (1970). On the generality of the laws of learning. *Psychol Rev,* 77:406–418.

Seligman MEP (1971). Phobias and preparedness. *Behav Ther,* 2:307–320.

Seligman MEP and Hager JL (1972). *Biological Boundaries of Learning.* New York: Appleton-Century-Crofts.

Skinner BF (1974). *About Behaviorism.* New York: Alfred A Knopf.

Steinberg SA, Klein E, Killens RL, and Uhde TW (1994). Inherited deafness among nervous pointer dogs. *J Hered,* 85:56–59.

Thompson WR (1957). Influence of prenatal maternal anxiety on emotional reactivity in young rats. *Science,* 125:698–699.

Thorndike EL (1911/1965). *Animal Intelligence: Experimental Studies.* New York: Hafner (reprint).

Thorne FC (1944). The inheritance of shyness in dogs. *J Genet Psychol,* 65:275–279.

Thorpe WH (1956/1966). *Learning and Instinct in Animals.* Cambridge: Harvard University Press (reprint).

Tinbergen N (1951/1969). *The Study of Instinct.* Oxford: Oxford University Press (reprint).

Tinbergen N (1953/1975). *Social Behaviour of Animals.* New York: Halsted (reprint).

Tolman EC (1924). The inheritance of maze-learning ability in rats. *J Comp Psychol,* 4:1–18.

Tomie A (1996). Locating reward cue at response manipulandum (CAM) induces symptoms of drug abuse. *Neurosci Biobehav Rev,* 20:505–535.

Tortora DF (1980). *The Right Dog for You.* New York: Simon and Schuster.

Tryon RC (1929). The genetics of learning ability in rats: A preliminary report. *Univ Calif Publ Psychol,* 4:71–89.

Tryon RC (1934). Individual differences. In FA Moss (Ed), *Comparative Psychology,* 409–448. New York: Prentice-Hall.

Uhde TW, Malloy LC, and Slate SO (1992). Fearful behavior, body size, and serum IGF-I levels in nervous and normal pointer dogs. *Pharmacol Biochem Behav,* 43:263–269.

Vollmer PJ (1977). The new puppy: Preventing problems through thoughtful selection. *Vet Med Small Anim Clin,* Dec.

Vollmer PJ (1978). The new puppy: 2. Preventing problems through thoughtful selection. *Vet Med Small Anim Clin,* Jan.

Von Frisch K (1953). *The Dancing Bees: An Account of the Life and Senses of the Honey Bee.* New York: Harvest.

Wahlsten D (1972). Genetic experiments with animal learning: A critical review. *Behav Biol,* 7:143–182.

Wallace FR, Osborne S, Norbor J, and Fantino E (1973). Stimulus change contemporaneous with food presentation maintains responding in the presence of free food. *Science,* 182:1038–1039.

Welker WI (1973). Principles of organization of

the ventrobasal complex in mammals. *Brain Behav Evol,* 7:253–336.

Wilcoxin HC, Dragoin WB, and Kral PA (1971). Illness-induced aversions in rat and quail: Relative salience of visual and gustatory cues. *Science,* 171:826–828.

Williams DR and Williams H (1969). Automaintenance in the pigeon: Sustained pecking despite contingent non-reinforcement. *J Exp Anal Behav,* 12:511–520.

Willis MB (1989). *Genetics of the Dog.* New York: Howell Book House.

Wright JC (1980). The development of social structure during the primary socialization period in German shepherds. *Dev Psychobiol,* 13:17–24.

6

Classical Conditioning

It is pretty evident that under natural conditions the normal animal must respond not only to stimuli which themselves bring immediate benefit or harm, but also to other physical or chemical agencies—waves of sound, light, and the like—which in themselves only signal the approach of these stimuli; though it is not the sight and sound of the beast of prey which is in itself harmful to the smaller animal, but its teeth and claws.

I. P. PAVLOV, *Conditioned Reflexes* (1927/1960)

THE CHANGING circumstances of the environment pose many behavioral and biological challenges for animals. The body is organized to accommodate many of these changes through physiological mechanisms that are directly or indirectly influenced by the action of reflexes. These reflexive actions facilitate a variety of behavioral adaptations and help to maintain biological homeostasis in the face of internal and external environmental change. The adaptive functioning of these various reflexive mechanisms depends on an active emotional, behavioral, and sensory interface between the animal and its environment. Just as the stimuli eliciting these reflexes are mostly outside of the animal's control, the responses involved are largely involuntary and occur irrespective of the animal's efforts.

Reflexes are comprised of unconditioned responses that are elicited by unconditioned stimuli having evolutionary significance for the animal and the ecological niche within which it is adapted to live. In addition, neutral stimuli that possess no such evocative capacity of their own may gradually become conditioned stimuli with the ability to elicit such reflex actions. This is accomplished by the neutral stimulus occurring regularly in close contiguity and proximity with the evocation of some unconditioned reflex. As a result, the previously neutral stimulus becomes a conditioned stimulus, with the power to elicit the target reflexive adjustment, originally only elicited by the unconditioned stimulus. This general arrangement of conditioned and unconditioned stimuli provides the raw data of classical conditioning. Associative processes translate such stimulus-response relations into predictive representations and encode them for future use. The result of this associative learning ability is enhanced behavioral flexibility, providing the animal with many advantages in terms of anticipating the occurrence or nonoccurrence of appetitive (attractive) and aversive events, such as the avoidance of danger. The appetitive usefulness of such learning is particularly significant in the case of predators, who rely on signs and traces left by the prey animal in order to track and secure a meal. The prey animal, on the other hand, is able to learn signals that regularly occur in advance of predatory attacks and, thereby, has a better chance of evading capture by the predator. In general, such acquired information about the environment optimizes an animal's access to essential resources and the maintenance of safety.

PAVLOV'S DISCOVERY

Ivan P. Pavlov (1927/1960) is credited with the discovery of *classical* or, in the terminology of behavior analysis, *respondent conditioning*. According to Pavlov, sensory inputs stimulate the nervous system in one of two opposing directions: excitation or inhibition. Normal nervous activity is the result of a harmonious interplay of excitatory and inhibitory processes mediated by afferent sensory inputs that are collected, organized, and interpreted by central neural mechanisms. Pavlov viewed the physiological significance of reflexive behavior in terms of *psychic* balance: "Reflexes are the elemental units in the mechanism of perpetual equilibration" (1927/1960:8). Classical conditioning is the most fundamental manner in which the animal learns about the changing stimulus contingencies in the surrounding environment, adjusting to them through the anticipatory action of various preservative and protective mechanisms. Through classical conditioning, innate reflexes are brought under the predictive control of causally independent (i.e., neutral) stimuli that are related to the unconditioned stimulus-response event by temporal contiguity and spatial orientation. Such learning is normally outside of voluntary control and is largely (but not entirely) independent of response-generated consequences (e.g., rewards and punishment).

Classical conditioning appears to have been discovered by chance. Pavlov, a physiologist, was occupied with an investigation of the dog's salivary response when he noticed that the more experienced dogs that he had been testing began to salivate before the samples of food were presented to them. This anticipation seriously confounded his physiological measurements of salivary flow in the presence of food but led him to make a much more important psychological discovery. He concluded that the alterations in salivary flow that he observed in his dogs were mediated by higher cortical mechanisms. Further, he hypothesized that the dog's salivary response could be used as an objective measure with which to investigate these higher nervous functions systematically "without any need to resort to fantastic speculations as to the existence of any possible subjective state in the animal which may be conjectured on analogy with ourselves" (1927/1960:16). By varying the stimulus event along several dimensions (e.g., intensity, duration, frequency, and contiguity) and carefully measuring and recording the amount of the dog's salivation, he believed that solid inferences could be drawn about associated brain activity and hypotheses tested with regard to the causal mechanisms at work.

The salivary response turned out to be an *overly* sensitive barometer of stimulus activity. The dog was not only affected by the test stimulus but also by many extraneous stimuli, like the presence of the experimenter or various ambient disturbances. Consequently, Pavlov had a special laboratory constructed in which the experimenter and dog were separated from each other in soundproofed rooms. Prior to testing, the dog's salivary ducts were surgically severed and passed through the cheek and attached to a fistula that conducted salivary secretions into a measuring device. Throughout the experiment, the dog was restrained in a harness attached to a sturdy frame that prevented it from moving about. While restrained in the harness, the dog was exposed to a wide variety of arbitrary stimuli (e.g., bell, light, metronome, and even electric current) presented contiguously with food powder.

BASIC CONDITIONING ARRANGEMENTS BETWEEN CONDITIONED STIMULUS AND UNCONDITIONED STIMULUS

All reflexes are composed of an *unconditioned stimulus* (US) and an *unconditioned response* (UR). Under ordinary circumstances, the US invariably elicits the UR. For example, Pavlov found that hungry dogs will almost always salivate when presented with food. Most

other stimuli falling on a dog's senses fail to elicit this stimulus-specific response—that is, they are neutral with regard to salivation. However, if one of these neutral stimuli (e.g., a tone) is repeatedly paired in close contiguity with the US (food), the previously irrelevant and *neutral stimulus* (NS) will begin to elicit the associated UR (salivation) independently of the reinforcing US. Conditioning transforms the originally neutral stimulus into a *conditioned stimulus* (CS) capable of eliciting a *conditioned response* (CR). Taken as a unit, the CS and CR are referred to as a *conditioned reflex*. The associative bond between the CS and the US is strengthened when the CS consistently occurs just before the presentation of the US and is weakened (extinction) when the CS and US occur independently of each other (Fig. 6.1).

Classical conditioning connects stimulus events together in an orderly way. An important function of associative learning is to provide dogs with predictive information about the occurrence or nonoccurrence of significant events. This information is derived from the regular concurrence or lack of concurrence between the CS complex (stimulus and context) and the occurrence of the US. Pavlov found that classical conditioning is strongly influenced by the temporal proximity and order of the conditioning stimuli involved (Fig. 6.2). Classical learning dictates that the CS closely precede the US in order for conditioning to occur. The optimal temporal relationship between the CS and US for practical purposes is obtained by presenting the CS approximately one-half second before the onset of the US. If the CS is presented after the US (*backward conditioning*) or separated by too much time from the US (*trace conditioning*), the associative bond between the CS and US will be weak or conditioning may not take place at all. An important exception to this general rule is found in a special conditioning phenomenon known as taste aversion, which is discussed in detail later in this chapter.

If the CS regularly occurs shortly before the US (*short-delay conditioning*), it gradually becomes predictive for the occurrence of the US. If the CS and US occur together (*simultaneous conditioning*), the arrangement is ana-

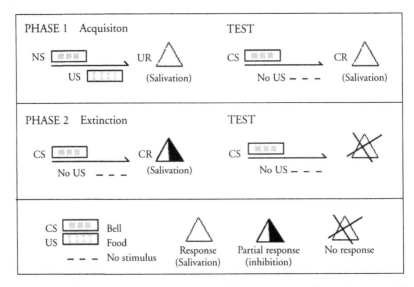

FIG. 6.1. Repeatedly following the connditioned stimulus (CS) with the unconditioned stimulus (US) results in acquisition of a conditioned response (CR), whereas, repeated presentation of the CS independently of the US results in extinction. NS, neutral stimulus; UR, unconditioned response.

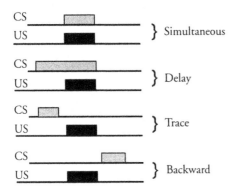

FIG. 6.2. Varieties of classical conditioning arrangement based on the temporal relation of the conditioned stimulus (CS) to the unconditioned stimulus (US). The least efficient forms of conditioning occur when the CS is presented simultaneously with the US or presented after it occurs.

lytical—the occurrence of the CS is temporally coextensive with the US. Finally, if the CS occurs after the US (*backward conditioning*) the cognitive correlate is inferential—that is, one can infer that the US has just occurred by the presence of the CS, but the CS fails to become predictive for the US. Although the latter two outcomes of classical conditioning may be of significance to hu-man reasoning and causal thinking, such analytical and inferential cognitions play a much less important role in understanding associative processes in animal learning.

COMMON EXAMPLES OF CLASSICAL CONDITIONING

A few everyday examples of classical conditioning will hopefully serve to illustrate how the process works. Most dogs respond readily to the sound of a doorbell ringing. For the first few times, however, the bell would probably produce little effect in a dog other than an orienting response and some curiosity. After several repetitions, though, in which the bell signals the arrival of someone at the door, the dog may begin to respond to the bell in anticipation of meeting the visitor at the door. In other words, the dog has learned to correlate a previously insignificant event with a significant one. Now when the doorbell rings, the dog dances with excitement anticipating the visitor's entry and greeting. However, if the owner decided that all this enthusiasm was a bit too much, he or she might endeavor to reduce it by repeatedly ringing the bell without opening the door.

After several daily sessions of nonreinforced exposures to the bell, the dog will gradually inhibit its anticipatory reactions and finally ignore the sound altogether. The ringing bell has been disconfirmed as a predictive cue and is now correlated with nothing special when it rings—that is, its conditioned effect has been *extinguished*. After a few of days without additional extinction trials, though, if an actual guest happens along and rings the doorbell, the owner may find that the dog's reaction had in the interim returned to nearly its original strength. This conditioning phenomenon is known as *spontaneous recovery*. More interestingly, though, is what occurs over the course of several hundred trials of differential reinforcement of the CS-US relationship. If the percentage of confirming rings (guest present) is exactly equal to the percentage of disconfirming rings (guest not present), the sum outcome is the neutralization of the doorbell as a predictive cue (the dog learns to ignore it). Stimulus neutrality results when the occurrence of the US is rendered independent of the occurrence or nonoccurrence of the CS—that is, the US is as likely to occur in the presence of the CS as it is in the absence of the CS (Rescorla, 1988). This formulation of classical conditioning has many implications for dog training and is discussed in greater detail below.

Classical conditioning mechanisms also play an important role in the development of fears and anxiety. A neutral stimulus is readily conditioned to elicit startle or fear by being paired with a fear-eliciting US. For instance, dogs frequently develop fears associated with the veterinary clinic, especially if they have undergone painful procedures there in the past. Such dogs may begin showing signs of anxiety as soon as they enter the hospital parking lot. Providing dogs or puppies with treats and other pleasurable experiences while being examined may help to prevent such negative associations, perhaps even leading the animals to look forward to the experience rather than fearing it. Lifelong phobic reactions can occur as the result of a single traumatic event. Dogs suffer a broad spectrum of phobic fears, most of which are established and reversed through classical conditioning procedures.

Many additional examples of classical conditioning could be cited, but a particularly useful one involves the conditioning of bridging stimuli or conditioned reinforcers. A *bridge stimulus* is a signal that connects the emission of a desired behavior with a delayed reinforcement. A bridge stimulus is also referred to as a *conditioned reinforcer*. During training, it is not always possible to reinforce a selected behavior directly at the exact moment when it is emitted. Still, it is very desirable that a dog be given positive feedback from the trainer at such times. The conditioned reinforcer takes the place of the unconditioned reinforcer (reward) until it can be given to the dog later. A common bridging cue used in dog training is the word signal "Good" or the sound made by depressing a tin clicker. By repeatedly pairing the word signal "Good" with food or other rewards, the previously neutral vocal sound or click is gradually transformed into a generalized reinforcer capable of strengthening selected actions, sequences, or patterns of behavior from a dog's instrumental repertoire. On the other hand, by carefully pairing aversive events or the absence of reinforcement with word signals like "No" or "Enough," then a *conditioned punisher* is produced. Experienced dogs quickly learn to avoid or abandon offending behaviors that trigger the onset of such conditioned punishers or reprimands. The foregoing discussion anticipates a more thorough treatment of conditioned reinforcement covered in the following chapter devoted to instrumental learning.

KONORSKI'S CONCEPTUALIZATION OF REFLEXIVE BEHAVIOR

J. Konorski (1967) extended Pavlov's excitatory-inhibitory paradigm of classical conditioning to include an analysis of the ethologically significant central mechanisms and drives underpinning the process. According to Konorski, a dog's reflexive behavior can be divided into two general biological categories—preservative or protective—depending on the reflex's adaptive function (Fig. 6.3). The term *preservative* denotes the set of reflexive behavioral adjustments employed to satisfy basic needs like nutrition, warmth, so-

Preservative preparatory	Preservative consummatory
Protective preparatory	Protective consummatory

FIG. 6.3. Konorski's (1967) classification of adaptive behavior.

cial contact, and reproduction, whereas the term *protective* denotes the set of reflexive behavioral adjustments that either direct the animal away from noxious or dangerous stimuli (flight) or cause the animal to attempt to destroy them (fight). Preservative reflexes are appetitive and elicited by attractive stimuli, whereas protective reflexes are defensive and elicited by aversive stimuli. These reflexive mechanisms are related to one another along an approach-withdrawal continuum based on a biological optimization of the organism's well-being and adaptation to the surrounding environment.

Preparatory and Consummatory Reflexes

This scheme of reflexive organization is further subdivided into two sequential and interdependent modes of expression that Konorski refers to as preparation and consummation. Both preservative and protective reflexes are expressed through these two sequencing modes. The term *preparatory* denotes all the drive and emotional factors compelling a dog to seek out attractive stimuli or to avoid aversive ones. *Consummatory* reflexes include all those reflex actions associated with the adaptive demands made by the environment upon a dog. Preservative consummatory reflexes include biological actions like salivation, mastication, drinking, and swallowing. Protective consummatory reflexes are composed of both defensive and offensive reactions. Defensive reflexes include escape-avoidance responses and various biological rejection reflexes like vomiting, sneezing, spitting, shaking, scratching, and blinking. Offensive consummatory reflexes include various forms of aggressive behavior directed toward the control or destruction of a threaten-

ing or harmful target.

Preparatory reflexes are composed of centrally organized motivational and evocative mechanisms arousing an animal to action in the mutually exclusive directions of attraction or repulsion. Alimentary reflexes, whether involving eating, urinating, or defecating, depend on the operation of a number of internal preparatory reflexes that provide the necessary motivational conditions for the specific consummatory actions to occur. The preservative action of eating, for example, is composed of preparatory reflexes related to hunger, which set the motivational occasion for the consummatory reflexes associated with the ingestion of food. The amount of hunger experienced by an animal directly affects the magnitude of the consummatory eating reflex finally expressed. Likewise, elimination is comprised of an interaction of preparatory and consummatory reflexes. As the result of pressure-sensitive receptors located in the bladder and bowel, preparatory reflexes are elicited that set the motivational occasions for the consummatory actions of urinating or defecating.

A similar cooperative arrangement between preparation and consummation mediates the expression of protective reflexes. Preparatory protective reflexes involve the escape-avoidance of painful or fearful internal states. Fear is essentially an autonomic response preparing the organism with appropriate emotional arousal for the occurrence of aversive stimulation:

> There is no doubt that most fear reflexes are closely correlated with pain. As a matter of fact, every living creature is afraid of pain, and a large part of its behavior is concerned with developing such preparatory activities as would prevent the occurrence of painful stimuli. It is, however, clear that preventing a noxious stimulus depends upon its anticipation, which is usually accomplished through conditioning. (Konorski, 1967:30)

Some fears, however, do not appear to depend on a conditioning process to develop. Such fears are, in the terminology of Seligman (1971), biologically *prepared* (or *hardwired*). Many dogs are innately fearful of loud, startling noises like fireworks or thunder. Some are emotionally reactive toward separation or isolation in an unfamiliar place, leading to intense preparatory reactions aimed at restoring contact. Virtually all normal dogs exhibit varying degrees of fear toward painful stimulation. The fearful experiences of loud noises, isolation, or pain are innately programmed reactions or URs to sufficiently salient and evocative unconditioned stimuli.

During fearful stimulation, animals will choose a strategy of active or passive defense. When faced with intense fear, dogs are thrown into a three-way dilemma, requiring them to decide whether or not to flee, freeze, or fight. Opting to freeze, a common defense choice among small prey animals, is a passive defensive reflex. Running away, as well as fighting, are both conceptualized as active defensive reflexes. Defensive reflexes are emotionally and centrally opposed by a *relief subsystem* that serves to counteract fearful effects when the fear-eliciting stimulus is withdrawn.

Besides the preparatory reflexes associated with increasing fear, animals are prepared for defensive and offensive activity through the elicitation of preparatory anger reflexes. The physiological and behavioral effects of anger are very different from those associated with fear. Angry feelings express themselves through frontally oriented displays, including intense facial threat gestures, stiff-legged body posturing with front legs prominent, and an overall enhancement of body size (piloerection and muscular tensing) and carriage in the direction of the target. During fearful displays, the direction of action tends to move toward the rear, with submissive fawning or preparations to flee.

Targeting Reflex

Another important group of consummatory reflexes are the so-called *targeting reflexes* or those reflexes that "denote the adjustment of a given analyzer to the better perception of a stimulus" (Konorski, 1967:17). All sensory organs exhibit a variety of targeting reflexes that assist in the efficient and accurate organization of sensory perception. For example, the visual targeting reflex includes orientation of the head and eyes on the object of interest,

the adjustment of the pupils and lenses, and converging of the eyes on a single item of focused attention. Similarly, audition is made possible through the operation of various auditory targeting reflexes, including turning the head toward the source of sound, pricking the ears, and various muscular actions occurring in the middle ear. Consummatory targeting reflexes are driven by preparatory arousal in the form of curiosity or a searching reflex.

Searching behavior is triggered and directed by motivationally significant needs and deprivation states (e.g., food, comfort, and sex), but many animals, including dogs, exhibit a general curiosity about the environment and a need for sensory stimulation in itself. Even under conditions where a dog is not driven to find a particular satisfaction, it may engage in general *undirected* or playful exploration of its surroundings. There may exist a physiological requirement for a certain amount of daily sensory and somatic stimulation that the animal needs in order to feel sufficiently content to abstain from exploratory activity. Sensory and social deprivation may result in the display of exaggerated compensatory reactions designed to satisfy an intensified need for stimulation and social attention.

RESCORLA'S CONTINGENCY MODEL OF CLASSICAL CONDITIONING

Pavlov viewed conditioning from the perspective of a physiologist, leading him to form a mechanistic interpretation of the cognitive and emotional dynamics governing the process. Rescorla questioned Pavlov's contiguity theory of classical conditioning and posited an alternative account that emphasized the importance of *contingency*:

> The notion of contingency differs from that of pairing in that it includes not only what events are paired but also what events are not paired. As used here, contingency refers to the relative probability of occurrence of US in the presence of CS as contrasted with its probability in the absence of CS. The contingency notion suggests that, in fact, conditioning only occurs when these probabilities differ; when the prob-

ability of US is higher during CS than at other times, excitatory condition occurs; when the probability is lower, inhibitory conditioning results. Notice that the probability of a US can be the same in the absence and presence of CS and yet there can be a fair number of CS-US pairings. It is this that makes it possible to assess the relative importance of pairing and contingency in the development of a CR. (1968:1)

Rescorla interprets conditioning from a cognitive viewpoint attributing both predictive and informative properties to the CS. The model places equal importance on the presence as well as the absence of the CS in relation to the occurrence of the US. According to Rescorla, associative conditioning depends on a predictive contingency (both positive and negative) holding between the CS and US. If the US occurs regardless of the presence or absence of the CS (i.e., the US occurs independently of the CS), then in spite of many *chance* pairings between the CS and US (all being offset by an equal number of US events occurring without the CS), no effective conditioning takes place. Under conditions in which the US occurs indepen-

dently of the presence or absence of the CS, the CS is neutralized (Rescorla, 1967). Rescorla's important discovery suggests that classical conditioning is a contingency-based process in which the CS functions as a statistically informative signal about the probability of the occurrence or nonoccurrence of the US (Fig. 6.4).

As a supplement or correction to the contiguity theory, the contingency theory provides a coherent and elegant way to describe what takes place during classical conditioning. Besides predicting the occurrence of the US, the CS also provides information about the type and size (magnitude) of the anticipated UR, as well as various significant contextual relations between the occurrence of the CS and CR. But, as Rescorla writes, "It is not only temporal and logical relations among events that are important to conditioning. Conditioning is also sensitive to relations involving the properties of the events themselves" (1988:153).

Formulating predictions about such information requires that the CS be somehow associatively linked with the US eliciting the UR. The so-called stimulus-stimulus (S-S)

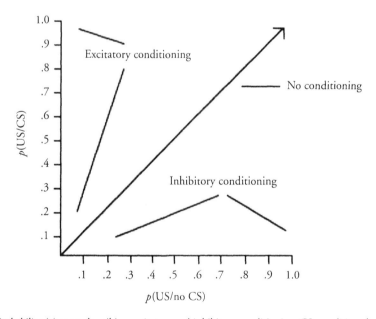

FIG. 6.4. Probability (*p*) space describing excitatory and inhibitory conditioning. CS, conditioned stimulus; US, unconditioned stimulus.

theory of classical conditioning asserts that the connection between CS and US events is mediated by control centers in the brain, perhaps corresponding to Gray's septal-hippocampal comparator system, "a system which, moment to moment predicts the next likely event and compares this prediction to the actual event" (Gray, 1991:112) (see Chapter 3).

Predictions about the size of the US are estimated along an excitatory-inhibitory dimension. If the CS underestimates the size of the pending US, excitatory learning takes place (*acquisition*). If the CS overestimates the size of the US, inhibitory learning occurs (*extinction*). If the CS accurately estimates the size of the US, no additional learning takes place (*steady state* or *homeostasis*). Classical conditioning is acquired, maintained, or extinguished on the basis of a variable correlation between a predictive CS and a corresponding US. Acquisition or extinction occurs when a dog's expectation of a pending event is different from what actually happens. Regarding this relationship, Rescorla and Wagner write,

> Organisms only learn when events violate their expectations. Certain expectations are built up about the events following a stimulus complex; expectations initiated by that complex and its component stimuli are then only modified when consequent events disagree with the composite expectation. (1972:75)

This cognitive view of conditioning is in sharp contrast to the emphasis traditionally placed on factors such as repetition and forward contiguity between associated CS-US events. Although factors like these are important, they are not sufficient alone to explain the laboratory findings reported by Rescorla and other contemporary investigators studying classical conditioning.

Information Provided by the Conditioned Stimulus About the Unconditioned Stimulus

As already discussed, more information is derived from the regular concurrence of the CS and US than simply the probability of the US. Besides calculating event probability, clas-

sical conditioning also yields information about the size and type of anticipated stimulation. According to Rescorla, the size or magnitude of the CR depends on the associative strength acquired by the CS together with the stimulus intensity of the original US. For instance, a CS paired with an electric shock will yield a stronger avoidance response than a similar CS paired with a light slap on the hands. Additionally, the magnitude of the CR is influenced by the salience of the eliciting CS. For instance, a softly spoken reprimand will yield only a small response from a dog, whereas the same signal spoken more loudly will elicit a correspondingly larger effect.

The context or situation where the CS occurs has a significant bearing on the magnitude of the CR elicited. Dogs, like children, can easily discern that "No" in one situation does not necessarily mean the same thing as it does in another. Dog owners exhibit predictably different behavior regarding the application of punishment, depending on the social milieu current at the time of the offending misbehavior. Dogs learn that "No" when guests are around only infrequently leads to the actual occurrence of the threatened outcome—an event that would more likely occur if guests were not present. Under such conditions, guests represent a *safety signal* informing dogs that the warning will not likely be followed by actual punishment. The lesson dogs learn here is that displaying unwanted behavior in the presence of guests is safe. Such mixed messages and differential treatment lead dogs into a frustrating and confusing game of probabilities and risk.

An interesting effect of context can be observed by comparing the speed and ease of acquisition taking place in a familiar environment versus an unfamiliar environment. New learning is most easily introduced within a familiar environment. However, at the point where the learning curve begins to flatten, further (sometimes dramatic) progress is easily achieved by moving the training activity into less familiar surroundings. This observation supports the opinion of many professional trainers that introductory training should be carried out first in the home and subsequently reinforced in a group setting.

Assumptions Derived from the Rescorla-Wagner Model

Classical Conditioning (S-S Theory)

Defined: Learning about stimuli or signals predicting the occurrence or nonoccurrence of significant events.

Three possibilities exist for each presentation of the CS:

1. The CS becomes excitatory.
2. The CS becomes inhibitory.
3. The CS exhibits no change.

The model attributes significance to an animal's *expectations* regarding anticipated stimulation, especially with respect to predictions about the occurrence or nonoccurrence of the US. However, the CS also makes predictions about the impending US, including its relative salience or intensity:

1. If the US is larger (i.e., more attractive or aversive) than expected, then excitatory conditioning of the CS occurs.
2. If the US is smaller than expected, then inhibitory conditioning of the CS occurs.
3. If the US is identical to the animal's expectation, then no additional conditioning takes place.

These predictions generate the following hypotheses concerning the S-S theory of learning:

1. An animal's ability to form accurate expectations regarding the size or intensity and type of the US event presumably entails that the CS and US are centrally linked through associative and cognitive processes. Through conditioning, a neural link or pathway is produced between the CS center (e.g., auditory center in the case of tone stimuli and visual center in the case of light stimuli) and the US center (appetitive center in the case of food and fear center in the case of aversive stimulation).
2. The strength of association between the CS and US is relative to the size or intensity of the expected US. For example, the word "Good" (CS) paired with a large and delicious portion of food (US) will generate a stronger associative link between the CS

"Good" (auditory center) and US food (appetitive center) than if the US presented were a small bit of stale bread. Of course, the relative effect of US size and type on associative strength will depend on the animal's degree of deprivation or satiation, as well.

3. The size or intensity of the US ultimately determines the strength or weakness of the CS-US association. When conditioning is complete (asymptotic), the strength of the association will be directly proportionate to the size or intensity of the US.

Example 1: CS (light) is paired with shock (US)

Characteristics of the US: The associative strength (S) supportable by the US at asymptote is arbitrarily denoted as superscript 1 (i.e., the amount of shock delivered). S^1, therefore, represents the actual size of the US (shock stimulus) presented.

Characteristics of the CS: The expectancy (E) is derived from the associative strength existing between the CS and US, that is, between light (^{L}) and shock (S^1). $E^{(L)}$ represents an expectation that has been formed by the association of the CS (light stimulus) occurring regularly and contiguously with the US event. Over the course of conditioning, predictions made by the animal [$E^{(L)}$] will gradually come to approximate or match the actual US event (S^1).

Example 2: Pairing a compound CS (light and tone) with a US,

$E^{(L)}$ = the associative strength of the light stimulus
$E^{(T)}$ = the associative strength of the tone stimulus

Over the course of several conditioning trials in which $E^{(L)}$ and $E^{(T)}$ are presented together in the presence of shock, both stimuli will increase in associative strength. However, neither the light CS nor the tone CS will independently progress to the associative strength supported by shock (S^1). In the case of compound conditioning, the sum of the two, that is, $E^{(L)} + E^{(T)}$, upon reaching asymptote, will approximate the associative strength supportable by shock.

1. If the auditory CS (tone) and the visual CS (light) are equally salient at the onset of conditioning (i.e., both stimuli elicit an equal orienting response), then the respective associate strengths $E^{(L)}$ and $E^{(T)}$ relative to the US will increase at an equal rate as conditioning progresses.

2. If one CS is weaker or less salient (e.g., a dim light versus a loud tone), the stronger of the two stimuli will obtain more associative strength relative to the US. Nonetheless, at asymptote, the sum of $E^{(L)}$ and $E^{(T)}$ will approximate, but not exceed, the value of S^1.

Acquisition, Extinction, and Asymptote (Fig. 6.5)

1. *Acquisition* occurs when S (associative strength supportable by the US) is greater than E (CS expectancy)—that is, the US is underpredicted by the CS, resulting in excitatory conditioning (the CS increases in associative strength relative to the US).

2. *Extinction* occurs when S is less than E—that is, the US is overpredicted by the CS, resulting in inhibitory conditioning (the CS decreases in associative strength relative to the US).

3. *Asymptote* occurs when S is equal to E—that is, the US is well predicted by the CS, resulting in no additional conditioning

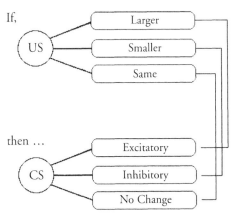

FIG. 6.5. Relationship between expectancy and classical conditioning. CS, conditioned stimulus; US, unconditioned stimulus.

(the associative strength of the CS is verified relative to the US).

STIMULUS FACTORS AFFECTING CONDITIONED-STIMULUS ACQUISITION AND MAINTENANCE

External Inhibition and Disinhibition

Even after a CS has been well established, it may undergo further potentiation or attenuation under the influence of various internal and external events impinging on the central mechanisms controlling it. Both excitatory and inhibitory conditioned stimuli are subject to such change. Dramatic examples of external inhibition and disinhibition can be observed among dogs fearful of loud noises or subject to separation distress when left alone. During thunderstorms or fireworks, such dogs are often overcome with fear and may lose control of many previously well-conditioned habits. A startling noise may cause otherwise well-trained dogs to pull frantically out of harm's way, even though danger never actually threatened them. Dogs reactive to separation may lose control of bladder and bowel functions, howl and bark continuously, or become destructive toward owner belongings. The effects of external inhibition or disinhibition can never be entirely eliminated. Well-trained dogs should be *proofed* against these influences through graduated exposure to diverse environments and by training them under progressively stressful conditions.

Conditioned Inhibition

Once a CS reliably predicts the occurrence of the US, it becomes an excitatory stimulus (CS+) for response properties controlled originally only by the US. Opposing inhibitory conditioning occurs when the CS is presented in the absence of the US. The inhibitory CS (CS−) predicts the nonoccurrence of the US. For instance, if a dog is differentially exposed to a light that always precedes food and a tone that always precedes the omission of food, the light will become an excitatory stimulus (CS+) for food and the tone an inhibitory stimulus (CS−) predicting the absence of food. Later, if the experimenter decided to reverse this arrangement by making the tone predictive for food instead of signaling its omission, the dog would learn this contrary association much more slowly than if the stimulus were neutral. This impediment results from previously learned stimulus associations competing with current training efforts. Dogs must first unlearn what they have already learned about the tone (i.e., the tone must first be disconfirmed as a predictor of no food) before it can become an excitatory stimulus predicting the presentation of food.

Pavlov studied conditioned inhibition as a phenomenon occurring between excitatory and inhibitory conditioned stimuli. Conditioned inhibition occurs when a previously acquired excitatory CS is presented in combination with an inhibitory CS. Take, for example, a dog that has been trained to respond to a bell as a CS for food. On all occasions when the bell is presented alone, it is followed by food. Now consider what happens if the bell is intermittently presented in combination with a tone, but whenever the bell and tone are presented together, the food is omitted. Over time, the tone (CS−) will restrain the excitatory effects of the bell (CS+) when the two stimuli are presented together as a compound stimulus:

bell (CS+) > food::salivation
bell (CS+) & tone (CS−) > no food::
    reduced salivation

The dog has learned that the presentation of a compound stimulus composed of a bell and tone stimulus predicts the absence of food. If the inhibitory tone stimulus (CS−) is now combined with some other previously conditioned excitatory stimulus (CS+), for example, a light, it will be found that the inhibitory effect obtained by presenting the bell and tone together without food transfers to control this remote CS+ (light). When the light (CS+) is presented with the tone (CS−), salivation normally elicited by the light CS+ is inhibited (Fig. 6.6).

Further, as just noted, if the tone (a conditioned inhibitor) is now paired with food to make it an excitatory CS, it is found that this is a rather more difficult process. It takes the dog longer to learn that the tone predicts food because this new association conflicts with a previously well-established contrary association—that is, the tone predicts the absence of food. This so-called *retardation of acquisition effect* can be observed in many training contexts. Dogs regularly exposed to CS events not followed by expected US events learn to treat such impinging signals and stimuli as irrelevant. Effective use of classical conditioning requires that dogs be exposed to clear and predictable occurrences of the CS preceding the US. Classical learning is never inactive: it provides inquisitive dogs with information regarding either the occurrence or nonoccurrence of important events—that is, the dogs are always learning to respond or not to respond.

Findings such as the foregoing suggest that both excitatory and inhibitory influences affect the CS. The excitatory CS (CS+) predicts the occurrence of the US, whereas the inhibitory CS (CS−) predicts the absence of the US (Fig. 6.7). These excitatory and inhibitory influences extend equally to attractive and aversive stimuli. Taken together, these various relations produce four types of classical conditioning (Fig. 6.8). Under natural conditions, the actual strength of the CS is a composite of CS+ and CS− influences, with the valence of the particular CS depending on the extent to which it predicts the presence or absence of the US.

Latent Inhibition

Repetitious presentation of a NS independently of the US results in the NS becoming associatively resistant to future classical conditioning. For example, if a dog's name is used casually (without evoking an appropriate attending response), the attention-controlling and orienting function of the name will be compromised and rendered more difficult to learn later on. Studies have shown that as few as 15 to 20 nonreinforced presentations of the NS prior to conditioning are sufficient to produce latent inhibition (Lubow, 1973). Animals exposed to such treatment fail to attend to the stimulus because its presentation has proven to be uneventful in the past, producing a cognitive interference effect that Baker (1976) refers to as *learned irrelevance*. If a dog has inadvertently learned that the CS is irrelevant, this interfering conviction must first be disconfirmed before new learning can take place. Classical learning appears to proceed most efficiently under circumstances where a completely novel CS occurs contiguously with a startling or surprising US.

Sensory Preconditioning

An interesting conditioning phenomenon occurs when neutral stimuli are paired together prior to conditioning (Fig. 6.9). For example, if the sound of a clicker occurs just prior to the word cue "Good" over several trials, an associative connection between these signals will occur even though the arrangement is not followed by a US. Evidence for the effectiveness of preconditioned associations becomes apparent only after the CS "Good" undergoes some actual conditioning with the US (e.g., food). Once such conditioning

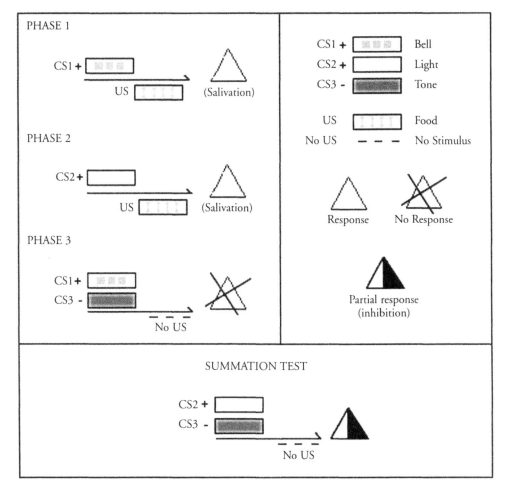

FIG. 6.6. Diagram demonstrating conditioned inhibition. CS, conditioned stimulus; US, unconditioned stimulus.

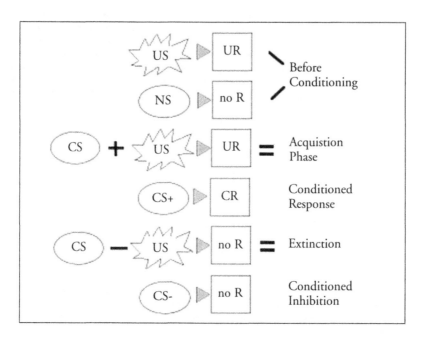

FIG. 6.7. Basic excitatory and inhibitory relations between the stimulus and response in classical conditioning. CR, conditioned response; CS, conditioned stimulus; NS, neutral stimulus; R, response; UR, unconditioned response; US, unconditioned stimulus.

CS+ Aversive excitatory	CS- Aversive inhibitory
CS- Appetitive inhibitory	CS+ Appetitive excitatory

FIG. 6.8. Matrix showing the four basic types of classical conditioning. CS, conditioned stimulus.

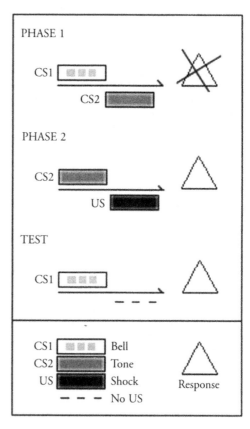

FIG. 6.9. Sensory preconditioning. CS, conditioned stimulus; US, unconditioned stimulus.

takes place, the clicker (which had not been previously paired with the US) spontaneously acquires associative strength derived through its previous presentation with the word cue "Good." This phenomenon readily occurs even in cases where the delay between the two preconditioning stimuli is as long as 4 seconds and after as few as 4 or 5 trials (Prewitt, 1967).

CONDITIONED COMPOUND STIMULI

The concurrent conditioning of more than one stimulus at a time has received a great deal of experimental attention. If two stimuli are paired simultaneously with a single US, both will share a portion of the acquired associative strength and predictive value. The amount of the portion acquired is determined by many factors. Certainly, a stimulus affected by conditioned or latent inhibition will get a lesser portion than a novel stimulus unaffected by such opposing conditioning. Some stimuli are simply more salient and command more attention than others—that is, they *overshadow* less salient stimuli with which they happen to occur (Fig. 6.10). In practice, the effect of overshadowing can be observed by raising or changing the tone of voice, which has the immediate effect of focusing a dog's attention by overshadowing other competing interests. A phenomenon known as the *blocking effect* occurs when one of the combined stimuli has already undergone previous conditioning with the US. That is, the previously established CS will block conditioning of the NS with which it is combined (Kamin, 1968) (Fig. 6.11).

Surprising effects sometimes occur when previously conditioned stimuli are presented together. For example, Woodbury (1943) trained dogs to lever press for food in the presence of a low-pitched buzzer sound and a high-pitched buzzer sound. In the presence of either of these stimuli, lever pressing was reinforced with food, but when both signals were presented together, food was never delivered when lever pressing occurred. The dogs consequently learned to lever press when either of the two signals were presented separately but refrained from responding when both signals were presented together. This finding is a little odd, since one would expect, if both the low-pitched and high-pitched buzzer sounds produce responding, that when both sound stimuli are presented together, responding should still occur. What appears to occur, however, is the formation of a distinct compound configuration composed of elements derived from both stimuli but sufficiently different from each to be easily discriminated and associated with the absence of reinforcement.

HIGHER-ORDER CONDITIONING

Once a CS has been established, it can be used to condition other stimuli to elicit the CR. This is accomplished by pairing the new stimulus with the CS but omitting the presentation of the US (Fig. 6.12). The previously conditioned stimulus takes the place of the US in this arrangement. In comparison to the associative strength acquired through

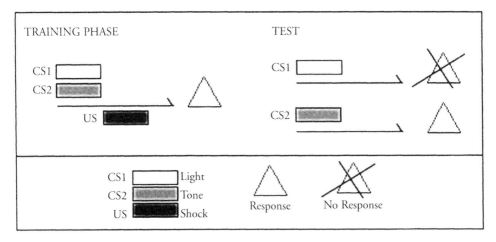

FIG. 6.10. The absence of conditioning in the case of the light stimulus (CS1) suggests that the tone (CS2) has a greater salience and overshadows the light stimulus when both light and tone are presented together as a compound stimulus. CS, conditioned stimulus; US, unconditioned stimulus.

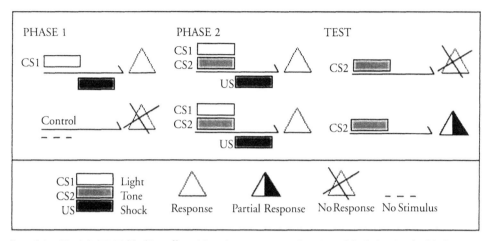

FIG. 6.11. Kamin's (1968) blocking effect. Note that previous conditioning of the light stimulus blocks acquisition of conditioning of the tone stimulus when the tone is presented together with the light. However, when the light and tone are presented together as neutral stimuli, the tone rapidly acquires the ability to produce the conditioned response (CR)—given that it is not *overshadowed* by the light. CS, conditioned stimulus; US, unconditioned stimulus.

first-order conditioning, higher-order conditioning is relatively weak. Pavlov was not able to establish appetitive excitatory conditioning beyond the second order, although aversive excitatory conditioning was taken to the third order when shock was employed as the original US (1927/1960). Although the existence of higher-order conditioning is of great importance theoretically, it has limited practical use in dog training. An area where it may have important implications is in case of phobic stimuli. Over time, the phobic-stimulus complex may widen to include remote stimuli not originally belonging to the traumatic situation itself. This extension of fear beyond the immediate fear-conditioning situation may be in part due to the effect of second-order conditioning taking place between the original CS and various novel stimuli with which it subsequently happens to come into regular contact.

GENERALIZATION AND DISCRIMINATION

An important property of the CS and CR is known as generalization. *Stimulus generalization* and *response generalization* provide the

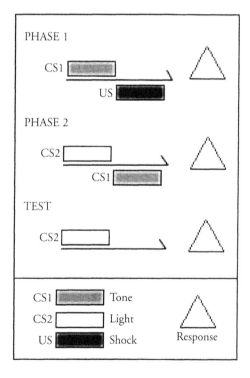

FIG. 6.12. Diagram of second-order conditioning. CS, conditioned stimulus; US, unconditioned stimulus.

means whereby information derived from one situation is made useful in others that are not exactly the same. Under natural conditions, animals are rarely exposed to identical stimulus events or situations; thus, the ability to generalize is a vital adaptation. Dogs easily generalize from one safe encounter with an object to many others sharing similar stimulus features. Similarly, startling or dangerous encounters are generalized with even greater facility over many objects, sometimes only remotely similar. Phobias and fears are extended by generalization to include a large number of objects and situations not directly associated with the original trauma. The ability to generalize enables the animal to draw conclusions about a whole set of objects and situations without having to take the time to test each one. However, such generalizations may not hold in at least two directions: (1) Not all items sharing known safe characteristics are actually safe. (2) Not all items sharing known dangerous characteristics are actually dangerous. For example, a puppy in the habit of tugging and chewing on its leash might generalize the safety of such activities to electrical cords. The electrical cord is similar in many ways to the leash, except for one very serious difference. If the puppy is tempted and unfortunate enough to get shocked by the cord, it will quickly learn to discriminate the cord from leashes and other items sharing a similar appearance. Yet, another possible consequence of the puppy's experience might occur—the development of a fearful generalization about items sharing characteristics belonging to electrical cords. In this case, the second excess of generalization may ensue. The puppy may now incorrectly consider all items sharing characteristics belonging to electrical cords as dangerous and consequently exhibit inappropriate fear toward leashes, ropes, strings, ribbons, and the like. Only through additional experience and discrimination learning will the puppy find that such items are different from electrical cords and gradually regard them as being safe. In contrast to stimulus generalization, response generalization refers to the concurrent elicitation of similar responses to the one being explicitly conditioned. Such generalization results in a loss of specificity but increases, within the confines of adaptive limits, the range of behavioral variability available to the animal.

Generalization and discrimination processes play an active role in all training activities. For example, the process of developing a conditioned reinforcer can be adversely affected by unanticipated generalization effects. A dog that has been trained to respond to the word signal "Good" as a positive conditioned reinforcer will also respond to great many other word cues spoken in a similar tone of voice. It is important, therefore, to differentiate clearly the reward cue from other voice signals used in training. Usually, a higher-pitched tone of voice is used to sound the reward cue, whereas a lower, more assertive tone is used to sound the reprimand or negative conditioned reinforcer. An alternative is to choose a conditioned reinforcer that is highly distinct and unique (e.g., a clicker or whistle).

Discriminative stimuli (S^D) or *command cues* are customarily spoken in a normal tone of voice. Stimulus control is established by training a dog to expect reinforcement to occur if it responds appropriately in the presence of the command cue. In cases where a specific command cue needs to be discriminated from other similar verbal sounds, explicit discrimination training efforts may be needed. During such training, the range of generalization and potential confusion is reduced by selectively reinforcing only responses occurring in the presence of the specific command cue or S^D. Responses occurring in the presence of similar (generalized) verbal cues are either blocked (response prevention) or extinguished by withholding reinforcement if they happen to occur. For example, in the case of the command cue "down," verbal sounds similar to "down" are presented (e.g., found, town, pound, clown, and sound) while unwanted down responses are prevented from occurring or simply not reinforced, that is, they are extinguished. This discussion anticipates a more thorough treatment of the topic of stimulus control and instrumental learning that is covered in Chapter 8.

EXTINCTION OF CLASSICAL CONDITIONING

Stimulus-response associations established through classical conditioning can be weakened by a process called *extinction*. If the occurrence of a CS is not regularly followed by the presentation of the reinforcing US, the associative bond between the CS and US will deteriorate. After many such nonreinforced trials, the CS will fail to elicit the CR—that is, the CS has been extinguished. For example, saying "Good" without occasionally following it with an actual reward will result in its extinction—that is, the dog will learn to ignore the bridging stimulus. Remember that the CS serves to predict future events. Whenever the CS fails to predict the accustomed US, it will begin to forecast the opposite— the absence of the US. In the case of the reprimand, habitual failure to follow the reprimand cue with an actual punitive event may inadvertently teach a dog to interpret the reprimand as a safety signal—a very undesirable outcome. Unfortunately, the typical learning experience of many dogs is one in which they are exposed to a stream of nonreinforced presentations of significant cues (essentially empty warnings and bribes) occurring independently of actual outcomes.

SPONTANEOUS RECOVERY AND OTHER SOURCES OF RELAPSE

Extinction is subject to *savings*, that is, influences from previous learning that persist and interfere with the permanent uncoupling of the associative link between the CS and US (Kehoe and Macrae, 1997). Despite many previous extinction trials, the CS may spontaneously recover and elicit the previously extinguished CR. In practice, the extinction process serves only to reduce the future occurrence of the CR, not eliminate it. The persistence of classically conditioned behavior is particularly evident and problematic in the case of fear conditioning, phobias, and aggression.

In addition to spontaneous recovery, the classical conditioning phenomenon known as *disinhibition* can interfere with extinction efforts. Disinhibition occurs when a startling or surprising event (a distraction sufficient to elicit an orienting response) is presented together with the extinguished CS. As a result of this arrangement, conditioned responding to the CS spontaneously reappears in spite of many previous extinction trials. Under natural conditions of dog training, these sorts of disinhibitory influences are impossible to avoid entirely, requiring instead that they be proofed against as part of the training process.

Several other sources of relapse have been identified in addition to spontaneous recovery and disinhibition (Bouton and Swartzentruber, 1991): renewal, reinstatement, and reacquisition.

Renewal

Renewal refers to the effect that a change of context has on the extinction of a CR. Contextual cues play a significant role in the learning and unlearning of behavior. In the typical renewal experiment, a conditioned fear response is first trained in one context and then extinguished in another. When the animal is placed back into the original context, the extinguished fear response is strongly renewed despite the intensive extinction efforts. Another variation on the renewal experiment involves testing the animal after extinction in a novel context. Fear is renewed in the novel context even though no previous conditioning has actually taken place there. These sorts of experiments indicate that the animal learns to express or inhibit fear depending on the degree of safety or danger associated with the situation—that is, extinction is to a significant extent context dependent.

Reinstatement

Reinstatement of an extinguished CS occurs when the original US is presented in the absence of the CS. Later (after a day or more), the CS is tested and found to have recovered its ability to elicit the previously extinguished CR. The reinstatement effect plays an important role in the recovery of phobias. For example, a dog exposed to a particularly fearsome sample of thunder may recover previously extinguished fear-eliciting conditioned stimuli associated with thunder (overcast skies, barometric pressure changes, and distant lightning flashes).

Reacquisition

Recovery effects are also evident during reacquisition training. When a previously extinguished CS is paired again with the US, the recovery of responding is much more rapid than when a NS is paired with the US. The degree of recovery during reacquisition training depends on the context and associated renewal effects. Contexts that have been associated with past aversive training tend to produce more rapid and robust reacquisition, whereas contexts that have been associated with safety tend to retard reacquisition.

These various recovery phenomena indicate that extinction does not entirely erase the associative link formed between the CS and US or degrade the encoded memory of previous emotional conditioning. Instead of being conceived as a means for erasing past learning, extinction is best interpreted as an active learning process, incorporating and consolidating previously acquired associative information about the CS and US with new input from the environment. As such, extinction is dependent on both stimulus-specific associations between the CS and US, as well as contextual *occasion setting* cues. Learning about specific stimulus relationships and the contexts in which they occur provides the organism with a flexible and discriminating associative interface with biologically significant events.

HABITUATION AND SENSITIZATION

Habituation is a nonassociative learning phenomenon that is often confused with extinction. Extinction results when the CS fails to predict the occurrence of the associated US, that is, the CS no longer elicits the CR. In contrast, habituation occurs when the US is repeatedly presented until the associated UR is no longer elicited. For instance, the occurrence of a strange loud noise will evoke a vigorous orienting response from most dogs. However, if the noise is repeated many times, dogs may learn to ignore it. In effect, they have learned that their original reaction is no longer appropriate, determining that the noise is irrelevant to them and that it can be safely ignored. If subsequently exposed to the same noise a day or two later, the dogs' reaction will have probably returned to nearly the same strength as it was prior to habituation. This effect is known as *spontaneous recovery*. Spontaneous recovery affects both habituated URs and extinguished CRs.

Sensitization produces the opposite effect of habituation. The sensitization effect is produced by exposing dogs to an intense sample of the US sufficient to elicit a startle or surprise reaction. Subsequent exposures to the US at lower intensities (perhaps previously ignored) will produce a noticeable increase in UR magnitude. Another method for sensitizing dogs to a US of low salience is to pair it with a different US of stronger intensity. Such US-US pairings are very useful in dog training. For instance, the vocal reprimand, while possessing some surprise/startle properties, is easily fatigued through repeated use but may be potentiated by being presented simultaneously (compound conditioning) with a startling US like the toss of a shaker can. Sensitization techniques are especially useful in training situations involving avoidance conditioning and aversive counterconditioning.

SPECIAL PHENOMENA OF CLASSICAL CONDITIONING

Classical conditioning usually depends on repeated contiguous pairings of the CS with the US. There exist, however, several examples involving classical conditioning that appear to violate these basic requirements: pseudoconditioning, one-trial learning, taste aversion, and imprinting. Another classical conditioning phenomenon not fitting neatly into the Pavlovian paradigm is what Solomon and Corbit (1974) has termed *opponent processing*, a special case of hedonic conditioning having pronounced (theoretical) effects on emotional learning and reactivity.

Pseudoconditioning

Pseudoconditioning is usually observed in classical conditioning situations, especially as a confounding influence that must be experimentally controlled against. As just discussed, the normal relationship between the CS and the US in Pavlov's paradigm depends on the forward and contiguous presentation of the CS followed by a US—a CS-US arrangement referred to as *pairing*. After repeated pairings (although sometimes one is enough), a conditional association between the two stimuli is established, so that the previously neutral stimulus (now a CS) is capable of eliciting a CR resembling the UR that had been originally elicited only by the US. In pseudoconditioning, the stimulus (neutral) elicits a response resembling a UR, even though it has never been paired with the US.

For example, if a dog receives an intense shock delivered by an electronic collar and then a few hours later a buzzer sound is delivered by the same collar, the dog may react to the sound as though it had been actually shocked rather than just buzzed. This behavioral change occurs even though the buzzer was never actually paired with shock in the past. The buzzer apparently acquires CS-like properties through sensitization and other association effects that do not strictly belong to the classical conditioning paradigm. In fact, any strong surprising or startling event may cause *pseudoconditioning*, that is, evoke responses to neutral stimuli that have never been paired with the eliciting US. Another important factor in the foregoing example is *generalization*—that is, the vibrating buzzer may seem similar in some particulars to shock, thus facilitating a connection between the two stimulus events. However, the similarities between the shock and buzzer sound are not the only factors involved. Although generalization is often present in pseudoconditioning, an even more important consideration is *context*. In the present instance, the buzzer occurs in close association with the source of electrical stimulation, with both stimuli being produced by a collar fastened around the dog's neck.

As the result of a particularly aversive event, the context in which the incident occurs may itself become conditionally linked to the aversive experience. When under the influence of a similar situation in the future, the dog may be more vigilant and alert for danger, exhibiting a much lower threshold for startle or escape behavior. Now an otherwise innocuous event may elicit a strong fear response (as occurs, by the way, in post-traumatic stress disorder and is commonly observed in abused dogs). For example, if a dog is attacked by another dog while out on a walk, on future occasions while walking in that same general vicinity at about the same time of day the dog may appear to be more cautious and defensive about its surroundings. Sounds and movements that might be ignored in other places now take on a new significance. A passing car with a loud muffler or a pile of leaves shifting abruptly in the wind might evoke a strong startle or panic reaction, even though there is no actual threat (past or present) associated with such occurrences themselves. For trainers working with emotionally motivated behavior problems (e.g., aggression, fears, or separation distress) behavioral effects associated with pseudoconditioning should be carefully assessed and taken into consideration when developing behavior modification programs.

One-Trial Learning

Many chronic phobias can be traced to a single event. There appear to be hardwired neurobehavioral mechanisms designed to facilitate rapid learning of information derived from particularly dangerous experiences or startling stimulus events. Under natural conditions, life-threatening or potentially injurious situations may not offer an animal the luxury of repeated exposures or close encounters in order for it to learn that the stimulus in question predicts danger. Consequently, some avoidance patterns appear to be innately programmed or prepared in advance so that they are easily learned with minimal exposure to the threatening situation (Seligman, 1971). Such preparedness is a natural safeguard, allowing the animal to identify especially dangerous associations quickly and efficiently without depending on repeated exposure.

One-trial learning frequently results when a strongly startling or threatening US is paired with a novel CS. The operative word here is *novel.* Positive or neutral past experiences (latent learning) with the CS may interfere with one-trial learning. This interference effect stems from competitive *safe* expectancies that must first be disconfirmed before new learning can take place. Many arrangements provide sufficient conditions for one-trial learning, but it is optimally evoked in situations where the environment itself produces the desired effect. For example, a puppy that has developed the dangerous habit of chewing on electrical cords can be discouraged by preparing electrical cords so that an intense startle or aversive event occurs whenever they are disturbed. A common method employed for this purpose is to booby trap the forbidden item so that an intense startle is produced if the cord is disturbed. The resulting effect provides a lasting aversive association and avoidance of electrical cords.

Taste Aversion

Taste aversion is another example of associative learning that does not fit neatly into the classical conditioning paradigm. A lasting taste aversion often results when an animal ingests a food item or flavor that is followed by a nausea-producing illness. As previously discussed in Chapter 5, Garcia and colleagues (1966) performed a series of experiments in which rats were presented with a compound stimulus involving flashing lights and noise while drinking saccharine-flavored water. While drinking the flavored water, the rats were simultaneously exposed to radiation. Such exposure to radiation causes nausea within an hour or so. Subsequent testing revealed that the exposed rats had developed an intense aversion toward the taste of saccharine but not toward the auditory and visual conditioned stimuli employed. A curious feature of taste aversion is that the effect can be

produced even if the inducement of nausea is delayed for several hours. Also, taste aversions can be reliably established after only a single trial. The conditions under which taste aversions are established are inconsistent with the requirements normally present during classical conditioning, that is, *repeated contiguous* pairings of the CS and US. There appear to exist special learning sensitivities connected with taste and nausea, aiding some animals in differentiating safe from poisonous food items. Seligman (1970) has postulated an internal *preparedness* facilitating the learning of such associations. Taste-aversion techniques have been used effectively to discourage predation on sheep by coyotes (Gustavson et al., 1974; Garcia et al., 1977). It makes biological sense that a foraging animal would evolve strongly prepared sensitivities for the development of taste aversions. As in other examples of one-trial learning, the food item being conditioned must be *novel,* that is, lack a history of safe ingestions. Food safely ingested in the past may require nausea-producing exposures before it is avoided.

A taste aversion procedure may be useful for controlling refractory coprophagia. Eating feces is a common canine vice, and, though not usually harmful to the offending dog's health, it is aesthetically objectionable to many owners. In cases where everything else fails, a taste-aversion arrangement might prove helpful (Houpt, 1991), although such methods have not been demonstrated consistently effective in dogs (Hart and Hart, 1985). The procedure is simple: as soon as the dog ingests feces, the owner is instructed to induce vomiting with a chemical emetic. Sometimes the feces itself is contaminated with the emetic. Gustavson (1996) has noted, however, that emesis per se is not sufficient to establish taste aversion, suggesting that common emetics such as ipecac are inappropriate for establishing such learning. The critical factor involved here is that the chemical being used is capable of eliciting nausea, that is, producing sensations of physical illness. One of the most common compounds employed to achieve this end is lithium chloride. Gustavson and coworkers have recommended the use of taste-aversion procedures for control-ling a variety of appetitive vices and excesses. In spite of the potential benefits of taste aver-sion, such treatment is not without potential risks, side effects, and discomfort for dogs. Consequently, the method should be per-formed only under close veterinary supervi-sion and reserved as a last-resort treatment for serious and refractory appetitive behavior problems.

Imprinting

Konrad Lorenz, credited with the discovery of imprinting in birds, early expressed the opinion that imprinting was not a learning phenomenon but an instinctive process of at-tachment to a social object: "This process cannot be equated with learning—it is the acquisition of the object of instinctive behav-ior patterns oriented toward conspecifics" (1970:124). Subsequent study, however, has shown that a great many classical condition-ing factors do play a role in the imprinting process (Sluckin, 1965). Imprinting may be interpreted as a variant form of classical learning in which several behavior patterns, attachments, and preferences are facilitated through brief exposures early in life. Imprint-ing is unique in that it takes place most effi-ciently (if at all) during narrowly defined sen-sitive periods occurring early in the animal's life. If this period of sensitivity passes without the occurrence of appropriate stimulation, then irreversible adjustment problems may develop (Scott and Fuller, 1965).

Imprinting is distinguished from most forms of classical conditioning along several different dimensions: speed of acquisition, permanence of associations, resistance to fu-ture learning effects, resistance to decay by disuse, and the reliance on sensitive periods early in life. Another significant difference between imprinting and other forms of classi-cal conditioning is that imprinting often in-volves complex behavior patterns, whereas most other stimulus learning involves more simple and discrete units of behavior. Studies designed to determine whether imprinting and social attachment involve instrumental components have demonstrated that positive reinforcement (food rewards) does not play a

significant role (Brodbeck, 1954; Scott, 1962). In fact, the effects of imprinting ap-pear to be enhanced by conditions adverse to instrumental learning. Animals appear to be even more strongly attracted to the imprinted object when they are forced to endure obsta-cles and aversive stimulation during the im-printing process (Hess, 1964).

CLASSICALLY GENERATED OPPONENT PROCESSES AND EMOTIONS

Emotional states are complicated and cannot be adequately explained by the simple asso-ciative model of classical learning. The Pavlovian model only accounts for responses occurring contiguously with the presented stimulus. But, actually a chain of stimulus-re-sponse events takes place, composed of some aspects that are not only inconsistent with the originally elicited response but actively antagonistic to it (Solomon and Corbit, 1974). According to the opponent-process theory, elicited emotional states (a-processes) are simultaneously counteracted by diametri-cally opposed affects (b-processes), a sort of af-fective shadow that remains outside of con-scious awareness during active stimulation (Fig. 6.13).

According to Solomon and Corbit, oppos-ing b-processes serve to maintain emotional balance and equilibrium by guarding against potentially overarousing stimulation from ei-ther hedonically pleasurable or aversive a-process experiences. The magnitude of any emotional response is regulated by a summa-tion of interactive components from both a-process and b-process affective input. This opponent processing determines the animal's state of emotional arousal at any given mo-ment. If affective states were not balanced by concurrent counterpoised opponent processes, emotional stimulation would be chaotic and uncontrollable. Instead, each a-process emotion is counteracted as it occurs by an antagonistic emotional b-process shad-owing it. Opposing b-process aftereffects are consciously experienced only after the source of a-process stimulation is withdrawn. For ex-ample, if the reader were to pinch himself or herself briefly and then observe introspec-tively the affects attending the cessation of

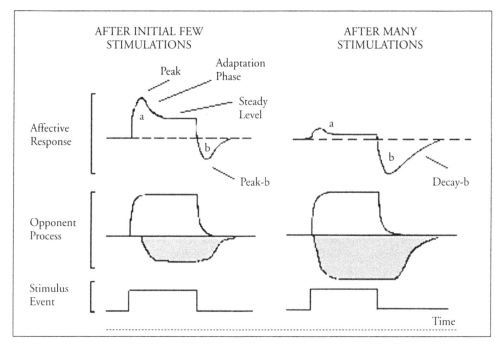

FIG. 6.13. Opponent-process effects resulting from emotion-eliciting stimulation. After Solomon and Corbit (1974).

pain, he or she would probably note a subtle, yet distinctively pleasurable, emotional aftereffect contrasting with the previous pain. In this case, the painful pinch (a-process) is followed by an opposing pleasurable sensation (b-process) when the pinch is terminated. Another interesting example of opponent processing occurs in vision involving color afterimages. If one steadily looks at a patch of color and then turns abruptly away focusing on a white wall, slowly the color's opposite or complement begins to appear.

A-Process and B-Process Attributes

A-processes and b-processes are contrasted on several dimensions. The following is a brief inventory of some of these differences.

A-Process Attributes

1. A-process affects are immediate and contiguous with the stimulating event.
2. A-process affects pass through three basic phases: a peak of emotional stimulation,

followed by an adaptation phase, and finally leveling off into a steady state.
3. Once emotional stimulation is terminated, a-process reactivity quickly returns to baseline levels (denouement).
4. Repeated stimulation of a-process reactions results in their weakening (habituation).

B-Process Attributes

1. Opponent b-process reactions are sluggish both in terms of initiation and decay.
2. Opponent b-process affects are entirely reactive, opposing a-process stimulation.
3. Opponent b-process affects are overshadowed by the a-state until stimulation is withdrawn.
4. Repeated stimulation results in the strengthening of b-process affects.

Practical Application of Opponent-Process Theory

Theoretically, whenever any hedonically significant event (producing pleasure or pain) takes place, both a-processes and b-processes are mobilized. Several interactive factors influence the final outcome and the relative strength of these opposed states. One of the most important of these factors involves the effect of repeated use. Frequent stimulation weakens a-process emotions while simultaneously strengthening b-process aftereffects. After frequent stimulation of a-process emotions, the b-process aftereffects begin to occur more rapidly and the denouement to baseline levels requires a much longer time to occur.

These various effects of frequent stimulation may be at work in a common behavioral disorder: separation anxiety. Separation-anxious dogs and puppies are unable to cope calmly with owner departures and separations (Voith, 1981). Instead of passively accepting such periods of loneliness, separation-reactive dogs become overly anxious (panic) and act out in a variety of destructive or maladjusted ways. Dogs predisposed to separation anxiety are typically highly dependent, exhibit excessive attention needs, are overly sensitive, and are prone to develop compulsive behavior disorders.

Opponent-process theory interprets attachment and separation-distress reactions in terms of a-processes and b-processes (Hoffman and Solomon, 1974). When a separation-anxious dog is with its human companion, the dog is comforted by social contact and security, but when the owner departs, the separation-vulnerable dog becomes distressed and worried. Even though apparently fully at ease when the dog is with the owner, actually underlying opposing b-process affects are already being generated, offsetting and balancing a-process affections and attachments. These opposing b-process emotions do not become obvious until after the owner departs, when shortly thereafter the dog is overwhelmed with fears of abandonment and loss of security. After many subsequent trials, a-process stimulation begins to wane, losing its ability to support the separation-anxious dog's growing attachment needs even when the owner is present.

The consequence is nervous or anxious attachment, a condition of perpetual social attention seeking and contact neediness that can never be fully satisfied (Bowlby, 1973). According to the opponent-process theory, such compensatory efforts are futile and counterproductive, since repeated stimulation of positive social affects merely causes the strengthening of underlying opposing fears of social isolation. On those inevitable occasions when the dog must be left alone, b-processed fears of abandonment and isolation will rise with even greater intensity than before, evoking ever-escalating levels of distress and panic until the cycle of attachment and fear of loss/abandonment is broken. Most separation-anxious dogs exhibit some form of nervous attachment toward their owners. To treat separation anxiety effectively, this vicious cycle of nervous attachment and panic must be systematically altered so that positive a-processed affects and attachment needs are normalized and negative b-processed anxieties are reduced through desensitization and counterconditioning efforts.

Another situation where opponent processing may play a significant role is in the case of long-term and excessive punishment. Many dog owners seek professional help only after many months of frustrated training efforts. In some cases, punishment was the primary method used to establish behavioral control. Such owners are often confused and profoundly discouraged by their dog's resistance to training. Even though routinely and severely punished, the offending dog quickly recovers and persists "doggedly" despite escalating harsh treatment. While such oppositional behavior usually involves a number of factors that need to be considered in their own right (e.g., unresolved dominance tensions, hyperactivity, and negative attention seeking), the trainer might also consider the possibility that the dog's resistance and apparent lack of responsiveness is due to the effects of frequent and excessive punishment. Punitive owners often comment on a decline in their dog's responsiveness to discipline, a progressive strengthening of general resistance and willfulness, and the development of armorlike thresholds against startle and pain. Some dogs actually wag their tails or may exhibit penile erection (a consternating result for an angry owner) immediately after punishment and happily come back for more. The opponent-process theory predicts such behavioral tendencies as a result of frequent punishment.

Physical punishment usually evokes two primary reactions: fear and pain. Initial stimulation elicits strong inhibitory reactions, autonomic activation, and escape. According to opponent-process theory, subsequent stimulations become progressively weaker as they fall under the opposing influence of underlying b-processes, which are essentially the hedonic opposite of fear and pain. In the case of frequent aversive stimulation, the a-process reactions become slower and weaker while the pleasurable b-processes become faster, stronger, and decay much more gradually. Paradoxically, over time and frequent use, punishment may actually become a rewarding event, since the effect of frequent aversive stimulation is the production of highly pleasurable and sustained b-processed emotions.

A possible neurophysiological cause of this acquired immunity to punishment may be attributed to the release of endogenous opioids (endorphins) resulting from chronic stress or punishment. Watkins and Mayer (1982) demonstrated that aversive events (shock) produce lasting analgesic aftereffects involving both opioid and nonopioid systems. Such analgesia can be produced directly by the aversive event itself or indirectly via the mediation of classically conditioned stimuli associated with it. Besides stimulating an analgesic effect, endorphins exhibit several psychotropic actions, including calming and antidepressant actions, as well as reducing aggressive reactivity and general fearfulness. Drugan and colleagues (1985) found that animals exposed to uncontrollable shock develop greater and longer-lasting analgesic numbing than animals able to escape shock. Exposure to chronic stress and punishment may activate physiological dependence or addiction to endogenous opiates, *perhaps* motivating dogs to act in ways that ensure sufficient dosing. Christie and Chesher (1982) reported that both the injection of naloxone

or the termination of noxious stimulation resulted in morphinelike withdrawal symptoms in their stressed animal subjects.

COUNTERCONDITIONING

Pavlovian conditioning plays a vital role in the learning and unlearning of emotional reactions through counterconditioning. To resolve fears and other problems involving emotional components (e.g., phobias, separation anxiety, and aggressiveness), classical conditioning may be required. Unlike instrumental behavior, classically conditioned responses are largely autonomous and independent of central control. Dogs never consciously choose to *feel* fearful or anxious; such emotions simply come over them as automatically as such feelings may come over us. This autonomic component is mostly outside the reach of voluntary control. Despite great effort and preoccupation, people suffering with phobias are unable to control their fearful arousal when in the presence of the eliciting stimulus. The inherent resistance of highly motivated emotions to voluntary control is especially evident in the case of well-established phobias. Behavior problems involving aversive emotional components like fear and anger must be treated with a two-pronged approach utilizing both classical and instrumental training methods.

Although dogs may learn to cope with emotionally distressful stimulation, they cannot directly control the onset and offset of autonomic affective arousal, except by moving out of the range of eliciting stimuli. To be controlled, an aversive emotion (e.g., anger or fear) must be countered by the elicitation of an even stronger and incompatible emotional response. The philosopher Spinoza precisely described the premise of counterconditioning in his *Ethics*: "An emotion can only be controlled or destroyed by another emotion contrary thereto, and with more power for controlling emotion." Similarly, William James emphasized the necessity of employing an emotional impulse to control the expression and magnitude of an opposing emotional impulse: "Reason, per se, can inhibit no impulse; the only thing that can neutralize an impulse is an impulse the other way" (1890/1950:393). This is an important basic principle and credo for dog trainers and behaviorists to keep foremost in mind when working with highly motivated behavior. Of course, James and Spinoza had humans in mind, but the same sort of behavioral flexibility exists in dogs.

Counterconditioning essentially involves opposing one response by the elicitation of another. To eliminate an unwanted CR, the CS controlling the response is paired with an US that elicits a contrary response. If the UR is sufficiently strong and incompatible with the undesired CR, the new connection between the CS and US will attenuate or block the unwanted response in the future. Counterconditioning is a powerful tool. Even very painful unconditioned stimuli can be counterconditioned by pairing them through gradual increments of intensity with a strong contrary US. Pavlov, for example, counterconditioned traumatic shock by pairing its presentation with food. A dog was shocked and then given a piece of food, and forced to eat it if he refused to take it voluntarily. Over the course of several sessions, the intensity of stimulation was gradually increased until the shock was so severe that it caused "severe burning." Even when stimulated with the maximum current, the dog showed no signs of fear but only turned his head toward the customary location of food, followed by profuse salivation, and chomping appetitive movements in anticipation of food.

In addition to appetitive counterconditioning, aversive counterconditioning is commonly used in dog training. For example, a dog may develop an interest or appetite that is dangerous or unacceptable for one reason or another. Such appetites can be very persistent and resist ordinary methods of deterrence. Just as counterconditioning can be used to reduce aversive associations and avoidance, it can also be used to generate or increase aversive associations and avoidance when necessary. Appetitive interest and attraction to a forbidden or dangerous item can be effectively decreased by pairing the item with a sufficiently aversive or startling stimu-

lus. During aversive counterconditioning, the US (startle) must closely follow the presentation of the CS (forbidden item) or US evoking undesirable interest. Many applications and a variety of conditioning arrangements in puppy and dog training use aversive counterconditioning. Aversive training procedures should always be avoided until less intrusive methods have been considered and implemented.

CLASSICAL CONDITIONING AND FEAR

Voluntary Versus Involuntary Behavior

Behavior can be roughly divided into two broad categories: *voluntary* (goal directed) and *involuntary* (reflexive). This division is not arbitrary but is based on the two fundamental ways behavior is modified. Voluntary behavior is highly goal directed and influenced by the consequences it produces. Involuntary behavior, on the other hand, is largely composed of automatic mechanisms operating outside of a dog's volition and ability to choose. In the case of involuntary behavior, the presentation of a sufficiently salient stimulus evokes the elicitation of a highly predictable response. Involuntary behavior is usually associated with simple reflexive and emotional responses. Although functionally independent of voluntary control, involuntary behavior is affected by antagonistic motivational states and modified through associative learning procedures. Together voluntary behavior and involuntary behavior provide an adaptive interface between a dog's changing biobehavioral needs and the surrounding environment.

Behavioral disorders are complex and problematical, consisting of both instrumental and reflexive (respondent) components. Defensive behavior involves two motivational processes, one under relatively more voluntary control (freeze, flight, and fight) and the other under relatively more involuntary or autonomic control (fear and anger). For example, individuals fearful of snakes cannot by an act of will persuade themselves not to feel afraid when confronted with a snake, but can, despite great apprehension and reluctance, possess enough self-control not to run away. Consequently, to attenuate fearful behavior properly, one must address both instrumental fearful responses as well as the underlying emotional concomitants. From the perspective of some forms of behavior therapy, fear is best reduced by simply strengthening instrumental behavior incompatible with fear while ignoring or blocking (response prevention) fearful behavior when it happens to occur. Sometimes, however, the underlying fear is so strong and pervasive that it must first be addressed and modified through direct means, including respondent counterconditioning, relaxation training, exercise, or medications. As the underlying fearful arousal is diminished, the instrumental behavioral expressions of it will spontaneously improve, thus making it easier to shape more confident behavior.

Three Boys and a Brief History of Fear

Among the earliest controlled studies on the development of conditioned fear were those carried out by the American psychologist John Watson (1924/1970) and coworkers. Watson, often called the father of behaviorism, successfully conditioned a stable fear response in an 11-month-old orphan infant named Albert (Watson and Rayner, 1920). Albert was exposed to a white rat and observed for his reactions. Prior to conditioning, he was accustomed to holding and playing with the animal and exhibited no signs of fear. The fear-conditioning stimulus used by Watson was a startling sound made by striking a hammer against a heavy steel bar held behind the infant's head. As the child reached for the rat, the bar was struck, causing Albert to recoil from the animal. Over the course of several similar trials, Albert's fear deepened and became progressively more reactive and generalized. It was found during subsequent tests that Albert's fear had generalized to include other furred animals (a rabbit and a dog) and inanimate objects such as a fur coat. Although there were plans to "uncondition" Albert, he was subsequently adopted by a family living out of town. No one knows what finally became of Little Albert.

Additional work was carried out by Mary Cover Jones (1924) in an effort to isolate the most effective training techniques for reducing fearful behavior in children. Jones studied several methods, but the one she called *direct unconditioning* is of particular interest to dog trainers and behavior consultants. Peter, a 3-year-old boy, already exhibited intense fears toward various animals and furry objects. After trying several methods with varying degrees of success, the researchers exposed Peter to an early prototype of graded counterconditioning that turned out to be extremely effective. The method involved feeding Peter in the presence of the feared animal (a rabbit). The rabbit was initially caged and then systematically presented to the child at closer distances. The progress of these graded exposures was regulated by Peter's willingness to eat, based on an observation that relative appetite was a sensitive indicator of fear. The rabbit was gradually moved closer to the child through progressive steps, until finally he was able to eat without signs of anxiety while at the same time petting the animal who had been placed on his lap.

A decisive shift in the study of fear occurred with the publication of an article written by Wolpe and Rachman (1960). In the article, they criticize the psychoanalytical perspective on phobias and their development, especially with respect to Freud's interpretation of one of his cases involving a child named Little Hans. Little Hans, who was a patient of Freud, had acquired a strong phobia of horses. In a lengthy report, Freud concluded that the boy's fear was fueled by an underlying Oedipal conflict with his father. He argued that the horse was symbolically linked in the boy's mind with his father—the true object of the boy's fear. As the result of the child's forbidden wish to possess his mother sexually coupled with an unconscious desire to kill his father, the boy experienced a profound sense of guilt and transferred his fear of retribution to the horse. Wolpe and Rachman argued that little evidence in Freud's case study actually supported an Oedipal interpretation of the boy's fear. In reading the material, they discovered that the boy had witnessed a tumultuous accident in which a horse had fallen in the street while pulling a bus. The experience was a traumatic one for Hans and, the researchers argued, one sufficient to explain the boy's subsequent fear of horses.

Phobic Cats and Systematic Desensitization

Wolpe's (1958) experimental work with conditioned fear was carried out with cats from 1947 to 1948. Several cats were exposed to conditioning procedures that resulted in neurotic fear reactions to a variety of stimuli and situations. One group was conditioned to respond to the "hoot" of a horn that was followed by shock delivered into the floor grid of the experimental cage. The second group of cats was first trained to go to a dispenser of food in response to a buzzer signal. Once this behavior was well established, shock was delivered just before the cat took the available food into its mouth. Both groups developed strong phobic reactions toward the conditioned stimuli. The latter method is very similar in effect to that used by Watson on Little Albert. Unlike Albert, however, who showed no signs of generalized fear involving the experimental setting, Wolpe's cats not only exhibited intense fear toward the eliciting conditioned stimuli, they also resisted entering the cage, exhibited various signs of fear while in the cage, and refused to eat even after several days of continuous food deprivation while in the cage where the shock too place.

Wolpe studied several methods for extinguishing fear in cats. Some of the fearful cats were encouraged to eat food by pushing it toward them with a stick. Wolpe theorized that the cats would see the hand as a conditioned appetitive stimulus, since they had been previously fed by hand. A few of the cats did, in fact, respond to this method. Cats who failed to respond to this first method were exposed to a directive training procedure in which they were forced into close contact with an appetizing food item. Under these conditions, several additional cats were eventually coaxed into eating. Since many of the cats not only exhibited fear in the experimental cage but also to the surrounding room, Wolpe attempted to feed the remaining cats in four separate rooms of increasing similarity to the one in which the shock took place. This method proved very effective, allowing the cats eventually to eat readily from within the experimental cage itself.

The next training problem was to devise procedures for reducing the cats' fearfulness and avoidance in the presence of the buzzer or horn sounds. This training goal was accomplished along two lines of conditioning. The first method was very similar to that used by Jones with the phobic child Peter. Wolpe determined that cats would remain relatively undisturbed if the hooter was sounded at a distance of at least 40 feet away. This distance could be progressively decreased by gradual successive approximations. This method was carried out until the cats accepted the sound of the horn and buzzer at full conditioning intensity. An alternative method he employed to attenuate the intensity of the eliciting CS was accomplished by truncating its duration to a fraction of a second. The first sample was presented at full volume for a fifth of a second. Under such conditions, the cats would initially react and, after a short delay (about 40 seconds), would consume the food pellet dropped into the cage. Gradually, over several trials, the delay between the CS sample and eating decreased until at last the cats were taking the food within a couple of seconds following the CS. The duration of the fear-eliciting CS was then gradually increased until the cats would continue eating under a continuous presentation of the CS for 30 seconds.

Reciprocal Inhibition

Wolpe attributed the effectiveness of his training efforts to *reciprocal inhibition*. Essentially, reciprocal inhibition postulates a hypothetical interference occurring when two opposing emotional states are simultaneously elicited. Two hedonically opposing emotional states cannot exist simultaneously: one overshadows or offsets the other. In the case of Wolpe's fearful cats, they could not be interested in food while at the same time feeling anxious; appetite in this case overshadows or reciprocally inhibits fear. This process of countering aversive emotional arousal by eliciting stronger appetitive arousal or relaxation in the presence of the aversive event is referred to as *counterconditioning.* Wolpe states the underlying principles facilitating the effects of counterconditioning as follows:

> If a response inhibitory of anxiety can be made to occur in the presence of anxiety-evoking stimuli it will weaken the bond between these stimuli and anxiety (1969:14).

Negative emotional reactions evoked by fear-eliciting conditioned stimuli can be systematically reduced, modified, or replaced with more adaptive and positive response patterns through counterconditioning. Many undesirable conditioned emotional reactions are traceable to some past event and are learned in a manner consistent with the experimental models devised by Watson and Wolpe. The goal of counterconditioning is to disassociate past learning from the eliciting CS and to establish new, more positive associations controlled by the same stimulus.

Graded Counterconditioning

Fearful emotional responses are subdued by the elicitation of competing incompatible emotional responses (e.g., appetite or relaxation). The central maxim informing this process is "contraries are cured by contraries," that is, two hedonically opposed emotional responses cannot exist at the same time—the elicitation of one reciprocally inhibits the other. For example, a strange noise occurring while a dog is happily chewing on a fresh bone is less likely to elicit fear than is a similar stimulus occurring at another time when the dog is not so preoccupied. In this case, the appetitive interest evoked by the bone reciprocally inhibits fear elicited by the strange noise. Other important factors affecting counterconditioning, as both Wolpe and Jones have demonstrated, is the intensity and proximity of the fear-eliciting CS. If the fear-eliciting CS is too strong or close, the incompatible counterconditioning stimulus may be overshadowed and the process impaired. For example, a xenophobic dog may not notice a stranger walking 100 feet away but will react with intense fear if the same person approaches too closely or attempts to make

physical contact. For effective counterconditioning to occur, the dog must be gradually exposed to strangers at progressively closer distances and under increasing levels of provocativeness while the dog is concurrently stimulated by a strong counterconditioning stimulus.

The best counterconditioning results are achieved by presenting stimuli that either relax a dog or satisfy it appetitively while systematically exposing it to the fear-eliciting target. Relaxation and eating are incompatible with fear—that is, a dog cannot be simultaneously fearful while relaxing or eating. Some activities like playing, running, and even walking can be used as counterconditioning stimuli to reduce mild fears and anxieties. For convenience, food is usually chosen as the primary counterconditioning stimulus, although massage can be used effectively in some situations. The course of systematic desensitization follows a regular pattern. A hungry dog is progressively exposed to the feared object through a series of defined steps (a hierarchy of fear-eliciting stimuli), which enables closer proximity and, finally, direct contact without eliciting fear at any point. Each step of this hierarchy is associated with food and reassurance, providing a secure foundation for the next step. The dog learns to associate good things with the feared object, gradually abandoning its fearful attitude in exchange for a more positive expectation.

Conditioned fear is frequently very resistant to normal extinction procedures. Since fears and anxiety may not be attenuated under normal conditions, special methods must be employed to achieve the desired effect. In addition to counterconditioning, a key element in the reduction of anxiety and fear is controlled exposure that allows the dog to engage in direct interaction with the feared object/situation.

Interactive Exposure and Flooding

The reduction of fearful behavior is facilitated by utilizing a combination of behavioral training methods. In addition to graded counterconditioning, several other fear-reducing techniques have proven efficacious in reducing fear. Jersild and Holmes (1935) provide an important historical study detailing the broad aspects of graded *interactive exposure*—a method that has proven complementary to Wolpe's model and, according to some authorities, should replace it as the treatment strategy of first choice (Marks, 1977). Jersild and Holmes observed that two primary methods of confronting fear are most commonly used by parents of fearful children: direct repeated exposure to the feared object and ridicule. Of the two methods, direct exposure appears to be the most effective, resulting in the reduction of fear in 50% of the cases studied. Ridicule and invidious comments (e.g., wimp, "scar'ty cat") yield no benefit in bolstering a child's courage. They found that common childhood fears could be systematically reduced by replacing avoidant behavior with confidence-building interactive skills, resulting in the progressive development of *competence* in the fearful situation. Their method emphasizes developing various coping skills and participatory activities that the child engages in while in direct contact with the feared object/situation. They utilized attractive counterconditioning stimuli, not intended to change associative responses directly but to provide additional incentives to the child for making such contact. The counterconditioning stimulus serves as a bait to lure the child into sustained interactive contact with the feared object/situation. Similar benefits may be derived in the case of moderately fearful dogs. In many particulars, the Jersild and Holmes method anticipates current methods for reducing fear in dogs.

Since Wolpe's discovery, many studies have been carried out to evaluate the therapeutic efficacy of the desensitization and the counterconditioning process. The results have often been critical of Wolpe's conceptualization on several grounds. For instance, the need for a hierarchy of fear-evoking conditioned stimuli presented systematically in the presence of hedonically antagonistic counterconditioning stimuli (eating or relaxation) has proven relatively unimportant under experimentally controlled conditions (Delprato, 1973; Delprato and Jackson, 1973). In fact, according to Delprato's study (1973), simple extinction proved more effective than both

systematic desensitization (graded counterconditioning) and graded exposure. Since the desensitization analogue used by Delprato differed from graded exposure only in terms of the presentation of food, it might even be further argued that the presentation of food actually interferes with the reduction of fear. One possible explanation he presented to explain this unexpected result is that the acquisition of food during graded exposure overshadows an animal's attention to the fear-eliciting stimulus. Unlike in the cases of graded exposure and simple extinction, the animal may have failed to learn that the CS no longer predicts a pending aversive event. Subsequently, when exposed to the fear-eliciting stimulus without food, the counterconditioned animal exhibited little or no improvement in comparison to controls.

The most important factor in the desensitization process appears to be sustained exposure to the fear-evoking stimulus until fear subsides (Marks, 1977). This procedure is commonly referred to as *flooding* through response prevention. Response prevention and direct exposure (flooding) can be carried out in the presence of full-intensity samples of the fear-eliciting stimulus or, more optimally, a progression of increasingly intense samples. A precaution needs to be carefully observed: if dogs are fearful when the flooding exposure is terminated, their fearfulness might be made worse. Also, there is some evidence that frequent brief exposures to the feared stimulus situation might actually strengthen the reaction rather than weaken it. Therefore, it is important that fearful exposures be of sufficient duration at each step to allow elicited fears to habituate before proceeding to the next step or before quitting.

Response Prevention and Directive Training

Whether counterconditioning or interactive exposure is used, additional supportive techniques may be required that force a dog into direct contact with the feared CS complex. At some point in the process, the dog may become overly reactive or attempt to escape from the situation. While care should be taken not to overwhelm fearful dogs with exposures that they are unable to tolerate, when avoidance responding does appear it must be blocked or corrected (Askew, 1997). In some situations, dogs may completely refuse to engage in some behavior as the result of competing avoidance responding, such as climbing stair steps or entering certain rooms or places. In such cases, directive exposure involving the use of a series of corrective prompts on the leash is often both expedient and very effective.

Various response prevention techniques can be selectively applied during counterconditioning and flooding efforts. Occasionally, dogs undergoing rehabilitative training will persist in phobic avoidance behavior despite gradual and patient efforts. One theory suggests that avoidance responding actually forestalls the unlearning of fearful responses (Levis, 1979). Persistent avoidance responding prevents dogs from coming into direct contact with the fear-evoking stimulus, thereby impeding the normal extinction process. Experiments designed to block or prevent avoidance responding have shown that extinction of such behavior is facilitated by such measures (Baum, 1970). Response prevention involves physically restraining a dog so that the avoidance response cannot be performed, requiring instead that the dog directly experience the avoidance-signaling CS while being prompted to perform some incompatible response (e.g., sitting or lying down) that is consequently rewarded. Such training provides the dog with coping options that supersede the avoidance response and may eventually take its place. The foregoing discussion of fear and its management anticipates a more thorough treatment of the subject in Volume 2.

REFERENCES

Askew HR (1997). *Treatment of Behavior Problems in Dogs and Cats: A Guide for the Small Animal Veterinarian.* Cambridge, MA: Blackwell Science.

Baker A (1976). Learned irrelevance and learned helplessness: Rats learn that stimuli, reinforcers, and responses are uncorrelated. *J Exp Psychol,* 2:130–141.

Baum M (1970). Extinction of avoidance responding through response prevention (flooding). *Psychol Bull,* 74:276–284.

Bouton ME and Swartzentruber D (1991). Sources of relapse after extinction in Pavlovian and instrumental learning. *Clin Psychol Rev,* 11:123–140.

Bowlby J (1973). *Attachment and Loss,* Vol 2: *Separation, Anxiety and Anger.* New York: Basic.

Brodbeck AJ (1954). An exploratory study on the acquisition of dependency behavior in puppies. *Bull Ecol Soc Am,* 35:73.

Christie MJ and Chesher GB (1982). Physical dependence on physiologically released endogenous opiates. *Life Sci,* 30:1173–1177.

Delprato DJ (1973). An animal analogue to systematic desensitization and elimination of avoidance. *Behav Res Ther,* 11:49–55.

Delprato DJ and Jackson DE (1973). Counterconditioning and exposure only in the treatment of specific (conditioned suppression). *Behav Res Ther,* 11:453.

Drugan RC, Ader DN, and Maier SF (1985). Shock controllability and the nature of stress-induced analgesia. *Behav Neurosci,* 99:791–801.

Garcia J, Ervin F, and Koelling RA (1966). Learning with prolonged delay of reinforcement. *Psychon Sci,* 5:121–122.

Garcia J, Rusiniak KW, and Brett LP (1977). Conditioning food-illness aversions in wild animals: *Caveant canonici.* In H Davis and HMB Hurwitz (Eds), *Operant-Pavlovian Interactions.* Hillsdale, NJ: Lawrence Erlbaum Associates.

Gray JA (1991). The neuropsychology of temperament. In J Strelau and A Angleitner (Eds), *Explorations in Temperament.* New York: Plenum.

Gustavson CR (1996). Taste aversion conditioning versus conditioning using aversive peripheral stimuli. In VL Voith and PL Borchelt (Eds), *Readings in Companion Animal Behavior.* Philadelphia: Veterinary Learning Systems.

Gustavson CR, Garcia J, Hankins WG, and Rusiniak KW (1974). Coyote predation control by aversive stimulation. *Science,* 184:581–583.

Hart BL and Hart LA (1985). *Canine and Feline Behavioral Therapy.* Philadelphia: Lea and Febiger.

Hess EH (1964). Imprinting in birds. *Science,* 146:1128–1139.

Hoffman HS and Solomon RL (1974). An opponent-process theory of motivations: III. Some affective dynamics in imprinting. *Learn Motiv,* 5:149–164.

Houpt KA (1991). *Domestic Animal Behavior.* Ames: Iowa State University Press.

James W (1890/1950). *The Principles of Psychology*, Vol 2. New York: Dover (reprint).

Jersild AT and Holmes FG (1935). Methods of overcoming children's fears. *J Psychol*, 1:75.

Jones MC (1924). A laboratory study of fear: The case of Peter. *J Genet Psychol*, 31:308–315.

Kamin LJ (1968). Attention-like processes in classical conditioning. In MR Jones (Ed), *Miami Symposium on the Prediction of Behavior: Aversive Stimulation*. Miami: University of Miami Press.

Kehoe EJ and Macrae M (1997). Savings in animal learning: Implications for relapse and maintenance after therapy. *Behav Ther*, 28:141–155.

Konorski J (1967). *Integrative Activity of the Brain: An Interdisciplinary Approach*. Chicago: University of Chicago Press.

Levis DJ (1979). The infrahuman avoidance model of symptom maintenance and implosive therapy. In JD Keehn (Ed), *Psychopathology in Animals: Research and Clinical Implications*. New York: Academic.

Lorenz K (1970). *Studies in Animal and Human Behavior*, Vol 1. Cambridge: Harvard University Press.

Lubow RE (1973). Latent inhibition. *Psychol Bull*, 79:398–407.

Mackintosh NJ (1983). *Conditioning and Associative Learning*. Oxford: Clarendon.

Marks I (1977). Phobias and obsessions: Clinical phenomena in search of a laboratory model. In JD Maser and MEP Seligman (Eds), *Psychopathology: Experimental Models*. San Francisco: WH Freeman.

Pavlov IP (1927/1960). *Conditioned Reflexes: An Investigation of the Physiological Activity of the Cerebral Cortex*, GV Anrep (Trans). New York: Dover (reprint).

Prewitt EP (1967). Number of preconditioning trials in sensory preconditioning using CER training. *J Comp Physiol Psychol*, 64:360–362.

Rescorla RA (1967). Pavlovian conditioning and its proper control. *Psychol Rev*, 74:71–80.

Rescorla RA (1968). Probability of shock in the presence and absence of the CS in fear conditioning. *J Comp Physiol Psychol*, 66:1–5.

Rescorla RA (1988). Pavlovian conditioning: It's not what you think it is. *Am Psychol*, 43:151–160.

Rescorla RA and Wagner AR (1972). A theory of Pavlovian conditioning: Variations in the effectiveness of reinforcement and nonreinforcement. In A Black and WF Prokasy (Eds), *Classical Conditioning: II. Current Theory and Research*. New York: Appleton-Century-Crofts.

Scott JP (1962). Critical periods in behavioral development. *Science*, 138:949–957.

Scott JP and Fuller JL (1965). *Genetics and the Social Behavior of the Dog*. Chicago: University of Chicago Press.

Seligman MEP (1970). On the generality of the laws of learning. *Psychol Rev*, 77:406–418.

Seligman MEP (1971). Phobias and preparedness. *Behav Ther*, 2:307–320.

Sluckin W (1965). *Imprinting and Early Learning*. Chicago: Aldine.

Solomon RL and Corbit JD (1974). An opponent-process theory of motivation: I. Temporal dynamics of affect. *Psychol Rev*, 81:119–145.

Voith VL (1981). Attachment between people and their pets: Behavior problems of pets that arise from the relationship between pets and people. In B Fogle (Ed), *Interrelations Between People and Pets*. Springfield, IL: Charles C Thomas.

Watkins LR and Mayer DJ (1982). Organization of endogenous opiate and nonopiate pain control systems. *Science*, 216:1185–1192.

Watson JB (1924/1970). *Behaviorism*. New York: WW Norton (reprint).

Watson JB and Rayner R (1920). Conditioned emotional reactions. *J Exp Psychol*, 3:1–14.

Wolpe J (1958). *Psychotherapy by Reciprocal Inhibition*. Stanford: Stanford University Press.

Wolpe J (1969). *The Practice of Behavior Therapy*. New York: Pergamon.

Wolpe J and Rachman S (1960). Psychoanalytic "evidence": A critique based on Freud's case of Little Hans. *J Nerv Ment Dis*, 131:135–147.

Woodbury CB (1943). Learning stimulus patterns by dogs. *J Comp Psychol*, 35:29–40.

7

Instrumental Learning

Now, whereas the gods have given to men the power of instructing one another in their duty by word of mouth, it is obvious that you can teach a horse nothing by word of mouth. If, however, you reward him when he behaves as you wish, and punish him when he is disobedient, he will best learn to do his duty. This rule can be stated in few words, but it applies to the whole art of horsemanship.

XENOPHON, *On the Art of Horsemanship* (1925/1984)

T HE DISCUSSION in the preceding chapter was mainly limited to an exploration
of the more or less involuntary mechanisms
and processes mediating stimulus-response
(S-R) learning. Behavioral change, however,
often involves much more complicated and
dynamic interactions between the animal and
the environment than the S-R model can adequately handle. Opposed to the involuntary
nature of reflexive behavior, a great deal of
what a dog does is highly motivated, organized, and goal directed. These more complicated aspects of dog behavior cannot be reduced to a simple chain of S-R events.

DIFFERENCES BETWEEN CLASSICAL AND INSTRUMENTAL CONDITIONING

The dog's ability to learn as the result of experience is a key factor ensuring its adaptive

success. In addition to the associative, infor-
mation-producing functions provided by
classical conditioning, dogs also depend on
various instrumental or operant means to secure control over the social and physical environment. Through the combined efficacy of
classical and instrumental learning processes,
dogs can reliably predict and control the occurrence of biologically significant events.
Classical conditioning provides dogs with
predictive information about the occurrence
of these events, while voluntary instrumental
efforts serve to optimize the dog's control
over them.

Instrumental learning differs from classical
conditioning in several significant ways. An
important distinction between these two
forms of learning is embodied in the different
uses of the terms *elicit* and *emit*. Reflexive or
respondent behavior is *elicited* by an appropriate stimulus event, whereas instrumental
or operant behavior is *emitted* without the
presence or necessity of an eliciting stimulus.
Another prominent difference between classical and instrumental learning is the relative
amount of voluntary control exercised by an
animal. In contrast to the largely involuntary
nature of reflexive behavior, instrumental
learning mostly involves goal-directed behavior that actively *operates* on the external environment to produce desirable consequences.
Unlike reflexive behavior, instrumental behavior does not depend on an eliciting stimulus, although it can be brought under the
control of a signal or discriminative stimulus.

As discussed previously, classical conditioning primarily involves conditioned and
unconditioned stimuli and the various responses elicited by them. In the case of classical conditioning, response strength depends
on various attributes belonging to the eliciting stimulus (e.g., its salience or intensity),
the animal's readiness to respond, and the existence of a contingent relationship between
the conditioned stimulus and the unconditioned stimulus. In the case of instrumental
learning, response strength depends foremost
on the presence of an established contingency
between the response and a reinforcing outcome regularly following its occurrence. As is
discussed later in this chapter, many other
motivational, biological, and cognitive factors

affect the strength of instrumental behavior.

Classical and instrumental learning also differs in terms of their respective functions. A vital function served by classical conditioning is the formation of reliable predictive representations about the occurrence or nonoccurrence of beneficial or dangerous events. Instrumental learning, on the other hand, provides the animal with information about how these events can be successfully controlled through various behavioral adjustments involving approach, escape, or avoidance. As the result of such learning, the animal gradually maximizes access and control over attractive outcomes while avoiding or minimizing the occurrence of aversive ones. The information and behavior derived from instrumental learning is goal directed and biologically purposeful, forming a flexible repertoire of adaptive behaviors shaped for the preservation and protection of the animal. In combination, classical and instrumental learning activities provide a fluid and adaptive interface between the animal and the surrounding environment. Tarpy writes,

> Response learning represents a mechanism by which animals can change the world to their advantage. Since strong biologically active stimuli usually represent either valuable resources or threats to survival, then these stimuli must not only be predicted (stimulus learning provides one mechanism), but they also must be controlled. Organisms who have evolved the mechanisms that permit response learning can change the environment to their own advantage. They can acquire expectancies about future outcomes based upon their own behavior; and the response they execute alter stimuli in ways that are important for survival. (1982:94–95)

Instrumental-like Conditioning of Reflexive Behavior

Some evidence suggests that classical conditioning may not be the only way autonomic behavior is modified. Instrumental control of reflexive behavior appears to be possible under highly controlled experimental conditions. For example, Miller (1969) demonstrated that many reflexes can be modified with instrumental conditioning, utilizing a complicated operant conditioning procedure. In these experiments, rats were paralyzed with curare, and intracranial electrodes were placed into the brain to stimulate reward sites. Miller's preparation allowed the researchers to shape visceral activities, like heart rate, urinary output, peristaltic activity, and other autonomic functions, without the confounding influence of voluntary striated muscle activity. In one study, heart rate was differentially accelerated or decelerated depending on the presence or absence of reinforcement (intracranial stimulation). Heart-rate increases were also brought under the control of a compound (light and tone) discriminative stimulus (Miller and DiCara, 1967). Miller's work shows that under conditions of paralysis (i.e., when voluntary control of striatal muscle is disrupted) many autonomic functions can be altered by instrumental consequences (i.e., reward and punishment). In another study (Miller and Carmona, 1967), the salivary reflex in dogs was enhanced or diminished according to the consequences that followed its emission. Food naturally elicits salivation, but water does not. In their experiment, water was used as a reinforcer for salivation. In water-deprived dogs, salivation increased when it resulted in access to water and decreased when salivation postponed the delivery of water.

Additional evidence for the central control of autonomic functions comes from many biofeedback studies with humans. As a result of biofeedback, human subjects can learn to control such functions as heart rate and blood pressure voluntarily, though this is not necessarily evidence that an operant factor is at work. A subject may simply learn to selectively stimulate opposing motivational substrates through cortical enervations of the limbic system and other subcortical mechanisms.

A Uniprocess Theory of Learning

Classical and instrumental learning activities are always functionally integrated, although, for some practical and experimental purposes, they are frequently treated as separate phenomena. Over the years, several experimental psychologists have attempted to extend

Pavlov's findings to the study of instrumental behavior (Watson, 1924/1970; Guthrie, 1935/1960; Konorski, 1967; Gormezano and Tait, 1976). Pavlov himself believed that his reflexology would ultimately show that all learning was under the central control of a single S-R mechanism—an ambitious expectation that has fallen short of realization in many ways. However, recent and ongoing efforts by Robert Rescorla and his associates at the University of Pennsylvania to study instrumental behavior in terms of a Pavlovian analysis and methodology have yielded promising results. They have found Pavlovian associative linkages and structures embedded in every major facet of instrumental conditioning. These *encoded* Pavlovian structures include S-R relations, predictive stimulus-outcome relations, and Pavlovian-like response-outcome expectations (Rescorla, 1987, 1991).

THEORETICAL PERSPECTIVES

Attempting to understand how voluntary behavior is modified produces many interrelated theoretical and practical questions. Whereas behavioral scientists are primarily interested in developing general laws and principles governing learned behavior, trainers focus on how voluntary behavior is most efficiently modified and turned to practical purposes. Many lines of theoretical reasoning inform modern training theory. To appreciate these various contributions, a brief theoretical overview is provided below. This overview is not intended as a complete historical representation of the development of learning theory, but rather an effort is made to delineate some of the more significant historical issues and to summarize them with emphasis on their relevance for the dog behavior consultant and trainer.

THORNDIKE'S CONNECTIONISM

Edward L. Thorndike (1911/1965) is credited with founding the study of instrumental learning and placing comparative psychology on an experimental foundation. He was specifically interested in the question of how performance improved through trial and error, and he performed numerous experiments involving problem solving in cats and other animals.

Basic Mechanisms of Behavioral Change: Stamping In and Stamping Out

In the typical experiment, a cat was confined inside a puzzle box equipped with various mechanisms that could be manipulated to gain escape. A piece of fish was placed just outside of the cage as an added incentive. Thorndike measured the amount of time it took for each cat to find a way out, for example, by pulling on a loop of string or stepping on a platform arranged to release the door. Typically, cats engaged in a great deal of anxious searching behavior until they happened upon the correct solution by chance. Over the course of succeeding trials, the cats *gradually* became more skilled at escape. Thorndike observed that cats did not learn through insight or discovery but struggled through a process of trial and error with successful behaviors being *stamped in*, whereas frustrating, unsuccessful behaviors were *stamped out*. He concluded that a response was directly connected or bonded to the associated stimulus complex through a process of stamping in. According to Thorndike, all "learning is connecting." The animal's trial-and-error learning is dependent neither on deliberate reasoning nor on the exercise of some specialized instinct but depends entirely on the selective stamping in or stamping out of relevant S-R connections.

Thorndike's Basic Laws

Thorndike sums up his experimental findings in three basic laws of learning:

1. The *law of effect* states that an S-R connection (or bond) is strengthened or weakened depending on the hedonic quality of consequences following it. A response followed by a reward or "satisfier" strengthens the S-R bond and is stamped in. A response followed by a punisher or "annoyer" is weakened and is stamped out.

2. The of *law of exercise* states that a response is strengthened through use and weakened through disuse.

3. The *law of readiness* is couched in a pe-

culiar language of conduction units. Hilgard and Bower (1975) suggest that what Thorndike means by such units is an objective *action tendency* or preparation for action. When an animal is motivationally prepared to act, then the performance of the action is satisfying. When an animal is ready to act but prevented from doing so, the animal is annoyed, i.e., mildly punished or frustrated. Annoyance is also experienced (expressed as resistance) when an animal is motivationally unprepared to act but compelled to do so anyway. Readiness to act is affected by an animal's mental set or attitude (i.e., personal motivations determining what will annoy or satisfy it at any given moment). The law of readiness anticipates in several details Premack's theory of reinforcer reversibility (Premack, 1962). What under one set of motivational conditions is reinforcing may be punitive under another. For example, a satiated dog may find the opportunity to go for a walk more satisfying than the chance to eat more food. Additional eating for a satiated dog is punitive, i.e., annoying. On the other hand, a well-exercised dog would more likely choose to eat than undergo additional exercise. Whether a particular activity is annoying or satisfying is relative to the animal's varying motivational state.

Thorndike's law of effect underwent significant modification in his later writings. As the result of studies involving the use of mild punishment such as the word *wrong* or brief isolation, he generalized (wrongly) that punishment did not weaken instrumental behavior as he had previously postulated in the second half of the law of effect (see Chapter 9). Although he still recognized the power of punishment to disrupt behavior, he no longer believed that it was sufficient to alter learned connections to the same extent that rewards do. He also revised the law of exercise. He now argued that learning was not substantially influenced by the mere effort of practice and repetition, although such practice may benefit the performance of an already learned connection. For practice to be effective (i.e., promote additional learning), the repeated behavior must be associated with re-inforcement—rote practice will not alter learned connections by itself.

Thorndike's emphasis on reward over punishment was an important contribution in the development of modern educational philosophy. Although subsequently proven wrong by a variety of studies, the rejection of punishment and the endorsement of more positive methods for behavioral control had a widespread and beneficial effect on animal training, child-rearing practices, and educational programs.

GUTHRIE'S LEARNING THEORY AND BEHAVIOR MODIFICATION

The writings of Edwin R. Guthrie (1935/1960) are distinguished among the literary efforts of the major learning theorists by the simple and accessible language used to describe complex behavioral processes. Guthrie presents his theories and supporting information in a minimally technical form and effectively illustrates his theoretical arguments with numerous anecdotes and stories, including many involving dog behavior and training. Most of the concepts and principles discussed in his book *The Psychology of Learning* are easily within reach of patient, nonacademic readers. Although theoretically oriented, the book is organized more like a manual of behavior modification than a theoretical treatise. It is filled with valuable insights for the everyday control of behavior, representing an important source of practical information for the professional trainer/behaviorist working with problem dogs.

Like Pavlov and Watson before him, Guthrie argued that all learning (classical and instrumental) takes place within the context of a simple S-R model of associative conditioning. It is not surprising, therefore, to discover that his theory of learning is based on a single, all-encompassing postulate: "A combination of stimuli which has accompanied a movement will on its recurrence tend to be followed by the movement" (1935/1960:23). In other words, behavior occurring in some given situation will tend to recur under the same or similar circumstances in the future. In place of Thorndike's conceptualization of reward and punishment (involving satisfying and annoying events) and B. F. Skinner's notion of operant reinforcement, Guthrie proposed a unique interpretation of reinforcing and aversive contingencies, arguing that either sort of event is sufficient to reinforce or suppress behavior, depending on the situation in which it happens to occur:

> I do not hold that all satisfiers tend to fix the associative connection that has just preceded them. When a satisfying situation involves breaking up the action in progress it will destroy connections as readily as punishment. In teaching a dog to sit up, tossing his rewarding morsel to a distant part of the room will prove a very ineffective method. There is no doubt of the satisfying character of the meat. The dog certainly "does nothing to avoid, often doing such things as attain and preserve," not, of course, the meat, but the eating of it. But the effect of the reward will be that the dog instead of sitting up stands ready for another dash across the room. ... Just as satisfiers do not always "stamp in" a connection, so annoyers do not, as Thorndike himself perceived, always "stamp out." What we can predict is that the influence of the stimuli acting at the time of either satisfaction or annoyance will be to reestablish whatever behavior was in evidence at the time. (1935/1960:127)

The hedonic value (i.e., relative pleasure/pain) of the reinforcing event is not intrinsically significant to the effect it has on behavior, although the emotional excitement generated by the event (punitive or rewarding) facilitates its reinforcing effect, i.e., excitement accelerates learning. In general, the event's significance is determined by what it *does* to behavior. Both rewards and punishers serve to interrupt ongoing behavior, thereby preventing subsequent behavior from interfering with the situation and competing with the emission of the target behavior. For example, throwing food on the floor just as surely suppresses jumping up as shoving the dog off does. At the moment of reinforcement, both procedures result in the dog having returned all four feet on the ground. According to Guthrie, the feeling states generated by such events are irrelevant to what is learned, what is relevant is what the animal does:

> It is not the feeling caused by punishment, but the specific action cause by punishment that determines what will be learned. In training a

dog to jump through a hoop, the effectiveness of punishment depends on where it is applied, front or rear. It is what the punishment makes the dog do that counts, or what it makes a man do, not what it makes him feel. The mistaken notion that it is the feeling that determines learning derives from the fact that often we do not care what is done as a result of punishment, just as long as what is done breaks up or inhibits the unwanted habit. (1935/1960:132)

Within the context of Guthrie's system, the adaptive function of learning is the formation of stereotyped and effortless habits. According to this view, such stereotyped habits serve the organism by refining and making more efficient its adaptation to the surrounding environment. Once established, stereotypic habits tend to persist and may resist being "broken" or "sidetracked" through training. One method described by Guthrie for breaking a habit involves isolating the initiating cues and associating them with other behaviors that are incompatible with the unwanted one—a process known to the contemporary behavior therapist as counterconditioning. This is not always an easy process, since many initiating cues may support a well-established habit. Although aversive punishment is a useful procedure, unless it is applied in a sufficiently intense form, it may not prove to be very effective but could instead inadvertently reinforce the unwanted habit by making its performance more exciting. Many negative attention-seeking behaviors are maintained under the control of such inadequate punitive contingencies. Further, although punishment can be an effective means for breaking unwanted habits, such treatment may, in addition, produce adverse side effects, like making the punishing agent (e.g., the trainer or owner) a cue for fearful behavior and avoidance. Guthrie points out that aversive punishment is not always necessary and notes that any external "interference that captures attention and introduces a new activity will be successful" (1935/1960:118). Again, punishment does not depend on how it makes the animal feel but on what it makes the animal do. To be effective, the distracting activity must be physically opposed to and incompatible with the unwanted behavior, so that "the muscle set of the obnoxious behavior which is the cause of its persistence is thoroughly changed" (1935/1960:118).

Counterconditioning or *response substitution* is an important procedure in Guthrie's system of behavior modification. In the process of illustrating this method, he tells the story of a horse that had been the subject of some mischievous training by two farm boys. The boys arranged themselves so that while one of them commanded the horse "Whoa," the other poked the poor animal with a pitchfork. The hoped-for result of their experiment was quickly obtained. When the hapless owner (a pastor visiting the boys' family) took his horse back from their care, he discovered to his discomfiture and terror what the boys had done in his absence. Upon issuing the command "Whoa," his erstwhile dependable and docile horse reared up and charged wildly out of control. Guthrie suggests that this incident dramatically exemplifies the process of response substitution in which a previously conditioned stimulus is associatively linked with a new and incompatible response:

> How do stimuli become distracters or inhibiters of an action? We may recall that in the case of the pastor's horse the sound of the word "Whoa" had previously been a signal for stopping. This had been in turn the effect of training in which the horse had been checked by the rein and the sound uttered a second or so before. The boys' efforts had substituted another reaction for the conventional one and in effecting this substitution the word became an inhibiter of the first response. ... A stimulus may thus be unconditioned by the very simple means of becoming a conditioner for an incompatible movement. Unlearning becomes merely a case of learning something else. And the rule which states whether conditioning or unconditioning will occur becomes simply the familiar principle of conditioning: Stimuli which are acting at the time of a response become conditioners of the response. In this case, *the response referred to in the rule is a response incompatible with the former response.* The horse can not lunge forward and stop at the same time. This is physically and neurologically impossible. The signal inhibits stopping because

it has become alienated from that response by a later association with the incompatible response. (1935/1960:55–56)

Guthrie also describes several other general and now familiar methods for breaking habits. Besides arranging for the evocation of incompatible substitute behavior in the presence of cues controlling the performance of an unwanted habit, habits can be systematically reduced or eliminated by gradual exposure. Guthrie refers to this general method as *negative adaptation.* In this procedure, a stimulus is presented at an intensity or form that remains just above threshold tolerances and is then gradually altered in intensity until the previously intolerable stimulus is readily accepted at full strength. Many fears and aversions are reduced through negative adaptation. Negative adaptation is particularly effective in cases where gradual exposure to the negative stimulus occurs in the presence of a more positive stimulus, like attention, food, or relaxation. This general method is referred to in the contemporary language of behavior modification as *systematic desensitization.* Guthrie illustrates the procedure of negative adaptation by recounting various techniques used by animal trainers to reduce fearful reactions in dogs and horses. For example, he describes the case of hunting dogs that are gradually exposed to increasingly loud and naturalistic gunshot reports until the dogs can react impassively to a shotgun blast at close quarters (Whitford, 1928). Similarly, a horse being trained to carry a rider is first exposed to the saddle and other gear gradually and systematically (e.g., starting with a light blanket and progressively adding more equipment and weight) until the horse can tolerate the full weight of the rider on its back. In addition to gradual exposure, Guthrie also favors the use of what is generally referred to today as *response prevention.* He writes in this regard that "when the cue occurs but the response *is prevented by any means,* negative adaptation of the response to that cue takes place" (1935/1960:63). Guthrie succinctly summarizes these basic methods for the breaking of unwanted habits:

Bad habits are broken by substituting them for good habits or innocuous habits. The rule for breaking an undesired conditioned response becomes this: So control the situation that the undesired response is absent and the cue which has been responsible for it is present. This can be accomplished by fatiguing the response, or by keeping the intensity of the cue below the threshold, or by stimulating behavior that inhibits the undesired response. If the cue or signal is present and other behavior prevails, the cue loses its attachment to the obnoxious response and becomes an actual conditioner of the inhibiting action. (1935/1960:65)

Another behavioral method discussed by Guthrie at some length involves *response fatigue* or *negative practice*. In the case of negative practice, the animal is required to repeat the offending behavior over and over again in the presence of the controlling cues. Guthrie describes the case of a little girl who had adopted the habit of playing with matches. As punishment failed to suppress the habit, the child's worried mother resorted to negative practice in an effort to break the habit. The procedure was simple: she simply required that her daughter strike dozens of matches in quick succession. The child soon bored of the activity and began actively to resist her mother's prodding. Instead of lighting matches, she began to push them away. As a result, a new set of responses incompatible with lighting matches was evoked in the presence of cues that were previously associated with lighting them. The last thing the child did in the presence of the matches was to push them away. Later, when the child was exposed to matches again, she showed no interest in playing with them. Theoretically, the escape or refusal response produced by negative practice became prepotent over "match lighting," thus causing the girl to abandon the dangerous habit. Such negative practice procedures can be effectively employed in the case of many intrinsically reinforced activities exhibited by dogs. An area of concern about negative practice is how it might impact on desirable behavior. For example, if one forces dogs to retrieve until they quit, their willingness to retrieve in the future will probably be negatively affected by the experience. Simi-

larly, excessively long and repetitive training sessions may not be as conducive to learning as shorter and more varied ones.

It is not within the scope of this discussion to cover in detail all of the major contributions of Guthrie to the current trends and methods informing behavior therapy and behavior modification, but it should be noted, as is rarely done in the pertinent literature, that most of these developments owe Guthrie a great deal (Malone, 1978). Many of the major contemporary therapeutic procedures, including in vivo exposure and response prevention, counterconditioning, systematic desensitization, negative practice, and overcorrection, are described in detail by this insightful psychologist.

TOLMAN'S EXPECTANCY THEORY

Edward C. Tolman (1934) adhered to many of the fundamental tenets of behaviorism but also introduced several new perspectives into the study of behavior and learning—some of which were highly controversial and inconsistent with the behaviorist platform. Tolman viewed the study of behavior both as an experimental process (fact finding, hypothesizing, and falsifying) but also emphasized an interpretative component that evaluated the meaning or purposiveness of the behavior being studied. Most behaviorists before him viewed behavior as a *molecular* phenomenon composed of individual S-R effects and relationships. Tolman believed that behavior had to be investigated in the context of the subject's intended purpose, thus extending the study of behavior to include an evaluation of its purpose, that is, its *molar* implications.

Tolman's scientific thrust aimed at developing hypothetical constructs inferred from concrete experimental observations of behavior. The study of purposiveness does not imply observations based on empathy or introspection (methods that Tolman rejected) but rather the formulation of inferences derived from observed behavior. In the scientific study of behavior, three experimental variables co-interact to arrive at significance:

1. *Independent variables.* The various controlled aspects of the experiment, especially the stimulus conditions and motivational state of the animal.

2. *Dependent variables.* All measured changes occurring in the behavior of the subject under the influence of controlled experimental conditions.

3. *Intervening variables.* Abstract constructs necessary to explain the observed S-R relationship.

The intervening variable is not a subjective interpretation but an objectively defined presumption arrived at by holding constant all independent variables except those hypothesized significant to it. The intervening variable is inferred from experimental evidence—that is, it helps make sense of experimental results. The validity and usefulness of the intervening variable is established by making predictions based on it and then designing experiments to systematically falsify those predictions. The intervening variable is operationally defined and delimited by the results of such experimental analysis and falsification.

For example, if a dog is presented with two bowls of food, one with meat in it and the other with dry food, the dog will most likely choose the one containing meat. A reasonable conclusion that one might draw from this experiment is that the dog "prefers" meat over dry food. Although this is a possible conclusion, however, it is not the only one possible from this experiment. To demonstrate preference some quantifiable correlation needs to be elaborated, defining *preference* (itself unquantifiable) as the most relevant variable controlling the dog's choice of meat over dry food. A hypothetical experiment might involve making the dog expend physical energy (jumping over a barrier of increasing difficulty) or mental effort (solving a difficult puzzle or maze) to acquire the meat as a goal and then comparing the dog's effort with respect to other food items. The assumption here is that the dog's preference for the food item is positively correlated with a willingness to work harder for it. Further-more, his preference can be quantified relative to other less preferred items of food.

A slightly more complicated situation occurs in a two-choice discrimination task. In this experiment, the dog is trained to choose between two cards, one patterned with a checkerboard pattern and the other left blank. Choosing the checkerboard pattern always results in the presentation of food, whereas the blank card is never reinforced. Within several trials, the dog learns to choose the patterned card when prompted to choose. In this case, many possible intervening variables may subsist between the presentation of the positive and negative cards and the pattern of subsequent choice making. One very general hypothetical construct is that the dog "thinks" about the choice options and then chooses according to cognitive rules of discrimination; another broad view might theorize that the dog "learns" to choose the correct card as the result of trial and error; another observer might claim that the dog is innately attracted to patterned objects and is more likely to attend to the checkerboard-pattern card over the blank card; another possible theory is that the positive choice is an outcome of the nonreinforcement of the blank card (extinction) rather than a result of reinforcement of the positive card; and another theorist might explain the dog's mastery as an outcome of classical conditioning—that is, the dog is attracted through associative learning to the positive card.

As the foregoing inventory of possible intervening variables shows, there are many possible ways to explain the dog's successful discrimination. To determine how the dog manages to learn such a discrimination task requires experiments that isolate one intervening variable at a time while controlling the effects of others. The theory that the dog is innately attracted to the positive card can be easily *falsified* by presenting the blank card as the positive stimulus and comparing relative rates of learning with the checkered card. But what about the relative importance of trial and error versus extinction-based learning, and the role of classical conditioning? What are the most important variables influencing discrimination learning? Answering such questions as these would require the design of several controlled experiments isolating significant from confounding variables.

Tolman placed a stronger emphasis on stimulus or sign learning than he did on response habit formation (i.e., Thorndike's stamping-in or stamping-out process). Instead of learning a response pattern, Tolman argued that an animal learns a cognitive map of significant relations or sign-gestalts (signs, significates, and behavior routes leading from sign to significate) in the environment, leading to the satisfaction of appetitive demands and goals. In a general sense, *signs* correspond to the classical conception of the conditioned stimulus and *significates* to the unconditioned stimulus:

> The sign-gestalt theory asserts that the conditioning of a reflex is the formation of a new sign-gestalt. It asserts that a conditioned reflex, when learned, is an acquired expectation-set on the part of the animal that the feature of the field corresponding to the conditioned stimulus will lead, *if the animal but waits* [behavior route], to the feature of the field corresponding to the unconditioned stimulus. (Tolman, 1934:393)

Hilgard and Bower (1975) described several experiments that tend to support Tolman's cognitive interpretation of learning. One of these experiments (Tinklepaugh, 1928) involved a delayed-response test in which a hungry monkey was shown a banana that was then hidden under one of two cans. The monkey quickly mastered this discrimination and easily found the concealed banana. Later, while the monkey was out of sight, the banana was secretly removed and replaced with a leaf of lettuce. When the monkey returned and discovered the change, he rejected the lettuce (a less preferred food item) and began searching for the hidden banana. This study implies that the animal had formed a definite expectation about finding a banana. Besides forming expectations about outcomes, animals learn from signs and place cues how to reach specific goals—that is, the animal is not learning a specific series of responses but exhibits behavior that implies that he *knows* where the goal is located and

uses various signs and routes to get there, which is a "what leads to what" theory of learning. Another study [Macfarlane (1930), reported by Hilgard and Bower (1975)] provided additional support for a connection between cognitive mapping and goal-directed behavior. Macfarlane first trained rats to wade through a flooded maze and then required that they swim the course instead. The swimmers were found to do equally well as the waders, indicating that the response sequence was not dependent on learning a set of specific motoric or kinetic actions but depended on a more general knowledge of place.

Thorndike (1946) proposed an experiment to test the role of learned expectancy versus habit formation and response reinforcement in instrumental learning. The experiment involved placing a rat on a cart and pulling it through a maze. After a number of such trials, the rat would than be tested for its ability to learn the maze route and the results compared with that of a naive rat not previously exposed. Thorndike predicted that both subjects would learn the task equally well. However, subsequent studies have contradicted Thorndike's prediction (Mazur, 1986). Experiments by Dodwell and Bessant (1960) found that such preexposure *did* affect learning rates in a positive direction. In their experiment, animals were pulled through a water maze in a little car. Subsequent tests demonstrated that the preexposed rats performed better than controls not exposed. Earlier studies demonstrated that rats that underwent pretraining exposure, by being permitted to explore the maze prior to training, did substantially better than controls not given such exposure. This latter evidence is somewhat confounded, however, since the benefit of such pretraining exposure may have been due to adaptation to the training environment rather than due to learning. On the whole, these results contradict Thorndike's view that instrumental learning is solely dependent on response-contingent connections.

Tolman's learning theory makes several theoretical distinctions between learning and performance. For Tolman, learning is independent of performance, but performance is not independent of learning. Motivational levels strongly impact performance by generating goal-directed tensions demanding satisfaction. In an important sense, performance is a composite of current motivational states and past learning experiences. Even though learning is not dependent on motivation, as seen in the aforementioned case of latent learning, it is not entirely independent of it either. Motivational substrates (appetite, fear, and aversion) define the specific details of the environment that an animal most alertly and selectively attends to. An animal pays greatest attention to and learns the most from items that possess significant motivational interest. Hungry dogs seek out signs of food, whereas fearful dogs search for routes of escape. The cumulative organization of all available signs and routes together with their corresponding significates forms a cognitive map of sign-gestalts representing the overall field of available expectancies (Tolman, 1948).

Perhaps Tolman's most significant contribution to the study of animal behavior is his emphasis on the cognitive aspects of learning. From this perspective, learning represents much more than the acquisition of a series of simple S-R outcomes or response-reward relationships. Tolman's view places learning within a much broader context or field. Learning takes place on an integrative, molar level where S-R events are interpreted and made meaningful by assimilation of the particular into the general, a mediation effected by "sign-gestalt expectations." Through learning, dogs are ever-forming predictive interpretations and expectancies about the occurrence of important stimulus events—a process that is both purposive and cognitive.

B. F. Skinner and the Analysis of Behavior

Undoubtedly, the most forceful and controversial figure in the history of behaviorism is B. F. Skinner (1938/1966). Many of the concepts and principles used by the professional trainer/behaviorist were originally developed in the laboratory of Skinner and subsequently elaborated by his many devoted followers, who refer to themselves as *behavior analysts.* Skinner's system is coherent and eminently

pragmatic, with direct and powerful applications for the modification of behavior in the practical setting. Like Thorndike before him, Skinner viewed the effects of reward and punishment asymmetrically, placing far greater emphasis on the use of positive consequences, rather than punishment, for altering and controlling behavior. Skinner derived his emphasis on behavioral consequences directly from the tradition of Thorndike and the law of effect. A publication of particular interest to trainers interested in becoming better acquainted with his system and terminology is the programmed text *The Analysis of Behavior* (Holland and Skinner, 1961), which is a well-designed presentation of the basic concepts of behavioral analysis provided in a user-friendly format. Another well-written and easily understood introduction is *A Primer of Operant Conditioning* (Reynolds, 1968). For a more thorough and detailed treatment of behavior analysis, the books *Learning* (Catania, 1992) and *Psychology of Learning and Behavior* (Schwartz, 1989) are highly recommended.

One of the most important experimental contributions made by Skinner to the study of behavior was the invention of special equipment for recording behavioral events. The *Skinner box* is composed of a bar lever (for rats) or a disc (for pigeons), a food magazine, and a light and sound source for the presentation of discriminative stimuli. The animals are trained to operate the manipulanda by either pressing the lever or pecking (in the case of pigeons) an illuminated disc. These responses are then recorded on a cumulative recorder that graphically displays the animal's rate of responding (number of responses per unit of time) on a rolling sheet of paper. Through the use of a cumulative recorder, the experimenter can track changes in the rate of behavior as it is related to various reinforcement schedules and the alteration of other significant independent variables. In the modern learning laboratory, these scheduling and recording functions are usually managed through computer automation. Skinner was primarily concerned with measuring changes in emitted behavior under the influence of varying conditions of reinforcement. The manipulation and analysis of reinforcement schedules remains Skinner's most important contribution to learning theory.

Skinner's system of operant and respondent conditioning consists of two sets of binary laws. The Type S laws that regulate respondent learning are inductive generalities derived from the studies of Pavlov:

1. *The law of conditioning of Type S:* "The approximately simultaneous presentation of two stimuli, one of which (the 'reinforcing' stimulus) belongs to a reflex existing at the moment at some strength, may produce an increase in the strength of a third reflex composed of the response of *the reinforcing reflex and the other stimulus.*"

2. *The law of extinction of Type S:* "If the reflex strengthened through conditioning of Type S is elicited without presentation of the reinforcing stimulus, its strength decreases" (1938/1966:18–19).

The Type R laws governing operant learning are very reminiscent of Thorndike's modified law of effect:

1. *The law of conditioning of Type R:* "If the occurrence of an operant is followed by presentation of a reinforcing stimulus, the strength is increased."

2. *The law of extinction of Type R:* "If the occurrence of an operant already strengthened through conditioning is not followed by the reinforcing stimulus, the strength is decreased" (1938/1966:21–22).

These are the basic laws of Skinner's system of learning. In many ways, they are little more than a reiteration of Pavlov and Thorndike. Skinner's contribution does not rest on the discovery of the general laws of learning but on the creative and productive ways that he applied them to the study of behavior.

Skinner refers to operant conditioning as Type R learning, emphasizing its independence from stimulus learning or Type S learning. In Type S learning, the stimulus *elicits* a response in the manner of Pavlov. In Type R learning, the animal *emits* a response in an effort to operate on the environment to produce desirable consequences. He denies that operant conditioning is an S-R system, claiming that the "stimulus occupied no special place among the independent variables" of his studies. Although stimuli play no part in the sense of response elicitors in operant conditioning, they do play important subsidiary roles in announcing conditions of reinforcement (discriminative stimuli)—that is, they inform an animal when reinforcement is available given that a particular response is emitted. Another stimulus used in operant conditioning is the conditioned reinforcer. When a desired behavior is emitted, the response is bridged to the unconditioned reinforcer by the presentation of a conditioned reinforcer. A conditioned reinforcer is a neutral stimulus that has been associatively linked with an unconditioned reinforcer (operant reinforcer) through respondent (classical) conditioning.

One of Skinner's most controversial positions was his rejection of most forms of scientific theorizing. For example, he consistently argued against extrapolating from behavioral observations and data back to some more original place in the brain or mind of the animal. He eschewed all theorizing that went beyond empirically founded predictions or guesses in anticipation of experimental results. In a seminal article, "Are Theories of Learning Necessary," Skinner (1950) outlined his experimental approach to learning. According to Skinner, the study of behavior should be strictly limited to observable behavioral events that are precisely described in objective behavioral terms only. He strongly rejected the hypothetico-deductive method in which hypotheses are formulated and tested as being wasteful and productive of much useless experimentation. In addition, he excluded physiological descriptions and theories as well as mentalistic and hedonic interpretations like expectancies and pleasures occurring inside of the subject. Finally, he rejected conceptual accounts that, although relying on operational constructs referring to observed behavior, make appeal to explanatory extrapolations and intervening variables not physically present in the observed event:

A science of behavior must eventually deal with behavior in its relation to certain manipulable variables. Theories—whether neural, mental, or conceptual—talk about intervening steps in these relationships. But instead of prompting us to search for and explore relevant variables, they frequently have quite the opposite effect. When we attribute behavior to a neural or mental event, real or conceptual, we are likely to forget that we still have the task of accounting for the neural or mental event. When we assert that an animal acts in a given way because it expects to receive food, then what began as the task of accounting for learned behavior becomes the task of accounting for expectancy. The problem is at least equally complex and probably more difficult. We are likely to close our eyes to it and to use the theory to give us answers in place of the answers we might find through further study. (1950:194)

Skinner also denies the usefulness of intervening variables (à la, Tolman):

The simplest contingencies involve at least three terms—stimulus, response, and reinforcer—and at least one other variable (the deprivation associated with the reinforcer) is implied. This is very much more than input and output, and when all relevant variables are thus taken into account, there is no need to appeal to an inner apparatus, whether mental, physiological, or conceptual. The contingencies are quite enough to account for attending, remembering, learning, forgetting, generalizing, abstracting, and many other so-called cognitive processes. (1938/1966:xii)

While the foregoing is ostensibly a logical argument against certain forms of theorizing, it falls short as a general methodological principle for the study of behavior. In spite of Skinner's objections against the study of mediational events, behavior is a mediated event that depends on a variety of internal cognitive and conative mechanisms for its purposeful expression. Furthermore, considering the many successes of other scientific disciplines employing the hypothetico-deductive method, it is hard to view Skinner's rejection of it very seriously. It is difficult to imagine where physics and chemistry would be today if physicists and chemists had depended on an experimental method in which hypothesis,

deduction, and falsification were preemptively excluded from the process of research.

Skinner has been referred to as a *radical behaviorist*—a term applied with no lack of contempt by detractors, but a name proudly adopted by some ardent enthusiasts of his method and brand of behaviorism. Contrary to a popular misconception, Skinner did not deny the existence of private feelings or individual purpose and meaning in the lives of people and animals. He did, however, reject such private experience as adequate subject matter for direct scientific observation and study. According to his viewpoint, internal experiences are controlled and modified in the same way that overt behavior is: by external contingencies of differential reinforcement and the law of effect. Furthermore, since private experiences do not submit to direct objective measurement, material like personal feelings and purpose can only be studied in the context of actual behavioral events. In other words, feelings like anger and love can be formally studied only by investigating their behavioral manifestations, that is, actual displays of aggressive or affectionate behavior occurring under various controlled circumstances.

BASIC CONCEPTS AND PRINCIPLES OF INSTRUMENTAL LEARNING

Terms and Definitions

Instrumental learning is regulated by what Thorndike has called the *law of effect*, which states that instrumental behavior is differentially strengthened (reinforced) or weakened (punished) by the consequences produced by its emission. Among behaviorists, the term *reinforcement* is preferred over the word *reward* for describing events or outcomes that increase the frequency/probability of instrumental behavior. Two common concerns are often expressed in defense of this preference: (1) The word *reward* implies that the animal itself is compensated for the emission of the selected behavior; however, such compensation does not necessarily mean that the emitted response is strengthened as a result. (2) Opposed to the vague meaning of reward, the term *reinforcer* is more precisely defined in terms of the measurable effect it has on behavior—that is, a behavior is reinforced when, other things being held equal, the future probability/frequency of the behavior it follows is increased by the presentation of the reinforcing event. A reward may or may not increase the future probability of the behavior it follows—if it does, it is a reinforcer.

The technical distinctions between reward and reinforcement are clear; however, the technical language becomes a bit more murky and forgiving when it comes to the term *punishment*. It is a little perplexing when one is admonished not to employ the word *reward* (because of the aforementioned reasons) but can, in the same breath, say correctly that a behavior is *punished*. There appears to be an obvious double standard at work in the way these two terms are scrutinized. Both words in common usage are typically directed toward the agent of behavior—not the behavior itself. The term *punishment*, therefore, appears to suffer the same sort of ambiguity as the word *reward*. In practice, this is not a very serious conceptual problem, since *punishment* is operationally defined as an event that lowers the probability of the behavior that it follows. Likewise, though, the word *reward*, given a similar operational definition, can be used as a synonym for *reinforcer*. For the sake of consistency, though, some other term would be preferable to the word *punishment*. It is unfortunate that we do not have a parallel word in English, like *suppressment*. For one thing the word *suppression* refers more explicitly to the effect that punishment has on behavior and, thereby, avoids the emotional connotations associated with this culturally loaded term. For future reference, the terms *reward* and *punishment* are used here in the more technical sense of events that differentially increase or decrease the future probability/frequency of the behavior they follow.

In general, there are two ways in which the probability/frequency of behavior is affected by the consequences it produces:

Reinforcement (R or S^R) increases the relative probability or frequency of the behavior it follows.

Punishment (P or S^P) decreases the relative probability or frequency of the behavior it follows.

In addition, there are two ways in which behavior is reinforced or strengthened:

1. *Positive reinforcement* (R+ or S^{R+}) occurs when a behavior is strengthened by producing or prolonging some desirable consequence.
2. *Negative reinforcement* (R− or S^{R-}) occurs when a behavior is strengthened by terminating, reducing, or avoiding some undesirable consequence.

Note: Both R+ and R− increase the future probability/frequency of the behavior they follow.

Finally, there are two ways in which behavior is punished or weakened:

1. *Negative punishment* (P− or S^{P-}) occurs when a behavior is weakened by omitting the presentation of the reinforcing consequence.
2. *Positive punishment* (P+ or S^{P+}) occurs when a behavior is *weakened* by presenting the previously escaped or avoided consequence.

Note: Both P− and P+ decrease the future probability/frequency of the behavior they follow.

In combination, these basic reinforcing and punishing contingencies provide four ways for modifying behavior, viz., R+/R− and P+/P− (Fig. 7.1).

Reinforcing Events

Dogs gain practical information about the physical and social environment through the consequences of their behavior. Such experiences teach them how to control and manipulate significant events vital to their interests. The exercise of control over important occurrences reinforces the learning process itself, both in terms of specific behavioral instances and in terms of general learning expectancies or sets. Learning is a cognitively organized pattern that must be mastered before com-

Frequency of Behavior			
Increase-reinforcement		Decrease-punishment	
R+	R−	P+	P−
Presentation of reward	Withdrawal or omission of aversive	Presentation of aversive	Withdrawal or omission of reward

FIG. 7.1. Various ways in which the frequency of behavior is influenced by the consequences it produces.

plex behavioral skills can be acquired. In an important sense, dogs are always learning *how* to learn.

Two complementary motivations drive instrumental learning: the maximization of positive outcomes and minimization of aversive ones. These complementary motivations correspond to the notions of positive and negative reinforcement. If a response becomes more probable as the result of its producing a desirable consequence (e.g., petting and food), then the potentiating effect is referred to as *positive reinforcement.* Conversely, if a response becomes more probable by its terminating or avoiding an aversive stimulus (e.g., leash correction), then the effect is referred to as *negative reinforcement.* Positive and negative reinforcement are the two primary ways in which goal-directed behavior is acquired and maintained.

Positive Reinforcement

Typical reinforcement events satisfy some physiological or psychological need. To hungry dogs, the opportunity to acquire a savory treat is worth effort and work. If the acquisition of food is made contingent on a dog sitting when requested to do so, the dog will quickly learn that sitting on cue results in the acquisition of the desired treat (positive rein-

forcer). After several such experiences, the probability that the dog will sit on cue is increased and will continue to increase as long as the performance is reinforced and the dog remains motivated or until additional learning is not possible (asymptote). In the foregoing case, the dog learns that a causal connection exists between the presence of a specific cue or discriminative stimulus (S^D), a response (R) and a resulting positive reinforcer (S^{R+}). Through this simple lesson, the dog not only learns how to sit, but, more importantly, the dog learns that its actions can control the environment—an outcome that makes learning itself intrinsically rewarding.

Negative Reinforcement

Negative reinforcement occurs when a dog discovers that a particular response terminates or avoids the presentation of an aversive stimulus. A natural example can be observed when a dog, having stayed too long in the sun, finds relief by moving to nearby shade. Moving out of the direct sunlight into the shade is a negatively reinforced behavior because it terminates the aversive condition of overheating. Traditional obedience training makes liberal use of negative reinforcement. For example, the sit exercise is often taught by applying an upward pull on the leash and collar coupled with a downward pressure on the rump. The forces involved are mildly aversive. Under such stimulation, most dogs will at first struggle and attempt to resist the pressure, but after several trials they usually learn to escape it by following the applied forces in the correct direction and successfully learn to sit under compulsion. If a word cue ("Sit") is presented before the onset of the pressure, the dog will learn to avoid the negative event by sitting in response to the cue alone. After several such trials, the dog will begin to recognize a causal linkage between the presentation of the avoidance cue, specific and timely action, and the avoidance of the anticipated aversive outcome. Such learning depends on anticipatory signals that reliably predict response-produced outcomes. This pattern is confirmed (acquisition) or disconfirmed (extinction) by repeated experience.

Intrinsic Versus Extrinsic Reinforcement

There are two general sources from which positive and negative incentives are derived: *intrinsic* (part of the task itself) and *extrinsic* (external to the task). Intrinsic incentives are those attractive and aversive motivational inducements that belong to the task itself. Intrinsic positive reinforcers are inherent to behaviors (e.g., playing ball, chasing a cat, or jumping on guests) that are enjoyed in and of themselves and maintained without additional external reinforcement. Intrinsic negative reinforcers, on the other hand, are inherent to the relief provided by behaviors that avoid or terminate situations that are annoying in and of themselves (e.g., growling or snapping when threatened or escaping confinement when left alone). Extrinsic incentives include all positive and negative inducements that derive from sources other than the behavior itself (e.g., various attractive and aversive events). Intrinsically reinforced behavior is acquired and maintained under natural reinforcement contingencies, whereas extrinsic incentives are provided contingently by the trainer. Both intrinsic and extrinsic incentives play important roles in dog training and behavior modification.

Timing and Repetition

Understanding that behavior is modified by its consequences is an important insight into how dogs learn. In addition, timing and repetition also play crucial roles in the training process. For a reinforcer to be effective, it must closely follow the target behavior. Optimally, the reinforcer should be presented immediately after the target behavior is emitted. Further, the connection between the reinforcer and the target behavior is strengthened by frequent repetitions. With practice, dogs learn to expect the eventual presentation of the positive reinforcer as the result of emitting the selected behavior.

Differential Reinforcement

Behavior is a fluid phenomenon with each event flowing seamlessly into the next. Under natural conditions, no edges or boundaries sharply separate one behavior from another. Behavioral differentiation occurs as the result of selectively reinforcing responses and sequences of the dog's behavior that are compatible with the trainer's objectives and ignoring or punishing behavior that is not. This process of selection strengthens certain tendencies and patterns while extinguishing or suppressing other aspects of the dog's behavior. As a result of such pressure and change, the dog's behavior is adjusted to fit and respond to the demands made upon it by domestic life.

The structuring of behavior is accomplished by the differential presentation and withdrawal of reinforcement or punishment. Since behavior is fluid, it is important that the reinforcing or punitive events coincide exactly with the behavior being strengthened or weakened. Unfortunately, dogs cannot be directly reinforced with most tangible rewards (e.g., food and petting) at the exact moment that they emit the target behavior, especially if the behavior occurs while they are some distance away. Also, in order to make punitive events effective, they must be timed to coincide with the occurrence of the target behavior.

Conditioned Reinforcement and Punishment

These problems are solved by using remote stimuli that temporarily take the place of the reinforcer or punisher until they can be delivered to the dog. On the one hand, the so-called *bridging stimulus* or *conditioned reinforcer* (S^r) serves to bridge the emission of the target response with the acquisition of a positive reinforcer. In contrast, the *conditioned punisher* (S^p) suppresses unwanted behavior by its being associated with the loss of an expected reinforcer or the impending presentation of a punishing aversive event. Conditioning the S^r is a Pavlovian process in which the bridging stimulus (e.g., "Good") is repeatedly paired with the presentation of the positive reinforcer or the termination of a negative reinforcer. On the other hand, a conditioned punisher is produced by pairing the bridging stimulus (e.g., "No") with the loss of positive reinforcement or the presentation of an aversive punishing event.

Additional Characteristics of Positive Reinforcement

The reinforcer is conceptualized as a contingent event capable of satisfying some biological necessity or drive that, when presented upon the emission of some behavior, will make the occurrence of that behavior more likely under similar circumstances and states of motivation in the future. For example, the presentation of a biscuit to a hungry dog after sitting will make the dog more likely to sit in the owner's presence in the future when hungry. But actually reinforcement is much more complicated than this reward paradigm suggests, exhibiting many irregular and, perhaps, unanticipated characteristics. For example, while the opportunity to eat represents a strong reinforcer for a hungry dog, the dog may also find just smelling the food reinforcing (Long and Tapp, 1967). There are several other characteristics of positive reinforcement that should be kept in mind: The incentive (or conditioned reinforcement associated with the work and the anticipation of reinforcement) may be more strongly reinforcing

than the actual reward or unconditioned reinforcer itself. Highly desirable rewards may generate faster acquisition of simple skills but retard the acquisition of more complicated ones. Large food rewards generate an enthusiastic performance while the food is available but result in learning that is more prone to extinction when it is withdrawn. Smaller rewards may not generate very much enthusiasm initially but learning acquired under the control of small rewards is more resistant to extinction. Finally, slow, steady learning is the most resistant to extinction (Tarpy, 1982).

MOTIVATION, LEARNING, AND PERFORMANCE

A dog's performance is a direct reflection of its past history of reinforcement and its current motivational state or readiness to act. For positive reinforcement to be effective, a dog must be in a state of need that can be satisfied only after the dog behaves in a predetermined way. The most commonly employed reward in animal training is food. As a reward, food is effective only so long as dogs are either hungry or sufficiently interested in the food item being used. Utilizing a dog's hunger drive together with its added willingness to work for special treats promotes the strongest effect. Although puppies will readily work for kibble, it is not usually sufficient to offer a dog the regular ration of food in a piecemeal fashion. Similarly, training dogs immediately after eating will negatively impact food as a positive reinforcer, as well as impede the development of classically conditioned appetitive associations. Combining food deprivation together with the presentation of special treats produces the best training results. The term *deprivation* means scheduling training sessions before meals rather than after them. The meal itself can be given to reinforce the overall training session as a sort of jackpot.

Although the provision of food is a powerful reward, it is not the only positive reinforcer available to trainers. In fact, anything the dog finds desirable can be used as a reinforcer. Although it has been argued that petting and praise may not possess sufficient reward value to strengthen newly acquired behavior (Romba, 1984), controlled studies by Fonberg and Kostarczyk (1980) contradict this view, demonstrating conclusively that petting and verbal praise are viable social rewards for dogs. These researchers trained dogs under experimental conditions to perform a series of simple exercises (sit, paw, and down) with great efficiency and rapidity using petting and praise alone. To some extent, the pleasure from petting is an acquired taste and dependent on the degree of attachment and familiarity between the dog and the trainer. Bacon and Stanley (1963) found that running speeds in puppies were differentially affected by the amount of social contact that they received prior to testing, with puppies exposed to "satiating" contact running slower than "deprived" counterparts. The authors note that these effects are analogous to the increased instrumental responsiveness of rats exposed to food or water deprivation prior to training. In addition to petting and praise, the opportunity to go for a walk, ball play, access to chew toys, bouts of play, and access to other dogs—all represent potentially reinforcing events for dogs interested in obtaining such activities. Each activity, however, yields only a limited reward quotient, depending on the dog's need for the offered activity. A dog that has just undergone a long ball-play session will probably find additional ball play less reinforcing than access to a chew toy or a moment of rest. Similarly, a dog that has been engaged in chewing will not likely choose additional chewing over an opportunity to go for a walk. Reward training should not be restricted to food reinforcement alone. In fact, the reward value of food is relative to a dog's momentary motivational state of hunger. Under certain circumstances of satiation, a dog might actually find food punitive in comparison to an opportunity to play.

ANTECEDENT CONTROL: ESTABLISHING OPERATIONS AND DISCRIMINATIVE STIMULI

The manipulation of motivational states conducive to learning is referred to as *antecedent control*. Some forms of antecedent

control remain outside the trainer's direct influence (e.g., genetic and biological factors such as breed-typical tendencies, inherited traits, and some behavioral thresholds). In addition to setting events such as hunger, thirst, biological condition, medications, and general social needs, several other forms of antecedent control are under the direct influence of the trainer. These include establishing operations (e.g., reinforcer sampling or priming and a variety of transient motivational changes conducive to instrumental learning); discriminative stimuli (e.g., signals and commands-setting occasions when reinforcement is most likely to follow some specified behavior); and conditioned stimuli (conditioned attractive or aversive establishing operations). An establishing operation (EO) is a motivational antecedent that influences the extent to which a particular outcome (reinforcer or punisher) will strengthen or weaken the behavior it follows. According to Michael, an EO is an "environmental event, operation, or stimulus condition that affects an organism by momentarily altering (a) the reinforcing effectiveness of other events and (b) the frequency of occurrence of that part of the organism's repertoire to those events as consequences" (1993:192).

Setting events and EOs are of great significance for behavior modification because their manipulation alters the relative effectiveness of reinforcement and punishment. For example, the presentation of food to a hungry dog may be highly reinforcing, whereas if the dog is sick or sated, the food reward may not function as a reinforcer at all. In fact, in such cases, the presentation of food may punish the behavior that it follows. Further, manipulating EOs increases or decreases the likelihood that some class of behavior associated with the reinforcer or punisher will or will not occur. In the case of a hungry dog offered a noncontingent treat (reinforcer sampling), the dog will be more likely to beg, increase activity levels, or emit other behavior that has successfully obtained food in the past. A similar effect is achieved by briefly giving the dog a ball to play with, then making continued access to it contingent on some required behavior.

A warning or threat may function as an

EO for avoidance behavior, thus making it more likely that the dog will respond to a command previously associated with negative reinforcement. A failure to sit, for example, followed by "No!" will raise the likelihood that the dog will sit when the command is repeated. In this case, the reprimand "No!" is an EO making the sit response more likely to occur in the presence of the vocal signal as well as enhancing the effect of negative reinforcement when the dog sits. Obviously, an EO and a discriminative stimulus (S^D) (e.g., "Sit") share a functional relationship as antecedent variables controlling the occurrence or nonoccurrence of both wanted and unwanted behavior. In the case of reinforcement, the EO raises the likelihood that some particular behavior will occur and be effectively reinforced, whereas the S^D precisely defines the occasion when the response is most likely to produce the reinforcer, that is, the EO exercises *motivational control* while the S^D exercises *stimulus control*. Identifying EOs and S^Ds controlling unwanted behavior is vital for effective behavioral intervention. By manipulating EOs and altering or eliminating controlling S^Ds associated with unwanted behavior, such behavior is rendered much more responsive to modification. Secondly, by properly manipulating motivational states, more desirable alternative forms of behaviors can be easily shaped and brought under control.

PREMACK PRINCIPLE: THE RELATIVITY OF REINFORCEMENT

The usual way reinforcement is described emphasizes its *stimulus* characteristics and their potentiating effects on behavior, but reinforcement can also be analyzed in terms of the potentiating effects that responses have on other responses. David Premack (1965), who performed a number of experiments supporting this sort of analysis, has demonstrated that behavior occurring at a high frequency or probability tends to reinforce behavior occurring at a lower frequency/probability. According to this perspective, the determination of whether any particular behavior is a reinforcer (or punisher) depends on its relative probability with respect to the behavior it follows. Premack states this relationship in terms of response probability: "For any pair of responses, the independently more probable one will reinforce the less probable one" (1962:255).

If one distributes the dog's behavior on a hierarchy or continuum ranging from low to high response probability, then, according to the *Premack principle*, behaviors ranked higher up on the hierarchy of probability will tend to positively reinforce ones ranked lower down. Alternately, if a response occurring lower on the probability hierarchy follows one ranked higher up, the relationship is punitive—that is, the higher-ranked antecedent response will be rendered less probable by the lower-ranked consequence. Therefore, reinforcers and punishers are relative and dependent on a dog's transient behavioral tendencies and motivational states.

Instead of conceptualizing the reinforcing event as a stimulus, Premack describes it in terms of an indivisible S-R composite. For example, a biscuit for the hungry dog is both stimulus (something to be eaten) and a response (the act of eating it). These observations emphasize an important difference between instrumental and classical conditioning. Responses reinforce responses in the case of instrumental learning, whereas stimuli reinforce stimuli in classical conditioning.

A significant factor in the foregoing paradigm of reinforcement is the role of response-activity deprivation (Timberlake and Allison, 1974). Any behavior can be made more valuable and, therefore, more probable by depriving the animal access to it. Similarly, any behavior can be made less valuable and punitive by satiating the animal with it, thus making it less probable. Further, the value of any given reward is dynamic and dependent on the animal's changing sensory needs and the attainment of what Wyrwicka (1975) has described as a *better state* of being.

During an ordinary training session, the dog is going to prefer performing some exercises more than others. Determining at any moment what the dog would prefer to do and then providing access to that activity on a contingent basis is a sound and efficient incorporation of the Premack principle. For instance, having a dog heel out of a down-stay is a reinforcing consequence for staying, regardless of what else is done to strengthen the down-stay exercise. Although there appears to be a natural inclination for active exercises to reinforce stationary ones, this is not always the case. For example, if a dog is made to heel for a long period without stopping, the dog's inclination to sit or lay down will gradually become stronger than its inclination to continue heeling. When the dog is finally permitted to sit or lay down, the opportunity to rest will tend to reinforce the previous heeling pattern.

Another example involves the trained habit of coming when called from the sit-stay. Most dogs find coming when called preferable to staying still in the sit position. Consequently, even in the absence of other rewards, the sit-stay is reinforced when the dog is called by its handler. However, having the dog come and then to sit-front may have a contrary effect. In this situation, the dog moves from a highly reinforcing activity (coming) into a less reinforcing one (sitting). The overall effect is mildly punitive. There-

fore, at the outset of recall training, it is better not to require that dogs perform the customary sit-front each time they come. Instead, it would be consistent with the Premack principle to follow the performance of coming with an even more exciting and reinforcing opportunity, for example, an immediate opportunity to play ball. An alternative approach would be to train the sit-front to a high degree of proficiency, thus making it highly probable, and then to chain the less probable recall response to it.

LEARNING AND THE CONTROL OF THE ENVIRONMENT

Just as expectancies are formed between a conditioned stimulus and the occurrence or nonoccurrence of a corresponding unconditioned stimulus in classical conditioning, a similar contingency relation appears to exist between the instrumental signal, response, and reinforcing outcome (Rescorla, 1987). Instrumental acquisition, schedules of reinforcement, and extinction can all be described and understood in terms of a rein-

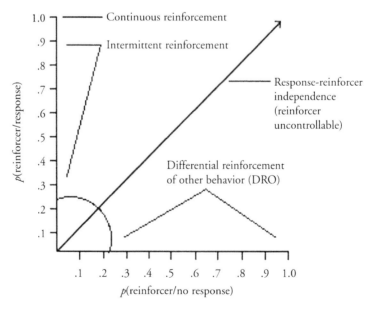

FIG. 7.2. Diagram showing various general contingency relations between the reinforcer and the occurrence or nonoccurrence of the instrumental response. After Seligman et al. (1971).

forcer-response contingency. Figure 7.2 illustrates various contingency relations between the reinforcer and response, ranging from a situation in which the reinforcer is certain to follow the response each time it occurs (continuous reinforcement), to intermittent reinforcement, and, finally, to a condition in which any response *other than* the specified one is followed by reinforcement (differential reinforcement of other behavior—see below). The most problematical contingency is represented by the diagonal line in the diagram. Here the animal is exposed to a situation in which reinforcement is equally likely to occur whether or not the specified response occurs—that is, the reinforcer and response occur independently of each other. Under conditions of appetitive training, the noncontingent presentation of food may result in various interference effects collectively referred to as *learned laziness*. On the other hand, under conditions in which aversive stimulation is presented on a noncontingent basis, a number of devastating interference effects called *learned helplessness* may ensue, impeding normal escape and avoidance learning.

The unpredictable or noncontingent presentation of rewards or punishers may adversely affect the learning process in many ways. Habitually providing dogs or puppies with gratuitous affection and treats without clearly defining a causal linkage between such rewards and the animals' behavior may lead them to conclude that their behavior does not play an instrumental role in obtaining such outcomes. Such "spoiled" puppies are more prone to develop adjustment problems and become more difficult to train as adults. Early training that encourages puppies to earn desirable resources and activities in exchange for appropriate behavior is fundamental to rearing well-behaved and adjusted puppies. Evidence supporting this view has been found by comparing rats that had obtained varying amounts of free food (i.e., food presented noncontingently with respect to their behavior) with rats who received food on a contingent basis (Seligman, 1975). When later tested and compared on a simple lever-press task, the spoiled or "lazy" rats learned the target response much more slowly than unspoiled controls:

Different groups of hungry rats had pellets of food dropped "from the sky" through a hole in the roof of their cage, independently of their responses; then they had to learn to get food by pressing a bar. The more free food they had received in pretraining, the worse they did at learning instrumental responses for food. Some of the rats just sat around for days, waiting for more food to drop in; they never pressed the bar. (Seligman, 1975:34–35)

Wheatley and colleagues (1977) performed a series of controlled experiments exploring the interference effects of noncontingent rewards on subsequent appetitive learning in rats. The results substantially support Seligman's observations. They found that rats exposed to noncontingent food during pretraining sessions performed at a much lower level in comparison to rats pretrained to perform a simple response to obtain the same food. Lack or loss of controllability of positive outcomes affects not only subsequent appetitive training but also the animal's ability to learn aversive contingencies—that is, the interference effect is cross-motivational (Sonoda et al., 1991).

Another source of concern regarding noncontingent rewards is the adventitious reinforcement of unwanted behavior and, perhaps, the development of superstitious behavior. Although B. F. Skinner's famous study and demonstration of superstitious behavior in pigeons has been widely cited as evidence for such learning, unfortunately it has not been experimentally duplicated. In fact, a more detailed study by Staddon and Simmelhag (1971) failed to show confirming evidence for the sort of bizarre and idiosyncratic superstitions observed by Skinner in his earlier experiment (Skinner, 1948). Although superstitious behavior may develop from time to time as the result of adventitious or noncontingent reinforcement, the form described by Skinner is probably not very common among animals.

In the case of unpredictable and uncontrollable aversive stimulation, the effects are even more pervasive and debilitating. Common sources of such stimulation include noncontingent punishment and negative reinforcement applied without adequate avoidance cues. Following the application of such improper punishment, the owner may futilely attempt to explain the cause of the "surprise attack" with meaningless verbal admonitions and directives. Of course, to the bewildered and frightened dog, all of this only adds to the confusion.

Sadly, many dogs are subjected to a daily round of punishment and affection based largely on an owner's shifting moods. In general, the loss of control over significant events via the noncontingent presentation of appetitive or aversive stimuli results in reduced operant initiative and retards associative learning processes. Dogs habitually exposed to excessive noncontingent punishment tend to become overly cautious, nervous, and insular. Their experiences with punishment have taught them that they can neither predict nor control such aversive events. Consequently, they learn to take punishment passively as an inevitable outcome rather than learning from it. They appear to be pain insensitive or extremely stubborn, sometimes failing to learn the most simple training exercises without exhibiting great difficulty, resistance, and struggle. They are often passively resistant and withdrawn. They appear to be mentally paralyzed; lacking normal voluntary initiative, they must be physically prompted or forced through every step of the training process. They are frequently stiff with muscular tension as though anticipating the worst and bracing for it. Because of their negative outlook, such dogs are very difficult and draining to work with, resisting every effort to increase their interest and enthusiasm. They often refuse food, reject invitations to play, and are unresponsive to petting. They are typically hypervigilant and suspicious. These behavioral effects of uncontrollable punishment are consistent with the symptoms of *post-traumatic stress disorder* (PTSD) and what Seligman has collectively termed *learned helplessness* (see Chapter 9).

SCHEDULES OF POSITIVE REINFORCEMENT

One of the most important contributions of B. F. Skinner to training theory was the elucidation of various reinforcement schedules and their differential impact on the performance of learned behavior (Ferster and Skinner, 1957). In dog training, reinforcement is provided according to various plans and schemes depending on the specific requirements of the training objective. During the early stages of training, a new behavior is reinforced every time it occurs. The new behavior is acquired on a continuous schedule of reinforcement (CRF). Once a stable operant level is obtained, the behavior is usually brought under the control of an intermittent schedule of reinforcement. Intermittent schedules require a dog to emit a prerequisite number of responses (ratio schedule), emit at least one response within a predetermined period of time (interval schedule) before reinforcement is delivered, or emit the target behavior continuously over some period of time (duration schedule). All three schedules can be either fixed or variable. In combination, therefore, three basic schedules of fixed and variable reinforcement are possible: (1) fixed and variable ratio (FR/VR), (2) fixed and variable interval (FI/VI), and (3) fixed and variable duration (FD/VD).

An FR schedule of reinforcement requires that a dog emit a fixed number of responses before reinforcement is presented. For example, requiring a dog to sit three times before giving it a treat is an FR 3 schedule of reinforcement. A VR schedule is set according to an on-average occurrence of reinforcement. For example, a dog reinforced randomly on the first, third, or fifth time it happens to sit would be maintained on VR 3 schedule of reinforcement. Interval and duration schedules are also applied on a fixed or a variable basis. For instance, an interval schedule only requires that the dog sit at least once during some fixed or variable period of time. On the other hand, a duration schedule involves a fixed or a variable length of time during which the response must be continuously emitted before reinforcement is delivered. A common example in dog training that utilizes a duration schedule is the stay exercise. A dog required to sit and stay for a period of 30 seconds before being reinforced is working on an FD 30s schedule of reinforcement. If the dog is required to sit for varying lengths of time, but on average for a 30-second duration, then the dog is working on a VD 30s schedule.

An important benefit of intermittent reinforcement is that it makes the selected behavior more resistant to extinction. While a CRF schedule will result in fast, steady acquisition, if reinforcement is suddenly withdrawn, the learned behavior will extinguish with a corresponding rapidity. The foregoing reinforcement schedules outlined require that a dog emit more responses for the same amount of reinforcement. The effect is to "immunize" the learned behavior against extinction should reinforcement not always be forthcoming. Not only do the various schedules (especially the VR schedule) cause instrumental behavior to become more resistant to extinction, they also stimulate dogs to work even harder for a comparatively smaller reinforcer. This added benefit allows for an easy transition from tangible rewards like food to less tangible social rewards like petting and praise. When food is used during the acquisition phase, it is usually *faded* as soon as possible and replaced with various social rewards sufficient to maintain the learned behavior. Finally, intermittent schedules are very important in shaping procedures where a previously established approximation must give way to the next step in the program of contingencies without causing the dog to quit.

EVERYDAY EXAMPLES OF REINFORCEMENT SCHEDULES

The influence of reinforcement schedules can be observed in many everyday situations. Imagine, for example, the behavior of a person who had just thrown the switch of a lamp and discovered that it did not work. What will he or she do to remedy the situation? Some reasonable efforts might include turning the light switch on and off a couple of times, checking whether the plug was properly inserted into the electrical outlet, or even looking for some other possible causes to explain the failure (e.g., a defective bulb, switch, or fuse). But one would not expect the person to turn the light switch on and off again repeatedly in a vain effort to make it

work. This latter option is unlikely because of the sort of reinforcement schedule controlling the "switch turning" behavior. The habit of turning the light switch on was acquired on a continuous schedule of reinforcement. In the past, the lamp had responded as expected on nearly every occasion the switch had been thrown. Under such conditions of reinforcement, a single failure of the light to work as expected disconfirms the entire pattern of reinforcement, resulting in its rapid extinction.

Similarly, if one were to insert a quarter into a pay phone and received neither a dial tone nor the coin in return, one would probably not continue to insert additional coins hoping that it might finally work. Both these examples illustrate the primary weakness of continuous reinforcement—the sensitivity of such schedules to the effects of extinction. Of course, extinction in these situations is only temporary. Both of these habits quickly recover as soon as they are reinforced again, that is, when the lamp is repaired or after a working pay phone is found.

A similar effect can be seen when dogs are trained on a CRF schedule. They, too, learn to "expect" the presentation of a reinforcer for each behavior they emit. If this pattern of continuous reinforcement is discontinued, dogs will refuse to emit the behavior. However, once the accustomed reinforcement schedule is reinstated, their willingness to perform will rapidly recover to previous levels. The foregoing observations suggest that dogs do not learn a *habit* per se, but rather a *set of instrumental contingencies* consisting of available outcomes, rules for their acquisition, correlated expectancies (given that they follow the rules), identification of the stimulus situations in which the rules apply, and an overall confirmation or disconfirmation of the learning set based on prior experience.

Comparing the foregoing example of switching on a lamp with that of starting a car reveals several important differences between continuous and intermittent schedules of reinforcement. While my car usually starts on the first attempt, I have learned to expect that occasionally it may take two or three additional efforts before starting. On some occasions, though, when it is extremely cold or wet outside, the car may require much more sustained effort and prompting to get started. Under these reinforcement contingencies, a warm sunny day has become a discriminative stimulus (S^D) under which circumstances my car usually starts easily on the first attempt. A cold dreary day, on the other hand, has become an S^D predictive of difficulty starting the car but usually promises success for sustained repeated effort. Under the conditions of warm and dry weather, I will be more likely to quit trying after only a few efforts and consider various mechanical failures instead. However, under weather conditions involving cold and heavy rain, I am more inclined to try many more times before giving up. The prevailing S^Ds in the first case cause me to *match* my efforts to predictions based on a CRF schedule, whereas in the second case my behavior is matched to predictions based on an intermittent VR schedule. As the

second case demonstrates, behavior under the control of intermittent scheduling tends to persist even under adverse reinforcement contingencies.

HOPE, DISAPPOINTMENT, AND OTHER EMOTIONS ASSOCIATED WITH LEARNING

Training events produce various expectancies and presumptive states of emotional arousal, ranging from frustration and disappointment to relief and hope (Fig. 7.3). In addition, anger, fear, and anxiety are commonly associated with aversive training techniques (see Chapter 8). As the foregoing examples illustrate, continuous reinforcement schedules tend to generate expectancies based on some degree of certainty (elation), whereas intermittent reinforcement schedules tend to generate expectancies based on probability

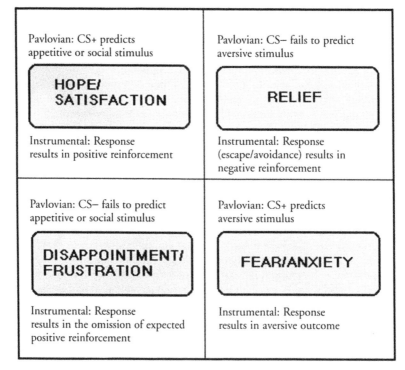

FIG. 7.3. Both classical conditioning and instrumental learning generate emotional arousal including hope, satisfaction, relief, disappointment, and fear. After Mowrer (1960).

(hope). When the light switch fails, I do not try over and over again hoping that it will eventually work. I may switch it on and off one or two times out of frustration or bang the broken pay phone out of anger (perhaps, with some hope of dislodging a sticky coin because of intermittent successes in the past by doing so), yet, almost as soon as my car fails to start on the first try, I begin to hope that it will start sooner rather than later.

Conditions of intense hope easily transport the subject into irrational realms of superstition and compulsivity. Hope is a controlling motivational factor in most games of chance. The actual outcome of gambling (the purse, etc.) is not as important as the associated elation of having won, an elation that is significant in terms of having avoided the disappointment of losing. Slot machines are programmed to pay off on a VR schedule. The behavior exhibited by players of such machines is virtually identical to the behavior of laboratory animals working under intermittent reinforcement. Individuals engaged in lever pulling for quarters are probably little interested in actually winning money (slot-machine players typically lose much more money than they win) as much as they are motivated to experience the sheer pleasure and elation of winning and avoiding the painful disappointment of losing.

Many of the effects occurring under ratio schedules can also be observed in behavior controlled by duration or interval contingencies. Dogs trained to sit-stay on an FD schedule will stay only as long as the duration to which they have been accustomed is not exceeded by too much time. For example, a dog trained to stay for a period of 5 seconds (FD 5s) will probably get up after 7 seconds or so if not rewarded. Rewards presented on an FD schedule establish an expectancy of certainty based on past learning experiences in which reinforcement always occurred within a fixed period of time. If this general expectancy is violated by making the dog stay longer without some transitional training, the stay performance will deteriorate under the influence of disappointment, at least until the previous duration contingency with which the dog is accustomed is reinstated.

FI schedules, like FR schedules, are very sensitive to extinction. For example, receiving a paycheck after a week of work is a common expectancy for the average working person. The strict regularity of this outcome may cause the worker to quit his or her job (depending on the presence or absence of other controlling reinforcers in the workplace) if the expected payment did not occur when promised. An employee working on a commission basis might be much more flexible, since he or she is accustomed to a VI schedule in which payments occur more randomly. A worker paid on a commission basis might persist for long periods between paydays based on the hope of an eventual payoff or a big bonus. Under normal circumstances, FI schedules are rare in comparison with VI schedules. FI schedules control behavior patterns based on expectancies of certainty, whereas VI schedules tend to generate expectancies of hope.

In general, behavior based on expectancies of certainty is vulnerable to disappointment, but behavior based on expectancies of hope is more persistent and motivationally *immunized* against the adverse influences of disappointment.

MATCHING LAW

The ability to choose between alternative courses of action is a behavioral imperative that enables an animal to adjust purposefully to the moment-to-moment demands presented by the environment. Choice behavior is influenced by the history of reinforcement produced by past choices made under similar conditions. The general pattern of choice-making is highly correlated or *matched* with the relative reinforcement value of the available alternatives presented to the animal from which to choose.

Expectancy and Matching

An important influence on choice behavior is *expectancy*—a cognitive construct—combining classical information (relative predictability) and instrumental information (relative controllability) derived from experience (Fig.

Expectancy Learning

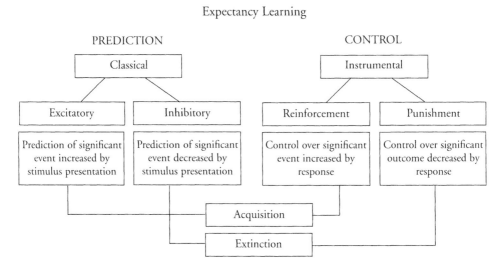

FIG. 7.4. Diagram showing various interactions between prediction and control in the formation of behavioral expectancies and learning.

7.4). Expectancy is constantly undergoing adjustment according to whether predictions have been accurate and whether control has been successful. This general process of confirmation and disconfirmation is a vital link between learning and performance. A learned behavior whose performance in the presence of a particular cue leads to an expected outcome is confirmed and its probability of future performance under similar circumstances is strengthened, whereas a behavior that fails to result in an expected outcome is disconfirmed and its probability of future performance correspondingly weakened. Confirmation promotes the acquisition of behavior, whereas disconfirmation promotes extinction.

Prediction-control expectancies are not necessarily "conscious" calculations, although in many animals (including the dog), they may be conscious to some extent. On a most basic level, such behavioral expectancies are cognitive representations, or *schema,* derived from experience. These expectancies appear to differentially stimulate internal motivational substrates, exciting or inhibiting behavior—substrate changes that may be felt or experienced (e.g., anxiety, frustration, relief, elation) and variously may impede or invigo-

rate behavior.

The statistical nature of expectancy is elegantly expressed in the tendency of animals to match their behavioral output to the relative reinforcement values offered by alternative choices. This ability to proportion behavior according to a matching rule was first described by Tolman and Brunswick (1935). According to them, the "causal texture" of the environment does not ordinarily produce firm expectancies; instead, an animal makes rough judgments based on probabilities of success or failure. This state of affairs entails a probability calculation based on the reinforcement history (reward and nonreward) of the particular class of behavior operating under particular conditions (cue-context relations). For example, Brunswick (1939) experimentally demonstrated that animals tend to apportion their behavior according to definite rules based on probability. In his early study of matching, rats were trained to run a T maze but were rewarded twice as often when they ran down one arm of the maze. That is, they were rewarded every time they ran down one arm but also received reinforcement every other time they ran down the opposite arm. An unexpected consequence occurred as the result of this experimental arrangement: the rats learned to apportion their choices based on the availability of rewards. A ratio of 2:1 was observed between the two available choices. This is an interesting finding, since it appears to violate the principle of least effort, stating that an animal prefers the shortest or easiest route to any given goal. Ostensibly, it would seem much more easy and efficient for the animal to simply run down the right arm for a 100% rate of reward and avoid the left arm altogether! More recent formulations of the *matching law* have been devised, and the phenomenon has been confirmed in a variety of animals. One possible explanation for the added work output is the acquisition of valuable information about a less than optimal source of food.

Concurrent Schedules

Over the years, many experiments have demonstrated that animals will reliably distribute their responses proportionally between the two sources of reinforcement according to the relative value of reinforcement made available by the respective alternatives. This propensity to apportion responding according to the relative value of reinforcement is governed by the matching law, which states that "the relative rate of responding equals the relative rate of reinforcement" (Rachlin, 1976:562). For example, consider a pigeon working in an operant chamber with two functioning disks producing food on different concurrent variable interval schedules. The right disc is programmed to present reinforcement on a VI 20s schedule, while the left disc is programmed to present reinforcement on a VI 120s schedule. The pigeon will likely choose to peck on the right disc six times as often as the pigeon responds on the left disc. This is a rather extraordinary learning phenomenon with a wide phylogenetic distribution among animals (Bitterman, 1965).

Extinction of Instrumental Learning

Extinction is a procedure whereby a posi-

tively or negatively reinforced response is decreased in strength or frequency by discontinuing the contingency of reinforcement maintaining it. During the acquisition phase, dogs learn that reinforcement or its omission depends on what they do. Under the extinction phase, they learn that the desired or expected consequence is no longer available for the same response. This does not imply that extinction is the functional opposite of learning, nor is it a passive effect based on response fatigue or some other such phenomenon (e.g., habituation), but rather extinction is the result of additional active learning about the relevant discriminative stimulus (S^D), response, and outcome ($S^{R+/-}$). Extinction results when the controlling S^D fails to predict the occurrence of the expected outcome for which the selected response is emitted, that is, to control the presentation of the positive reinforcer (S^{R-}) or to escape or avoid the occurrence of the negative reinforcer (S^{R-}). Consequently, during extinction, dogs learn not to respond in the presence of the signal since it no longer adequately predicts the occurrence or nonoccurrence of the anticipated attractive or aversive stimulus. However, extinguishing a response under the control of one S^D or signal does not mean that it will be adversely affected in the presence of other signals that still adequately predict reinforcement. In fact, if the previously disconfirmed signal again becomes predictive of reinforcement, the erstwhile extinguished response will quickly recover to its original strength.

Extinction procedures are often used to reduce attention-motivated disruptive behavior that is under the control of social contingencies of reinforcement (Ducharme and Van Houten, 1994). For example, many puppies rebel against being restrained in their crate at night, often exhibiting strong protestations in the form of barking and persistent efforts to escape. A concerned owner may reinforce this behavior by either attending to the puppy or, worse yet, by releasing the puppy from confinement. In cases where such a history of reinforcement is evident, extinction by simply ignoring the puppy often proves very effective. An interesting parallel case has been described by Williams (1959), in which a dramatic reduction of "tyrant-like tantrum behavior" was expressed by a 2-year-old child whenever he was put to bed. The child quickly responded to the extinction efforts carried out by the family, until one night the child exhibited a period of tantrum behavior (spontaneous recovery) while an aunt was watching him. This single reinforcing event caused the tantrum behavior to recover, requiring that another series of extinction trials be carried out. After a few days, the behavior was fully suppressed.

As mentioned previously, the rate of extinction depends to a great extent on the reinforcement history controlling the targeted behavior. Behaviors maintained under an intermittent schedule of reinforcement tend to be more resistant to extinction than ones maintained under a CRF. Characteristically, intermittent reinforcement also tends to produce higher rates of responding than does reinforcement occurring on a continuous schedule. In some cases, therefore, especially involving difficult-to-extinguish behavior, it may make sense to place the unwanted behavior on a continuous schedule before proceeding to the extinction phase of training. At first, this sort of behavioral intervention may seem highly questionable (i.e., deliberately reinforcing unwanted behavior), but the evidence is fairly clear—such an approach tends to reduce the overall rate of responding while rendering the behavior more vulnerable to subsequent extinction efforts. Lerman and colleagues (1996) have successfully tested and confirmed the efficacy of a similar approach with human subjects exhibiting disruptive and aggressive behavior.

Extinction Burst

When an instrumental response undergoes extinction, it may actually intensify before beginning to decrease in strength. For example, if one wishes to extinguish begging behavior by withholding food treats, the frequency and magnitude of begging behavior may initially increase to levels exceeding pre-extinction operant levels. This so-called *extinction burst* or frustration effect is usually followed by a gradual decrease in response strength until the behavior is finally extinguished over the course of several non-reinforced trials.

Spontaneous Recovery

After a day of rest following a series of extinction trials, a trainer may find that the behavior that he or she thought was extinguished the day before had meanwhile returned to nearly its full original strength. This phenomenon is referred to as *spontaneous recovery*, which frequently occurs after a rest period between extinction sessions. However, such recovered behavior is usually much more sensitive to subsequent extinction efforts, yielding more rapidly than before. Over the next several days, the begging behavior is apt to recover periodically but with progressively weaker strength and persistence. If the owner remains steadfast, the begging behavior will be eventually extinguished without further episodes of spontaneous recovery. If, however, the owner becomes lax or forgetful and gives the dog a *single* treat (intermittent reinforcement), future extinction efforts will be adversely impacted.

While extinction can be usefully employed to reduce the strength of an unwanted behavior, competing phenomena like bursts and spontaneous recovery make it an impractical training tool for many situations. Further, because extinction is essentially a punitive measure (the withdrawal of positive reinforcement is punishment), the dogs or puppies are not learning anything new—they are only learning that the behavior under extinction no longer produces the expected reinforcement. In the case of simple extinction, it is important to introduce and differentially reinforce an alternative or incompatible behavior to replace the one being extinguished.

DIFFERENTIAL REINFORCEMENT

There exist many ways to reduce the occurrence of unwanted behavior besides punishment and extinction. Perhaps the best initial approach to decrease unwanted behavior is to reinforce some competing alternative behavior differentially while simultaneously simply ignoring the unwanted one (Skinner, 1953; Kazdin, 1989). There are three basic schedules of differential reinforcement: (1) differential reinforcement of other behavior (DRO), (2) differential reinforcement of incompatible behavior (DRI), and (3) differential reinforcement of low rate (DRL).

Differential Reinforcement of Other Behavior

The schedule for differential reinforcement of other behavior (DRO) provides reinforcement for any behavior provided that the unwanted one does not occur during a fixed period of time. DRO scheduling is especially suited to nuisance behaviors occurring at a high frequency. For example, puppies exhibiting excessive mouthing tendencies might accept petting for 5 seconds or so before engaging in the undesirable habit. It is important to determine this baseline interval accurately before beginning the training process. The first step is to reward the puppy after 5 seconds regardless of what he is doing as long as he is not mouthing and has not mouthed for at least 5 seconds. Once the 5-second requirement is mastered, the DRO schedule can be lengthened through gradual increments of duration, until he accepts longer periods of attention without mouthing. The DRO schedule directly impacts on the mouthing behavior by reinforcing other behavior occurring in its absence.

An important drawback of the DRO schedule is that an equally unwanted behavior might be inadvertently reinforced (Foxx, 1982a). The puppy in the foregoing example is reinforced at the end of a fixed period, provided that he does not mouth regardless of other behavior that might be going on. At the moment of reinforcement, the puppy may not be mouthing but he might be barking or jumping up, undesirable behaviors that could be easily strengthened as a result of reinforcement. Another drawback of the DRO schedule is that it does not require that the puppy learn anything new to replace mouthing—it only requires that the puppy

not mouth or bite.

Differential Reinforcement of Incompatible Behavior

These problems can be mitigated by introducing a schedule for differential reinforcement of incompatible behavior (DRI) after the DRO schedule has reduced the frequency of the unwanted behavior into workable dimensions. Under the DRI schedule, the puppy is rewarded only if it performs an incompatible target behavior that is both motivationally and physically opposed to the unwanted behavior. In the aforementioned case of excessive mouthing, the target behavior might be licking. DRO and DRI schedules can be implemented together. For instance, the puppy can be reinforced after a predetermined interval of time, provided that no mouthing has occurred and that it licks at the end of the period.

The selection of reinforcement can help make this strategy even more effective. In many cases, the most desirable reinforcer is an opportunity to perform the unwanted behavior in a more acceptable form. This could be arranged by substituting an alternate object and activity in place of biting on hands. In the case of excessive mouthing, providing the puppy with a tennis ball, together with gentle tug and fetch games, is a quite satisfying outlet and alternative to mouthing on one's hands. This is a very constructive alternative, since ball play serves an important role in the puppy's future training. Excessive or persistent mouthing is often associated with dominance testing and may require additional training efforts to fully resolve.

Differential Reinforcement of Low Rate

The schedule for differential reinforcement of low rate (DRL) is similar to the DRO schedule in that a certain interval of time must pass between opportunities for reinforcement. In the case of DRL, the dog must emit a predetermined number of targeted responses over a fixed interval period or the entire interval is reset, thus further delaying reinforcement. The DRL schedule is also similar to a fixed interval schedule, except that any responses exceeding the required contingency reset the interval. DRL schedules are sometimes used in controlling excessive social behaviors that need to be reduced in frequency but not eliminated altogether. Though of technical interest in the laboratory, the DRL schedule is rarely employed in the management of dog behavior.

ATTENTION CONTROL

For most training purposes, attention can be divided into two broad categories: *orienting* and *attending*. Both forms of attentional behavior are controlled by a dog's name and other similar signals. The orienting response is governed by classical conditioning processes, as well as by the more primitive adjustment mechanisms involved in sensitization and habituation; Pavlov referred to it as the "What is it?" reflex. Although influenced and modified by learning, the orienting response actually precedes and makes possible learning in the first place—without the activation of the orienting response, no new learning is possible. Orienting behavior can be divided into four types of responses, depending on their strength: strong, moderate, weak, and no response. Typically, strong orienting reactions are evoked by the presentation of startling or surprising unconditioned stimuli. Moderate orientation is evoked by cues previously associated with appetitive or aversive events, weak orientation is stimulated by cues associated with highly predicted and controlled appetitive or aversive events, and, finally, no orientation is likely to occur in the presence of irrelevant or insignificant events.

Some stimuli unconditionally elicit an orienting response, whereas others develop the strength to do so only after conditioning. Commonly employed unconditioned orienting stimuli used in dog training include clapping, whistling, kissing sounds, clucking, yelling, and stomping. Note that many of these orienting stimuli involve the production of different kinds of sound. Audition is a particularly favorable sensory modality for attention training because it can be stimulated

at a considerable distance and from any direction. The other sensory modalities (especially sight and touch) are not quite as accessible to stimulation as hearing but are nonetheless commonly used. Visual orienting stimuli used in attention training include changing body postures, waving the hands, running away from or toward the dog, tossing a ball or other object, or moving a laser pointer. Tactile orienting stimuli are commonly used, as well. Besides the use of touch as a physical prompt to get a dog's attention, various throw tools (chains or rings) are used in the case of dogs unresponsive to auditory and visual orienting stimulation.

To condition the dog's name as an orienting cue, it is paired with one of these unconditioned orienting stimuli. For example, just before clapping the hands to capture a distracted dog's attention, the dog's name is shouted out. After several pairings with a variety of orienting stimuli, the name becomes a generalized orienting signal. Unconditioned orienting stimuli can be strengthened by a process of sensitization. For example, the sharp clap of hands may after many repetitions become habituated. Its strength can be recovered by pairing it with a stronger unconditioned orienting stimulus like the crash of a shaker can. In this example, the trainer claps his or her hands and immediately thereafter tosses the shaker can in the direction of the distracted dog. After one or two such pairings, the dog will respond much more strongly to a clap alone.

The attending response requires that the dog exhibit sustained eye contact toward the trainer. One method for obtaining such control (described in more detail below) involves prompting the dog to look up by making a kissing or clucking sound and then appropriately bridging and reinforcing the response. At first, the dog is only required to look up briefly, but as training proceeds the requirement of duration is increased until the dog is holding eye contact for 3 to 5 seconds. Once the attending response is well conditioned, the dog's name is spoken just before the clucking sound is made. Gradually, the clucking prompt is faded and the dog learns to attend with sustained eye contact to his or her name alone.

TRAINING AND STIMULUS CONTROL

An important aspect of dog training involves bringing learned behavior under the control of cues and commands or what learning theorists call discriminative stimuli. Essentially, *stimulus control* refers to a process whereby a learned response is rendered more probable in the presence of some arbitrary stimulus. For example, once a dog has learned that some instrumental response is regularly associated with a specific outcome, the response-outcome relationship can be readily associated with a discriminative stimulus (S^D). The S^D functions similarly to a CS in classical conditioning, serving to establish a correlation between its presence and the occurrence of an associated instrumental response and reinforcer (Rescorla, 1991). The S^D is a signal that both selects the desired behavior and announces the moment when its emission will most likely result in reinforcement—that is, either producing a positive reinforcer or avoiding the occurrence of a negative one.

SHAPING: TRAINING THROUGH SUCCESSIVE APPROXIMATIONS

Sometimes a behavior that is unlikely to occur spontaneously will need to be trained in gradual steps. This sort of training is called *shaping*. Shaping is a process in which a selected behavior is obtained by differentially reinforcing successive approximations of it. Shaping involves breaking down the training objective or target behavior into more manageable and easily learned parts. Many otherwise difficult behaviors can be efficiently trained by carefully arranging these component parts of the target behavior according to a plan or program of instrumental shaping contingencies. Shaping has many applications in dog training. Almost any response or behavior pattern within a dog's behavioral capability can be shaped as long as a few basic rules are followed. An excellent introduction to shaping dog behavior through differential reinforcement of successive approximations is provided by B. F. Skinner (1951).

The first step in the process is to prepare a conditioned reinforcer (S^{r+}, notice the little "r") by pairing a stimulus (e.g., "Good" or clicker/tone) with an unconditioned reinforcer (S^{R+}). The S^r is often referred to as *bridging stimulus*. Effective conditioning of the bridging stimulus is crucial to the shaping process. Before shaping can be effective, a dog must recognize that the bridging stimulus communicates at least two messages: (1) that its presentation is contingent on the emission of a particular behavior and (2) that its occurrences are linked with a remote but forthcoming reinforcer. Murphree (1974) recommends that 50 to 100 pairings between the S^r and food be carried out before using it as a bridging stimulus for operant-shaping procedures. In the case of ordinary training activities, far fewer pairings are needed.

Once the S^r has been conditioned, it should be tested to confirm that it meets the aforementioned criteria. The test can be carried out by using the S^{r+} to teach a simple behavior dependent on conditioned reinforcement for its acquisition. Normally, the behavior used to test the S^{r+} is the orienting or attending response—that is, the bridge stimulus is used to reinforce the behavior of following the hand prompt or looking into the trainer's eyes. Another possible shaping objective might be to train the dog to move toward an opposite corner of the training room. While this behavior is fairly simple, it will help illustrate the most salient features of shaping.

Step 1: Define the Goal or Target Behavior

It is important to define precisely the target behavior before training begins. *Training objective*: To train the dog to leave the handler's side on signal and walk to a predetermined corner of the room.

Step 2: Design a Plan or Program of Instrumental Contingencies

The target behavior should be broken down into as many simple parts as is practical. The plan for shaping the foregoing target behavior might include the following components:

1. The dog turns its head away.
2. The dog turns its head away and in the general direction of the corner.
3. The dog turns and moves its whole body away.
4. The dog turns and moves its whole body toward the corner.
5. The dog is required to move farther away.
6. The dog moves farther away and in the general direction of the corner.
7. The dog moves closer to the corner.
8. The dog enters the corner.

During the early stages, progress may be rapid, but as the requirements become more difficult, the acquisition curve may flatten out. Shaping is a dynamic process controlled by a feedback loop between the dog's progress and the program of instrumental contingencies. If progress is slow, renew momentum by going back a step or two. If the step still proves too difficult, break it down into even simpler elements. A program of instrumental contingencies should be flexible and opportunistic but never vague and capricious. Such adjustments to the plan, therefore, should not be made hastily or without good purpose. Each preceding step should receive enough training to make it a reliable foundation for the next step.

Once a step has been mastered, further requirements must be introduced that compel the dog to experiment with closer approximations to the target behavior. This transition is accomplished by reinforcing the previous step on an intermittent basis. This shift in reinforcement scheduling causes the dog to emit other related behaviors (response generalization) that might offer a higher rate of reinforcement. Placing previously mastered steps on an intermittent schedule is also important to prevent their extinction when selection pressures are made more demanding. Care should be taken, however, to avoid shaping transitions that cause the dog to quit, become overly anxious, or frustrated. When anxiety or excessive frustration appear, the trainer should go back to a previously successful step. Always end each training session on a positive note.

Step 3: Bring the Shaped Behavior Under Stimulus Control

Once the dog has reliably learned to go to the correct corner of the room, the new behavior can be brought under stimulus control. By overlapping the behavior with a hand gesture pointing in the same direction as the dog's movement, he will soon associate the gestural prompt with the movement of walking toward the designated corner. After many repetitions, a new contingency can be introduced requiring that the dog move toward the corner only when signaled to do so. All attempts to move toward the corner not initiated on cue are not reinforced. Such attempts can be overlapped with an S^{p-} "No," indicating to the dog that reinforcement is not forthcoming for the behavior. By reinforcing only those behaviors controlled by the gestural prompt, the dog soon learns to move only when prompted to do so. Once the gestural prompt controls the behavior, it is easy to bring the behavior under the control of a verbal S^D, for example, "Move." Pairing the S^D "Move" with the prompt results in the former acquiring the ability to control the shaped behavior. Once a sufficient number of trials have taken place, the gestural prompt can be gradually faded out, with the verbal S^D "Move" alone controlling the newly learned behavior.

The foregoing method of shaping is intended to provide the reader with a formal and structured approach. Under actual training situations, however, shaping is often carried out much more informally. The basic principles of breaking down the training goal into simple parts, organizing and teaching them in the most easily learned order, and carrying out training in a positively oriented manner are common features of all training activities. Shaping techniques provide the skilled trainer/behaviorist with powerful and efficient tools for orchestrating behavioral change through positive reinforcement. Pryor (1975, 1985) wrote at length on the use of operant-shaping techniques in the training of sea mammals and other animals, including dogs.

ADDUCTION

Adduction refers to a training procedure in which a novel response is produced by combining two or more previously learned component repertoires. More specifically, adduction occurs when two previously learned behaviors are evoked by presenting their respective discriminative stimuli together. The resulting adducted response is reinforced and subsequently brought under stimulus control. For example, although training a dog to crawl can be accomplished by gradually shaping the crawling behavior through successive approximations or by utilizing appropriate physical prompts or props (e.g., a low table), the crawling behavior can also be obtained by signaling the evocation of two previously learned behaviors whose combined emission results in crawling. In this case, the dog might first be taught to heel and to lay down on signal. Once both behaviors are under stimulus control, the dog is signaled to lay down while heeling. In response to this arrangement, the dog may start to lay down but continue moving forward at the same time and, perhaps, begin to crawl. As a result, crawling behavior has been adducted from the combined occurrence of laying down and heeling. If the crawling response is reinforced under such circumstances, gradually it can be brought under stimulus control and then trained to occur independently of the antecedent component repertoires.

CHAINING: ORDERING COMPLEX PERFORMANCES

Training often requires that a sequence of arbitrary behaviors be structured so that they occur in a specific order. This order of occurrence is based on a predetermined continuity in which one behavior must always precede the next in a set sequence. Orderly sequencing is accomplished by making the advancement of the series contingent on the emission of a predetermined response occurring before the next one in the series is selected. To accomplish this goal, each task in the chain is brought under the stimulus control of a dual-functioning signal serving both to reinforce the correct antecedent behavior conditionally and to simultaneously select the next response in the series. This pattern is repeated until the entire sequence of behaviors is emitted and terminally reinforced.

Within the chain, each discriminative stimulus (S^D) provides conditional reinforcement for the behavior that it follows and simultaneously selects the next response. The S^D's dual function is an outcome of the way in which a chain is constructed. The chain is built up by connecting the final response with the terminal reinforcer and then adding on successive behaviors up to the origin of the chain. To obtain reinforcement, dogs must perform each response in the chain at the proper time. Each S^D in the chain not only selects the next behavior in the chain but also reinforces the preceding behavior because it advances the dog one step closer to the terminal reinforcer (S^{R+}).

Perhaps the easiest way to show how chaining works is to use a common example. The recall pattern involves a six-part chain: sit, stay, come, sit-front, finish, and sit. Both the terminal response and the origin are sit responses. Between the origin and the terminal response are four chained responses: stay, come, sit-front, and finish. These various components are linked through shared stimulus control and conditioned reinforcement. The chain is terminated with a sit response and final reinforcement at the trainer's left side. The terminal response is under the stimulus control of the S^D "Sit." "Sit" not only selects the terminal response, it also conditionally reinforces the preceding finish behavior. The next link is the finish behavior, which is brought under the stimulus control of the S^D "Heel." "Heel" not only selects the behavior of moving to the trainer's side but also conditionally reinforces the previous link in the chain—sit-front. Sit-front is under the stimulus control of the S^D "Sit," which not only selects the sit response but also conditionally reinforces coming. Coming is under the stimulus control of the S^D "Come," which also conditionally reinforces the dog for staying. The S^D "Stay" selects staying behavior and conditionally reinforces the sit response. The sit response is the origin of the chain and is under the stimulus control of the S^D "Sit" (Fig. 7.5).

A far more common form of chaining in everyday dog training is called *forward chaining*. Although forward chaining lacks the behavioral elegance of backward chaining, it does offer many valuable features and several distinct advantages. Forward chaining requires only that a series of responses be performed on cue for a single reward. The forward chain is built up by placing each response component on an intermittent schedule of reinforcement and randomizing its occurrence in the chain sequence. Such a strategy of intermittent reinforcement and randomization results in the development of a hoped-for expectancy occurring equally with each link in the chain—a result that usually translates into a general strengthening of the chain, as well as immunizing component responses against extinction. It should be noted in the case of *backward chaining* that behaviors near the end of the chain are the most strongly reinforced, since they are the closest to the terminal reinforcer. In the case of forward chaining, responses near the origin of the chain are the strongest with the lure of reinforcement rapidly declining as the chain of responses is extended. Care must be taken, therefore, not to extend the forward chain too rapidly, perhaps causing a dog to quit. An important advantage of forward chaining is that it provides a means to place acquired behavior on an intermittent schedule. For example, instead of reinforcing a dog on every occasion for sitting, forward chaining might require the dog to perform any combination of the series stand, sit, down, sit from the down, and sit-stay for a single re-ward. Individual responses comprising the foregoing chain are conditionally reinforced at each step with praise ("Good"), but the final reward is presented only after the required sequence is performed or the whole series is completed successfully. Forward chaining teaches dogs to expect reinforcement after a certain amount of work, regardless of the actual behaviors performed. Also, the order of responses can be easily altered without significantly affecting the viability of the chain. The response order of a backward chain is locked in without much room for variability or change, other than shortening the chain by assigning the origin to a response closer to the terminal reinforcer. Also, if any of the behaviors in the backward chain fail (a highly likely outcome with responses near the origin of a long chain), the whole chain breaks down. Although carefully constructed backward chains can be immunized against extinction, the sheer complexity of the chain and the repeated occurrence of individual component responses without direct reinforcement make backward chains very sensitive to breakdown under natural training conditions.

PROMPTING, FADING, AND SHADOWING

One way of developing stimulus control is to first bring the target behavior under the control of a prompt (Foxx, 1982b). Kazdin defines a *prompt* as an event that initiates behavior to be reinforced:

> Prompts are events that help initiate a response. They come before a response has been performed and are designed to facilitate its per-

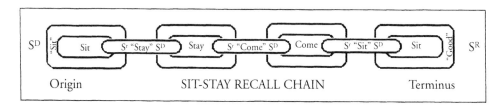

Origin   SIT-STAY RECALL CHAIN   Terminus

FIG. 7.5. Diagram showing the relationships linking together discriminative stimulus, response, and conditioned reinforcement in a chain of interdependent events.

formance. When a prompt results in the response, the response can be reinforced. Without the prompt, the response might occur infrequently or not at all. Prompts serve as antecedent events (e.g., instructions, gestures) that help generate the desired response. (1989:42)

Prompting is divided into two broad categories: physical and gestural. A physical prompt involves actively manipulating a dog's behavior into the form desired, for example, pushing a dog's rump into a sit or guiding him into a starting position at heel with the leash. Physical prompting sometimes involves props such as walking a dog along a fence line to encourage him to stay close at heel. Physical prompts often become gestural prompts by being *faded.* The movement of the hand guiding a dog into the sit position can be gradually faded as a physical prompt and become a hand signal or gestural prompt. The transition between the faded physical prompt and the gestural prompt is facilitated by a technique referred to as *shadowing*. Shadowing is employed during the last stages of fading. Instead of touching a dog to make it sit, the hand is held slightly above, that is, *shadowing* over its rump.

Controlling hand signals are often established in conjunction with orienting prompts. The orienting prompt is developed by training a dog to follow the movement of the hand closely, sometimes even requiring that the dog actually touch the moving hand with its nose. Also, orienting lures, like a ball or stick, are frequently used to guide the dog into the desired behavior. Once the behavior is mastered, it is then brought under the control of a word cue or gesture while the orienting lure is simultaneously faded out.

REHEARSAL AND STAGING

Successful modification of many behavior problems requires the use of rehearsal and staging techniques. *Rehearsal* involves having a dog master and repeatedly perform behavioral components needed for some later situation or remote context not present at the time of training. Although the situation or context itself may not be represented during rehearsal, each of the behaviors required can be independently shaped and ordered in the specific sequence needed. For instance, a socially overexuberant dog can be taught more appropriate manners independently of the presence of an actual guest. Of course, the actual situation when the guest arrives will be much more strained and charged than when the dog is home alone with the owner. It is important, therefore, that conditions be staged that more closely resemble the actual greeting as training proceeds. The effectiveness of rehearsal depends to a large extent on positive transfer and generalization. *Staging* allows previously rehearsed behavior to be performed under more natural conditions before exposing the dog to the actual situation. In the case of greeting behavior, someone familiar to the dog can play the role of the guest, making repeated entrances and exits under the control and direction of the trainer or owner. Rehearsal and staging have many applications in a broad variety of training and problem-solving situations, ranging from separation distress and fears to severe aggressive behavior.

TRANSFER OF LEARNING

It is important that training readily transfer from one situation to another. Such transferability should not be taken for granted, especially in cases involving complex skills and discriminations. Learned behavior tends to *bond* with the training context in which it is conditioned and may not readily move to other situations without additional work. The relative familiarity or novelty of the training context exercises an important influence on learning. New tasks are most easily learned under familiar conditions, whereas already learned tasks can be improved upon by moving training activities into progressively more and more unfamiliar and distracting surroundings. Learning plateaus are most efficiently counteracted by varying the training environment. These observations strongly support the benefit of introducing general behavioral training as an in-home process and only later graduating into the more distractive group-training situations. Further, newly acquired behavior is often state dependent, available only under the motivational states in which it was originally learned—for example, a dog trained to work for food might quit when no longer hungry. It is important, therefore, that training activities be carried out under a wide variety of motivational states in addition to changing the environmental contexts under which training takes place. Occasionally, a dog may be medicated with psychotropics or tranquilizers while undergoing training. Drug-dependent learning is a potential problem that must be carefully guarded against to ensure that a dog's ostensible progress is not dependent on a drug-induced motivational state.

Positive and negative transfer of training is a complex area of learning theory. Previous training that facilitates the acquisition of subsequent training is said to produce *positive transfer*. On the other hand, the effect of earlier learning that impedes subsequent acquisition is referred to as *negative transfer*. An interesting and paradoxical example involving transfer of training can be seen in a learning phenomenon known as the *overlearning-reversal effect* (Hall, 1976). The simplest experiment demonstrating this phenomenon would involve two groups of animals that are each taught a simple two-choice discrimination task. After achieving equal criterion levels, one of the two is given several additional training trials while the other one rests. Afterward, the discrimination is reversed so that the negative stimulus now becomes positive, and both animals are then tested on this new discrimination problem. One might guess that the animal receiving the additional trials would find it more difficult to learn the reversal (negative transfer) than the one receiving less training on the previous (now reversed) discrimination. Surprisingly, however, the effect of additional training facilitates learning of the reversal—that is, the animal receiving the extra training learns the new discrimination more quickly than its counterpart. The overtrained animal's success may have been due to added discriminatory skill developed as the result of its additional training. The overlearning studies tend to support a cognitive interpretation over a traditional S-R interpretation of discrimination learning.

Positive transfer is observed in situations where previous learning experiences facilitate the acquisition of new behaviors. For instance, a dog that has been trained not to jump up on its owner will be much more easy to train not to jump up on guests. Negative transfer often occurs in cases where previous learning is antagonistic to the acquisition of the target behavior. For example, puppies that have been exposed to a history of chase and evasion games will be much more difficult to train to come than counterparts without such experience. In the design of training systems, it is important to always keep in mind the influence of negative and positive transfer when ordering training events, so that it is organized in the most efficient and synergistic way possible.

BEHAVIORAL CONTRAST AND MOMENTUM

Behavioral contrast (matching) and momentum exercise powerful indirect influences on the overall effects of training, its transfer, and degree of permanence (Chance, 1998; Nevin, 1998). Behavioral contrast refers to the tendency of a target behavior undergoing reinforcement in one situation to occur less often in other situations where reinforcement is less likely to occur. Conversely, in comparison to baseline levels present prior to the onset of training, a behavior undergoing punishment in one situation will tend to occur relatively more frequently in other situations where it is less likely to be punished. Such effects are related to the matching law as already discussed. For example, if a dog's sitting behavior is exclusively rewarded only during formal obedience classes and practice sessions, the dog will be less likely to sit in everyday situations where reinforcement is not as likely to be forthcoming. Similarly, if a dog's social excesses (e.g., jumping up) during greetings are undergoing punishment in one situation but are permitted to occur at other times without consequence, the target excesses may significantly increase in those situations where punitive contingencies are not consistently in place.

Behavioral momentum is an important consideration when evaluating a particular behavior's resistance to change and its tendency to recover at the conclusion of therapy or training. Such momentum is represented in terms of the target behavior's operant baseline levels present at the outset of training, its relative resistance to change (as measured by its responsiveness to modification), and its tendency to persist, that is, its proclivity to recover after training is discontinued. Some undesirable activities of dogs are affected by powerful momentum influences that adversely compete with training efforts, thus making such behavior highly prone to recovery at the conclusion of training. For example, jumping up, playful biting on hands, and pulling on the leash are all influenced by a high degree of behavior momentum. Not only do they occur at a high operant level, they also resist disruption by behavioral means and tend to recover when training is discontinued. To overcome the detrimental influences of behavioral momentum, alternative behaviors must be adequately practiced and reinforced until they acquire sufficient momentum of their own to offset the recovery of unwanted behavior simultaneously undergoing behavioral suppression or extinction.

SOCIAL LEARNING

The effect of others exercises a tremendous influence on the efficient acquisition of learned behaviors and their performance. A dog's social dependency makes it keenly aware of the behavior of others. This perceptual tendency or bias to attend to the behavior of conspecifics (and non-conspecific others like ourselves) provides a vital cognitive interface for coordinating social interaction, regulating purposeful group activities important for survival (e.g., hunting) and maintenance of the group (e.g., reproduction), and for modulating social contagions conducive to unified group actions appropriate to the changing environmental circumstances operating on the group—ranging from the calming yawn and sleep to the alarm bark stimulating enhanced group arousal in preparation for effective social defense.

Although there can be little doubt that a dog's social tendency to attend to the activity of others contributes to what it does and broadly limits what it is likely to learn (an inclination reflected in a dog's willingness to accept obedience training and perform reliable services), the question of how these social influences affect learning by contact, coaction, and observation is a conceptual minefield, containing numerous pitfalls that require careful observance of subtle detail and logical distinctions if one is to navigate safely around them. This is especially the case with the question of observational learning. Indeed, before commenting on whether or not a dog learns via observation or imitation, it would seem advisable first to describe three other closely related behavioral phenomena, all of which have been confounded with observational learning in the dog behavior literature and elsewhere. These imitation-like phenomena include allelomimetic behavior, social facilitation, and local enhancement.

Allelomimetic Behavior

Allelomimetic or group-coordinated behavior depends on an innate social inclination to follow the lead of conspecifics and do the same thing, appearing to adjust to the locomotor pace and motivational intention of the other in the process. Puppies show signs of allelomimetic behavior from an early age onward, and many socially significant behaviors are learned as a secondary result of socially coordinated behavior. For example, coming when called is easily encouraged by having a puppy chase after the handler as the latter runs away and rewarding the puppy for following along. Similarly, walking along close at the handler's side is an allelomimetic tendency that can be rapidly shaped and brought under stimulus control, especially if the puppy is provided numerous walks early on that include appropriate reinforcement of such heeling behavior whenever it occurs.

Social Facilitation

A related concept in animal behavior is social facilitation. Scott (1968) carefully distinguishes allelomimesis from social facilitation, noting that the former is a purely descriptive term, whereas the latter refers to the potentiating effect that one animal has on the behavior of another. Although allelomimetic behavior is responsive to social facilitation, the terms are not the same and should not be confused with each other. In fact, social facilitation affects both allelomimetic and non-allelomimetic behavior. To emphasize this important distinction, Zajonc (1965) divided social facilitation into two general subtypes—coactive effects and audience effects—depending on whether the facilitator is performing the same behavior or is merely present in the situation.

Coactive social facilitation is observed in dogs doing something together, such as running, barking, greeting a guest, or defending against an intruder. When coactively engaged in some activity, they may reciprocally stimulate one another to run faster or bark louder than they might otherwise if alone. Many common examples of coactive effect can be observed (e.g., fence running). Similarly, two dogs fed together will usually eat more and eat faster than if fed apart. Social facilitation is something that many of us are likely to experience (and suffer) over holidays as we feast and wax merry with friends and family!

Social facilitation does not necessarily require that the other animal actually participate in the facilitated behavior. For example, the mere presence of a nearby dog will typically cause a dog that is eating to eat more rapidly or to eat even when it is no longer hungry. The facilitator need only be present as an "audience" to stimulate or enhance the other dog's eating behavior. These effects are common among humans, as well. Consider, for example, the effects of cheering fans on the behavior of athletes at a sporting event or even the gaping and awing of bystanders observing a street brawl (or dog fight, for that matter).

The potentiating effects of social facilitation appear to result from a state of generalized arousal (*nonspecific drive*) stimulated by the presence of another animal. This arousal tends to increase the magnitude of whatever the animal happens to be doing, especially if the ongoing behavior is well learned or motivationally dominant at the moment (e.g., eat-

ing, greeting, running, barking, or threatening).

Although social facilitation is often beneficial and desirable for enhancing performance [e.g., a sled dog's performance is enhanced (facilitated) by the presence of other dogs pulling in the same direction], it may interfere with learning new behavior, especially the acquisition of arbitrary or complex skills that require steady concentration to learn. In such cases, the effect of others is referred to as *social interference*. For example, the presence of other puppies playing nearby is apt to interfere with an observing puppy's ability to hold a sit-stay for long before breaking off and joining the fun. Such interference effects are a common obstacle in the process of modifying unwanted behavior in a home containing more than one dog.

Local Enhancement

Local enhancement is a special form of social facilitation that is sometimes interpreted as evidence of observational learning (Thorpe, 1956). Local enhancement appears to include aspects of allelomimesis, social facilitation, and trial-and-error learning. The term, however, specifically refers to the tendency of animals to orient and attend to the same environmental cues and stimuli as others with which they are interacting. This coordinated tendency to attend to the same environmental stimuli encourages them to behave in similar ways. For example, one dog may draw the attention of another to a hole in the fence by going through it, thus causing the other to approach the spot and quickly escape in a similar way without needing to search for a way out. Teaching a dog to hop into a car may be enhanced by allowing a more experienced dog to jump in first, followed by the less experienced dog. It is likely that the inexperienced dog will learn the action much more rapidly than if he had to figure it out by himself.

Learning by Observation: Myth or Fact?

Although the coordinating effects of allelomimesis, social facilitation, and local enhancement on learning often look like observational (i.e., imitative) learning or copying, they are not, at least, insofar as observational learning is defined by experimentalists working with such problems. Observational learning is operationally defined and limited by constraints that exclude these social learning phenomena. Typically, such experiments include a demonstrator in one compartment and an observer looking on from a similar adjacent compartment. An arbitrary behavior is selected by the experimenter that is learned through trial and error by the demonstrator. The test phase involves measuring and comparing differences in the rate of acquisition exhibited by observers versus nonobserver controls when presented with the same problem previously solved by the demonstrator.

Early efforts to quantify observational learning in dogs were carried out by Thorndike, who performed a number of studies but was unable to show evidence of observational learning in the dog, leading him to conclude,

> It seems sure from these experiments that the animals were unable to form an association leading to an act from having seen the other animal, or animals, perform the act in a certain situation. Thus we have further restricted the association process. Not only do animals not have associations accompanied, more or less permeated and altered by inference and judgment; they do not have associations of the sort which may be acquired from other animals by imitation. What this implies concerning the actual mental content accompanying their acts will be seen later on. It also seems sure that we should give up imitation as an *a priori* explanation of any novel intelligent performance. To say that a dog who opens a gate, for instance, need not have reasoned it out *if he had seen another dog do the same thing,* is to offer, instead of one false explanation, another equally false. Imitation in any form is too doubtful a factor to be presupposed without evidence. (1911/1965:95)

Thorndike's assessment all but closed the book on observational learning in dogs. This effect still echoes today, with remarks like those by Reid on the topic being fairly typical. Prefaced by an interesting flyball experiment for falsifying the notion of observational learning, she writes,

> Having described that hypothetical experiment, let me conclude by saying there is virtually no evidence that animals, except for humans and the great apes (gorillas, orangutans, and chimpanzees), are capable of pure imitation. Some researchers have devoted their entire professional lives to devising ways to demonstrate imitation, without success. Sorry to rain on your parade, but dogs just don't seem to be able to manage learning by imitation. (1996:169)

This statement is overly strong and not consistent with the available scientific evidence regarding observational learning in animals (see Vauclair, 1996). Observational learning has been demonstrated in many species other than the great apes, including a variety of birds, rodents, dolphins, and dogs (at least young dogs). Several studies have demonstrated evidence of observational learning in rats (Heyes and Dawson, 1990; Heyes et al., 1994).

Pryor (1975) reported an interesting example of observational learning in a pair of porpoises she had trained as part of her famous "creativity" study (Pryor et al., 1969). The two animals had worked in close proximity with each other but had learned separate routines. The performance followed a set order with one porpoise regularly preceding the other. When not performing, the remaining porpoise was restrained in a separate gated area from where it could look on and observe its cohort. One day during an actual performance, the two porpoises appeared unusually nervous and their performances were somewhat awkward, disorderly, and strained; nonetheless, each performed the behaviors required sufficiently well to not raise suspicion about what had happened. It was not until after the show was over, and the audience was beginning to leave, that the trainer realized the cause of the problem: the two animals had been mistakenly switched and put in the wrong holding tanks. The remarkable result was that each had performed the repertoire of the other. Apparently, working closely together over the preceding several months, each had learned the routine of the other, even though they had not received any explicit training to do so.

Observational learning is also apparently operative in young dogs. Adler and Adler (1977), for example, have shown that such abilities (i.e., response learning without direct reinforcement) are exhibited by puppies. The experiment employed was of a very simple and straightforward design. Observers were permitted to watch demonstrators learn by trial and error to secure a ribbon and pull a small cart with food on top of it into their cages. After five sessions, the observers were given access to the ribbon and timed. Significant benefit accrued to the observers, especially when comparing first-trial results. At 38 days of age, demonstrators took 697 seconds compared with observers, who solved the problem in 9 seconds. At 60 days, demonstrators took 595 seconds, with observers requiring only 40 seconds. These studies indicate several operative cognitive implications that extend well beyond simple S-R learning, including the ability to learn by observation and imitation. More recently, Slabbert and Rasa (1997) gathered fairly strong evidence indicating that dogs might benefit from observational learning. They found that when puppies between 9 and 12 weeks of age were permitted to observe their narcotic-detecting mothers search for hidden sachets containing narcotics, they generally proved more capable of learning the task at 6 months of age than controls not permitted to observe their mothers at work.

Observational learning remains a controversial topic. Further, before any blanket statements can be safely made about whether dogs learn via observation or not, there remains much to be studied in the area of animal cognition and learning. Although puppies clearly appear to learn through observation, the existence of observational learning in adult dogs remains in doubt, at least until more conclusive research is available. No experiment to date (that I know of) demonstrates observational learning in adult dogs.

HIGHER-ORDER CLASSES OF BEHAVIOR

The simple instrumental paradigm of learning discussed above is frequently insufficient in terms of explanatory value and practical control when applied to complex naturalistic situations. Estes drew attention to the important role of higher-order routines and classes of behavior in an effort to account for such problems with reinforcement theory. He notes that "the frequency with which animals and men in nonlaboratory situations repeat punished acts and fail to repeat rewarded ones is so great that, as a statistical generalization, the empirical law of effect is all but vacuous" (1971:26). Estes's observation does not imply that reinforcing and punitive events are without effect on behavior, but that the effects of such events appear to be vitiated by interference stemming from the collective influence of the higher-order class of behavior to which the response belongs. That is, the higher-order class of behavior may compete with the contingencies of reinforcement controlling specific instances belonging to it, sometimes rendering them, in the words of Catania, "insensitive to the contingencies arranged for them" (1992:377).

There are many examples of higher-order behavior exhibited by dogs, for example, attention seeking, fear-related behavior, dominance-related behavior, play, and attachment behavior. A couple of examples should help to illustrate and clarify the importance of higher-order classes in routine behavior modification. Many persistent behavior problems are driven by higher-order affiliations. For example, although extinction may be an effective procedure for the reduction of some excessive behaviors, it is rarely effective for attention-seeking behaviors like jumping up. Ignoring the jumper infrequently helps to reduce the frequency of the habit. Even when punishment is applied (e.g., time-out), the habit can be surprisingly persistent. One reason for this failure of extinction is that the higher-order class of *attention-seeking* is maintained by the reinforcement of other attention-seeking behaviors belonging that class. Another example of some practical significance is dominance-related behavior, especially involving aggression exhibited toward the owner. Despite the most conscientious efforts to suppress aggressive displays, unless all instances of competitive behavior are simultaneously treated as a group, such efforts will not yield much lasting benefit. According to Catania, "When a class of responses seems insensitive to its consequences, ... we must entertain the possibility that we have improperly identified the class and that it is part of a larger class the members of which continue to have their former consequences" (1995:196).

These general relationships between higher-order classes and subclasses have been examined in terms of expectancy theory. Rotter (1975) has divided expectations of reinforcement into two forms of expectancy: specific and generalized. *Specific expectancies* refer to a simple contingency between an emitted behavior and an associated reinforcing event. *Generalized expectancies*, on the other hand, develop as the result of a functional similarity between situations that typically result in reinforcement. Generalized expectancies are very similar in effect to learning sets or the process of "learning how to learn." Dogs exposed to previous training tend to generalize expectations from past successes or failures to current training demands. Consequently, specific and generalized expectancies form complex and dynamic interdependent relationships influencing both trainability and performance. Although generalized expectancies profoundly affect new learning situations, with repeated exposure generalized expectancies are typically weakened while specific expectancies based on experience with the training situation are strengthened. Returning to the previous example of jumping up, the jumper learns after repeated corrections or time-outs that the generalized expectancy is now being disconfirmed with regard to the higher-order class (attention-

seeking) operative in this specific case (jumping up). As a result, jumping is weakened, thus making the reinforcement of some other behavior incompatible with jumping up possible.

ATTENTION AND LEARNING

A dog's ability to concentrate selectively on specific aspects of the environment and to exclude others is a faculty of tremendous importance for effective dog training and behavior modification. Historically, the study of attention was neglected due to a widely held belief that the scientific investigation of behavior ought to be restricted to the study of measurable units resulting from the interaction of external events (i.e., stimuli and responses). This general doctrine known as *radical behaviorism* rejected cognitive phenomena like *attention* as inaccessible and irrelevant to a scientific understanding of animal behavior. Radical behaviorists also rejected explanations that employed physiological hypotheses and constructs.

The artificial dissection of behavior from its cognitive and physiological underpinnings was an unfortunate stratagem—one that logically precluded from the outset the possibility of a complete and holistic theory of behavior and learning. Interestingly, though, in spite of the outward rejection of attention as a worthy subject of scientific psychology, the radical behavioristic tradition has indirectly provided a rich and useful foundation and methodology for its investigation by contemporary cognitive psychologists (Cohen and O'Donnell, 1993). It should be stressed, however, that not all learning theorists historically rejected attention as a subject for study. Thorndike, for example, posited a subordinate law that he called the *prepotency of elements* in which certain features of the environment are selectively attended to by an animal on the basis of their prepotency or usefulness for solving a problem. Also, many modern learning theorists have contributed significantly to the study of attention; especially relevant here is the work of Rescorla, Kamin, and Macintosh (Hall, 1991). In addition, the dogmatic viewpoint regarding attentional behavior has yielded to some thoughtful revisions in recent textbooks covering the topic of attention and attending behavior (Schwartz, 1989; Catania, 1992; Lieberman, 1993).

Attention is perhaps the most basic class of behavior in which both classical and instrumental elements closely cooperate in the mediation of effective perception and action. What a dog pays attention to from moment to moment involves the participation of a complex cognitive gateway or interfacing mechanism processing information from within the animal (e.g., motivational states) and coordinating it with events and opportunities occurring outside of the animal within the changing circumstances of the environment. This cognitive gateway is regulated by a variety of motivational, perceptual, and motor components in constant interaction. In a broad sense, attentional activities specify a dog's intentions, reveal a dog's motivational state, and to some extent define what a dog is prepared to learn—that is, attentional activities reflect a dog's overall disposition to learn.

At the most basic level, all learning requires that an animal exhibit an active attention toward the training situation. As noted in the previous chapter, surprising or startling reinforcers produce the strongest effect on behavior. Such events also evoke the keenest interest and attentional focus—that is, startle and surprise serve to emotionally mediate and potentiate attentional behavior. Lieberman (1993) has called such events *markers*, suggesting that surprising/startling events produce dramatic effects on learning. Stimuli that lack surprising or startling qualities tend to drift into the background, become progressively irrelevant, and are eventually ignored. In the case of classical conditioning, conditioned stimulus (CS) salience or interest depends on its predicting some element of surprise. Once a CS exactly predicts the extent of the unconditioned stimulus (US), interest in the CS as a source of information gradually diminishes. This does not mean that the CS is considered to be *irrelevant* (ir-

relevance occurs when the CS occurs independently of the US), but that it is no longer actively followed or paid much attention to because there is not much more to be learned from its occurrence. Instead of actively attending to the CS, such well-conditioned stimuli are responded to in a progressively mechanical and automatic way. However, if suddenly a larger-than-expected US (e.g., consider the case of a bonus or jackpot) occurs in the presence of the diminished CS (e.g., "Good"), then new interest and attention will be generated by the future presentation of the conditioned reinforcer "Good."

Besides facilitating classical conditioning, markers also appear to play a very significant role in instrumental learning. Surprising events potentiate learning abilities, even promoting learning occurring under adverse conditions. As has been previously discussed, any delay of reinforcement usually has a deleterious effect on learning. However, Lieberman and his associates (1979) studied various situations in which these adverse effects could be overcome by utilizing a *marking* event. For example, they placed rats in a T maze where a food reward was delivered after a minute delay, provided that the rat chose the right arm of the maze. If the rat chose the left arm instead, no reward was delivered. The rats, as one might predict, failed to learn the correct response required to obtain the belated reward. However, the experimenters found that if the subjects were picked up immediately after they made their choice (whether correct or wrong) and were then placed back into the maze to complete their chosen route, the handled subjects learned the correct route much more effectively than nonhandled controls. During testing, the handled rats chose the correct arm in 90% of the trials, whereas the controls were only correct 50% (chance) of the time. Similar effects were observed in the case of other surprising/startling stimuli (e.g., light or noise) that were presented immediately after the rat's choice (correct or wrong) was made. Again, the food reward associated with the correct choice was always delayed. Lieberman and colleagues speculate that markers enhance the functioning of attentional processes and memory coding of relevant cues, with the marker evoking extra attention to events occurring immediately prior to its presentation. The overall effect is to make *marked* events more likely to be remembered and associated with remote outcomes, such as the delay of reinforcement as in the foregoing experiment.

Obviously, stimulating and controlling attentional behavior is of considerable interest to the trainer/behaviorist. Dogs pay attention to occurrences that are significant to them and learn to ignore occurrences that are irrelevant. Stimuli that have been associated with hedonically significant events or fear tend to attract more attention than neutral stimuli not having undergone such conditioning. In addition, previously conditioned stimuli tend to overshadow neutral stimuli occurring coincidentally in the training situation, thus blocking an associative connection from developing between them and the relevant US—a classical conditioning process that has been investigated in detail by Kamin (1968). Those elements of the environment that do not hold a dog's active attention are of little significance to the learning process. In short, selective attention allows dogs to focus on relevant stimuli while ignoring irrelevant occurrences competing for their attention. Without this ability to attend selectively to environmental events, dogs would not only be unable to learn, they would be thoroughly incapacitated by a disorganized influx of chaotic stimulation. Clearly, attention plays a very significant role here in terms of transforming raw experience into informative input about the environment.

Since attention is highly correlated with reinforcement (both positive and negative), it follows that animals should become more attentive with experience. This analysis implies that reinforcement of attention in one situation should improve attending behavior in other more remote training situations. Attending behavior may be reasonably interpreted, therefore, as a higher-order class of behavior that contains a large subclass of behaviors in which attention plays an instrumental role. In addition, since attending behavior is present in most successful learning situations, it may be considered the most

dominant class of higher-order behavior, under which all other classes of instrumental behavior are subsumed according to their relative frequency and probability. According to this line of analysis, the most likely behavior in any given learning situation is an attentional orientation (physical and perceptual) toward significant training stimuli. It is astonishing to consider that the most dominant class of instrumental behavior—attending—has been the least carefully studied.

The sort of stimuli that attracts a dog's attention frequently reveals an underlying biological significance and purpose being served by them as well as past learning. Many of these stimuli and events naturally attract and hold a dog's attention even prior to learning. For example, the vaginal discharge produced by an estrous female attracts the intense attention of an intact male even before his first sexual experience. The discharge contains pheromones (i.e., chemical signals) that trigger or mediate interest via olfactory stimulation of appropriate brain centers controlling sexual activity. These *hardwired* connections are established prior to actual sexual contact with a receptive female. A dog's sensory faculties also predispose it to react to certain stimuli in a relatively fixed manner. Visual cliff-avoidance reactions can be observed in young puppies (reliably after 28 days of age) prior to their experiencing any actual falls. Also, loud noises elicit intense startle reactions as soon as the ear canals open at about 3 weeks of age. The startle reaction to noise occurs without actually having been associated with previous aversive stimulation. Some sensory stimuli are attended to more keenly than others. Clearly, while color perception is of some usefulness to dogs, they are more apt to attend visually to movement, shapes, and shades of gray than to discriminate objects based on their color. Also, dogs appear to select certain classes of stimuli preferentially over others as cues when learning discrimination tasks. For example, Lawicka's (1964) discrimination studies have demonstrated that dogs prefer spatially lateralized discriminative stimuli or cues when learning a directional task and qualitatively differentiated cues (different tone frequencies) when learning go/no go discriminations. Also, McConnell (1990) has reported that dogs selectively respond to auditory stimulation depending on its characteristics. Her studies suggest that active behaviors such as coming when called may be more easily associated with signals composed of rapidly repeated sounds (e.g., hand claps and smooches), whereas staying in place may be more easily obtained with continuous, drawn-out signals (see Chapter 5).

Another important influence on a dog's attending behavior is the dog's changing motivational state. Motivation has a pronounced influence on the class of stimuli that will attract and maintain a dog's attention. Hungry dogs are especially attracted to odors and conditioned stimuli that have been associated with food in the past. Highly social or socially deprived dogs will likely search the environment for opportunities to make contact with other dogs or people. Aggressive dogs scan the environment for evidence of people or other dogs that they might challenge or attack. Fearful dogs often engage in hypervigilant searching behavior in an effort to identify and avoid potential threats.

A Brief Critique of Traditional Learning Theory

The principles of learning theory have been derived from the experimental study of behavior. This research has been based on a small set of empirical assumptions and beliefs. Perhaps the most central and pervasive of them is the *law of effect,* that is, behavior is modified by its consequences. If a behavior is rendered more likely to occur in the future as the result of its consequences, it is said to have undergone reinforcement. Reinforcement is divided into two categories depending on whether the behavior involved produces the reinforcer (positive reinforcement) or avoids/terminates the reinforcing event (negative reinforcement). The theory also posits punishment as producing an effect opposite to that of reinforcement. When an anticipated positive reinforcer is omitted, the effect is negative punishment (P−). Conversely,

when a negative reinforcer is presented positive punishment occurs (P+). In both cases, punishment is defined as an event that lowers the future probability of the punished behavior. The term *punishment* is also used more generally to designate any outcome that suppresses behavior—regardless of the target behavior's reinforcement history.

This general system of analysis has been extremely productive. Many thousands of studies have been performed ostensibly confirming these basic assumptions and postulates. Further, there is also little doubt that the paradigm works as a practical system for the control and modification of behavior. Despite such heuristic and practical value, however, these most fundamental assumptions are vulnerable to theoretical criticism, especially with regard to issues involving parsimony and logical coherence (i.e., how the theory relates to behavior).

Reinforcement and the Notion of Probability

The *notion of probability* is central to the traditional behavior analytical interpretation of reinforcement (Johnson and Morris, 1987; Catania, 1992). Despite the central importance of "probability" in science, and, in particular, behavior analysis, it has not received a great deal of independent attention. Curiously, in Murray Sidman's important book (the "Bible" of many experimental behavior analysts) *Tactics of Scientific Research: Evaluating Experimental Data in Psychology* (1960), *probability* as a scientific concept is left to the reader's imagination. This lack of analysis is especially surprising and troubling considering the generally vague meaning of the term *probability* in science. These various shortcomings appear to have prompted Bertrand Russell to sardonically comment: "Probability is the most important concept in modern science, especially as nobody has the slightest notion what it means" (quoted in Johnson and Morris, 1987:107).

Nonetheless, reinforcement is defined (as has been frequently reiterated above) in terms of the effect it has on the future *probability* or *frequency* of the reinforced behavior. *Response probability* is typically defined as a proportional relation between the number of opportunities for the response to occur and the number of times it actually occurs. For example, if a dog is signaled to sit 15 times but only sits on 9 of those occasions, the probability that he will sit on signal is 0.6 (calculated by dividing 9 by 15).

However, with this definition of response probability in mind, how can one determine whether a given response has undergone reinforcement, unless one knows in advance the effect of reinforcement. Let us say, for example, that a dog were to receive a reinforcer as the result of sitting on a single occasion, can an objective observer really make any predictions from that one event about the future probability of the sit response? How about after two, three, four, or five reinforcements? In fact, nothing very definite can be said about the response's future probability after a single exposure to reinforcement. Consequently, since it is not possible to calculate probabilities from the first reinforcing event onward, how can one say of these early events whether they were reinforcing? Obviously, it is only after the habit of sitting becomes highly predictable and regular that one might infer (or speculate?) that the sit response had undergone previous reinforcement.

Another problematical area regarding response probability as the defining characteristic of reinforcement is observed in cases where no additional improvement in response probability is evident as the result of continued reinforcement. Take, for example, a dog that has undergone several hundred trials of training, until the dog has achieved an almost errorless proficiency or fluency at sitting on signal. Reinforcement in this case may have some effect on the behavior of sitting, but, assuming that the sit response's probability of occurrence cannot be *measurably* improved upon, in what sense can one say that the behavior is reinforced? If the behavior's probability cannot be improved upon

(or worsened) through reinforcement, then what is the event to be called? (By the way, I have chosen the term *verifier* for such instances; see Chapter 8 for a more detailed discussion). In conclusion, it appears that the probability theory of reinforcement breaks down in cases involving single and many (asymptotic) reinforcing events.

The probability account of reinforcement also appears to break down in the case of shaping (Catania, 1992). During shaping procedures, no particular response is repeated in exactly the same way. Behavior operating under a shaping contingency is emitted with a high degree of variability, with differential consequences gradually narrowing instrumental efforts to progressively approximate the target response—a process in which response probability (e.g., frequency or rate) is rather irrelevant. It is evident during the shaping process that the dog optimizes its chances of obtaining the offered reinforcer by changing its behavior along several dimensions at once. In general, the dog becomes more active and exploratory, especially if it is hungry. When, as the result of discovering that some behavioral change improves its control over the reinforcer, the dog's effort in that direction is intensified.

Efforts to analyze the relationship between reinforcement and response probability in terms of the foregoing definition (i.e., reinforcement increases the future probability/frequency of the behavior it follows) are dependent on the size of the response/reinforcer sample being observed. The belief that response probability is improved as the result of reinforcement is an uncertain assumption in the case of small samples, but one that becomes progressively more certain (to a point) as the sample size increases. The assumed overall effect of reinforcement on response probability does not appear to be measurable on the level of individual responses and reinforcing events. If it is not measurable at the level of individual responses and reinforcing events, can one be sure that the effect is not a statistical myth?

Probability appears to be evident only in cases where patterns and molar relations (classes of behavior) are studied as the basic unit of analysis. Furthermore, the usual definition of reinforcement in terms of increasing response probability only begs the question about the effect that reinforcement has on discrete units of behavior—it says nothing about how or why increased predictability and regularity result from reinforcement. The usual definition only asserts that the response's increased predictability and regularity (as a function of probability) is predicated upon reinforcement. One might conclude that the relationship between reinforcement and response probability as it is characterized by behavior analysis is a post hoc interpretation of reinforcement—certainly not a causal account of how reinforcement affects the probability/frequency of behavior. Perhaps the strongest statement that can be made about the relationship between reinforcement and response probability is that the two are correlated—that is, reinforcement is positively correlated with an increased response probability/frequency.

A variety of experimental and conceptual considerations led Johnson and Morris to question the value of probability theory in the analysis of behavior: "If the concept of probability does not enhance the description, prediction, and control of behavior, then perhaps its role in behavior analysis should be re-evaluated" (1987:124). An alternative discussed by them is to replace the notion of probability with that of *propensity*, which is defined in terms of the experimental arrangement or context in which behavior occurs:

> "Propensity," then, makes clear the importance of context in affecting the outcomes that probabilities are taken to predict, whether of the behavior of coin tosses or organisms. With respect to the behavior of coins, for example, a biased coin will produce different outcomes depending on the strength of the gravitational field in which it is tossed. In a weak gravitational field, the bias will have little effect; in a strong gravitational field, the bias will be enhanced. Likewise, with respect to the behavior of organisms, a propensity interpretation emphasizes the contextual nature of behavior and takes probability to be a characteristic of the experimental arrangement as a whole, not just

a property of a sequence of events without reference to other conditions. (1987:124–125)

Positive and Negative Reinforcement and Ockham's Razor

The term *reinforcement* is further complicated by its division into positive and negative categories. On many levels, these distinctions appear arbitrary and confusing (Michael, 1975; Iwata, 1987). Positive reinforcement is distinguished from negative reinforcement by the manner in which the reinforcing event is operated upon by the animal. In the case of positive reinforcement the animal's behavior is reinforced by producing the presentation of an event, whereas in negative reinforcement the animal's behavior is reinforced by either terminating or avoiding the presentation of an event. In a certain sense, all instrumental learning can be reduced to one or the other of these categories. It simply depends on how the events are viewed and interpreted. An animal escaping and subsequently learning to avoid aversive stimulation may not in the first place "view" his success as escape-avoidance but, instead, frame the learning situation in terms of the acquisition of safety (a positive reinforcer) from aversive stimulation. Thus, under similar future circumstances of impending threat, the animal will likely select the successful behavior resulting in the acquisition of safety and relief in the past. Conversely, an animal that is deprived of free access to food and starved to 80% of its ad lib feeding weight may find the general physiological state aroused by deprivation aversive and attempt to terminate or avoid it by performing various arbitrary behaviors (e.g., key peck) to obtain food. Thus, from this perspective, working for food may be interpreted as escape-avoidance behavior aimed at reducing or terminating the aversive condition of starvation. Unfortunately, the terms positive reinforcement and negative reinforcement—although of some practical value in the everyday control of behavior—are highly subjective and appear to depend on an experimenter's point of view and bias.

In an important sense, the bifurcation of reinforcement into positive and negative categories is a rather unfortunate violation of Ockham's razor: *Entia non sunt multiplicanda praeter necessitatem* ("Entities are not to be multiplied beyond necessity"). Whether an animal's behavior produces or terminates/avoids the reinforcing event, the bottom line is that reinforcement is contingent on the successful prediction and control of significant impinging events. Whether these events are appetitive, sexual, social, agonistic, playful, or aversive is of only secondary interest. Regardless of an animal's disposition to learn, the goal of purposive behavior is to predict and control outcomes. Locating food when hungry and finding a successful route of escape when threatened are behaviors that are both strongly reinforced in the same general way. The reinforcement of such behavior does not depend on a hypothetical enhancement of probability but on the more immediate and real outcome of having successfully exercised decisive control over the occurrence of such events (i.e., finding food when hungry and locating a route of escape when threatened). Essentially, reinforcement occurs when an animal successfully controls any event in such a way that the animal's self-interests are served (survival) and its well-being enhanced.

An Alternative Theory of Reinforcement

According to the foregoing line of reasoning, instrumental reinforcement occurs when any behavior successfully controls a significant event or situation impinging on an animal. In other words, reinforcement does not stand apart from the reinforced behavior. In the case of classical conditioning, reinforcement occurs when a significant event is adequately predicted by anticipatory stimuli associated with its occurrence. Functionally speaking, sharp lines of distinction between instrumental and classical phenomena do not exist except under the artificial conditions of the laboratory and not really there either. The synthetic relationship and interdependency existing between these two classes of behavior

(instrumental and classical) results in the necessary conclusion that perhaps only one general form of reinforcement exists for both paradigms. *Successful control depends on adequate prediction and adequate prediction depends on successful control.* When significant events are adequately predicted and controlled, the consequence is adaptive success—an enhanced state of well-being, confidence, and power.

Within this general framework, the biological and motivational inclinations driving behavior (e.g., hunger, fear, and other homeostatic needs) together with past learning experiences form an animal's *disposition to learn.* The disposition to learn can be fairly characterized by the sort of environmental events the animal seeks to predict or control, that is, events that the animal treats as significant. For instance, the presentation of food to a hungry dog has a far greater significance to that dog than to another dog that is satiated. In the case of learning to sit, the disposition to learn is characterized by a dog's effort to control several basic needs, including contact (affection), food (appetitive), and, perhaps, the escape-avoidance of aversive stimulation (fear). The need to predict and control the environment is directly related to the maintenance of biological, emotional, and psychological homeostasis and security. The overall goals of the disposition to learn are survival, adaptive success, enhanced power, and, ultimately, reproduction.

In any instrumental learning situation, at least three basic elements interact with one another: a signal (S), a response (R), and an outcome (O). The primary function of the S is to announce a moment when a particular behavior will most likely result in reinforcement. However, the S is much more complicated than this simple description indicates. In addition to announcing the moment and the sort of behavior most likely to result in reinforcement, the S also makes other predictions. One such prediction concerns the type (quality) and size (quantity) of the probable reinforcer available. This prediction has a pronounced effect on how the response will be affected by reinforcement. Three general variations are possible, depending on the kind of prediction involved: (1) The S underpredicts the type or size of the reinforcer (acquisition). (2) The S overpredicts the type or size of the reinforcer (extinction). (3) The S exactly predicts (verifies) the type or size of the reinforcer (maintenance).

Relations Between the Signal, Response, and Outcome

On a basic level, most behavioral and training events are organized and structured in terms of triads. The most obvious triadic structure is composed of the signal (S), response (R), and outcome (O). Each element in this triadic compound depends on and influences the others, forming several binary relations. These several interdependent binary relations between S, R, and O provide a great deal of information to dogs (Rescorla, 1987). For example, S (cue or command) tells dogs what to do (S-R) as well as designating the contingent outcome available (S-O), provided that it responds. Several other relations between S, R, and O become progressively apparent as the response is repeated in the presence of the predictive signal and the confirming occurrence of the predicted outcome during the course of training. These intertrial effects are influenced by the repetitive occurrence of the basic pattern. For example, O confirms the prediction S (R-O) while simultaneously designating the end of the trial and the possibility of another. Thus, O has a link with S as part of a general confirming relation (O-S)—that is, the outcome confirms the predictions of S, concludes the trial, and signals the possibility of a new one. The outcome of the preceding trial also affects R of the succeeding trial by making it more or less likely to the extent that the previous emission of R confirmed or disconfirmed the predictions made by S. These intertrial relations and effects extending from trial to trial are summarized thus:

1. S (R-O) produces the predictive binary relations S-R and S-O, such that O will occur, if and only if R occurs in the presence of S.

2. O (S-R) produces the confirming binary relations O-S and O-R, such that R will be more likely, if and only if S adequately predicts the presentation of O given that R occurs. Conversely, if the prediction of O given S and R is disconfirmed (e.g., reinforcement is omitted), then R will become less likely in the future.

Finally, R is also connected to S and O in terms of the control R exercises over the presentation of the predictive signal and outcome. Under circumstances of repeated practice, a dog gradually learns that R controls the reoccurrence of the predictive signal and outcome or R (S-O). This last set of relations summarizes the operative or controlling effect that the dog's behavior has on the handler's behavior. In an important sense, the handler's training behavior is controlled by the dog's recognition (as evident in his behavior) of a contingent relation between its behavior and the presentation of the predictive signals and confirming outcomes controlled by its behavior. From the handler's point of view, the dog is successfully controlled by the presentation of the predictive signals and the confirming outcomes. In other words,

3. Provided that the predictive relations S (R-O) are confirmed by O (S-R), then R (S-O) produces the operative or controlling binary relations R-S and R-O, such that R sets the occasion for the presentation of the predictive S (R-O) contingency, producing the opportunity for R to produce O again, thus further strengthening R while reinforcing the entire chain of events.

In summary, the interdependent relations produced by repeated reinforcement include prediction, confirmation, and control:

1. S(R-O): A predictive relation between the signal and the response (S-R) and the signal and the outcome (S-O).
2. O(S-R): A confirmative relation between the predicted outcome and the signal (O-S) and the predicted outcome and the mediating response (O-R).
3. R(S-O): The operative relation between

the controlling response and the repeated confirmation of the predictive signal (R-S) and the predicted outcome (R-O).

Besides the foregoing functions, the S also formulates predictions about the ability of the target behavior to control available outcomes. Outcome control is operationally defined in terms of the dog's relative ability to predict and control significant outcomes (see Fig. 9.3).

The prediction and control of significant events result in the formation of various expectancies regarding the effectiveness of behavior to anticipate and control such events in the future. These expectancies or instrumental cognitive sets are derived from past learning experiences and are of great importance for both facilitating or retarding learning. An expectancy is confirmed or disconfirmed by the degree of correspondence between what the animal expects to occur and what actually occurs. A high degree of correspondence results in confirmation, whereas a low degree of correspondence results in disconfirmation. For example, if a dog expects to be reinforced each time it sits, but on some occasion it is not reinforced (i.e., the dog is *disappointed*), the generalized expectancy that sitting always results in reinforcement is disconfirmed. The disconfirmation of a generalized expectancy results in its revision into a *probable* or statistical expectancy—that is, the dog no longer expects to be reinforced each time it sits. Similarly, if a dog has never been reinforced as the result of sitting but happens to receive a treat on some occasion after sitting, the novel reinforcing event disconfirms the previously held expectancy that sitting is not followed by the presentation of food. In the future, the dog may now anticipate or *hope* for the presentation of food when it sits.

The revision of expectancies occurs in order to secure a more perfect match between past experience and current reinforcement contingencies, thus continuously refining and adjusting an animal's ability to predict and control significant events occurring within the flux impinging upon it. In an important sense, the cognitive function of expectancy is

the exercise of a reality principle, establishing an informative feedback loop between the animal's past experiences with current sensory and behavioral efforts to predict and control the occurrence of significant events. The most dramatic examples of *dissonance* occur in cases in which highly regular and generalized expectancies are disconfirmed. The least dramatic change or dissonance occurs in cases where the disconfirmation is statistically significant but remains consistent with the animal's overall expectations. For example, a dog that is accustomed to receiving reinforcement after sitting two or three times will notice, and adjust accordingly, when it is instead reinforced only on every fifth or sixth occasion. The change in this case would be merely statistical and not nearly as dramatic as the resultant dissonance would be if the dog were all of a sudden punished each time it sat, for example.

Punishment

What is the relationship between reinforcement and punishment? Traditionally, behavior analysis defines punishment in terms of the effect an event has on behavior insofar as its presentation (positive punishment) or omission (negative punishment) suppresses or lowers the future probability/frequency of the behavior it follows. However, defining punishment as a suppressive event is to describe it in terms of its most superficial and general attributes. As it stands, this definition of punishment might be construed to include events that are clearly not intended as punishment. For example, when dogs are reinforced with food, other possible behaviors, except those directly facilitating access to food and eating, are suppressed and made less likely to occur in the future by the reinforcer's presentation. Similarly, aversive stimulation suppresses all concurrent behavior at the moment except the response that results in the termination of aversive stimulation.

An alternative definition of punishment may be stated in terms of prediction and control. According to this interpretation, punishment is defined as occurring whenever a behavior fails to anticipate and control a significant event adequately. Punishment is not something done to a behavior or to an animal but rather something that the behavior itself does or fails to do—that is, it fails to appropriate an important resource or escape or avoid an aversive or dangerous situation. The cause of this failure can be causally traced to any number of factors. Instrumental punishment often results when stimulus events are inadequately predicted or when correct predictions are not followed into effective action. For example, if a hungry dog fails to obtain a piece of food for sitting because it misses a signal or fails to sit in a timely fashion, the dog is punished—not indirectly as the result of the withdrawal of the appetitive opportunity—but directly as the result of its failure to control the opportunity to obtain food. Conversely, if the same dog fails to terminate or avoid an aversive event by sitting because it misses a signal or fails to sit in a timely fashion, the dog is punished—not indirectly as the result of the presentation of the aversive event—but directly as a result of its failure to control the presentation of the aversive event.

Punishment is associated with the elicitation of various concomitant emotional states, especially fear and frustration. Punishment resulting from a failure to predict a reinforcing event results in fear/anxiety, whereas a failure to control the occurrence of a reinforcing event results in frustration. These emotional reactions facilitate adaptation in cases where prediction and control are compromised. Fear/anxiety serves to heighten vigilance and, thereby, improves the likelihood of anticipating future stimulus events associated with reinforcement. Frustration, on the other hand, serves to invigorate or amplify behavioral efforts aimed at restoring instrumental control over available reinforcers.

Within certain limits, both anxiety and frustration contribute beneficially to the efficiency of the learning process. However, in cases involving high levels of fear or frustration, learning may be adversely affected by these otherwise potentiating and useful states. Under conditions involving high levels of anxiety (unpredictability) and high levels of frustration (uncontrollability), a variety of conflict-driven learning dysfunctions are pre-cipitated. Learning situations in which significant events are both unpredictable and uncontrollable are prone to produce pathological emotional states (e.g., PTSD) and abnormal behavior patterns (e.g., learned helplessness—see Chapter 9). On the other hand, a high degree of control and predictability over significant resources and stimuli occasioning their presentation or escape-avoidance (as may be appropriate from moment to moment) fosters successful adaptation and a sense of well-being.

To a considerable extent, it boils down to a matter of whether one views punishment from the perspective of an event produced by behavior (the animal's perspective) or as an event done to behavior (the trainer's perspective).

PREDICTION-CONTROL EXPECTANCIES AND ADAPTATION

The central control of approach and escape-avoidance behaviors depends on various prediction-control expectancies and cost-benefit appraisals. Prediction and control expectancies share a common cognitive axis mediating reinforcement and punishment. Together, such expectancies guide all purposive behavior, including appetitive and escape-avoidance behavior. These various expectancies are either confirmed (verified) or disconfirmed. Disconfirmation of an instrumental expectancy results when the attractive outcome produced is more (reinforcing) or less (punishing) than expected. Taken together, efforts to control and predict the occurrence of significant events form expectancies such that, given some set of antecedent circumstances, an effortful behavior *a* will result in producing a consequence or outcome *b*. If the expectancy is confirmed, it is kept in tact, whereas if the expectancy is disconfirmed, both predictive assumptions and control efforts are altered, thereby making them more accurately fit the given circumstances. Predictive disconfirmation involving attractive outcomes results in increased arousal in the opposing directions of surprise or disappointment, depending on whether the outcome was more (surprise) or less (disappointment) than expected. In the case of aversive outcomes, disconfirmation results in arousal in the opposing directions of startle or relief, depending on whether the event was more aversive (startle) or less aversive (relief) than expected. Surprise and relief serve to mobilize learning efforts and represent an important source of reinforcement. Predictive disconfirmation involving disappointment is correlated with need-anxiety, whereas disconfirmation involving startle is correlated with threat-anxiety. Both need- and threat-anxiety internally prompt a preparatory adjustment (e.g., increased vigilance and autonomic arousal) and a reappraisal of the working circumstances. As a result, the dog forms new expectancies and behavioral strategies that better conform to the new information that it possesses.

Disconfirmation of control expectancies results in related behavioral and motivational changes in the dog. When the dog's efforts to control attractive resources exceed its control expectancies, then enhanced acquisitiveness or satiation ensues. On the other hand, when behavioral efforts fail to achieve what is expected, frustrative-loss occurs, and the behavior is adjusted in the opposing directions of invigoration-persistence or despair, depending on the dog's motivational state and relevant past experience with the situation. The appraisal of frustrative situations depends on the dog's disposition to persist in the face of frustrative nonreward—a control strategy that reflects its past success in controlling difficult working situations by persisting or trying harder. Repeated control disconfirmations involving attractive outcomes result in motivational changes in the opposing directions of hope or loss-anger. In the case of disconfirmed control expectancies involving aversive outcomes, behavioral adjustment efforts move in the opposing directions of courage (aversive event required less effort than expected) or threat-anger (aversive event required more effort than expected). Aversive events present other problems for the dog. When faced with a situation involving potent aversive events, failure may instigate disorganized efforts involving anger-anxiety loops and aggression. When both aversive and attractive outcomes are under a high degree of predictability and control, security and safety

prevail—a state of affairs that continues unchanged until a prediction-control expectancy is *disconfirmed*. Finally, under circumstances in which significant aversive and attractive outcomes are both unpredictable and uncontrollable, pathological helplessness and behavioral disorganization may ensue (see Chapter 9).

Expectancy Disconfirmation and Learning

Behavior is modified as the result of producing attractive or aversive outcomes that *disconfirm* previously established prediction-control expectancies concerning the relative frequency, size, quantity, or quality of those outcomes. At first glance, this may seem paradoxical, until one considers what occurs when a prediction-control expectancy is *confirmed*. Under circumstances in which significant events are both highly predicted and controlled, there is no need for the dog to adjust or change—successful confirmation simply "verifies" and maintains the prediction-control expectancy without modification. Neither the behavior nor the prediction-control expectancy controlling its expression needs to be changed (nor should they be changed) as the result of confirmatory experiences. Confirmation may be rewarding for the dog in the sense of enhancing efficacy beliefs and feelings of well-being, but such confirmation results in little additional adaptation in terms of behavioral acquisition or extinction.

Functionally speaking, reinforcement and punishment do approximately the same thing: They both variably influence the prediction-control expectancies regulating instrumental behavior, thereby optimizing the dog's adaptation and control over the environment, at least insofar as the environment is significant to the dog, that is, represents a potential threat or opportunity. Reinforcement occurs when an instrumental effort succeeds in achieving *more* control over some attractive or aversive event than predicted by the operative expectancy, whereas punishment occurs when an instrumental effort achieves *less* control over some attractive or aversive event than predicted by the operative expectancy (Fig. 7.4). In both reinforcement and punishment, the operative expectancy is disconfirmed by either increasing or decreasing control over the relevant attractive or aversive event. As a result of such disconfirmation, the prediction-control expectancy is reappraised and modified to render it more fully in accord with circumstances, thus making the dog's future behavioral efforts more accurately fitted to relevant opportunities or threats. Prediction-control expectancies are modified to agree with the cumulative behavioral successes or failures of the dog's behavioral efforts to access available attractive opportunities and to escape-avoid aversive threats.

These countless behavioral efforts and their modification continue until both prediction and control expectancies most adequately and fully provide behavioral control over significant attractive and aversive events. Part of the motivational impetus for these cognitive and behavioral changes is distressful emotional arousal: (1) when prediction expectancies prove inadequate, anxiety ensues, resulting in augmented behavioral vigilance and autonomic arousal; (2) when control expectancies are inadequate, frustration ensues, resulting in behavioral invigoration and persistence; and (3) when, in spite of behavioral effort, significant events remain both unpredictable and uncontrollable, the result is either depression (learned helplessness) or dysfunctional impulsive or compulsive behavioral excesses. Small amounts of anxiety and frustration are highly conducive to learning, whereas excessive amounts of such arousal may profoundly disturb learning and disorganize instrumental behavior.

Practical Example

The following simple experiment seems to confirm that dogs sometimes rely more on their expectations about future events than on immediate information obtained through their senses. The first part of the experiment consists of giving the dog a dozen or so treats exclusively with the right hand. After this preliminary conditioning is carried out, a treat is taken between the thumb and index fingers of each hand and held just in front of the dog's nose, thus giving the dog a clear view of its location. Next, with the treat shifted from the right into the left hand, but still held in full view, both hands are slowly moved laterally apart from one another, forcing the dog to choose between the left or right hand to get the food. Surprisingly, the vast majority of dogs trained in this way choose the empty (right) hand expecting to find the food in it, rather than track the plainly visible biscuit held in the left hand.

One is tempted to speculate that a dog in this case has formed a cognitive expectation about the likely location of food—one that overshadows the immediate and contrary sensory information that indicates otherwise. This effect is often very persistent, with the incorrect "belief" only gradually being disconfirmed and modified to fit the altered circumstances. As dogs recognize that their expectations about the food's location are no longer reliable, they appear to turn their attention away from the faulty cognitive appraisement to focus on local sensory information in an effort to restore or improve their control over the food's presentation.

A general two-part hypothesis is deducible from these observations: (1) When expected outcomes are highly regular and more or less anticipated, dogs may be more likely to make choices based on expectations than on immediate sensory information. (2) When significant outcomes occur on an irregular basis, however, dogs may rely more on sensory information than on expectations derived from past experience. Ultimately, the goal of sensory reappraisal is to adjust a dog's expectations so that behavioral operations are more efficient and neatly fitted to the actual contingencies and demands placed upon it by the environment. As noted above, dogs that base their actions on well-confirmed expectancies are less anxious or frustrated (less stressed) than dogs exposed to uncertain events. In the latter case, dogs must rely on moment-to-moment sensory input and are unable to relax because dependable expectations about the future are not available. The disruptive influence of an unpredictable and uncontrollable environment exercises a destructive influence on a dog's adaptation and welfare.

Diverters and Disrupters

An important key to successful training is to identify what the dog is attempting to accomplish by its behavioral efforts. A dog working hard to get food may not find the opportunity to play ball to be an adequate substitute—ball play is irrelevant to the control-prediction expectancies at work. Similarly, giving the dog a biscuit when it wants to play fetch may not represent a reinforcing event, although it may momentarily dampen or replace the dog's interest in chasing the ball. Presenting a ball to a dog who is momentarily interested in food represents a special kind of *surprise*—a diverter. Unlike a surprise, a diverter does not function as a reinforcer, even though it may become a reinforcer as the dog makes *efforts to control* its occurrence. Similarly, behavioral efforts can be disrupted by the presentation of special startling events called disrupters (e.g., a burst of air). The disrupter is presented independently of the dog's ability to control or predict it and is irrelevant to the control-prediction expectancies regulating the behavior occurring at the moment of presentation. The disrupting event is not punishment because the dog is not engaged in behavioral efforts aimed at avoiding or escaping its occurrence. The event serves only to momentarily disrupt behavior. Since there is no effort to control the presentation of diverters or disrupters in advance of their occurrence, such events result in neither punishment nor reinforcement. Their effects are primarily diversionary and disruptive. Both diverters and disrupters are used to initiate novel patterns of behavior that are subsequently brought under the influence of new control-prediction expectancies. Diverters and disrupters are means for initiating new behavior without first punishing or extinguishing already established behavior. Both diverters and disrupters are marking events that set the stage for establishing a new set of control-prediction expectancies with which to organize new behavior.

Another way of appreciating the function of diverters and disrupters is in terms of attractive and aversive establishing operations. Offering a ball to the dog in the above example motivationally diverts the dog from its appetitive interests and raises the likelihood that it will exhibit behavior aimed at controlling the ball. As this transition occurs, the contingent presentation or omission of the ball can then function as a reinforcer or punisher. Noncontingent reinforcement and punishment function in a similar way. For example, giving the dog noncontingent food during greetings turns its attention away from controlling social reinforcers to the possibility of controlling appetitive reinforcers. The initial presentations of food in such situations function as a diverting establishing operation, making it more likely that the dog will emit behavior aimed at controlling the food presentations (e.g., sitting instead of jumping up), thereby making reinforcement or punishment possible through the contingent delivery or omission of the food reward. Diverting and disrupting establishing operations play important roles in the management of a wide variety of behavior problems.

CONCLUSION

The foregoing methods of analysis and behavior modification are crucial for effective problem solving and routine training efforts. Such methods provide the trainer/behaviorist with a flexible and creative repertoire of alternatives to reactive force and punishment. Dogs trained with behavioral methods take to learning much more actively and exhibit a confidence and optimism that dogs trained with force alone never exhibit. The ideal outcome of behavior modification is the development of a system of communication between owner and dog based on a shared interface of understood expectancies, mutually cooperative and constructive mediational behaviors, and a shared set of common needs served by such interaction. Proper training establishes a foundation of interactive harmony based on realistic boundaries and cooperative exchange.

REFERENCES

Adler LL and Adler HE (1977). Ontogeny of observational learning in the dog (*Canis familiaris*). *Dev Psychobiol*, 10:267–280.

Bacon WE and Stanley WC (1963). Effect of deprivation level in puppies on performance maintained by a passive person reinforcer. *J Comp Physiol Psychol*, 56:783–785.

Bandura A (1977). Self-efficacy: Toward a unifying theory of behavior change. *Psychol Rev*, 84:191–215.

Bitterman ME (1965). Phyletic differences in learning. *Am Psychol*, 20:396–410.

Brunswick E (1939). Probability as a determiner of rat behavior. *J Exp Psychol*, 25:175–197.

Catania AC (1992) *Learning*, 3rd Ed. Englewood Cliffs, NJ: Prentice-Hall.

Catania AC (1995). Higher-order behavior classes: Contingencies, beliefs, and verbal behavior. *J Behav Ther Exp Psychiatry*, 26:191–200.

Chance P (1998). *First Course in Applied Behavior Analysis*. New York: Brooks/Cole.

Cohen RA and O'Donnell BF (1993). Attentional dysfunction associated with psychiatric illness. In RA Cohen, YA Sparling-Cohen, and BF O'Donnell (Eds), *The Neuropsychology of Attention*. New York: Plenum.

Dodwell PC and Bessant DE (1960). Learning without swimming in a water maze. *J Comp Physiol Psychol*, 28:83–95.

Ducharme JM and Van Houten R (1994). Operant extinction in the treatment of severe maladaptive behavior. *Behav Modif*, 18:139–170.

Estes WK (1971). Reward in human learning: Theoretical issues and strategic choice points. In R Glaser (Ed), *The Nature of Reinforcement*, 16–36. New York: Academic.

Ferster CF and Skinner BF (1957). *Schedules of Reinforcement*. New York: Appleton-Century-Crofts.

Fonberg E and Kostarczyk E (1980). Motivational role of social reinforcement in dog-man relations. *Acta Neurobiol Exp*, 40:117–136.

Foxx RM (1982a). *Decreasing Behaviors of Severely Retarded and Autistic Persons*. Champaign, IL: Research Press.

Foxx RM (1982b). *Increasing Behaviors of Severely Retarded and Autistic Persons*. Champaign, IL: Research.

Gormezano I and Tait RW (1976). The Pavlovian analysis of instrumental conditioning. *Pavlov J Biol Sci*, 11:37–55.

Guthrie ER (1935/1960). *The Psychology of Learning*, Rev Ed. Gloucester, MA: Peter Smith (reprint).

Hall G (1991). *Perceptual and Associative Learning*. Oxford: Clarendon.

Hall JF (1976). *Classical Conditioning and Instrumental Learning: A Contemporary Approach*. Philadelphia: JB Lippincott.

Harlow HF (1949). The formation of learning sets. *Psychol Rev*, 56:51–65.

Heyes CM and Dawson GR (1990). A demonstration of observational learning using a bidirectional control. *Q J Exp Psychol*, 42B:59–71.

Heyes CM, Jaldow E, Nokes T, and Dawson GR (1994). Imitation in rats (*Rattus norvegicus*): The role of demonstrator action. *Behav Processes*, 32:173–182.

Hilgard ER and Bower GH (1975). *Theories of Learning*, 4th Ed. New York: Appleton-Century-Crofts.

Holland JG and Skinner BF (1961). *The Analysis of Behavior*. New York: McGraw-Hill.

Iwata B (1987). Negative reinforcement in applied settings: An emerging technology. *J Appl Behav Anal*, 20:361–378.

Johnson LM and Morris ED (1987). When speaking of probability in behavior analysis. *Behaviorism*, 15:107–129.

Kamin LJ (1968). Attention-like processes in classical conditioning. In MR Jones (Ed), *Miami Symposium on the Prediction of Behavior: Aversive stimulation*. Miami: University of Miami Press.

Kazdin AE (1989). *Behavior Modification in Applied Settings*. Pacific Grove, CA: Brooks/Cole.

Konorski J (1967). *Integrative Activity of the Brain: An Interdisciplinary Approach*. Chicago, IL: Univ of Chicago Press.

Lawicka W (1964). The role of stimuli modality in successive discrimination and differentiation learning. *Bull Pol Acad Sci*, 12:35–38 [reported in Mazur (1986)].

Lerman DC, Iwata BA, Shore BA, and Kahng SW (1996). Responding maintained by intermittent reinforcement: Implications for the use of extinction with problem behavior in clinical settings. *J App Behav Anal*, 29:153–171.

Lieberman DA (1993). *Learning: Behavior and Cognition*. Pacific Grove, CA: Brooks/Cole.

Lieberman DA, McIntosh DC, and Thomas GV (1979). Learning when reward is delayed: A marking hypothesis. *J Exp Psychol Anim Behav Processes*, 5:224–242.

Long CJ and Tapp JT (1967). Reinforcing properties of odors for the albino rat. *Psychon Sci*, 7:17–18.

Macfarlane DA (1930). The role of kinesthesis in maze learning. *Univ Calif Publ Psychol*, 4:277–305 [reported in Hilgard and Bower (1966)].

Malone JC (1978). Beyond the operant analysis of behavior. *Behav Ther,* 9:584–591.

Mazur JE (1986). *Learning and Behavior.* Englewood Cliffs, NJ: Prentice-Hall.

McConnell PB (1990). Acoustic structure and receiver response in domestic dogs, *Canis familiaris. Anim Behav,* 39:897–904.

Michael J (1975). Positive and negative reinforcement: A distinction that is no longer necessary—Or a better way to talk about bad things. *Behaviorism,* 3:33–44.

Michael J (1993). Establishing operations. *The Behavior Analyst,* 16:191–206.

Miller NE (1969). Learning of visceral and glandular responses. *Science,* 163:434–445.

Miller NE and Carmona A (1967). Modification of a visceral response, salivation in thirsty dogs, by instrumental training with water reward. *J Comp Physiol Psychol,* 63:1–6.

Miller NE and DiCara LV (1967). Instrumental learning of heart rate changes in curarized rats: Shaping and specificity to discriminative stimulus. *J Comp Physiol Psychol,* 63:12–19.

Most K (1910/1955). *Training Dogs.* New York: Coward-McCann (reprint).

Mowrer OH (1960). *Learning Theory and Behavior.* New York: John Wiley & Sons.

Murphree OD (1974). Procedure for operant conditioning of the dog. *Pavlov J Biol Sci,* 9:46–50.

Nevin JA (1998). Choice and Behavior. In W O'Donohue (Ed), *Learning and Behavior Therapy.* Boston: Allyn and Bacon.

Premack D (1962). Reversibility of the reinforcement relation. *Science,* 136:255–57.

Premack D (1965) Reinforcement theory. In D Levine (Ed), *Nebraska Symposium on Motivation.* New York: University of Nebraska Press.

Pryor K (1975). *Lads Before the Wind.* New York: Harper and Row.

Pryor K (1985). *Don't Shoot the Dog: The New Art of Teaching and Training.* New York: Bantam.

Pryor K, Haag R, and O'Reily J (1969). The creative porpoise: Training for novel behavior. *J Exp Anal Behav,* 12:653–661.

Rachlin H (1976). *Behavior and Learning.* San Francisco: WH Freeman.

Reid P (1996). *Excel-erated Learning: Explaining How Dogs Learn (in Plain English) and How Best to Teach Them.* Oakland, CA: James and Kenneth.

Rescorla RA (1987). A Pavlovian analysis of goal-directed behavior. *Am Psychol,* 42:119–129.

Rescorla RA (1991). Associative relations in instrumental learning: The eighteenth Bartlett Memorial Lecture. *Q J Exp Psychol,* 43B:1–23.

Reynolds GS (1968). *A Primer of Operant Conditioning.* Atlanta: Scott, Foresman.

Romba JJ (1984). *Controlling Your Dog Away from You.* Aberdeen, MD: Abmor.

Rotter JB (1966). Generalized expectancies for internal versus external control of reinforcement. *Psychol Monogr Gen Appl,* 80:1–28.

Rotter JB (1975). Some problems and misconceptions related to the construct of internal versus external control of reinforcement. *J Consult Clin Psychol,* 43:56–67.

Schwartz B (1989). *Psychology of Learning and Behavior,* 3rd Ed. New York: WW Norton.

Scott JP (1968). Social facilitation and allelomimetic behavior. In EC Simmel, RA Hoppe, and GA Milton (Eds), *Social Facilitation and Imitative Behavior* (1967 Miami University Symposium on Social Behavior). Boston: Allyn and Bacon.

Seligman MEP (1975). *Helplessness: On Depression, Development and Death.* San Francisco: WH Freeman.

Seligman MEP, Maier SF, and Solomon RL (1971). Unpredictable and uncontrollable aversive events. In FR Brush (Ed), *Aversive Conditioning and Learning.* New York: Academic.

Sidman M (1960). *Tactics of Scientific Research: Evaluating Experimental Data in Psychology.* New York: Basic.

Skinner BF (1938/1966). *The Behavior of Organisms.* New York: Appleton-Century-Crofts (reprint).

Skinner BF (1948). "Superstition" in the pigeon. *J Exp Psychol,* 38:168–172.

Skinner BF (1950). Are theories of learning necessary? *Psychol Rev,* 57:193–216.

Skinner BF (1951). How to teach animals. *Sci Am,* 185:26–29.

Skinner BF (1953). *Science and Human Behavior.* Toronto: Macmillan.

Slabbert JM and Rasa OAE (1997). Observational learning of an acquired maternal behaviour pattern by working dog pups: An alternative training method? *Appl Anim Behav Sci,* 53:309–316.

Sonoda A, Okayasu T, and Hirai H (1991). Loss of controllability in appetitive situations interferes with subsequent learning in aversive situations. *Anim Learn Behav,* 19:270–275.

Staddon JER and Simmelhag VL (1971). The "superstition" experiment: A reexamination of its implication for the principles of adaptive behavior. *Psychol Rev,* 78:3–43.

Tarpy RM (1982). *Principles of Animal Learning and Motivation.* Glenview, IL: Scott, Foresman.

Thorndike EL (1911/1965). *Animal Intelligence.* New York: Macmillan (reprint).

Thorndike EL (1946). Expectation. *Psychol Rev,*

53:277–281.

Thorpe WH (1956). *Learning and Instincts in Animals.* Cambridge: Harvard University Press.

Timberlake W and Allison J (1974). Response deprivation: An empirical approach to instrumental performance. *Psychol Rev,* 81:146–164.

Tinklepaugh OL (1928). An experimental study of representative factors in monkeys. *J Comp Psychol,* 8:197–236.

Tolman EC (1934). Theories of learning. In FA Moss (Ed), *Comparative Psychology,* 367–408. New York: Prentice-Hall.

Tolman EC (1948). Cognitive maps in rats and men. *Psychol Rev,* 55:189–208.

Tolman EC and Brunswick E (1935). The organism and the causal texture of the environment. *Psychol Rev,* 42:43–77.

Vauclair J (1996). *Animal Cognition: An Introduction to Modern Comparative Psychology.* Cambridge: Harvard University Press.

Watson JB (1924/1970). *Behaviorism.* New York: WW Norton (reprint).

Wheatley KL, Welker RL, and Miles RC (1977). Acquisition of barpressing in rats following experience with response-independent food. *Anim Learn Behav,* 5:236–242.

Whitford CB (1928). *Training the Bird Dog.* New York: Macmillan.

Williams CD (1959). The elimination of tantrum behavior by extinction procedures. *J Abnorm Soc Psychol,* 59:259.

Wyrwicka W (1975). The sensory nature of reward in instrumental behavior. *Pavlov J Biol Sci,* 10:23–51.

Xenophon (1925/1984). On the art of horsemanship. In EC Marchant (Trans), *Xenophon: VII Scripta Minora.* Cambridge: Harvard University Press (reprint).

Zajonc RB (1965). Social facilitation. *Science,* 149:269–274.

8

Aversive Control of Behavior

As we know, however, the dog does not spontaneously perform all the services we require of him. We are often asked whether we should train a dog by kindness or compulsion. A kind heart is certainly an advantage to a trainer, but this alone will not induce the dog to perform reliable service, nor will treatment by those who are inclined and who constantly see "sullen resistance" on the part of the dog and inflict "punishment" accordingly. Good training needs a kind heart as well as a cool and well-informed head for the proper direction of the indispensable compulsion.

KONRAD MOST, *Training Dogs* (1910/1955)

THE AVERSIVE control of behavior plays an important role in dog training and behavior modification. In many training situations and applications, aversive techniques are not only necessary but sometimes even preferable to the various positive reinforcement procedures discussed in the previous chapter. Unfortunately, aversive training methods are often inadequately understood or applied in cases where positive methods would suffice. Although avoidance learning and punishment appear simple on the surface, as one probes the processes involved, it quickly becomes evident that they are far from simple.

FEAR AND PAIN

The most common source of fear is related to the experience of pain. Most dogs show a very strong fearful response toward pain, and the fear of pain is commonly used to study how fear is learned and affects behavior. The power of pain to evoke fear and facilitate fear-related learning is so highly prepared that it is often treated as though fear is simply a conditioned response to stimuli that predict pain. However, the threat of pain is only one of many potential elicitors of fear; other nonpainful stimuli such as loud noises, sudden movements, and isolation (among others) may also elicit fear and support avoidance learning. All of these various fear-eliciting events can also serve to augment or sensitize an animal's response to other sources of fear. Many conditioning accounts seem to presume that fear and pain are coextensive events. This does not appear to be the case. According to current neurobiological research, the widespread assumption that fear is simply a conditioned response to cues associated with pain is not a viable position (Panksepp, 1998). Pain is one of many experiences that is capable of eliciting fear, and the fear of pain is a strong behavioral motivator that plays a valuable role in an animal's successful adaptation. Fear is also a very common source of maladaptive aversive arousal underlying the development and expression of many behavioral disturbances.

NEGATIVE REINFORCEMENT AND AVOIDANCE LEARNING

Negative reinforcement occurs when the probability of a behavior's future emission is increased by (1) escape from ongoing aversive stimulation or (2) avoidance of an anticipated aversive outcome. Notice that the first part of this definition does not require that a dog respond to any predictive stimuli foreshadowing an aversive event. The definition only calls for an escape response terminating ongoing aversive stimulation—that is, the reinforcing event is both *response correlated and response contingent*. In this case, one response turns on the aversive event while another one turns it off. For example, many dogs exhibit a persistent habit of pulling on the leash when being walked. Discouraging such behavior often requires the use of leash prompts applied when the dog starts pulling. After several such corrections, the dog learns to avoid pulling on its leash because pulling behavior has been correlated with the correction. In this case, pulling on the leash is gradually suppressed through punishment and not pulling strengthened through negative reinforcement. After many walks under the influence of these instrumental contingencies, the pulling response itself gradually becomes an avoidance cue signaling the dog to stop pulling.

On the other hand, the second part of the foregoing definition does require that an antecedent signal occur before the onset of the aversive event, thus giving the dog an opportunity to avoid it—the arrangement is *stimulus correlated and response contingent*. For example, dogs being taught not to pull might be signaled just before the delivery of correction by letting loose of the leash slack, thus causing them to avoid the correction by attending to the avoidance cue (the abrupt giving way of leash slack when pulling) that signals them to stop pulling. In this case, the training event is stimulus correlated (the advent of abrupt leash slack while pulling) and response contingent (the anticipated leash prompt can be avoided by slowing down).

Avoidance training requires that contingent aversive stimulation be sufficiently strong to motivate dogs to avoid its presentation in the future. In the case of an unwanted behavior under the control of extraneous reinforcement, the intensity of the aversive event needs to be approximately correlated with the reward value of the positive reinforcer supporting the competing operant. For example, a dog bolting after a fluttering leaf might require a much smaller correction than the same dog chasing after a fleeing squirrel—a behavior that may require a fairly strong correction to suppress. Gentle leash tugs will not usually cause a pulling dog to give up the habit. From the pulling-dog's perspective, the occasional and mildly irritating tug on the leash is worth the opportunity to freely investigate and pull along as it pleases. In addition to such instrumental considerations, pulling against the leash elicits thigmotaxic reflexes that cause dogs to increase their efforts in an opposite direction to the force applied. The opposition reflex is always a competing or problematic factor in training activities that physically compel dogs to do something against their will.

The opportunity to acquire extraneous reinforcers or to engage in self-reinforcing activities may sometimes be worth even intense aversive outcomes in exchange. Frequently, naive and overly sympathetic owners only gradually intensify the amount of aversive stimulation, believing that such a procedure is fairer than starting at an appropriately intense level for the situation. The problem with such a method is that it systematically habituates dogs to the most important aspect of the correction—its startle effect. The effectiveness of punishment and negative reinforcement depends not so much on its pain-eliciting characteristics as on the elicitation of a startle response. Fear is the central motivational substrate regulating avoidance learning. Dogs learn to fear the presentation of the aversive stimulus or correction and, consequently, learn ways to avoid its onset. Further, the fear-eliciting event serves to reduce the potential reward value offered by competing extraneous reinforcers. Since the elicitation of fear is incompatible with positive reinforcement, attractive distractions are aversively counterconditioned as something

to be avoided rather than pursued.

Under response-correlated and response-contingent (Rcl/Rct) avoidance learning, one response turns on aversive stimulation while another one turns it off. As already discussed, pulling on the leash turns on a leash check or some other aversive event, whereas ceasing to pull marks the offset of the correction and possibly the onset of a reward for walking properly. During the early stages of such training, fear elicitation or the discomfort of the correction potentiates intraresponse components readying the dog for avoidance maneuvers (e.g., not pulling). Fear and discomfort occur simultaneously and are reduced together with the cessation of the aversive event. Because fear and its object (e.g., startle or pain) occur closely together, fear cannot serve a predictive function until an anticipatory signal is assigned to it, occurring just prior to the correction. In the case of response-correlated avoidance learning, the affected behavior itself becomes the avoidance cue.

The close relationship between fear and pain raises a number of important considerations for understanding avoidance learning. The only component deriving from the fear/pain response that can support conditioning is fear. The conditioning of pain itself as a conditioned response is not possible. For example, sounding a tone just before self-administering an electric shock will not, even after many trials of painful conditioning, produce an effect in which the tone is capable of eliciting painful electrical sensations. (Some components of the sensation may be conditioned but not the pain itself.) The conditioning of pain as a sensation is apparently blocked by the more pertinent conditioned response of fear elicitation. Even after a single pairing of the tone preceding the shock event, one might be seized with an intense foreboding of the forthcoming shock that the tone predicts. Pain or discomfort appear to be more closely linked with escape from aversive stimulation once it occurs, whereas fear serves to predict, anticipate, and avoid such hedonistically undesirable experiences.

Stimulus-correlated and response-contingent (Scl/Rct) avoidance learning depends on dogs learning an avoidance signal that predicts a forthcoming aversive event and selects the specific behavior needed to avoid it. Many theoretical issues stem from such learning (Mowrer, 1960; Seligman and Johnston, 1973). One problem is that animals trained to a high proficiency (asymptote) on avoidance contingencies do not typically show signs of fear prior to the emission of the required avoidance response. Instead, they are often very happy and relaxed workers. They appear to know what is expected of them and do it without hesitation and ostensibly without fear. This effect is obvious in the confident performance of an advanced competitor in the obedience ring. So, if avoidance learning is based on fear, why do avoidance-trained dogs not appear to be fearful? Another problematic (and sometimes highly desirable) feature of avoidance learning is its resistance to extinction (Solomon et al., 1953). Once dogs have been trained to sit on command to avoid a leash correction, they may not require another leash correction for many dozens of trials. One would think that after many presentations of the conditioned stimulus (CS) without actual reinforcement with the aversive unconditioned stimulus (US), that the former would rapidly lose its power to elicit fear and fail to motivate avoidance behavior. In fact, it appears as though the fear originally elicited by the avoidance signal gradually undergoes extinction but not the cue's ability to control avoidance responding. For example, during the early stages of avoidance training, dogs may back away or show other signs of fearful arousal, but after many additional trials, they will simply perform the exercise in a relaxed manner, exhibiting no signs of fear whatsoever.

MOWRER'S TWO-PROCESS THEORY OF AVOIDANCE LEARNING

O. Hobart Mowrer (1960) found that many phenomena observed during avoidance acquisition and extinction could not be adequately explained by previous theories of learning. For instance, Thorndike's *law of effect* postulates that behavior followed by reward is *stamped in*, whereas behavior followed by punishment is *stamped out*. The effects of punishment, however, are often more complicated than Thorndike's assessment indicates. Mowrer argued that two direct features are added to the training situation as a consequence of punishment: (1) punishment does not simply suppress an ongoing behavior, it also strengthens behavior directly associated with its termination, and (2) antecedent stimuli and cues occurring prior to the onset of punishment become emotionally conditioned with fear.

Startle devices like the shaker can are commonly used in dog training. Their purpose is to generate a startle effect immediately and directly associated with an unwanted behavior. For example, a common behavior complaint presented for modification is the habit of jumping on countertops in search of food. Since it is intermittently reinforced (sometimes with very large rewards), it can be a very persistent habit and resist suppression. One means of suppressing the tendency is to booby trap the countertop with a suspended shaker can or something else that causes a significant startle. Sometimes, forbidden items themselves are attached directly to the shaker can by a length of fishing line or dental floss. Dogs that attempt to steal a snack are very much startled by the resounding crash caused by their efforts.

Several things happen during such training. Both external cues (the tabletop and tempting food), internal cues (the desire to jump up for food), and the behavior of jumping itself are all associatively linked with the startling event. Also, dogs learn to escape the startling event by excitedly leaping away from the table (if the startle is sufficiently intense, and they are sufficiently sensitive to it). After a few trials, dogs learn to stay clear of tabletops (unless the potential reward of jumping up offsets the threat of punishment). In the foregoing case, a dog's tendency to jump up is conflicted by competing conditioned emotional responses (CERs) and two learned instrumental components: the tendency to jump off has been strengthened by successful escape and not jumping up rewarded with continued safety from the feared event.

In the laboratory, animals are often

trained to jump over a barrier dividing the experimental chamber into two identical compartments. The grid floor is attached to a shock generator. This arrangement is called a shuttle box and is commonly used in the study of punishment and escape-avoidance learning. During the escape phase of training, an electric charge is passed into the grid work of the floor. Animals learn by trial and error to escape the shock by jumping over the barrier into the safety of the other side. After several trials, they learn to escape more and more efficiently by jumping over the barrier as soon as the shock occurs. The avoidance phase of training involves pairing a neutral stimulus (e.g., a light or tone) with the delivery of shock. If a tone is presented just prior to the onset of shock, animals quickly learn to anticipate the occurrence of shock and avoid it by jumping over the barrier as soon as the auditory cue is heard. In the beginning this association may need periodic reinforcement, but as training progresses the animals respond almost without error. Once established, avoidance training is extremely resistant to extinction. Solomon and Wynne (1953) found that dogs trained to avoid traumatic shock under such conditions persisted in the habit long after the threat of shock was eliminated. Resistance to extinction is a peculiar feature of avoidance learning—a feature it shares with learned fears and phobias.

Although the foregoing scenario sounds straightforward enough, several perplexing aspects about avoidance learning prompted Mowrer's attention. One theoretical issue is how avoidance learning is maintained, since the avoidance response is rarely reinforced with shock. Mower proposed a two-factor theory of avoidance learning to account for it. His theory is composed of two distinct parts: a Pavlovian component involving conditioned emotional reactions and a Thorndikian component involving habit formation. The tone in the foregoing arrangement possesses no aversive or fear-eliciting properties until it is classically associated with shock. The tone signal gradually acquires motivational properties originally belonging only to shock itself. Consequently, the tone becomes a CS eliciting various fearful emotional responses and concomitant physiologi-

cal changes like accelerated heart rate and respiration. Mower theorized that animals find such emotional reactions aversive and learn to escape them in precisely the same way they learn to escape direct aversive stimulation— negative reinforcement. Since jumping the barrier reduces an aversive tension generated by the CS, the response is negatively reinforced. An experiment that is often cited in support of this view of avoidance learning was carried out by Kamin (1956), who found that if the CS was continued beyond the emission of the avoidance response, avoidance learning would be disrupted—that is, the extended CS *punished* the avoidance response. If the termination of the CS were delayed for as long as 10 seconds, avoidance learning was seriously impeded.

Subsequently, Rescorla and LoLordo (1965) performed a series of experiments that provided additional support for the two-factor theory of avoidance learning. In their study, dogs were trained to jump over a barrier without the aid of external avoidance cues (Sidman avoidance task). During this initial avoidance training, the dogs were exposed to regularly spaced shocks that they could avoid with well-timed responding. Once a strong pattern of avoidance responding was established, they were exposed to a classical conditioning procedure. Some of the dogs were presented a tone stimulus (CS1) that was regularly followed by shock after a variable delay. Another group of dogs was exposed to the same CS1, but instead of receiving shock, they were exposed to another tone stimulus (CS2)—a stimulus that was never followed by shock. The dogs' differential rate of avoidance responding in the presence of each CS arrangement was then measured. Dogs exposed to CS1 and shock were significantly more active avoidance responders. Their rate of jumping over the barrier was significantly increased whenever the tone stimulus was turned on. The other group in which CS1 was followed by another tone (but never shock) made fewer avoidance responses. The first preparation (CS1-shock) augmented avoidance responding while the latter (CS1-CS2) depressed such responding. In a sense, the dogs were less worried about the occurrence of shock in the presence of the CS1-CS2 arrangement. CS1 followed by CS2 predicts the absence of shock—that is, it is a "safety signal." These experiments demonstrate that some variable emotional factor alleviates or potentiates avoidance responding. In the presence of inhibitory CS1-CS2 (predicting the absence of shock) avoidance responding decreases, whereas in the presence of the excitatory CS1-shock (predicting the presence of shock) avoidance responding increases.

Mowrer progressively refined his analysis of avoidance learning and gradually modified his theoretical interpretation of two-factor learning. The bulk of these changes leaned in the direction of the cognitive learning theory of Tolman (1934). The two parts of his avoidance paradigm, corresponding to classical and instrument conditioning, were referred to, respectively, as *sign learning* (or the *what* to escape) and *solution learning* (or the *how* to escape). He viewed two-factor learning theory as a *creative synthesis* bridging traditional views of learning with Tolman's cognitive viewpoint:

> Reflexology (used here to include Thorndikian habit theory as well as Pavlovian conditioning) and cognition are, in some ways, poles apart—one being behavioristic and the other mentalistic—but two-factor theory represents an effort to bring about a creative synthesis thereof. We discard the notion that behavior itself is learned, whether as habit or as conditioned reflex; but we retain the concept of conditioning and, with Tolman, use it to explain how certain internal events get attached to new (extrinsic or intrinsic) stimuli. But whereas Tolman identified these internal events as "pure cognition," we see them, simply but more dynamically, as hopes and fears. And these then guide, select, or control behavior along lines which are, generally speaking, adaptive—a phenomenon which both Thorndike and Pavlov, in their different but equally oversimplified ways were also attempting to account for. (Mowrer, 1960:323)

The expectancy theory of avoidance has received a great deal of scientific interest, with many experiments having been carried out to determine the relative contribution and importance of emotional conditioning versus cognitive information in the formation of avoidance signals.

A COGNITIVE THEORY OF AVOIDANCE LEARNING

Seligman and Johnston (1973) articulated a cognitive theory of avoidance learning. According to this viewpoint, avoidance signaling results from both emotional conditioning and cognitive information processing of a form roughly corresponding to that outlined by Tolman. Although the acquisition phase of avoidance learning undoubtedly involves the conditioning of fear-eliciting avoidance cues, according to Seligman and Johnston (1973) this emotive phase is slowly subsumed under a more cognitive one. Avoidance training depends on dogs acquiring an expectation that their behavior controls the occurrence of such aversive events. This expectancy is confirmed (negatively reinforced) whenever a dog performs the assigned task within the time frame allotted for its emission. Essentially, the dogs learn to control the incidence of aversive stimulation by responding appropriately to available avoidance cues, thereby confirming the operative expectancy underlying the avoidance behavior.

According to Mowrer's two-factor theory of avoidance learning, fear reduction is viewed as the active reinforcing substrate maintaining avoidance behavior. However, as has been noted, this scenario is inconsistent with what actually appears to occur during avoidance training. In particular, this view conflicts with the relatively anxiety-free character of behaviors acquired through such learning and their unique resistance to extinction. Both factors suggest that the dynamics maintaining avoidance acquisitions do not depend exclusively on fear reduction. According to Seligman and Johnston's cognitive theory, instead of reducing fear of impending aversive stimulation, the learned avoidance behavior is maintained because it consistently confirms an expectancy that such behavior will successfully avoid the aversive event. As additional successful avoidance trials take place, this expectancy and its reinforcing confirmation produce increasing levels of confidence in the presence of fear-eliciting stimuli, and, as long as this expectancy is not disconfirmed by punishment (i.e., the presentation of the negative reinforcer), the behavior will be maintained at a high operant level on the basis of confirmation alone.

In effect, the avoidance signal functions in an identical manner to that of the discriminative stimulus (S^D) during positive instrumental learning. The S^D announces a moment where a reward is forthcoming, given that the dog emits the selected behavior in a timely manner. Dogs learn over several trials to expect a reward when they respond appropriately. When this expectation is confirmed by reinforcement, the linkage between the S^D and the behavior is strengthened or stamped in and extinguished or stamped out when the expectation is disconfirmed by the omission of reinforcement. For example, if a dog was trained to sit under two different signals and then exposed to a situation in which one of the signals is followed by the omission of reinforcement while the other continues to be associated with its presentation, the dog will subsequently learn to sit under the signal confirmed by reinforcement but not sit under the signal predicting the omission of reinforcement. The instrumental response of sitting per se is not affected by this training arrangement. What is affected is the stimulus control exercised by the two signals over the emission of the sit response. In the case of positive reinforcement, learning is based on the acquisition of a promised or hoped-for outcome in the form of a reward. In avoidance training, learning is based on behavior that successfully avoids the presentation of an aversive stimulus together with the concurrent production of emotional *relief* or relaxation as the result of having removed (postponed or avoided) the impending threat. Both positive and negative reinforcement paradigms depend on learned expectancies based on a history of confirmatory outcomes. These paradigms of learning are usually considered as two separate ways in which learning takes place. Viewing them as two sides of a single process within a broader context of expectancy and confirmation helps to clarify the nature of learning itself, and the respective role each reinforcement paradigm plays in the learning process.

SAFETY SIGNAL HYPOTHESIS

Another theoretical account of avoidance learning that has many adherents is the safety signal hypothesis. The aforementioned experiment by Rescorla and LoLordo (1965) is frequently referred to in support of this theory. Recall that as a result of the differential conditioning of CS1 (correlated with shock) and CS2 (correlated with the absence of shock), the rate of jumping over the barrier was increased in the presence of the stimulus previously associated with shock (CS1) and depressed in the presence of the tone stimulus that had been previously conditioned to predict the absence of shock (CS2). In the presence of the CS2 or safety signal, the dogs appeared to feel more relaxed or *safe* even though the signal had no real relevance to the actual arrangement of the avoidance contingencies involved.

The safety-relaxation theory suggests that dogs experience stimuli associated with relief from aversive stimulation as though they were positive reinforcers. These observations are relevant to traditional dog-training methodology. In addition to establishing various conditioned associations with rewards (e.g., food and ball play), praise represents a safety signal of some importance and usefulness. Interestingly, within the context of behavioral training, *praise* appears to derive a significant portion of its associative strength and reward value from its being paired regularly with the pleasurable relief occurring immediately after the corrective event. Because praise consistently *predicts* the absence of aversive stimulation and is paired with emotional relief from aversive stimulation, it gradually becomes highly desirable in itself and may be treated as a kind of conditioned positive reinforcer.

A leading proponent of the safety-relaxation theory of avoidance learning is M. Ray Denny (1971). His theory owes heavily to the stimulus-response contiguity theories of Pavlov and Guthrie. According to Denny, avoidance responding is acquired through the antagonistic dynamics of fear and relief-relaxation. Within the context of aversive situations in which fearful withdrawal or escape reactions result in the termination of the fear-eliciting stimuli involved, relief or relaxation responses are subsequently elicited that mediate approach behavior. These successive relief and relaxation responses serve to reinforce avoidance behavior. Relief and relaxation are differentiated along two primary dimensions: (1) Relief occurs shortly after the offset of the aversive stimulus and decays rapidly, whereas the onset of relaxation is both delayed and longer lasting. (2) Relief involves a strong autonomic factor, whereas relaxation involves striatal muscles and various motoric components. Relief begins approximately 3 to 5 seconds after the withdrawal of aversive stimulation and continues for 10 to 15 seconds. Relaxation, on the other hand, is a more sluggish response, requiring approximately 2.5 minutes to produce full benefits. Ideally, avoidance training should include conditioned safety or relief signals that are presented 2 to 5 seconds after the termination of aversive stimulation and continued for several seconds thereafter (Denny, 1976). The intertrial interval between exposures should be at least 2.5 minutes for optimally efficient avoidance training. Denny noted that "the effects of safety appear to double when both relief and relaxation, rather than one of them, are associated with a particular stimulus" (Denny, 1983). Such safety signals take on conditioned positive-reinforcing properties. Experimental support for this general idea has been reported by Weisman and Litner (1969), who demonstrated that behavior maintained on a Sidman avoidance schedule could be differentially increased or decreased by presenting a CS that had been previously associated with relief from aversive stimulation.

Not only does relaxation positively support avoidance learning, it also simultaneously results in its gradual extinction. Extinction occurs as the result of *backchaining* and counterconditioning effects originating in the safe, relaxed situation and generalizing step by step back to the original aversive situation.

After many trials of avoidance learning, previously feared stimuli belonging to the aversive situation are backchained and counterconditioned by the relaxation and comfort associated with safety.

Tortora (1983) applied the principles of safety training to the treatment of avoidance-motivated aggression in dogs. According to his assessment, aggressive behavior commonly diagnosed as dominance related is often the result of dysfunctional avoidance responding:

> The dogs in this study initially behaved as if they "expected" aversive events and that the only way to prevent these events was through aggression. The consequent reaction of the victim and the family, that is, withdrawal, turmoil, and belated punishment, confirmed the dog's "expectation" and reinforced the aggression. This positive feedback loop produced progressive escalation of the aggressive response, and the avoidance nature of the aggression presumably retarded or prevented its extinction. (1983:209)

The dogs were trained under a variety of conditions to perform 15 behaviorally "balanced" exercises or, as he calls them, operands. An important aspect of Tortora's study was the systematic pairing of a 3-second safety tone with the offset of shock delivered by an electronic collar. The training trials were spaced according to a variable interval of 5 minutes (ranging from 2 to 8 minutes), well within the 2.5-minute intertrial interval recommended by the relaxation theory. Between trials, the dogs were engaged in play. As a result of safety conditioning, the tone gradually became classically associated with relief and relaxation, becoming a conditioned positive reinforcer sufficient to strengthen cooperative prosocial behavior—behavior incompatible with aggression. According to Tortora, an important aspect of intensive avoidance and safety training is that it provides dogs with an alternative nonaggressive coping pattern when exposed to provocative or aversive situations. Tortora noted that dogs appeared to become more and more confident as they progressed through the various stages of training from avoidance to safety.

Another source of theoretical support for

the safety-relaxation theory of avoidance learning comes from opponent-process theory (Solomon and Corbit, 1974), which postulates that the offset of any hedonically significant stimulus results in a recoil of opposing emotional reactions (see Chapter 6). The withdrawal of aversive stimulation evokes opposing pleasurable emotional reactions. When an aversive stimulus is terminated, the opposing pleasurable recoil provides a source of covert reinforcement, either strengthening desirable alternative behavior or inadvertently reinforcing undesirable behavior.

Following the application of aversive stimulation, it is vital that some positive behavior be selected and prompted. Applying aversive stimulation without providing dogs with an opportunity to perform some alternative option risks the possibility that an undesirable competitive pattern, like running away or avoiding the owner, might be strengthened. The somewhat common practice of isolating or ignoring dogs after punishment is counterproductive from this perspective and should be assiduously avoided. The most efficient aversive events are those that simultaneously suppress an unwanted behavior while evoking a more desirable or incompatible alternative to take its place. This arrangement is commonly used during formal obedience training where unwanted behavior is suppressed by timely correction, which in turn prompts the desired response. A well-designed correction always functions in this dual manner.

Relief may by usefully employed in conjunction with aversive counterconditioning. A common behavior problem seen among puppies and dogs involves inappropriate appetitive interests, that is, attraction to some forbidden object as a chew item. By exposing a dog to a sufficiently aversive-startling stimulus at the moment the object is approached, the dog will quickly acquire a negative conditioned association with the item (determines that it is unsafe) and avoid it in the future. Interest and approach are replaced by distrust and avoidance as a result of the startling experience. Recognizing that a corresponding degree of pleasurable relief is bound up with the event, it is advisable to present the dog with an alternative, safe chew item shortly after applying the startle. Opposing the startle response are opponent approach-appetitive recoil affects associated with relief that help to make the alternative item more attractive and desirable.

SPECIES-SPECIFIC DEFENSIVE REACTIONS AND AVOIDANCE TRAINING

Some interesting speculation on avoidance learning has advanced the idea that animals undergoing aversive stimulation respond in species-specific ways, thereby facilitating some forms of avoidance learning while impeding others (Bolles, 1970, 1973). According to Bolles (1970), animals are innately prepared to react to novel or startling stimuli with a limited set of defensive behaviors. These species-specific defensive reactions (SSDRs) do not depend on learning for their expression: they are motivationally and topographically stereotypic, possess an evolutionary significance, and exhibit a low threshold for expression:

> What keeps animals alive in the wild is that they have very effective innate defensive reactions which occur when they encounter any kind of new or sudden stimulus. ... The mouse does not scamper away from the owl because it has learned to escape the painful claws of the enemy; it scampers away from anything happening in its environment, and it does so merely because it is a mouse. The gazelle does not flee from an approaching lion because it has been bitten by lions; it runs away from any large object that approaches it, and it does so because this is one of it species-specific defensive reactions. Neither the mouse nor the gazelle can afford to learn to avoid; survival is too urgent, the opportunity to learn is too limited, and the parameters of the situation make the necessary learning impossible. The animal which survives is one which comes into its environment with defensive reactions already a prominent part of its repertoire. (1970:33)

Bolles has argued that SSDRs can either facilitate or impede avoidance training. Depending on the species involved, aversive stimulation evokes varying degrees of immobilization, flight, or active defensive reactions.

Avoidance or escape responses that are similar to an animal's natural defensive repertoire are most easily learned; in the language of Seligman (1970), the responses are *prepared*, whereas those avoidance responses that are dissimilar or incompatible with the animal's natural defensive repertoire are either *unprepared* or *contraprepared* for such training. For instance, teaching rats to lever press to avoid shock is relatively hard to accomplish. In comparison, training rats to jump over a low hurdle or to run to the opposite side of a training compartment is much more easily attained. Ostensibly, jumping and running are high-priority defensive reactions in rats, whereas lever pressing is not. The latter response may be more directly associated with appetitive-consummatory activity associated with the search for food and eating it.

Hineline and Harrison (1979) challenged Bolles's theory of prepotent species-specific avoidance responding. In a series of experiments, they compared the differential acquisition of lever pressing with that of lever biting in rats. The operative assumption was that lever biting should prove innately prepotent over lever pressing and, therefore, be learned more rapidly. Instead, they found that rats actually learned lever pressing more rapidly than lever biting. Their findings, however, are not inconsistent with predictions based on Bolles's SSDR theory of avoidance learning. The study simply demonstrates that lever biting is not prepotent over lever pressing in rats. The researchers appear to have been misled by a presumption that defensive aggression ought to be prepotent over other escape-avoidance actions, such as lever pressing. In fact, under conditions of aversive stimulation, attack may not be prepotent over other escape possibilities. Azrin and colleagues (1967) found that escape was typically dominant over attack in rats and was only likely to occur when (1) escape was otherwise not possible or (2) when the escape requirements were too difficult. Also, although attack behavior tended to interfere with escape behavior during the acquisitional phases of training, this early attack behavior quickly diminished as the escape response was mastered.

In dogs, many competing SSDRs occur during the early stages of obedience training. According to Bolles, "The trick in the avoidance situation is to punish all of the wrong responses so that the right response will occur" (1973:299). Dogs being trained with forceful methods typically react by systematically experimenting with various defensive postures and reactions that are prepotent to the dog as a species. These defensive behaviors range from bolting and jumping up, to dropping down and freezing; balking and struggling to pull away, or biting the leash. Some dogs exhibit a wide variety of passive submissive displays or, in the opposite extreme, occasionally threaten or snap at the handler. The early stages of avoidance training (really punishment training) involve systematically suppressing these innate defensive reactions and replacing them with forcefully prompted alternatives. Only once all defensive reactions are punitively suppressed or reduced to the *obedient* target response does systematic and formal avoidance training begin.

PUNISHMENT

Punishment is an inescapable fact of life. From a behavioral perspective, punishment is everywhere, defining what will and will not occur without discomfort or disappointment. Taken together, the escape-avoidance of aversive events and the acquisition-maximization of rewarding ones form the yin and yang of behavior. Confucius discerned the importance of difficult trials in one's life: "The gem cannot be polished without friction, nor man perfected without trials." Similarly, Aristotle extolled the virtues of pleasure and pain for achieving the "happy life." In his *Nicomachean Ethics* (1985), he writes,

> For pleasure is shared with animals, and implied by every object of choice, since what is fine and what is expedient appear pleasant as well.
>
> Further, since pleasure grows up with all of us from infancy on, it is hard to rub out this feeling that is dyed into our lives; and we estimate actions as well [as feelings], some of us more, some less, by pleasure and pain. Hence, our whole inquiry must be about these, since

good or bad enjoyment or pain is very important for our actions. (1985:38)

Later, he expands on this general theme:

> The next task, presumably, is to discuss pleasure. For it seems to be especially proper to our kind, and hence when we educate children we steer them by pleasure and pain. Besides, enjoying and hating the right things seems to be most important for virtue of character. For pleasure and pain extend through the whole of our lives, and are of great importance for virtue and the happy life, since people decide to do what is pleasant, and avoid what is painful. (1985:266)

Properly understood, reward and punishment are morally neutral, the one being neither better nor worse than the other. Both outcomes serve equally vital functions in perfecting an animal's adaptation to the social and physical environment. Learning to respond and cope appropriately with the treats and trials of life is an important part of normal development for dogs and humans alike. One need but think about walking into the path of a moving car, cheating on one's spouse, approaching a snarling dog, or stepping on a pin to feel the inhibitory and protective benefits of punishment. Although punishment is unpleasant, precisely that aspect makes it so beneficial and useful. It is far better to experience a little fear or pain than to be severely injured or utterly destroyed as the result of its absence.

Definition

The terms *punishment* and *negative reinforcement* are often used vaguely or interchangeably with each other. However, punishment and negative reinforcement operate in quite different ways and serve entirely different functions. Although punishment and negative reinforcement often occur together, by definition, punishment is functionally the opposite of negative reinforcement. A behavior is negatively reinforced when its emission is made more likely in the future as a result of its either avoiding or terminating the presentation of an aversive event. In contrast, punishment occurs when the emission of a behavior is made less likely by the presenta-

tion of an aversive event (positive punishment) or by the withdrawal of a desirable one (negative punishment). *Negative punishment* (P−) causes an effect opposite to that of positive reinforcement. Conversely, *positive punishment* (P+) results in an effect opposite to that of negative reinforcement. Both positive and negative reinforcement function to strengthen behavior, whereas the function of punishment is to weaken it. With this functional consideration in mind, Azrin and Holz (1966) defined *punishment* as "a consequence of behavior that reduces the future probability of that behavior" (1966:381). Punishment has one functional purpose: the suppression of the punished behavior. Through punishment, dogs learn that performing a particular act turns on an aversive event (P+) or results in the loss of a desirable one (P−). Given that the punitive event (positive or negative punisher) is sufficiently aversive or costly, dogs will be less likely to emit the punished behavior in the future—that is, the behavior has been suppressed.

Critics of Punishment

Unfortunately, not only is punishment often poorly understood as a behavioral procedure, it is just as often bogged down in dire warnings of serious side effects and, more importantly, the false view that it does not work. Understanding how these criticisms and myths developed begins with a look at how Thorndike viewed punishment. Initially, Thorndike (1911/1965) believed that the effects of reward and punishment were symmetrical opposites, with the former strengthening behavior while the latter weakened it. In his later writings, this original formulation of the *law of effect* underwent significant modification (Hilgard and Bower, 1975). These changes came about as the result of additional animal and human studies that Thorndike carried out using mild (annoying) punishment. Briefly, for example, in one study with human subjects learning a vocabulary task, he found that the social reward or satisfier "right" helped participants to learn correct verbal responses, but the punisher or annoyer "wrong" failed to produce a corresponding decrease in the overall number of mistakes made by the subjects. In another study involving punishment of animals, he trained chicks to choose between three arms of a simple maze. Choosing the correct arm led to a compartment containing other chicks eating grain (strong social and appetitive incentives). Choosing the wrong arm resulted in social isolation for 30 seconds. He found that correct choices were stamped in, but incorrect ones, contrary to predictions based on the original law of effect, were not stamped out. These findings led him to conclude that punishment was less efficacious than reward. Unfortunately, as will be recognized by astute readers, the foregoing experiments prove only that the punishers used in his experiments were insufficient to suppress the target behaviors being punished. Neither experiment says anything very significant about the effects of punishment per se, but only that the punishment procedures employed were not very effective. Despite the absence of much in the way of strong evidence, Thorndike (1931) and his colleagues eagerly generalized from such findings as the foregoing to conclude that punishment, as a rule, did not weaken instrumental behavior. While he still recognized the power of punishment to disrupt behavior, he no longer believed that punishment was an adequate and efficient means for altering learned connections:

> Annoyers do not act on learning in general by weakening whatever connection they follow. If they do anything in learning, they do it indirectly, by informing the learner that such and such a response in such and such a situation brings distress, or by making the learner feel fear of a certain object, or by making him jump back from a certain place, or by some other definite and specific change which they produce in him. (1931:46)

Thorndike and his followers subsequently collected and published numerous testimonials and tracts in support of the superior effectiveness of reward to bolster this somewhat extreme and counterintuitive position with respect to punishment (Hilgard and Bower, 1975).

Following in the tradition of Thorndike, B. F. Skinner (1974) also viewed the effects of reward and punishment asymmetrically, placing far greater emphasis on the use of positive reinforcement for altering and controlling behavior than he attributed to punishment and negative reinforcement. Despite a large body of contrary evidence, Skinner believed that punishment exercised a temporary influence over behavior and was loaded with negative side effects. He argued along with Thorndike that punishment only transiently disrupts behavior, causing emotional disturbances and behavioral disorganization—not suppression. According to Skinner, punished behavior tends to recover quickly once the punitive contingency is withdrawn, and the animals are given time to recover their shaken composure. This position has been criticized by leading behavior analysts, including Hineline:

> Within behavior analysis, Skinner has consistently advocated keeping punishment in a separate domain. Initially, the balance of data supported that view. ... However, Skinner has continued to argue—in the face of accumulating contrary data—that punishment procedures produce only indirect effects on behavior, and has emphasized temporary effects of punishment when punishment procedures are discontinued. Of course reinforcement procedures are similarly temporary when reinforcement procedures are discontinued. (1984:496)

Perhaps, the most important consideration influencing Skinner's rejection of punishment was a concern about its potential for producing private (distress) and social adverse side effects, especially evasion or retaliation. Although aversive stimulation is capable of evoking serious side effects, they usually occur under specific conditions and as the result of abusive treatment—not punishment. Murray Sidman (1989) has written at length regarding the various side effects and problematic features associated with *coercive* methods of control. In the tradition of Thorndike and Skinner, Sidman argues (sometimes convincingly, sometimes emotionally) that most behavioral manipulations and modifications can be achieved without resorting to aversive methods. There can be little disagreement with the selection of training methods that utilize positive reinforcement whenever possible, but to exclude punishment arbitrarily from a trainer's armamentarium would be counterproductive and artificial.

Although Thorndike's revised opinions about punishment were subsequently repudiated, his emphasis on reward training provided a propitious rebuttal against an equally extreme distortion about the superior efficacy of punishment current at the turn of the century. The primacy and effectiveness of punishment was vigorously defended by many parents, educators, and dog trainers. According to S. T. Hammond, dog training during this time was often an unpleasant and grueling process for dogs; he lamented over the severity of his contemporaries and their excessive reliance on force for *breaking* their hunting dogs:

> Nearly all writers upon the subject of the dog agree that there is but one course to pursue; that all knowledge that is not beaten into a dog is worthless for all practical purposes and that the whip, check-cord and spike-collar, with perhaps an occasional charge of shot or a vigorous dose of shoe leather, are absolutely necessary in order to perfect his education. (1894:1)

Since this early call for reform, a tremendous amount of progress has been made in the art and science of dog training, making it both more rational and humane. Similarly, Skinner's positive contribution to rational training methodology cannot be overly praised and should be the object of intensive and thorough study by anyone aspiring to become a professional dog trainer. However, and with all due respect for the accomplishments of both Thorndike and Skinner, some of their more extreme views about punishment must be questioned in the light of scientific advances and the empirical findings derived from practical experience.

Since Thorndike's time, the pendulum has swung from a stubborn reliance on punishment and negative reinforcement to an equally unnatural extreme in which the use of punishment and negative reinforcement (in some quarters) is shunned to embrace a so-called "positive" approach to training and behavioral control. Extreme positions, whether based on good intentions or not, are typically based on irrational beliefs and assumptions—not scientific knowledge and experience. The adoption of an exclusive reliance on punishment or reward alone reflects a core of misunderstanding about how dog behavior is most efficiently modified. Such positions are doomed to miss the mark, since they are based on a distortion of the subject matter and basic facts. Montaigne, in his essay *Of Moderation*, wrote correctly with respect to extremist positions: "The archer who overshoots his mark does no better than he who falls short of it. My eyes trouble me as much in climbing upward toward a great light as in going down into the dark." Despite the current wave of vocal enthusiasm and polarizing debate about the virtues of positive reinforcement and the evils of punishment, the vast majority of dog trainers and behaviorists remain pragmatic opportunists about the use of reward and punishment—that is, they do what *works* within the context of practical considerations and ethical standards. Punishment is unpleasant (both for dogs and for trainers) and, whenever possible, reward-based instead of punishment-based methods should be used, but sometimes the effects of punishment are simply more expedient, reliable, and enduring than the results of positive reinforcement alone. Certainly, there are occasions when punishment and other aversive training procedures simply cannot be avoided, where "punishment procedures even provide the most effective basis for humanely achieving social good" (Hineline, 1984:496). Punishment is especially beneficial in cases in which a dog's unwanted behavior endangers either the dog itself or others with whom the dog comes into contact. In such cases, where an immediate and more or less permanent change is needed, punishment has many advantages over positive reinforcement. Of course, humane trainers select the least intrusive punishment necessary to achieve their behavioral objectives and strive to minimize its use whenever possible. The aim of punishment is to eliminate the use of punishment in the future. Instead of extreme positions, accusatory innuendo, moralizing, and half-truths, what is needed is a balanced and informed attitude regarding the practical use, misuse, and abuse of punishment.

A similar controversy is ongoing among applied behavior analysts and other practitioners using *gentle teaching* procedures to instruct persons suffering mental retardation and other debilitating disorders (Jones and McCaughey, 1992). Advocates of gentle teaching emphasize the importance of bonding, mutual change, trust, and accommodation—that is, the formation of a fulfilling and reciprocal relationship between clients and caregivers. There is nothing inherently inconsistent with these worthy goals and behavior modification, except that *gentle teachers* believe that such goals should be attained through nonaversive means *only*. Consequently, they reject any use of aversive training measures as "sinful" and dismiss the behavioral approach as a "culture of death" based on "deliberate torture." This sort of divisive polarization of views is also evident in some camps of quarreling dog-behavior modifiers, especially those regarding a similarly one-sided gentle-training approach as the only humane approach to dog training.

Does Punishment Work?

In Lewis Carroll's "The Hunting of the Snark," the Bellman woos his crew to believe that truth is sanctioned by his earnest repetition of some statement—no matter how false or ludicrous it happens to be:

> "Just the place for a Snark!" the Bellman cried,
> As he landed his crew with care;
> Supporting each man on the top of the tide
> By a finger entwined in his hair.
>
> "Just the place for a Snark! I have said it twice:
> That alone should encourage the crew.
> Just the place for a Snark! I have said it thrice:
> What I tell you three times is true."

Many critics of punishment seem to be guided by a similar criterion of truth, believing that the heartfelt repetition of a falsehood is enough to make it true. Despite the lingering historical influences already discussed and contemporary efforts to misrepresent its usefulness, the efficacy of punishment is not really in doubt, especially if science is accepted as the final arbiter of the debate. The facts are clear and indisputable: When applied properly (promptly and in the correct measure), punishment works, it works quickly and, in many cases, the suppressive effects of punishment are permanent. Among several hundred

scientific studies demonstrating the efficacy of punishment, Azrin and Holz state the situation in certain and unambiguous terms:

> One of the most dramatic characteristics of punishment is the virtual irreversibility or permanence of the response reduction once the behavior has become completely suppressed. Investigators have noted that the punished response does not recover for a long period of time even after the punishment contingency has been removed. ... How quickly does punishment reduce behavior? Virtually all studies of punishment have been in complete agreement that the reduction of responses by punishment is immediate if the punishment is at all effective. When the data have been presented in terms of the number of responses per day, the responses have been drastically reduced or eliminated on the very first day in which punishment was administered. (1966:410)

Although it is true, as Skinner noted, that mildly punished behaviors tend to recover when the punitive contingency is discontinued, a comparable effect is also observed in the case of behavior under the control of positive reinforcement. Both punished behavior and rewarded behavior tend to recover or extinguish when the punitive or reinforcing contingency is withdrawn. The main difference between positive reinforcement and punishment in this regard is that the latter appears to exert a much more rapid and permanent modification of behavior than produced by the former. In response to Skinner's assertion that "punishment is ineffective," John Staddon writes,

> Well, no, it isn't. Common sense aside, laboratory studies with pigeons and rats (the basis for Skinner's argument) show that punishment (usually a brief electric shock) works very well to suppress behavior, as long as it is of the right magnitude and follows promptly on the behavior that is to be suppressed. If a rat gets a moderate shock when he presses a bar, he stops pressing it more or less at once. ... Does the punished behavior return when the punishment is withdrawn? That depends on the training procedure. An avoidance procedure called shock postponement, in which the rat gets no shock so long as he presses the bar once in a while, produces behavior that can persist indef-

initely when the shock schedule is withdrawn. (1995:92)

Besides misrepresenting and confusing the facts, excessive moralizing about the use of punishment and other aversive training procedures may have a very undesirable effect on the dog-owning public, making responsible owners feel guilty about exercising the necessary aversive prerogatives needed to establish constructive limits and boundaries over a dog's behavior. Many of the basic facts of life that all dogs must learn to accept (if they are to become successful and welcome companions) are won through the mediation of directive training, combining a balanced application of behavior modification—not just positive reinforcement. Instead of grinding away at a very dull ax, a dog's welfare is better served by teaching the owner when punishment is necessary and how to use it effectively and humanely.

Punishment and "Neurosis"

A reasonable concern underlying the rejection of punishment is its potential role in the etiology of *neurosis* in dogs. This concern is validated by a considerable body of experimental literature. Numerous studies (e.g., by Pavlov, Wolpe, Masserman, Liddell, Maier, and Seligman) have confirmed the dangers of aversive stimulation under certain conditions—concerns that are discussed in detail in the following chapter. Puppies exposed to excessive physical punishment may be more difficult to manage later as the result of the lasting effects of traumatic stress. Abusive treatment and stressful rearing practices are associated with many of the following symptoms, all of which have a direct relevance for the welfare and development of dogs: (1) hypervigilance and irrational fear, (2) heightened irritability, (3) impulsive-explosive behavior, (4) hyperactivity, (5) aggression evoked with minimum provocation, (6) withdrawal and social avoidance, (7) anhedonia (loss of sensitivity to pleasure and pain), and (8) depressed mood. Most cases in which punishment is associated with serious side effects involve rather special applications of punishment. Especially important are such

factors as intensity, predictability, and control—vital factors in the effect and side effects of punishment. Solomon (1964) noted four specific conditions that are necessary for punishment to result in maladaptive behavior: (1) the stimulation generates vigorous and sustained emotional arousal, (2) the stimulation is unpredictable, (3) the stimulation is uncontrollable, and (4) the stimulation is inescapable. All of these criteria are often satisfied by a common form of aversive stimulation: *noncontingent punishment*. The habit of "punishing" a dog long after the behavioral event has occurred does little more than confuse the dog, while quite possibly damaging the dog's trust and affection for the owner. Horace Lytle deftly summarized the adverse effects of unpredictable and uncontrollable aversive stimulation long before the concept of *learned helplessness* was formally articulated: "A dog which is always expecting punishment—never quite sure when it is going to come, and never quite sure why it is being administered—that sort of a dog never amounts to much. And he isn't given a chance to amount to much" (1927:xvi). Such treatment is not punishment at all; it is simply irrational and ineffectual abuse that should be strictly abstained from by professional dog trainers and behaviorists.

Positive Side Effects

Although negative side effects obviously occur and should be carefully assessed before employing punishment, most of these side effects can be minimized. Some side effects of punishment, however, may actually be beneficial (Kazdin, 1989). Punitive events often help to set and enforce social boundaries, promote impulse control, reinforce social status, and provide various other generalized effects that assure an optimal adaptation to the social and physical environment. Many researchers have reported a variety of beneficial side effects directly resulting from the use of punishment, including improved social behavior and cooperation, increased emotional responsiveness and positive mood, the appearance of more appropriate play behavior and other constructive activities, and improved attentional behavior (Newsom et al.,

1983). Even side effects that might be considered adverse may have a beneficial aspect to them, as Azrin and Holz point out:

> When we punish a response, our primary concern is to reduce the frequency of that response. If we have not overlooked the effects of the reinforcement variables or the discriminative variables, there is every reason to believe that our punishment procedure will be completely effective in eliminating the undesired response. The emotional state or enduring behavioral disruption of the punished subject are not necessarily undesirable outcomes of punishment; nor are the severity of the response reduction or the behavioral generalization of the punishing effects undesirable. In fact all of these effects are probably quite useful where a physical punishment is concerned, from an evolutionary point of view, in reducing the future likelihood of painful and possibly destructive events. (1966:442)

The primary negative side effects of punishment are related to its improper use and various disruptive social effects (e.g., fear or aggression directed toward the punishing agent/situation), but punishment is not alone in its potential for producing troubling side effects. Staddon points out that positive reinforcement can produce similar problems:

> Positive reinforcement also provokes counterattack. Every student who cheats, every gambler who rigs the odds, every robber and thief, shows the counterattack provided by positive reinforcement schedules. (1995:93)

Coercive Compulsion and Conflict

Not unexpectedly, aversive events frequently generate high levels of conflict and generalized arousal; effects that may lead to problems if not carefully managed. Problematical aversive compulsion is most commonly found in two general dog-training applications, what Konrad Most (1910/1955) called *compulsive inducement* of action or abstention from action:

Inducing action. Compulsion is applied to *induce* a dog to execute an *action* that it does not want to perform. Under the influence of compulsion, the dog is wedged between two opposing possibilities: performing an undesirable action or being compelled by force (primary inducement) or threat of force (secondary inducement) to perform it. This sort of aversive situation may trigger an avoidance-avoidance conflict, requiring the dog to choose between two equally undesirable alternatives.

Compelling abstention. Compulsion is applied to *compel* a dog to *abstain* from executing an action that the dog wants to perform. In this case, the dog is conflicted between its desire to consummate the forbidden action and the pending threat of aversive stimulation if it fails to abstain from doing so. When the aversiveness of compulsion is motivationally equal to the reward value of the forbidden activity, then a disruptive approach-avoidance conflict may ensue.

These two uses of compulsion correspond to what most trainers refer to as a *correction*. When properly applied in practical dog training, such methods can be efficient and useful. However, such procedures are often used improperly or abusively. Compulsion may produce severe conflicts as the result of a collision of opposing motivational interests. Since conflict has been implicated in the development of experimental neurosis and displacement stereotypies, such treatment as abusive compulsion should be avoided.

Another potential hazard with the use of compulsion is that it may block or interfere with the natural functioning and satisfaction of the targeted behavioral system, possibly generating some degree of internal disruption (stress) and homeostatic imbalance. Behavioral outlets for drive satisfaction are necessary for healthy emotional development and equilibrium in dogs. Often, however, these innate drives are expressed in undesirable behavior that must be modified or redirected for the sake of domestic harmony. Although aversive techniques are often relied upon to achieve such ends, they are not always necessary or desirable. Seven other possible behavioral techniques should be considered before resorting to punishment: (1) modify the unwanted behavior into an acceptable form, (2) modify the environment so that the unwanted behavior cannot be performed, (3) redirect the unwanted behavior into a more acceptable outlet, (4) bring the behavior under stimulus control and then signal for it only under acceptable conditions, (5) modify the reinforcement contingencies maintaining the behavior (extinction), (6) select and reinforce an alternative behavior that is incompatible with the undesirable behavior, and (7) in the case of intrinsically reinforced behavior, bring the behavior under the control of an extrinsic reinforcer and then extinguish it. When punishment must be used, it is most effectively employed in a training context where the punished behavior is replaced by an alternative behavior that is subsequently brought under the control of positive reinforcement. Unless the punished behavior is replaced with an adequate substitute, the effect of punishment may be temporary, requiring that it be applied over and over again with diminishing net results.

Another important factor is the strength of the aversive event employed as punishment. The punitive event should be strong enough to evoke an incompatible response to the behavior being punished. Insufficiently strong punishment may only excite dogs, perhaps serving more as a reinforcing event (i.e., negative attention) than a punitive one. Ideally, the cessation of the punitive event and the emotional *relief* associated with its withdrawal ought to coincide with the emission of an appropriate alternative behavior. Therefore, an efficient punishment should consist of at least two elements: (1) punishment should result in the dog emitting some behavior incompatible with the one being punished and (2) the emission of this alternative behavior should occur with the onset of relief from punishment. Unfortunately, sometimes relief from punishment reinforces an equally unwanted behavior. For example, a jumping dog might be successfully punished for jumping up during greeting only to learn to urinate submissively instead when the owner comes home.

Finally, above all other training procedures, punishment requires great knowledge, practical experience, compassion, refined and expert skills, and, most importantly, self-mas-

tery. C. B. Whitford pretty much sums things up with the following sage advice about punishment in a chapter entitled "Breaking the Breaker":

> The rule to follow is: Do as little breaking as possible; try to encourage the dog to do the proper things and develop him as much as possible with the least amount of control. As a final word to the breaker, it may be said that he should so educate himself that he will know that it is always wise, when in doubt, to give the dog the benefit of that doubt. Not only should he know this, but he must have such complete control of his feelings as to give his knowledge effect. The breaker who spends much time in considering his own weaknesses will profit by his effort. (1908/1928:20–21)

P+ AND P−: A SHARED EMOTIONAL AND COGNITIVE SUBSTRATE?

As discussed previously in Chapter 6, Konorski (1967) proposed that classical conditioning be analyzed in terms of preparatory and consummatory components. The *preparatory component* includes all the various drive and emotional factors underlying the event, whereas the *consummatory component* refers to the specific appetitive or defensive actions elicited. He argued that preparatory or emotional factors are prepotent over consummatory elements during the conditioning process—that is, learning depends more on emotion than consummatory reflexive actions. This raises a question regarding the emotional substrates underlying punishment. As previously discussed, punishment takes two basic forms: the withdrawal of rewards or the presentation of aversive stimulation. Studies utilizing Kamin's (1968) blocking effect indicate that a similar emotional substrate is involved during both forms of punishment, whether the punitive event is the withdrawal of reward (negative punishment) or the presentation of an aversive event (positive punishment). The blocking effect refers to a phenomenon observed when a compound stimulus is presented (CS1 and CS2) where CS1 has been previously paired with the reinforcing US (e.g., shock). Under an arrangement where CS1 (tone) and CS2 (light) are subsequently presented together, the tone will *overshadow* the light stimulus, causing the latter to remain neutral with regard to the reinforcing US (shock). CS1 is said to absorb all the associative strength that the US can support.

To determine whether negative punishment and positive punishment function similarly, the following experiment could be performed. First a clicker (CS) is paired with food (US) until a strong conditioned response is evident. The second part of the experiment involves presenting a light stimulus together with the previously conditioned clicker, but this combination is never followed by food. Pairing the clicker with the presentation of food generates a strong conditioned response to the sound of the clicker. In the second case, however (where the clicker and light are presented without food), conditioned inhibition (no response) occurs—that is, the compound stimulus composed of the light and clicker predicts no food. Let's take this analysis one step further. Returning to the aforementioned blocking experiment where shock was used as the US, what would occur if the light stimulus previously compounded with the clicker (predicting the absence of food) was compounded with a neutral tone stimulus and paired with shock? This is precisely what Dickinson and Dearing (1979) set out to determine in a similar experiment. Interestingly, the researchers found that the light CS1 blocks conditioning of the tone CS2. This is a rather astonishing result, since the light stimulus had never been actually associated with shock, yet it was able to block conditioning of the neutral tone stimulus.

How might this result be interpreted? It appears as though at some level the animal experiences the loss of reward in much the same way it experiences the presentation of an aversive stimulus. Mackintosh (1983) considered this possibility and argued, using Konorski's paradigm, that the preparatory emotions experienced during aversive stimulation are actually very similar to those experienced during the withdrawal of an anticipated food reward—that is, the feelings elicited by the withdrawal of reward are emotionally analogous to those elicited by aversive stimulation. Although the preparatory emotions associated with the two forms of punishment are not identical, their significant emotional impact is identified as though they were the same—that is, they are associatively linked or identified with the same emotional substrate. Theoretically, such a linkage between positive and negative punishment is a very important finding. These distinct modes of punitive stimulation are obviously differentiated on a physiological level. The only way to identify the two is via an independent organizing concept or shared hedonic category, like "not good" or "disappointment" (i.e., a mediating cognitive construct). If the foregoing interpretation is accurate, it may be misleading to view negative punishment (e.g., extinction) as being significantly "better" emotionally than positive punishment (e.g., shock). Both forms of punishment can cause great anxiety, frustration, and distress if not skillfully employed. On the level of emotional integration, punishment is punishment. Panksepp, while discussing various distinctions between hedonic affects and true emotions from psychobiological perspective, speculated along similar lines of analysis:

> Certainly at the broad functional level, pleasure is a property of external stimuli which help sustain life, while feelings of aversion arise from stimuli which tend to be incompatible with survival. In the simplest brain scenario, it may turn out that the affective properties of various stimuli funnel into a few, perhaps just two, primary affective processes—generalized pleasure (such as might be mediated by brain opioids and/or dopamine) and generalized aversion (perhaps by anti-opioids and anti-dopaminergics)—with the multitude of apparent distinctions being the result of non-affective sensory details. (1988:44)

PUNISHERS, REWARDS, AND VERIFIERS

Whether a given stimulus event is interpreted by a dog as a punitive one or a rewarding one depends on the dog's moment-to-moment motivational state and learning history. As previously discussed in Chapter 7, giving a fully satiated dog a treat may actually function punitively—that is, the dog may experience the ingestion of food when not hungry as an aversive event. Similarly, a dog that has been exercised to the point of exhaustion will view an opportunity to play very differently than at some other time when the dog is well rested. In general, the provision of anything that the dog would rather be doing at any given moment may function as a reward. On the other hand, anything that the dog would rather not be doing at any given moment might be used as an effective punisher. This general motivational interpretation of reward and punishment has been elegantly described by Premack (1962).

It is useful to interpret ongoing behavior in terms of a *field* of learned *expectations* and controlling *signs*. Dogs make fine predictions from moment to moment based on past experiences, including the identification of signs anticipating future events. In the words of Tolman (1934), "A conditioned reflex, when learned, is an acquired expectation-set on the part of the animal that the feature of the field corresponding to the conditioned stimulus will lead, *if the animal but waits*, to the feature of the field corresponding to the unconditioned stimulus" (1934:393). A common example of classical conditioning in dog training involves the bridging stimulus. Consistently saying "Good" just before giving the dog a piece of food teaches the dog to expect a treat on each occasion it hears the vocal signal. What happens, however, if the vocal signal "Good" is presented independently of the presentation of food—that is, when it is randomly paired or not paired so that the animal cannot predict the actual outcome on any given trial?

Rescorla's (1968, 1988) laboratory findings indicate that if an animal is exposed to random shocks that are signaled only 50% of the time by a tone stimulus but unsignaled the remaining 50% of the time, the result is that the tone will fail to develop as a CS— that is, the animal will fail to respond to the tone as a predictive signal for the occurrence or nonoccurrence of the US (shock). Such stimulus neutrality occurs in spite of many positive pairings between the tone and the US, since the positive pairings are offset by an equal number of US events occurring in the absence of the tone. In this case, the tone equally fails to predict the absence or the presence of the US—that is, it occurs independently of the US. Rescorla's studies prove that the animal forms an expectancy derived from a contingency of probability existing between the occurrence and nonoccurrence of the CS and the US (see Chapter 6). Furthermore, in addition to making predictions about the probable occurrence of the US, the dog also makes predictions about its size and quality. In this regard, associative expectancies between the CS and US yield three general possibilities:

1. The CS exactly predicts the size and quality of the US (*no new learning results*).
2. The CS underpredicts the size and quality of the US (*acquisition*).
3. The CS overpredicts the size and quality of the US (*extinction*).

In terms of conditioned reinforcement, these various relationships between conditioned and unconditioned stimuli result in the following outcomes: (1) If the word signals "Good" or "No" are always followed by the same amount of unconditioned stimulation (the same reward or aversive event), then no new learning takes place (i.e., the strength of the S^{r}s "Good" and "No" remains the same). (2) If the word signals "Good" or "No" are sometimes followed by a larger-than-expected reward (e.g., a bonus) or an unexpected punisher, then additional associative conditioning takes place. Such stimulus learning is facilitated under conditions of appetitive surprise (Blanchard and Honig, 1976) or aversive startle (Kamin, 1968). (3) If the CS overpredicts the size of the reward or punisher, then extinction occurs. For instance, if dogs have learned to expect a piece of steak each time they hear the word signal "Good" and are then given a biscuit instead, they will quickly adjust their expectations to reflect the disappointment. In the case of punishment, if dogs have learned to expect aversive punishment every time they hear the word signal "No" while engaging in some unwanted behavior but are then exposed to a series of mild physical prompts instead, the fearful emotional and avoidance responding previously controlled by the reprimand will undergo extinction.

During the training process, dogs definitely form certain predictions and expectations about outcomes associated with their behavior. Extrapolating from the foregoing analysis of classical conditioning to instrumental learning, if a dog receives a reward that is significantly smaller than expected, the outcome is perceived as punitive (disappointment), resulting in the trial rendering the response weaker. If, on the other hand, the reward exactly matches the dog's expectations, then the instrumental response that resulted in reward is neither rendered stronger nor weaker than it was before reinforcement. A reinforcer that does not result in additional learning (acquisition or extinction) might aptly be termed a *verifier*, serving to confirm the status quo but not resulting in any new learning. This general theory suggests that a third instrumental outcome exists in learning besides rewards and punishers (i.e., verifying events that function to maintain behavior at the same level of probability). For new instrumental learning to take place, the reward must exceed a dog's expectation—that is, additional positive learning depends on a surprise element. According to this viewpoint, instrumental behavior is strengthened only to the extent that the anticipated reward exceeds the dog's predictions about the reward's size, quality, or context.

Similarly, in the case of punishment, an aversive event that exactly matches a dog's expectations should not alter or weaken the behavior that the aversive event follows—such a well-predicted event serves only to verify the status quo. That the dog anticipates the aversive outcome and still performs the targeted behavior at a steady rate is empirical evidence for such an interpretation. However, if the punitive event exceeds the dog's prediction, then a corresponding degree of suppression will occur. Finally, if the punitive event is less than the dog has predicted, one would likely observe extinction of punishment effects.

Several general outcomes can be anticipated from the reciprocal relationship between the probability of punishment and its intensity:

1. If the probability of punishment is high but intensity low, the degree of suppression will be correspondingly mitigated.
2. If the probability of punishment is low but the intensity high, suppression should likewise decline over time. [This case finds some trouble when compared with findings from traumatic escape-avoidance experiments (Solomon et al., 1953) and *one-trial learning events*. Avoidance learning is typically very resistant to extinction.]
3. The highest degree of suppression occurs when both the intensity of punishment and its probability of occurrence are high.
4. The lowest degree of suppression occurs when both the intensity of punishment and its probability of occurrence are low.

When the effects of expectancy are factored into the foregoing cases, the following additional predictions are obtained:

5. If the expectation of punishment is matched exactly with the aversive event's actual probability and intensity, no additional suppression will occur.
6. If the expectation of punishment is underestimated in either the direction of probability or intensity, then additional suppression will occur.
7. If the expectation of punishment overestimates the aversive event's probability or intensity, then the degree of suppression controlled by punishment will be correspondingly attenuated.

DIRECT AND REMOTE PUNISHMENT

Punishment is applied in a direct or remote manner, depending on the relative distance of the trainer from the punitive event. During direct punishment, in which the trainer applies punishment to a dog, the trainer becomes part of a punitive stimulus complex. The most common form of direct interactive punishment is corporal (i.e., punishment that is inflicted upon a dog's body). The use of severe corporal punishment is rarely necessary and should be eschewed, except in cases of self-defense against an otherwise uncontrollable aggressor. The routine use of slapping, hitting, punching, or kicking has no place in professional dog training and should be shunned both on technical as well as humane grounds. Corporal punishment is provocative and may elicit additional aggressive behavior and agonistic tensions, thereby compounding the situation. Such physical punishment may cause the hands or feet to be associated with fear and pain, thus resulting in an increased risk for defensive or preemptive biting whenever dogs are surprised by hands or feet moving quickly toward them. Although the individual delivering such punishment may intimidate a dog sufficiently to suppress immediate retaliation by the dog, other less imposing figures, like children or strangers, may become the victims of redirected aggression. Another significant side effect of interactive corporal punishment is that it may cause dogs to fear and avoid their owners. Although certain forms of interactive punishment may be necessary to establish control and dominance over some dogs, as a general rule direct interactive punishment should be used sparingly and only after other methods have been considered and exhausted. Procedurally, physical punishment should be delivered, when necessary, through the modality of a leash and collar, with hands being reserved for the delivery of prompts and affection or other rewards for compliant behavior.

When punitive intervention is necessary, it is preferable to incorporate a remote strategy. Remote punishment separates the owner's presence from the punitive event. Another preferable aspect of remote punishment is that the event can be arranged so that the unwanted behavior triggers the aversive event. A common form of remote punishment is a startle-producing booby trap. Many behavioral complaints (e.g., destructiveness and digging) can be corrected with a little ingenuity through booby-trap arrangements.

USING TIME-OUT TO MODIFY BEHAVIOR

Time-out (TO) is a useful tool for the management of a number of common behavior problems and excesses, especially those driven by strong affiliative motivations, such as at-tention-seeking and competitive play. The effectiveness of TO depends on a number of procedural constraints: timing, bridging, duration, repetition, provision of a reward-dense training situation, and immediate reinforcement of a suitable alternative behavior to replace the one being suppressed. Besides being effective, TO has relatively few negative side effects compared with other punitive methods commonly used for the control of socially disruptive excesses.

Several biological, psychological, and social factors contribute to TO's effectiveness:

1. TO possesses psychobiological significance for dogs.
2. TO avoids stimulating generalized arousal and related adverse side effects associated with interactive punishment.
3. TO has direct relevance to the underlying motivations (e.g., enhanced social contact and control) driving intrusive social excesses and disruptive competitive behavior.
4. TO temporarily removes the dog from the problem situation, thereby preventing inadvertent reinforcement of the unwanted behavior.
5. TO minimizes competitive interaction between the owner and dog, thus avoiding undesirable escalation of dominance tensions.

Loss of Social Contact

From an early age onward, emotional arousal is likely to occur whenever a dog is left alone, especially if the dog is restricted to an unfamiliar place. During periods of isolation, varying degrees of distress (ranging from worry to panic) are predictably stimulated, often together with intense and persistent efforts to regain social contact. Separation-distress reactions may disrupt bioregulatory functions, as well as trigger a variety of undesirable behavioral manifestations, including distress vocalizations, inappropriate elimination, or destructive behavior. Separation-reactive dogs are quieted only after the lost object of affection is finally restored or they exhaust themselves trying to secure such contact.

These primitive separation-distress reactions reflect the dog's psychobiological need for close contact with other dogs and people with whom the dog has formed a strong attachment.

J. P. Scott, who was the first researcher to describe in detail these motivational aspects of canine social behavior, clearly recognized the potential value of separation-related distress for the control of dog behavior:

> In dogs there is an ever-present desire for the company of familiar places and animals, whether human or canine. A dog will work very hard and undergo much inconvenience and discomfort in order to obtain this goal, and will struggle violently if confined away from familiar places or even if isolated in a familiar one. Not only can we use this motivation to direct a dog's behavior toward what we consider desirable ends, but also we can control its development by choosing the places and individuals to which a puppy is allowed to form primary social attachments. (Scott, 1967:128)

As a result of the dog's innate desire to maintain relatively constant social contact, even a very brief period of isolation can be enough to evoke significant emotional distress. TO is based on the finding that mild separation distress can be contingently applied to control undesirable social excesses.

Loss of Social Control

Besides the dog's need for close social contact, its behavior is also strongly influenced by agonistic motivations and tensions, that is, social control. Playful disruptive excesses are often composed of both attention-seeking and competitive components. TO targets both of these motivations by teaching dogs that certain social impulses and excesses regularly result in an abrupt and annoying temporary loss of social contact and control over the situation. In addition, the directive handling used during TO helps to define and enforce appropriate social boundaries.

Where playful competitive tensions are involved, TO is less likely to generate confusion about an owner's intentions. Besides removing a dog from a potentially reinforcing situation, TO signals unequivocally that the dog

must refrain from such inappropriate behavior in the future or risk losing contact and control. In addition, other relevant reinforcers (e.g., affection, treats, and toys) can be contingently offered in exchange for more appropriate behavior, thereby providing dogs with alternative means to establish limited control over the situation. The best way to reform a manipulative and controlling dog is to teach the dog how to secure control over the owner by employing socially acceptable and cooperative behavior.

Loss of Positive Reinforcement

Besides withdrawing social contact and control, TO also removes reward opportunities that might otherwise be available to dogs if they had remained in the training situation. The response-dependent withdrawal or omission of positive reinforcement is a strong form of punishment (negative punishment), especially in contexts providing valuable and frequent reinforcement opportunities. TO as loss of positive reinforcement is aversive, and animals work hard to escape or avoid TO from positive reinforcement (Leitenberg, 1965). In fact, under laboratory conditions, TO compares favorably with shock as a punitive contingency. McMillan (1967), for example, found that animals responded to TO and shock similarly, with a TO of 60 to 90 seconds producing nearly the same level of suppression as a brief shock (30 milliseconds at 1 to 2 mA).

HOW TO USE TIME-OUT

Bridging

The effective use of TO requires that the behavior modifier adhere closely to several procedural constraints. Foremost among these considerations is the need for the TO to be well timed and *bridged* with the occurrence of the unwanted behavior. For TO to be effective, a direct connection must be established and maintained between the occurrence of the target behavior and the TO consequence. This is accomplished by immediately following the unwanted behavior with a conditioned punisher (e.g., "Enough!—

Time-out"), seizing the leash firmly, and posthaste hauling the dog off to the TO room. These closely connected events are necessary to form an adequate connection or bridge between the unwanted behavior and the TO consequence.

The bridging stimulus serves two complementary functions: (1) Bridging explicitly identifies the target behavior responsible for turning on TO. (2) Bridging helps link the occurrence of the target behavior with the delayed TO outcome. The vocal conditioned punisher or bridging stimulus identifies the exact behavior triggering the TO event. This signal is immediately followed by an abrupt upward pressure on the leash that is maintained until the dog reaches the nearby TO room or TO station. Alternatively, a loud continuous tone can be substituted as the bridging stimulus or used in conjunction with a taut leash. The continuous bridging stimulus (the taut leash or tone) helps to connect the emission of the unwanted behavior with the remote TO consequence. Without adequate bridging, the specific target behavior may not be adequately identified and connected with the belated TO. By acting quickly and emphatically, there is a much greater chance of a functional relationship being formed between the occurrence of the unwanted behavior and the TO consequence.

Repetition

Besides timing and bridging, repetition is another vital ingredient influencing the effectiveness of TO. A dog may require several repetitions of TO before a strong connection is established between the unwanted behavior and the TO consequence. An exceptionally persistent behavior may take many repeated TOs before it is possible to reinforce an alternative substitute behavior effectively. Also, training should focus on one specific item at a time, with TO following the unwanted behavior whenever it occurs—at least in the beginning stages. Although TO is most effective when it is presented on a continuous basis, the suppressed target behavior is also more prone to recover (extinction) after punishment on a continuous schedule is withdrawn (Kazdin, 1989). Consequently, it is recom-

mended that TO be initially scheduled on a continuous basis, but once an adequate level of suppression has been achieved, an intermittent schedule of TO is introduced and adjusted—as needed—to maintain low levels of responding (Clark et al., 1973; Calhoun and Lima, 1977; Lehrman et al., 1997). In addition to introducing an intermittent contingency of TO, it is important that desirable behavior be actively prompted and reinforced to facilitate the training process.

Duration

The duration of TO is also important (Kaufman and Baron, 1968). Most dogs respond to repeated 1- or 2-minute TOs, but even shorter periods of 30 seconds can be very effective. Nobbe and colleagues (1980) recommend a 3-minute TO period for punishing aggressive behavior, but this longer TO does not appear to be necessary for most nonaggressive social excesses. Polsky (1989) suggests isolating the dog in a darkened closet and then ignoring the dog for an additional 5 minutes after the TO period is over. These and similar aversive embellishments of the basic procedure (e.g., excessively long TOs lasting from 5 to 10 minutes or more) are unnecessary and should be avoided. Instead of ignoring the dog following TO, the dog should be routinely taken back to the original situation, where an appropriate substitute behavior is prompted and reinforced; or, if the unwanted behavior occurs again, the TO can be reinstated and repeated until a sufficient level of suppression is achieved to permit reinforcement of the selected substitute behavior.

Time-in Positive Reinforcement

The effectiveness of TO also depends on the relative value and frequency of positive reinforcement opportunities yielded by time-in and lost by TO. TO from a reward-dense situation will have a stronger effect over the unwanted target behavior than TO from a punishment-dense situation (Solnick et al., 1977). Consequently, the time-in environment should offer dogs abundant opportunities to obtain positive reinforcement, while excluding other forms of punishment besides TO (if possible). Emphasis on positive training efforts provide two complementary benefits: (1) positive reinforcement encourages more desirable behavior, and (2) the presence of ongoing positive reinforcement maximizes the punitive effect of TO over the unwanted behavior. If, on the other hand, the time-in environment is reward lean, providing insufficient opportunities for the dog to obtain reinforcement, punishment dense, or (worse still) saturated with uncontrollable aversive contingencies, the net effect of TO will be correspondingly diminished. In cases where excessive interactive punishment is used, the TO period may be *welcomed* by dogs as an opportunity to escape from the situation, possibly reinforcing the unwanted behavior rather than punishing it.

Positive and Negative Feedback

Ideally, the unwanted behavior turning on TO is replaced by an incompatible substitute behavior overlapping the termination of TO. For example, TO is often applied in the case of nuisance barking or excessive activity (e.g., jumping up). During the TO period, dogs typically become more quiet and subdued, behavior that is reinforced because it is associated with release from isolation. Once out of isolation (time-in), a dog's continued social contact depends on its willingness to remain quiet or by exhibiting appropriate social restraint and impulse control. A dog that happens to bark or jump up after being released is immediately timed-out again and released only after calming down. The objective is to train dogs to recognize that being quiet and less demanding results in their being freed from TO, whereas barking or excessive attention seeking results in its reinstatement. The TO is designed to work optimally under such conditions of positive and negative feedback.

TYPES OF TIME-OUT

The TO is arranged so that the target behavior triggers the loss of social contact/control or the withdrawal of positive reinforcement. The two general types of TO used to modify

dog behavior are referred to as *exclusionary* and *nonexclusionary* (Foxx, 1982).

Exclusionary Time-out

TO often involves removing dogs from the training situation. The most common way to confine a dog for TO is to place the dog in a lighted bathroom or some other separate room. As the door is closed, the dog's leash is pinched in the doorjamb, leaving just enough slack so that the dog can comfortably stand and sit but not wander about the room. The common practice of punishing a dog by isolating it in a crate is inconsistent with proper crate training and should be avoided. When first exposed to TO, dogs may complain by barking or scratching at the door. Releasing them at this point would reinforce and encourage such undesirable behavior in the future. Sometimes, merely kicking firmly at the base of the door is enough to discourage the behavior. Many dogs require a stronger message, however. Persistent protests are responded to by abruptly opening the door and delivering an assertive reprimand, "Enough!" If necessary, this later procedure is followed by a sharp rattle of a 7-penny shaker can.

A dog that is still complaining after the TO period has elapsed should be ignored and released only after being quiet for at least 10 to 15 seconds. If the dog has remained quiet during the TO, he is praised ("Good boy/girl") through the door, released with reassuring affection, and taken back to the training situation. Additional TOs are applied as needed, until the unwanted behavior is sufficiently weakened to permit instrumental counterconditioning. Exclusionary TOs can also be carried out by confining the dog in the room where the unwanted behavior occurs. This is accomplished by closing the door on the leash as the owner exits the room, leaving the dog restrained on the other side.

Nonexclusionary Time-out

TO sometimes involves withdrawing reinforcement without socially isolating or removing the dog from the training situation. Nonexclusionary TOs are especially effective in cases where reward training is ongoing. Such TOs can be carried out by simply turning away from the dog, withdrawing the opportunity to earn rewards, or by ignoring the dog. For example, to discourage undesirable behavior occurring during an active training session, a mild version of nonexclusionary TO is carried out by suspending the opportunity to earn rewards for 15 to 30 seconds. This brief *in-training TO* is initiated by saying "time-out" and placing one's hands up and across the chest at shoulder level and turning away from the dog. The overall effect is akin to a "cold shoulder." This particular variation is useful for the control of many mild playful excesses. Another useful nonexclusionary TO involves tying the dog to a doorknob or post so that the dog can comfortably stand and sit but not lay down. A variation of this method is used to apply TO outdoors, where the dog is tethered to a tree or post. The restrained dog is left alone by walking a short distance away.

TIME-OUT AND SOCIAL EXCESSES

Many common behavior problems are driven by attention-seeking or playful competitive motivations. Using harsh physical punishment to control such behavior is questionable on a number of grounds but especially because punishing one behavior might simultaneously affect other closely related (but desirable) behaviors belonging to the same functional or motivational class. For instance, physically punishing a greeting excess (e.g., jumping up) will probably suppress the unwanted behavior; however, such aversive procedures could unintentionally dampen a dog's overall willingness to approach or play with family members or visiting guests in more socially acceptable ways, as well. Furthermore, punitive handling during greeting exchanges might encourage the development of an even worse behavior problem, such as submissive urination. Considerations like these warrant the use of techniques that gradually shape alternative patterns of social behavior with positive reinforcement over methods that rely too heavily on interactive punishment.

Some social excesses may be resistant to physical punishment because they are partially or totally shielded from the effects of such punitive treatment. During greetings, for example, and at other times of increased social arousal, affectionate emotions may overshadow the aversive effects of interactive punishment. This effect is clearly evident in the now classic study performed by Fox (1966) in which puppies tended to persevere in their efforts to approach a handler in spite of the delivery of approach-dependent shock. Similarly, Hess (1973) found that young animals would persistently follow and become strongly attached to a punitive imprinting object. This social "immunity" to punishment and pain may be mediated by the endogenous opioid system. Many studies have demonstrated that physical pain evokes the release of modulatory endorphins, morphine-like neuropeptides that produce an analgesic effect. Knowles and coworkers (1987) have shown that dogs exhibit increased tail-wagging and attention-seeking behavior under the influence of naloxone (an opioid antagonist), whereas such affiliative behavior is reduced by the administration of low doses of morphine. Perhaps as a result of the opioid response to pain, some attention-seeking excesses may be maintained by an "addiction" to opioids secreted during punitive interaction with the dog. Further, it has been demonstrated that endorphin activity can be brought under the control of classical conditioning (Watkins and Mayer, 1982), suggesting the additional possibility that the owner's mere presence might elicit a potent opioid cascade, thereby numbing the dog to pending aversive stimulation.

Impulsive social excesses may be potentiated by punitive stimulation failing to reach an effective aversive threshold. Rather than suppressing an unwanted behavior, ineffectual punishment may actually excite increased arousal of the prevailing motivational system, thereby stimulating more—not less—of the target excess. Besides the risk of arousing the dog further, interactive punishment may inadvertently reinforce the unwanted behavior. Again, unless punitive stimulation is sufficiently aversive, it may be overshadowed by incompatible affectionate or playful emotions present at the same time punishment is delivered. After repeated exposures in which punishment is paired with a pleasurable internal state, the punitive stimulus may be gradually transformed via counterconditioning into an hedonically pleasurable stimulus, thus potentially serving to reinforce the unwanted behavior rather than suppressing it as intended. Punishment under such circumstances may become a discriminative stimulus that evokes considerably more target responding than if it had not be applied at all.

A similar pattern of escalating punishment is very common among dog owners. Fearing to alienate their dog's affections by using harsh methods, owners may choose instead to correct social excesses with an assortment of mild aversives, gradually increasing the level of aversive stimulation over several weeks or months before realizing the futility of their method. In addition, such owners may attempt to reassure and calm the dog after delivering punishment, thereby making punishment a discriminative stimulus for reinforcement. Such interaction between punishment and reinforcement has been demonstrated to exert a tremendous mitigating influence on the effect of punishment (Holz and Azrin, 1961). Consequently, as a combined result of gradual escalation and adverse discrimination effects, aversive stimulation may need to be presented in very intense doses to achieve very modest effects.

Interactive punishment can become a discriminative stimulus (cue) controlling negative attention seeking or aggressive play. Many dogs appear to misinterpret their owner's punitive intentions, viewing their most sincere efforts as little more than a "rough" invitation for play. Attention from the owner is often highly desirable for the dog, regardless of its positive or negative valence, with each form of attention controlling a relatively exclusive set of instrumental behaviors. Positive attention (e.g., affectionate interaction) tends to promote harmonious interaction and strengthen cooperative behavior, whereas negative attention (e.g., ineffectual punishment) tends to reinforce socially disruptive and competitive behavior.

Besides the risk of increased generalized arousal, counterconditioning, and confusion, interactive punishment directed against social excesses may inadvertently facilitate the rise of dominance tensions between an owner and dog. If the owner is not convincing during such contests, the dog may surmise by default that he has won. Such "victories" may be a significant source of reward for some dogs. Establishing one's dominance over another is strongly reinforcing for most animals, including humans, who frequently report experiencing a euphoric sense of well-being or elation after winning a hard-fought battle of wits or brawn. For the subordinate, losing is correspondingly distressing and aversive— just ask any dog owner despondent over a problem of this sort!

Although not necessarily leading to full-blown aggression, playful competitive behavior may be reinforced by a similar elation-mediating mechanism. Competitive dogs often take great delight in vying with and besting their beleaguered owners, sometimes to the point of appearing "silly drunk" on the power derived from such interaction. In dogs predisposed to exhibit aggressive behavior, impulsive competitive interaction with the owner may anticipate more serious dominance-related conflicts appearing later on in life, especially as they reach social maturity.

It should be emphasized that TO is an adjunctive procedure that is most effectively employed in the context of other behavior modification and management activities. Unless fears, frustrative influences, social confusion, impulse-control deficits, and various other contributory factors are reduced or removed, punitive measures are not likely to be lastingly effective. Disruptive behavior is complex and requires careful evaluation and assessment. Treatment includes behavior therapy/modification, formal obedience training, and physiological interventions when indicated by veterinary examination. In this overall context of training, TO should be viewed as an effective "damage control" option rather than a primary leverage point of change.

NEGATIVE PRACTICE, NEGATIVE TRAINING, AND OVERCORRECTION (POSITIVE PRACTICE) TECHNIQUES

Negative practice is a behavioral technique in

which an unwanted behavior is decreased by requiring dogs to repeat it over and over again, until its performance becomes aversive in itself. For example, jumping up is a common behavior problem. In addition to appropriately discouraging dogs from such behavior through more conventional means (e.g., TO and counterconditioning a sit or stand response), owners might subject persistent jumpers to a regimen of negative practice. Negative practice in this case would involve having such dogs jump up again and again, perhaps as many as 15 to 20 times per session, or until they begin actively to resist the prompting. At this point, negative practice is abandoned and replaced with negative training. Negative training is a process in which a dog's tendency to resist performing an unwanted behavior is negatively reinforced. For example, in the case of a jumper, the dog is pulled upward but with insufficient force to break the dog's resistance, a resistance that is negatively reinforced by letting go of the leash pressure. The consequence of several such trials of negative training is that a tendency to resist jumping up is encouraged. Negative practice and negative training procedures are very useful for controlling a wide spectrum of persistent behavior problems. As with all aversive techniques, such methods should be used only in a context where reward-based training activities have been proven ineffective as a means to decrease the unwanted behavior.

Another useful punitive tool is *overcorrection* (Foxx and Azrin, 1973; Ollendick and Matson, 1978), a procedure that incorporates positive practice—that is, having a dog repeatedly perform a behavior that is incompatible with the unwanted behavior being suppressed. The usual pattern involves vocally correcting the dog for the infraction and then requiring that the dog repeat some series of related but incompatible behaviors over several minutes. Frequently, the dog must be physically guided through these responses in the beginning. For example, in the case of jumping up, the dog is reprimanded with the vocal cue "Off" and pushed off and prompted to sit. Following this initial correction, the dog is required to perform a series

of general exercises like sit/sit-stay and down/down-stay over 3 to 5 minutes (some dogs may require more or less positive practice time). Subsequently, on every occasion that the dog attempts to jump up, the dog is reprimanded and subjected to positive practice. Overcorrection can also be used in cases involving mild aggression problems: dogs that behave aggressively are given a sharp vocal reprimand, followed by a brief TO, and then required to assume a subordinate position while undergoing several minutes of relaxing massage or provided with food treats as long as they remain quiet. TO and overcorrection are highly compatible and work well in conjunction with each other.

REMOTE-ACTIVATED ELECTRONIC COLLARS

A device for delivering remote punishment that has considerable usefulness is the remote-activated electronic collar. Remote electronic stimulation provides a means for delivering a well-timed and measured aversive event. In many ways, it represents an ideal positive punisher, having many potential applications in dog training. In addition to intractable barking problems, dangerous habits such as chasing cars and bicyclists, various predatory behaviors, persistent recall problems, and refractory compulsive habits—all are often responsive to training efforts utilizing an electronic collar. Tortora (1983) has advocated the use of electronic training in the management of certain forms of aggression.

Ideally, the electronic collar should possess several operating features: (1) a variable shock intensity adjustable from the transmitter and collar, (2) a warning and safety tone built into the collar, and (3) reliable operation and range. Little in the dog-behavior literature has been written on the use of shock in dog training or behavioral management, perhaps reflecting the stigma attached to its use, yet limited professional use of such collars is definitely warranted and justified (Vollmer, 1979a, 1979b, 1980; Tortora, 1982, 1983). There are many potential complications in the use of shock for the suppression of behavior, including the possibility of evoking redirected and pain-elicited aggression (Azrin et al., 1967; Polsky, 1998). Notwithstanding the potential for abuse and undesirable side effects, limited professional use of remote electronic collars is definitely warranted and justified. What may not be justifiable is their current widespread use by dog owners with little behavioral background or experience. There is a considerable risk for abuse when such collars are placed into naive and inexperienced hands.

MISUSE AND ABUSE OF PUNISHMENT

Punishment and other forms of aversive control (e.g., aversive counterconditioning and negative reinforcement) can be humane and effective behavioral tools in the hands of competent trainers, but noncontingent (after the event) punishment and excessive physical punishment or brutalization (e.g., beating, hanging, or kicking) have no legitimate place in the armamentarium of professional trainers. That such methods exist today and are employed in the name of dog training is a blemish on the profession.

Noncontingent Punishment

Perhaps the most frequently misused form of aversive control is noncontingent punishment. Procedures involving such treatment are often recommended for the control of behavior problems that occur while the owner is away from home. Unfortunately, this abuse of punishment has been defended by a number of highly regarded authors (Koehler, 1962; Benjamin, 1985; Evans, 1991). The influence of this popular literature is compounded by many dog owners honestly believing that their dog's misbehavior is motivated by spiteful intentions.

"Spite" and Pseudoguilt

Dog owners who believe that their dog's misbehavior is motivated by *spite* point to the dog's appearance of *guilt* as proof of a premeditated purpose underlying the dog's undesirable behavior. The dog's guilty appearance during homecomings suggests to them that the dog knows and is behaving in a way calculated to somehow injure them. This rationalization provides a basis (at least in their minds) for the delivery of harsh punishment long after the behavior has occurred. Such treatment is targeted against the dog's bad attitude and the dog's need for discipline. The owner's urge to hurt the dog in such cases is rarely constructive but rather the outcome of an angry reaction to the presence of a soiled area or destroyed personal belonging—anger and frustration that is subsequently directed in the form of physical abuse toward the dog.

When such abusive treatment fails (as it inevitably does), the owner may interpret the failure as recalcitrance on the dog's part and point to growing levels of guilt on homecomings as additional evidence of such an interpretation, thereby justifying an ever-escalating cycle of abusive interaction. Konrad Most long ago repudiated this faulty interpretation, arguing that the dog may never know the reasons for punishment but only learn that some modes of behavior result in aversive outcomes:

> It has to be constantly borne in mind that the animal can never learn the reason for a disagreeable experience, but only that certain modes of behavior result in disagreeable experiences. (1910/1955:17)

Later, he stresses, regarding the dog's appearance of guilt,

> The "guilty conscience" is caused simply and solely by the so-called fear inspired by the menacing noises and gestures of the human being. In fact, the dog's "conscience" is quite "clear." Such fear is always aroused in the dog by hostile behavior on the part of its master. For, as a rule, the animal has had it knocked into his memory from puppyhood that hostile human attitudes are accompanied, or quickly followed, by some disagreeable experience. But the cause of fear in the presence of the master is never awareness in the dog of any present, let alone any past, behavior to which the man objected. (1910/1955:72)

Although it is impossible to know for sure, dogs probably do not reflect much on the past or future significance of their behavior. "Every dog," as Hans Tossutti (1942) once noted, "considers his acts as right."

Instead of worrying about the past or future significance of what they do, dogs are content with the here and now, living in a perpetual present where time flows like the Heraclitean river into which "we step and do not step." Although dogs can encode experiences and retrieve memories, they are most likely unable to form conceptual constructs and symbolic representations of events from which to deduce causal inferences about the distant past or future. Consequently, appealing to a canine ability to extrapolate from a present consequence to a past action does not help to explain the dog's appearance of guilt. Although a dog may be able to associate the presence of a destroyed item with the owner's anger, it is unlikely that the culpable action is directly influenced by the owner's disapproval or abusive efforts. Unfortunately, however, the owner reads the dog's guilt as if it was related to a remote action present in the dog's mind at the time of punishment. Dogs do not appear to have such cognitive abilities. To dogs, threats of future punishment are as useless and meaningless as punishment is for long past actions. Actually, most of what we do and value as humans is probably lost on dogs. William James offers a bit of sobering analysis regarding the situation:

> Our dogs, for example, are in our human life but not of it. They witness hourly the outward body of events whose inner meaning cannot, by any possible operation, be revealed to their intelligence—events in which they themselves often play the cardinal part. My terrier bites a teasing boy, for example, and the father demands damages. The dog may be present at every step of the negotiation, and see the money paid, without an inkling of what it all means, without a suspicion that it has anything to do with him; and he never can know in his natural dog's life. (1896/1956:57–58)

The Persistent Belief that Noncontingent Punishment Works

Another factor contributing to the popularity of noncontingent punishment is the appearance that it somehow works. Since noncontingent punishment is often directly associated with the object or area where the offending behavior took place, any appear-

ance of effectiveness is probably due to the influence of aversive counterconditioning. In other words, the ostensible benefit of such treatment is not due to the remote suppression of the unwanted behavior, but rather such methods probably work by indirectly conditioning fear toward the object or location where punishment took place in the past. One of the most repugnant examples of noncontingent punishment in the dog-training literature illustrates this effect:

> If you come home and find your dog has dug a hole, fill the hole brimful of water. With the training collar and leash, bring the dog to the hole and shove his nose into the water; hold him there until he is sure he's drowning. If your dog is of any size, you may get all of the action of a cowboy bull-dogging a steer. Stay with it. I've had elderly ladies who'd had their fill of ruined flower beds dunk some mighty big dogs. A great many dogs will associate this horrible experience with the hole they dug. ... It is not necessary to "catch the dog in the act" in any of the above instances of correction. Be consistent in your corrections and your dog will come to find the smell of freshly dug earth quite repugnant. (Koehler, 1962:200)

Pressing a dog's nose into water is irrelevant to digging per se, but, as the author points out, the terrifying sensation of drowning causes the dog to acquire a repugnance to the smell of soil, to say nothing of how it affects the dog's attitude toward the owner. Instead of suppressing the tendency to dig, chew, or eliminate in the owner's absence, such extreme methods cause the dog to avoid the item or place where aversive stimulation took place. Along with Koehler, Benjamin (1985) and Evans (1991), using much more restrained aversives, also emphasize the need to present evidence or proof to the dog to make the "disciplinary" event effective. Such treatment does nothing to deter destructive behavior or inappropriate elimination, but it may instill a fear of the object, place, or person associated with "punishment."

Although aversive counterconditioning has a useful place in dog training, such variants as the aforementioned method are ill-conceived and excessive. One concern about the method is that dogs may learn to associate aversive stimulation, not only with the surrounding area or object, but with the abusive owner applying it. Because of this risk, aversive counterconditioning is best carried out through remote means utilizing booby traps and other procedures by which the object or area itself appears to deliver the aversive stimulus. Such methods require comparatively mild aversives, with far less risk of producing side effects, while at the same time promising a much greater likelihood of success.

Interpreting Pseudoguilt

If dogs are unable to connect punishment with the behavior occurring in the remote past, what causes their appearance of guilt? A frequently cited analysis of guilty behavior interprets *guilt* as a ritualized submission display aimed at avoiding noncontingent punishment (Borchelt and Voith, 1985). This theory holds that *pseudoguilt* is maintained by a triadic structure of conditioned associations involving three components: (1) evidence of a destroyed object or soiled area, (2) the presence of the owner, and (3) a history of previous punishment under similar conditions in the past. Many anecdotal reports support this sort of interpretation. For example, it is not uncommon for an adult dog who is kept with a puppy to show guilt when the owner returns home, especially if the puppy happens to eliminate during the owner's absence. It is the adult dog who exhibits guilt, even though the puppy's action was responsible for the offending mess. There are other potential causes of pseudoguilt that ought to be investigated. One possibility is that emotional cues current at the time of the unwanted behavior persist until the occurrence of remote aversive stimulation. These internal emotional cues may subsequently predict pending punishment. Whatever the cause, pseudoguilt is most likely not due to a lingering bad conscience over a past deed.

Negative Side Effects of Noncontingent Punishment

Noncontingent punishment is often harsh and sustained, with the dog often being

beaten immediately after homecomings. Most normal dogs are very enthusiastic about greeting their owners after a long separation. The active emotions are intensely affiliative, and the dog naturally seeks reciprocation— that is, the expectant dog anticipates an equally friendly reply. Instead, its affectionate efforts are met with an unexpected and aggressive assault. The result is a collision of violently opposed and conflicted emotions, a situation structurally similar to the procedures used to induce experimental neurosis in the laboratory. As will be seen in the following chapter, from the perspective of experimental neurosis, the collision of opposing and mutually incompatible emotional reactions predispose dogs to develop neurotic conflict. Because of the intensity of the emotions involved, coupled with the inescapable character of the stimulation, the potential for serious side effects is extremely high.

Adult dogs exhibiting separational distress frequently develop a number of persistent behavior problems such as barking, destructive behavior, and inappropriate elimination whenever they are left alone. This group of dogs is at a particularly high risk of becoming the hapless target of abusive and escalating brutalization as part of their "reform." That such treatment is harmful should be obvious, but it is commonly employed on the recommendation of authors such as Koehler (1962), who interpret separation-related behavior as deriving from sullen vengefulness— a condition that must be tortured out of a dog's character through repeated "spankings." This fraudulent view reinforces the popular interpretation of such behavior, which erringly implicates spite as its primary cause, but Koehler takes matters to an all time low in the following useless and cruel prescription for the "revenge piddler":

> For the grown dog who was reliable in the house and then backslides, the method of correction differs somewhat. In this group of "backsliders" we have the "revenge piddlers." This dog protests being alone by messing on the floor, and often in the middle of the bed. The first step of correction is to confine the dog closely in a part of the house when you go away, so that he is constantly reminded of his

obligation. The fact that he once was reliable in the house is proof that the dog knows right from wrong, and leaves you no other course than to punish him sufficiently to convince him that the satisfaction of his wrong-doing is not worth the consequences. If the punishment is not severe enough, some of these "backsliders" will think they're winning and will continue to mess in the house. An indelible impression can sometimes be made by giving the dog a hard spanking, of long duration, then leaving him tied by the mess he's made so you can come back at twenty-minute intervals and punish him again for the same thing. In most cases, the dog that deliberately does this disagreeable thing cannot be made reliable by the light spanking that some owners seem to think is adequate punishment. It will be better for your dog, as well as the house, if you really pour it on. (1962:196)

There is no reasonable behavioral justification for this form of mental and physical abuse, but, every single day across America, hundreds of frustrated dog owners are carrying out similar rituals of confusion and cruelty in the name of dog training. After several weeks or months of such abusive interaction, besides irreparably damaging the owner-dog relationship, such treatment inevitably results in the elaboration of more serious behavior problems.

The Need for Close Temporal Contiguity

A brief review of basic learning principles will help to underscore the importance of response-dependent punishment. As has already been repeatedly emphasized, learning depends on the timely and regular presentation of relevant stimuli. This holds equally true for both classical and instrumental types of learning. In the case of classical conditioning, the CS (e.g., whistle) must immediately precede the US (e.g., food) for a conditioned association between the CS and US to be established. Similarly, in instrumental learning, reinforcers and punishers must closely follow upon the emission of the target behavior. The behavior-modifying effects of reinforcement and punishment are both significantly diminished to the extent that their delivery is delayed or delivered independently of the oc-

currence of the target behavior. In the case of punishment, effective use depends on its prompt delivery whenever the unwanted behavior occurs. Under these experimentally established constraints, "punishment" occurring long after the event is a wasted effort that unnecessarily exposes dogs to aversive stimulation. Such interactive punishment serves no purpose, other than providing owners with an outlet to discharge anger and frustration.

Hitting and Slapping: Okay?

The routine hitting and slapping of puppies and dogs are also inappropriate forms of punishment, especially when they are delivered on a noncontingent basis. Sensitive dogs exposed to such treatment may develop a negative expectation about hands moving abruptly or startlingly in their direction. Voith and Borchelt have noted a significant correlation between abusive house-training measures and an increased incidence of fear-related aggression in adult dogs:

> Direct physical punishment from the owner, even if the dog is "caught in the act" can lead to fearful and defensive behaviors. Punishment unrelated to "the act" results in even more-intense defensive reactions to being approached, reached for, or touched by a person. Although dominance aggression is the most commonly diagnosed behavior problem presented to animal behaviorists, fear-induced aggression is probably the most common type of aggression among pet dogs. Fearfully aggressive housedogs almost invariably have a history of difficulties in housetraining and were inappropriately and unpredictably punished by the owners. (1996:176)

Under conditions of heightened distress or even momentary distraction, the startling approach of a child or stranger with outstretched hands may be interpreted as a threat, resulting in a preemptive attack aimed at controlling it. Further, the transition from a smack on the rear or chops to Koehler's method is one of degrees, not kind. Physical sorts of punishment rarely yield lasting suppression of behavior, unless they are delivered strongly. This characteristic often causes the "spanking" to escalate gradually into a periodic beating. Ethical trainers and behaviorists should draw the line firmly and exclude all forms of corporal punishment from routine training, except as might be needed in the case of self-defense.

Finally, uncontrollable painful stimulation occurring under some social circumstances may simultaneously elicit fear and anger as unconditioned responses. Where fear and anger are elicited together by the threat of inescapable pain (e.g., inappropriate physical punishment), the possibility of lasting irritability, vigilance, anxiety, and lowered thresholds for aggression may occur in the presence of the punishing agent. Under the influence of such abusive handling occurring early in a dog's life, fear and anger may become motivationally linked together as a conditioned response to pain or threat of pain and, over the course of the animal's development, "incubate" until the dog reaches maturity, by which time a highly intractable aggression problem may express itself.

ABUSIVE PUNISHMENT: THE NEED FOR UNIVERSAL CONDEMNATION

The use of corporal punishment to control dog behavior is very problematical and should be avoided. Not only are such methods dangerous for inexperienced owners to employ, they are probably ineffective (certainly in the sense of lasting and generalized behavioral control) and are fraught with potentially serious side effects. Physical punishment of aggressive behavior can easily result in an escalation of aggression or produce a more severe and difficult problem to control. For example, although an intimidated dog may not dare to threaten or snap at the person applying such abusive treatment, other family members of less social rank or unsuspecting guests may become the victims of redirected attacks or attacks following momentary disinhibition. Further, excessive punishment may suppress vital threat displays, making future attacks more difficult to anticipate and avoid safely. In the long run, such misguided training efforts may produce a much more difficult and dangerous situation to control.

Despite the criticism and growing pressure exerted by leading dog trainers, applied animal behaviorists, and veterinary behaviorists, corporal punishment remains deeply entrenched in the dog-training culture. Some advocates of extreme measures (e.g., beating and hanging) argue that it should be used only as a last resort for the control of incorrigible behavior problems. Many are simply ignorant and do not know any better. A national task force of animal behaviorists, dog trainers, and veterinarians was convened in March 1998 to address such problems by defining humane dog training and to set the groundwork for developing a professional standards and practices document. The efforts of the task force have been enthusiastically received and endorsed by many dog-training, humane, service-dog, and veterinary organizations. It remains to be seen how effective these efforts will be in curtailing abusive practices in dog training.

Although punishment is an important tool for the control of dog behavior, its use should be tempered by informed judgment, ethical restraint, and compassion. Dog trainers and behaviorists alike would do well to follow the spirit of the Hippocratic oath to "do no harm" and to avoid methods that so obviously "do harm" dogs and the human-dog relationship.

GENERAL GUIDELINES FOR THE USE OF PUNISHMENT

Punishment and other aversive training techniques are complex and require careful assessment and implementation. The following is offered as a general, but by no means exhaustive, set of guidelines for the effective use of punishment.

1. Punishment should be used only after other positive training options have been carefully considered or exhausted.

2. The trainer should never punish out of anger or frustration. Punishment should be used as a constructive training option, not as a means to vent negative emotions. Punishment should be performed with a pronounced sense of moral responsibility and

honest commitment to the dog's well-being and happiness.

3. Punishment delayed for even a second or two after the event should be avoided. Some behavioral authorities have made insupportable claims suggesting that a window of effectiveness for punishment exists ranging from 30 seconds to several hours after the event. The effect of punishment is progressively attenuated with every second elapsing between the emission of the target behavior and its belated application. This so-called delay of punishment gradient fades to nearly zero after a delay of only 30 seconds (Kamin, 1959; Camp et al., 1967). The best suppressive effects result when punishment overlaps the target response.

4. Punishment should occur at the earliest point in the behavioral sequence targeted for suppression. Ideally, punishment should be applied against intentional movements—the weakest and easiest links to break in the behavioral chain of events.

5. An alternative substitute behavior should always be prompted and reinforced immediately after the termination of punishment. Ideally, the behavior emitted with the cessation of punishment should be desirable and incompatible with the target behavior undergoing suppression.

6. Avoid excessively harsh punishers: never hit, kick, slap, hang, or beat a puppy or dog.

7. An antecedent signal or reprimand should be consistently paired with the punitive event. The reprimand will gradually become a conditioned punisher, perhaps, eventually taking the place of actual punishment. In general, training events should be presented in an orderly manner, allowing the dog to achieve a degree of predictive control over their occurrence.

8. Whenever possible, avoid interactive punishment. Many punitive events can be controlled remotely through indirect means and booby traps.

9. Select punishers that are relevant to the underlying motivation driving the unwanted behavior. For example, brief time-outs are best suited to attention-seeking and playful competitive behavior, whereas a physical as-

sertion of control may be more appropriate in situations involving dominance challenges.

10. Select punishers on the basis of their significance to the sensory modality most directly linked to the unwanted behavior being suppressed. For example, in the case of excessive barking, a startling sound can be used. Lunging into the leash is appropriately countered by an opposing leash correction sufficient to break the dog's forward momentum while knocking the dog slightly off balance.

11. Fit the punishment to the dog's temperament and behavior: do not "kill a mosquito with a sledgehammer" and, likewise, do not "attempt to stop an elephant with a squirt gun." A punitive event that is excessively intimidating for one dog may be barely effective or ineffective for another one possessing a bolder temperament and greater determination to persist in the unwanted behavior.

12. The most effective positive reinforcers possess an element of surprise. Likewise, aversive punishment is most effective when it generates a strong startle at the moment of its delivery. The infliction of pain is not a necessary component of effective punishment, but startle is necessary to maximize punitive effects.

13. Punish one behavior at a time. Novice trainers frequently error by attempting to do too much at once. Correcting more than one behavior at a time often results in confusion and inefficient use of training time.

14. Do not escalate punishment incrementally but use a sufficiently strong punisher from the beginning. The gradual escalation of punishment results in its systematic habituation. Such efforts ultimately result in the need to use a more aversive punisher than would have been necessary had a sufficiently strong one been used in the first place.

15. Vary the type of punishment. One punisher may work in one situation but not work as well in another.

16. A punisher that does not work within three to five trials should be reevaluated and possibly abandoned.

17. Make certain that the behavior being punished is not being inadvertently rein-

forced, especially if it tends to recover or resists suppression.

18. Always remember that the target of
punishment is the dog's behavior, not the dog.

19. Try to understand the dog's motivation and behavior from a canine point of
view. If in doubt about punishing a dog, give
the dog the benefit of doubt.

20. Be consistent.

REFERENCES

Amsel A (1971). Frustration, persistence, and re-
gression. In HD Kimmel (Ed), *Experimental
Psychopathology: Recent Research and Theory.*
New York: Academic.

Aristotle (1985). *Nicomachean Ethics,* T Irwin
(Trans). Indianapolis, IN: Hackett.

Azrin NH and Holz WC (1966). Punishment. In
WK Honig (Ed), *Operant Behavior: Areas of
Research and Application.* Englewood Cliffs,
NJ: Prentice-Hall.

Azrin NH, Hutchinson RR, and Kake DF (1967).
Attack, avoidance, and escape reactions to aversive shock. *J Exp Anal Behav,* 10:131–148.

Benjamin CL (1985). *Mother Knows Best: The
Natural Way to Train Your Dog.* New York:
Howell Book House.

Blanchard R and Honig WK (1976). Surprise
value of food determines its effectiveness as a
reinforcer. *J Exp Psychol Anim Behav Processes,*
2:68–74.

Bolles RC (1970). Species-specific defense reactions and avoidance learning. *Psychol Rev,*
77:32–48.

Bolles RC (1973). The comparative psychology of
learning: The selective association principle
and some problems with "general" laws of
learning. In G Bermant (Ed), *Perspectives On
Animal Behavior,* 280–306. Glenview, IL:
Scott, Foresman.

Borchelt PL and Voith VL (1985). Punishment.
Compend Contin Educ Pract Vet, 7:780–788.

Calhoun KS and Lima PP (1977). Effects of varying schedules of time-out on high- and low-
rate behaviors. *J Behav Ther Exp Psychiatry,*
8:189–194.

Camp DS, Raymond GA, and Church RM
(1967). Temporal relationship between response and punishment. *J Exp Psychol,*
74:114–123.

Clark H, Rowbury T, Baer A, and Baer D (1973).
Time-out as a punishing stimulus in continu-
ous and intermittent schedules. *J Appl Behav
Anal,* 6:443–455.

Denny MR (1971). Relaxation theory and experi-

ments. In R Brush (Ed), *Aversive Conditioning
and Learning,* 235–295. New York: Academic.

Denny MR (1976). Post-aversive relief and relaxation and their implications for behavior therapy. *J Behav Ther Exp Psychiatry,* 7:315–321.

Denny MR (1983). Safety catch in behavior therapy: Comments on "safety" training: The elimination of avoidance-motivated aggression in
Dogs. *J Exp Psychol Gen* 112:215–217.

Dickinson A and Dearing MF (1979). Appetitive-
aversive interactions and inhibitory processes.
In A Dickinson and RA Boakes (Eds), *Mechanisms of Learning and Motivation.* Hillsdale,
NJ: Erlbaum.

Evans JM (1991). *People, Pooches, and Problems.*
New York: Howell Book House.

Fox MW (1966). The development of learning
and conditioned responses in the dog: Theoretical and practical implications. *Can J Comp Vet
Sci,* 30:282–286.

Foxx RM (1982). *Decreasing Behaviors of Severely
Retarded and Autistic Persons.* Champaign, IL:
Research.

Foxx RM and Azrin NH (1973). The elimination
of autistic self-stimulatory behavior by overcorrection. *J Appl Behav Anal,* 6:1–14.

Hammond TS (1894). *Practical Dog Training:
Training vs Breaking.* New York: Forest and
Stream.

Hess EH (1973). *Imprinting: Early Experience and
the Developmental Psychobiology of Attachment.*
New York: D Van Nostrand.

Hilgard ER and Bower GH (1975). *Theories of
Learning,* 4th Ed. New York: Appleton-Century-Crofts.

Hineline PN (1984). Aversive control: A separate
domain? *J Exp Anal Behav,* 42:495–509.

Hineline PN and Harrison JF (1979). Lever biting
as an avoidance response. *Bull Psychon Soc,*
11:223–226.

Holz WC and Azrin NH (1961). Discriminative
properties of punishment. *J Exp Anal Behav,*
4:225–232.

James W (1896/1956). "Is life worth living?" In
The Will to Believe. New York: Dover (reprint).

Jones RSP and McCaughey RE (1992). Gentle
teaching and applied behavior analysis: A critical review. *J Appl Behav Anal,* 25:853–867.

Kamin LJ (1956). Effects of termination of CS
and avoidance of the US on avoidance learning. *J Comp Physiol Psychol,* 49:420–424.

Kamin LJ (1959). The delay-of-punishment gradient. *J Comp Physiol Psychol,* 52:434–437.

Kamin LJ (1968). Attention-like processes in classical conditioning. In MR Jones (Ed), *Miami
Symposium on the Prediction of Behavior: Aversive Stimulation.* Miami: University of Miami

Press.

Kaufman A and Baron A (1968). Suppression of behavior by timeout punishment when suppression results in loss of positive reinforcement. *J Exp Anal Behav,* 11:595–607.

Kazdin AE (1989). *Behavior Modification in Applied Settings.* Pacific Grove, CA: Brooks/Cole.

Knowles PA, Conner RL, and Panksepp J (1987). Opiate effects on social behavior of juvenile dogs as a function of social deprivation. *Pharmacol Biochem Behav,* 33:533–537.

Koehler W (1962). *The Koehler Method of Dog Training.* New York: Howell Book House.

Konorski J (1967). *Integrative Activity of the Brain.* Chicago: University of Chicago Press.

Lehrman DC, Iwata BA, Shore BA, and DeLeon IG (1997). Effects of intermittent punishment on self-injurious behavior: An evaluation of schedule thinning. *J Appl Behav Anal,* 30:187–201.

Leitenberg H (1965). Is time-out from positive reinforcement an aversive event? *Psychol Bull,* 64:428–441.

Lytle H (1927). *How to Train a Bird Dog.* Dayton, OH: AF Hochwalt.

Mackintosh NJ (1983). *Conditioning and Associative Learning.* Oxford: Clarendon.

McMillan DE (1967). A comparison of the punishing effects of response-produced shock and response-produced time out. *J Exp Anal Behav,* 10:439–449.

Most K (1910/1955). *Training Dogs.* New York: Coward-McCann (reprint).

Mowrer OH (1960). *Learning Theory and Behavior.* New York: John Wiley and Sons.

Newsom C, Favell JE, and Rincover A (1983). The side effects of punishment. In S Axelrod and J Apsche (Eds), *The Effects of Punishment in Human Behavior.* New York: Academic.

Nobbe DE, Niebuhr BR, Levinson M, and Tiller JE (1980). Use of time-out as punishment for aggressive behavior. In B Hart (Ed), *Canine Behavior.* Santa Barbara, CA: Veterinary Practice.

Ollendick TH and Matson JL (1978). Overcorrection: An overview. *Behav Ther,* 9:830–842.

Panksepp J (1988). Brain emotional circuits and psychopathologies. In M Clynes and J Panksepp (Eds), *Emotions and Psychopathology.* New York: Plenum.

Panksepp J (1998). *Affective Neuroscience: The Foundations of Human and Animal Emotions.* New York: Oxford University Press.

Pavlov IP (1927/1960). *Conditioned Reflexes: An Investigation of the Physiological Activity of the Cerebral Cortex,* GV Anrep (Trans). New York: Dover (reprint).

Polsky RH (1989): Techniques of behavioral modification: "time-out": An underemployed punishment technique. *Bull Comp Anim Behav Newsl,* 3(4).

Polsky RH (1998). Shock collars and aggression in dogs. *Anim Behav Consult Newsl,* 15(2).

Premack D (1962). Reversibility of the reinforcement relation. *Science,* 136:255–257.

Rescorla RA (1968). Probability of shock in the presence and absence of the CS in fear conditioning. *J Comp Physiol Psychol,* 66:1–5.

Rescorla RA (1988). Pavlovian conditioning: It's not what you think it is. *Am Psychol,* 43:151–160.

Rescorla RA and LoLordo VM (1965). Inhibition of avoidance behavior. *J Comp Physiol Psychol,* 59:406–412.

Scott JP (1967). The development of social motivation. In *Nebraska Symposium on Motivation,* 111–132. Lincoln: University of Nebraska Press.

Seligman MEP (1970). On the generality of the laws of learning. *Psychol Rev,* 77:406–418.

Seligman MEP and Johnston JC (1973). A cognitive theory of avoidance learning. In FJ McGuigan and DB Lumsden (Eds), *Contemporary Approaches to Conditioning and Learning.* Washington, DC: Winston-Wiley.

Sidman M (1989). *Coercion and Its Fallout.* Boston: Authors Cooperative.

Skinner BF (1974). *About Behaviorism.* New York: Alfred A Knopf.

Solnick JV, Rincover A, and Peterson CR (1977). Some determinants of the reinforcing and punishing effects of time out. *J Appl Behav Anal,* 10:415–424.

Solomon RL (1964). Punishment. *Am Psychol,* 19:239–253.

Solomon RL and Corbit JD (1974). An opponent-process theory of motivation: I. Temporal dynamics of affect. *Psychol Rev,* 81:119–145.

Solomon RL, Kamin LJ, and Wynne LC (1953). Traumatic avoidance learning: The outcomes of several extinction procedures with dogs. *J Abnorm Soc Psychol,* 43:291–302.

Solomon RL and Wynne LC (1953). Traumatic avoidance learning: Acquisition in normal dogs. *Psychol Monogr,* 67:1–19.

Staddon JER (1995). On responsibility and punishment. *Atlantic Monthly,* Feb:88–94.

Thorndike EL (1911/1965). *Animal Intelligence.* New York: Macmillan (reprint).

Thorndike EL (1931). *Human Learning.* New York: Appleton-Century-Crofts.

Tolman EC (1934). Theories of learning. In FA Moss (Ed), *Comparative Psychology,* 367–408. New York: Prentice-Hall.

Tortora DF (1982). *Understanding Electronic Dog Training.* Tucson, AZ: Tri-Tronics.

Tortora DF (1983). Safety training: The elimination of avoidance-motivated aggression in dog. *J Exp Psychol Gen,* 112:176–214.

Tossutti H (1942). *Companion Dog Training.* New York: Orange Judd.

Voith VL and Borchelt PL (1996). *Readings in Companion Animal Behavior.* Trenton, NJ: Veterinary Learning Systems.

Vollmer PJ (1979a). Electrical stimulation as an aid in training: Part 1. *Vet Med Small Anim Clin,* Nov:1600–1601.

Vollmer PJ (1979b). Electrical stimulation as an aid in training: Part 2. Bark training collars. *Vet Med Small Anim Clin,* Dec:1737–1739.

Vollmer PJ (1980). Electrical stimulation as an aid in training: Part 3. Conclusion. *Vet Med Small Anim Clin,* Jan:57–58.

Watkins LR and Mayer DJ (1982). Organization of endogenous opiate and nonopiate pain control systems. *Science,* 216:1185–1192.

Weisman RG and Litner JS (1969). Positive conditioned reinforcement of Sidman avoidance in rats. *J Comp Physiol Psychol,* 68:597–603.

Whitford CB (1908/1928). *Training the Bird Dog.* New York: Macmillan (reprint).

9

Learning and Behavioral Disturbances

One can conceive in all likelihood that, if these dogs which became ill could look back and tell what they had experienced on that occasion, they would not add a single thing to that which one would conjecture about their condition. All would declare that on every one of the occasions mentioned they were put through a difficult test, a hard situation. Some would report that they felt frequently unable to refrain from doing that which was forbidden and then they felt punished for doing it in one way or another, while others would say that they were totally, or just passively, unable to do what they usually had to do.

I. P. PAVLOV, *Conditioned Reflexes and Psychiatry* (1941)

The studies that are reviewed in this chapter raise serious ethical issues about the treatment of experimental animals. Many of these experiments, as well as others previously cited in this book, obviously caused the animals involved considerable distress and pain. Recent progress in the care and treatment of laboratory animals would make some of these experiments impossible to perform under current rules and ethical constraints. Contemporary experimental psychologists would certainly have a difficult time obtaining formal approval and public funding for the more aversive procedures used by workers in the past investigating experimental neurosis and traumatic aversive learning. Notwithstanding the obvious suffering and sacrifice extracted from the animals used in such study, the information obtained by these studies does provide practical information that may prove beneficial for dogs, both in terms of promoting welfare concerns and saving lives. Although the following accounts may be disturbing for sensitive readers, ignoring such information would only add insult to the already lamentable injury.

LEARNING PROCEEDS most efficiently under circumstances where relevant events occur in a more or less predictable and controllable manner. Unfortunately, these basic requirements of order are not always satisfied. In severe cases, such shortcomings result in long-term disturbances of behavior and learning. Behavioral disturbances range from compulsive disorders and phobias to generalized anxiety and depression. Abnormal behavior is often observed in dogs as the direct result of dysfunctional learning experiences.

EXPERIMENTAL NEUROSIS

A great deal of experimental attention has been focused on the etiology of abnormal behavior and neurosis in animals (Patton, 1951; Broadhurst, 1961). The term *neurosis* is used here in a narrow sense, not to be mistaken for the condition described in human psychiatry, although parallels do exist between human and animal neuroses. To limit confusion, a working definition of neurosis is needed. In the *Oxford Companion to the Mind*, Gregory defines neurosis as a maladaptive habit: "Neurosis is a habit that is either maladaptive in some obvious respect and/or distressing, yet more or less fixed and resistant to modification through the normal process of learning" (1987:549). The value of this definition is its conceptualization of neurotic behavior in terms of habit and learning. It falls short of being a complete definition because it fails to emphasize the role of emotional disturbance in the etiology of neurotic habits. In general, neuroses result from underlying emotional disturbances collectively impacting on various behavioral, cognitive, and somatic systems. Therefore, the definition is supplemented to include a recognition of the emotional aspect of neurotogenesis: *A neurosis is an emotionally maladaptive and persistent habit or compulsion that resists modification through normal processes of learning.*

Neurotic disturbances are most likely to occur in situations where an animal's ability to predict and control the environment is rendered by varying degrees independent of what actually happens (Mineka and Kihlstrom, 1978). Like many human neu-

rotics, neurotic animals seem to be "possessed by" a negative expectation that causes them to "believe" that what they do or intend to do will have little discernible impact on what occurs. In extreme cases, the effect can be described as a generalized state of powerlessness or futility, or what Seligman has called *learned helplessness*. Knowing that neuroses are precipitated by cognitive or behavioral failures to adequately predict and control significant events, it is not surprising to find that most neurotic disorders present comorbidly with chronic *anxiety* (a generalized emotional state associated with inadequate prediction) or *depression* (a generalized emotional state associated with inadequate control).

The laboratory induction of disturbed behavior is referred to as *experimental neurosis*. Most experimental neurosis studies have been based on the prevailing assumption that neurotic behavior disorders are of a learned origin. Several animal models based on this premise have been developed (Keehn, 1986), with the aim of clarifying the etiology and treatment of neurotically disorganized behavior. The discovery of experimental neurosis is credited to Pavlov's laboratory, in particular, to the Russian researchers Yerofeyeva and Shenger-Krestovnikova, who observed that some dogs when confronted with certain experimental arrangements exhibited dramatic disturbances of previously conditioned behavior. The dogs also exhibited a variety of collateral deviations from the norm both inside and outside the experimental setting. Pavlov considered these disturbances to be of a neurotic origin, that is, elaborations of internal conflict arising from the dysfunctional collision of excitatory and inhibitory processes.

The first example of experimental neurosis produced in Pavlov's laboratory was obtained by Yerofeyeva. In this instance, a dog was shocked and then presented with food, which the dog was forced to eat if necessary. The intensity of shock was gradually increased over several conditioning trials, until it was strong enough to cause "severe burning and mechanical destruction of the skin." Following conditioning, the dog showed no signs of defensive behavior or autonomic changes in respiration or heart rate, even when stimulated with the maximum level of current. The experimenters observed that the dog simply salivated and approached the food to eat when shock was turned on. This state of affairs persisted for several months, until the site of stimulation was moved to other places on the dog's skin. When the number of sites increased to a certain saturation point, the previously conditioned response to shock drastically changed. The dog now exhibited an explosive defensive reaction whenever and wherever the shock stimulus was delivered. Even electrical stimulation of the original location resulted in uncontrollable defensive behavior, with no sign of appetitive interest or salivation. The conditioned alimentary reflex to shock was permanently lost, and the previously calm dog became extremely agitated and hyperactive.

Pavlov's workers employed many other experimental methods to induce neurosis (Cook, 1939; Kurstin, 1968). The procedures included the following: (1) The repeated presentation of a conditioned stimulus (CS) that simultaneously elicits both an excitatory and a competing inhibitory reflex. Presumably, the effect is a collision of opposing emotional intentions, producing motivational conflict. (2) Difficult discrimination tasks in which similar stimuli control mutually incompatible responses (e.g., the experiment by Shenger-Krestovnikova discussed below). (3) Exceptionally long presentations of conditioned stimuli before being followed by unconditioned stimulus (US) reinforcement of excitatory conditioned reflexes—that is, disturbances produced by overstrain of anticipatory processes. Petrova (Pavlov, 1927/1960), for example, trained two dogs (one tending toward excitability and the other a more inhibited type) to respond to six different stimuli as salivary conditioned stimuli. Initially, the interstimulus interval between the CS and US was very brief, but as training proceeded this interval gradually increased by 5 seconds daily. Disturbances (in the excitable dog) began to appear after 2-minute intervals were reached. Dramatic disturbances of behavior were observed with 3-minute delays between the CS and US. Pavlov writes that the excitable dog "became quite crazy, unceasingly

and violently moving all parts of its body, howling, barking, and squealing intolerably. All this was accompanied by an unceasing flow of saliva, so that although the secretion increased during the action of the conditioned stimuli all traces of the delay completely disappear" (1927/1960:294). The more inhibited dog was able to cope with the delay without signs of behavioral disturbance. (4) An abrupt shift from an excitatory stimulus to an inhibitory one and vice versa. (5) Unpredictable expectancy reversals—for example, a CS that had been previously associated with food is followed by shock instead. (6) The occurrence of any intense, unusual, or traumatic stimulation—for example, the effect of the Leningrad flood reported by Pavlov or the laboratory dog fight reported by Gantt (see the following section on post-traumatic stress disorder).

The disturbances produced by the foregoing procedures can be divided into three general categories: (1) disturbances of normal learning abilities (e.g., some previously learned habit is no longer exhibited, loss of conditioned inhibition, or an impairment of an animal's ability to reacquire the lost habit or association); (2) autonomic disturbances (e.g., cardiac, respiratory, sexual, and secretory changes), and excessive emotional displays, like fear and aggression; and (3) elaboration and generalization of unusual behavioral changes, both inside and outside of the experimental context (e.g., increased shyness and aggressiveness toward other dogs and people as well as long-term autonomic disturbances). Hebb (1947) argued that many of these symptoms of neurosis could actually be viewed as adaptive species-typical responses to traumatic stimulation and nervous overstrain. He argued that true neurotic disturbance led to persistent learning deficits (e.g., a failure to perform acquired discriminations).

Shenger-Krestovnikova induced neurotic symptoms by exposing a harnessed dog to a series of difficult visual discriminations. In her famous experiment, she alternately presented the dog with a circle and an ellipse. The shapes were projected onto a screen located directly in front of the dog. The appearance of the circular shape was immediately followed by the presentation of food. After several trials, the circle became a conditioned excitatory stimulus (CS+) capable of eliciting salivation. Next, the elliptical shape was introduced. On each occasion that the ellipse appeared, food was withheld. Gradually, the ellipse became a conditioned inhibitory stimulus (CS−) predicting the absence of food. As the experiment proceeded, the ellipse was progressively modified, so that it gradually approximated the shape of a circle. At a critical point where the *susceptible* dog could no longer consistently differentiate the circle from the ellipse, it was either seized by hyperactive reactivity or despondency. The response exhibited depended on the dog's temperament and predisposition. Pavlov described the disorganized behavior of a dog exposed to this experimental arrangement:

> After three weeks of work upon this differentiation not only did the discrimination fail to improve, but it became considerably worse, and finally disappeared altogether. At the same time the whole behaviour of the animal underwent an abrupt change. The hitherto quiet dog began to squeal in its stand, kept wriggling about, tore off with its teeth the apparatus for mechanical stimulation of the skin, and bit through the tubes connecting the animal's room with the observer, a behaviour which never happened before. On being taken into the experimental room the dog now barked violently, which was also contrary to its usual custom; in short it presented all the symptoms of a condition of acute neurosis. (1927/1960:291)

A few dogs exhibited cataleptic immobility. This behavior was often associated with the refusal of food and with aggressiveness toward familiar persons with whom the dogs were previously friendly. Some dogs moved from a stupor into a state of furious rage. Others exhibited a cyclic, bipolar alternation of intense excitability followed by pronounced inhibition. Astrup (1965) noted that such symptoms are similar to those exhibited by human psychiatric patients with bipolar mood disorders.

Thomas and DeWald (1977) performed a series of experiments employing Shenger-Krestovnikova's procedure with cats. The cats were exposed to light and tone discrimina-

tion tasks in which the CS+ and CS− became progressively similar. They were trained under both classical and instrumental paradigms. Special controls and methods of quantification were also added to obtain more objective data of experimental neurosis. Their results are consistent with the aforementioned results reported by Pavlov, both in terms of dysfunctional learning symptoms (especially nonresponding) and collateral behavioral disturbances:

> All subjects in both paradigms [i.e., classical and instrumental] showed a very similar sequence of collateral behavior concomitant with the interruption of responding. As a rule subjects discontinued responding and suddenly became aggressive and attempted to escape. Many attacked objects within the chamber, such as the house light. The degree of emotionality may be inferred from the urination and defecation that often occurred in the chamber only during the specific periods of nonresponding. A number of animals developed diarrhea after at least two days of experimental neurosis. The initial symptoms, then, may be characterized as severe agitation. However, over a period of several successive days in the apparatus, the agitation abated and generally yielded to depression. Animals sat or lay immobile with their shoulders rigidly hunched in a distinctively depressive posture that is characteristic of experimental neurosis. Some animals crouched as if to urinate and remained in this position for long periods of time. ... Three animals refused food when the food magazine was operated. The other three animals approached the food very lethargically and often waited for several minutes after the food was presented before approaching and eating. (1977:222)

Pavlov found that not all dogs were equally susceptible to develop neurotic symptoms. A dog's degree of vulnerability to neurosis was dependent on its temperament. Pavlov divided dogs into four broad types, two of which he believed were particularly prone to the elaboration of neurotic disturbances. The temperament types that he recognized are (1) *sanguine*: very active, socially demonstrative and flexible; (2) *phlegmatic*: less active, socially retiring and stable; (3) *choleric*: highly unstable, manic, and prone to develop neuroses involving excitatory processes; and (4) *melancholic:* low activity, socially withdrawn and susceptible to neuroses involving inhibitory processes. Dogs with weak, unbalanced temperaments (choleric and melancholic) were found to be more easily stressed and at greater risk of developing learning and behavior disturbances than sanguine and phlegmatic dogs possessing balanced and flexible temperaments (Fig. 9.1). Pavlov believed that dogs were at an increased risk of developing neuroses during puberty and following castration (Windholz, 1994). Surprisingly, young puppies were found to be the least affected by adverse conditioning. Combining these basic temperament types with Eysenck's introversion (socially withdrawn, reserved, and passive) and extraversion (socially outgoing, impulsive, and active) dimensions (see Gray, 1971) produces a number of interactions of interest for understanding some aspects of dog behavior (Fig. 9.2). Traits on the upper half of Fig. 9.2 show signs of progressive neuroticism, with *dysthymic* (Eysenck's terms) instability affecting melancholic introverts (introverted neuroticism), whereas *hystericopsychopathic* instabilities present in the case of choleric extraverts (extraverted neuroticism) (see Gray, 1971).

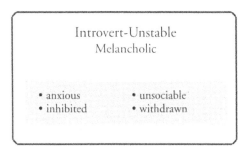

Introvert-Unstable
Melancholic

- anxious
- inhibited
- unsociable
- withdrawn

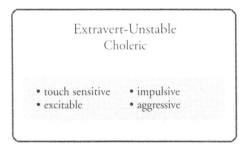

Extravert-Unstable
Choleric

- touch sensitive
- excitable
- impulsive
- aggressive

FIG. 9.1. Temperament types and traits most often associated with behavior problems.

Note that sanguine and phlegmatic temperament types combine with introversion and extroversion to form more stable traits.

GANTT: SCHIZOKINESIS, AUTOKINESIS, AND EFFECT OF PERSON

W. Horsley Gantt (1944) viewed Pavlov's discovery of experimental neurosis as a useful animal model for understanding human psychopathology. As a result, he performed a series of longitudinal studies of experimentally induced neurosis in dogs. One of the dogs he studied—Nick—was observed for over 12 years. His methods for inducing neurosis were similar to those used in Pavlov's laboratory. In addition, he studied the effect of strong emotional stimuli on conditioned behavior and the development of postconditioning neurotic sequelae—results that appear to parallel post-traumatic stress disorder (see below). These procedures included presenting intense and startling stimuli (e.g., setting off a loud explosion while the dog was restrained in the experimental harness), social restriction, fighting (both accidental and provoked), and sexual stimulation (a female in estrus was brought into the experimental chamber while conditioning was taking place). Some of the neurotic symptoms observed included anorexia, disorganized behavior, restlessness, abnormal breathing and heart rate patterns, fearfulness (especially toward persons associated with the experiments), elimination disturbances, and abnormal sexual excitement.

Gantt's work has been sharply criticized (Broadhurst, 1961). Although his experimental method may be wanting in scientific rigor and his data inconclusive, his work is nonetheless thought provoking and deserving of careful study. Gantt's general findings can be grouped into three basic categories: schizokinesis, autokinesis, and the effect of person.

Schizokinesis

Gantt has argued that classical conditioning occurs on more than one level at a time, with some conditioning (especially involving fear)

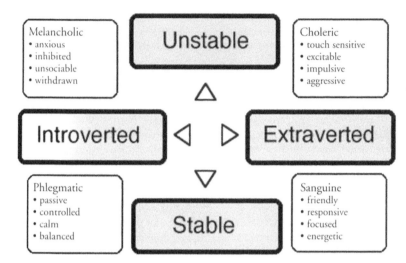

FIG. 9.2. Matrix of temperament types and traits associated with introversion and extraversion. After Pavlov and Eysenck (see Gray, 1971).

affecting remote emotional and endocrine systems in unexpected and sometimes destructive ways. Gantt referred to this cleavage between behavioral and emotional systems as *schizokinesis*. He observed that within these different response systems, respondent learning was acquired and extinguished at different rates. For example, he found that the cardiorespiratory system was particularly responsive to the effects of fear conditioning. Even after a single CS-US trial, a measurable effect could be detected in the dog's heart rate when the CS was presented alone. This pattern of rapid acquisition is in sharp contrast to the sluggish way most alimentary conditioned responses like salivation are acquired. Not only is the cardiorespiratory system sensitive to conditioning, once such conditioning is established it is very resistant to extinction.

These variable rates of acquisition and extinction have a pronounced effect on an animal's general adaptation. The schizokinetic effect sets into motion a physiological expression of psychological conflict and distress. An important corollary to be drawn from this apparent schizokinetic breach between current circumstances and an animal's emotional adaptation to them is that all psychobiological systems are, at any given moment, only partially adapted to the environment and are always homeostatically distressed to some extent. That is, all psychobiological systems (to some degree) are in a state of general disequilibrium, conflict, and distress.

Many fears and persistent anxieties may be interpreted in terms of schizokinesis. The phobic may rationally know that there is nothing to fear, but his or her body is unable to adjust to the known facts. Gantt's observations regarding schizokinesis are especially relevant to the etiology of chronic psychosomatic disorders like high blood pressure and gastric ulcers.

Autokinesis

Not only does neurotic behavior resist extinction (schizokinesis), it also undergoes various self-perpetuating processes. Gantt (1962) observed that—once established—neurotic behavior tended to take on a life of its own, spontaneously elaborating into different forms and gradually recruiting distant behavioral systems. This process of spontaneous elaboration Gantt called *autokinesis*. Frequently, these changes assume a destructive character with a progressive deterioration of the dog's condition (*negative autokinesis*). However, under the influence of beneficial conditions (e.g., appropriate training and therapy), such elaborations tend to follow a more adaptive course (*positive autokinesis*). The direction of autokinetic change is determined by a combination of temperament factors and environmental influences. For example, Gantt noted that dogs that were housed under the stressful conditions of the laboratory tended to worsen over time, whereas dogs that were retired to the more therapeutic conditions of a country farm tended to improve.

Effect of Person

During social encounters, dogs selectively respond to different people with varying degrees of approach or avoidance. Obviously, many factors, like a dog's temperament and past experiences, have a powerful effect on such social preferences and aversions. Gantt speculated that dogs respond differently, not only as a result of such influences, but also because of other less well-understood factors:

> The effect of person may take two forms: (1) He may act as a signal for some past experience in the same way as any other conditional signal acts. Thus, the person who has mistreated a child or dog may elicit anxiety, fear, or aggression. This is the more evident effect of person. (2) There is another less understood, obscure influence of one individual upon another. Without knowing its mechanism we see the profound effect. Whether it depends upon some undiscovered information-transmission relationship remains to be seen. Here is a vast field for investigation, but adequate methods are presently lacking. (1971:39)

Gantt attempted to quantify the effect of person by measuring and comparing heart and respiration rates under various social conditions. The results of these studies indicate that the mere presence of a passive person in the same room was sufficient to accelerate a dog's heart rate, whereas gentle petting had a decelerating effect. Gantt's observations emphasize the important role of touch and massage in the treatment of behavior problems and for the alleviation of emotional distress.

Of special significance in this context is the role of touch for the reduction of anxiety and other stressful emotional states. Gantt observed that neurotic dogs were particularly sensitive to the calming effect of touch. Nick, whose standing heart rate prior to petting was 167 beats per minute, could be soothed into 97 beats per minute through petting. Three general effects of person are observed among neurotic dogs: (1) extreme agitation and pronounced acceleration of heart rate, (2) a calming effect in which heart rate is decelerated, and (3) an autistic immunity to the effect of person, with little or no change in cardiorespiratory activity—a characteristic exhibited by many of Murphree's fearful pointer dogs (see Chapter 5).

Lynch and McCarthy (1969) performed a study to evaluate the effect of person on a classically conditioned cardiac/motor response to shock. The dogs in the experiment were divided into three groups according to the social circumstances current during testing: person absent, person present, and person present and petting. All animals were exposed to identical aversive conditioning in which a tone CS was paired with shock. Two activities were measured: heart rate and foot flexion. These measurements were taken before, during, and after the presentation of the tone CS. Dogs exposed to the tone while alone or while in the presence of the experimenter (without petting) exhibited the strongest amount of cardiac acceleration (tachycardia) and motor flexion. The dogs exposed to the tone in the presence of the experimenter were slightly less reactive than the dogs tested alone. The group of dogs exposed to the tone CS while being petted exhibited a significant *deceleration* (bradycardia) of heart rate relative to baseline levels taken prior to testing. The petted dogs also exhibited weaker foot-flexion response. An interesting incidental finding was the observation that female dogs exhibited a stronger benefit from petting than did males. In another experiment performed by Gantt, the acceleration of heart rate stimulated by shock was reduced by as much as 50% if a dog was in the presence of a comforting person. In general, petting appears to be an effective way to moderate fear in dogs. Petting is commonly employed with other counterconditioning stimuli (especially food) during desensitization efforts.

LIDDELL: THE CORNELL EXPERIMENTS

Howard S. Liddell (1954, 1956) studied experimental neurosis in farm animals, especially sheep and goats. Liddell's experiments involved exposing these animals to repeated simple and difficult discrimination tasks involving various stimuli and mild shocks while they were restrained in a Pavlovian frame and harness. The level of shock used by Liddell was very weak (barely perceptible to a finger moistened with salt water) but sufficient to elicit a vigorous unconditioned withdrawal response in the test animals. He utilized various conditioned stimuli ranging from somatic (a rhythmic pressure remotely applied to the skin) to auditory (metronome, bell, buzzer) and visual (dim and bright light) signals.

The typical animal was trained to perform various discrimination tasks involving conditioned stimuli predicting the presence (CS+) or absence (CS−) of shock. The behavior of one of these animals, a sheep named Robert, was described in detail by Liddell in his book *Emotional Hazards in Animals and Man* (1956). Robert had undergone extensive training over 3 years involving simple and difficult discrimination tasks. For example, he had been trained to respond positively to the sound of a buzzer and also to a metronome set to click once per second. The metronome or buzzer was presented 10 seconds before shock was delivered through electrodes attached to the animal's right front leg. Negative conditioned stimuli (those associated with the absence of shock) were also conditioned. Whenever the sound of a bell was presented, for example, it was never followed by shock. This sort of discrimination was easy for the sheep to master. Other negative (inhibitory) conditioned stimuli were also employed that were more difficult for Robert to differentiate from the positive or excitatory conditioned stimuli. This was especially the case with discriminations involving various metronome beats—some rates being associated with shock while others were predictive of its absence. These more difficult discriminations progressively resulted in the elicitation of greater distress and behavioral disturbance. Negative responses were conditioned to metronome rates of 120, 100, 92, 84, 78, and 72 clicks—all of these rates of clicking predicted the absence of impending shock. Robert easily learned to discriminate the metronome set at 60 clicks per minute (positive CS predicting shock) from the metronome set at 120 clicks (predicting the absence of shock). As the rate of clicking neared the positive stimulus, however, the sheep became progressively reactive and disturbed. Exposure to the 72-click rate followed a minute later by the presentation of the positive CS (metronome set at the 60-click rate) resulted in Robert failing to respond appropriately as he had done many hundreds of times in the past to the positive CS. His failure to predict the impending shock resulted in an exaggerated and inappropriate response when shock was finally delivered. Liddell describes this demonstration and the result:

> Exactly one minute after metronome 72 has ceased we sound the metronome at 60 beats per minute and for the first time during the hour Robert fails dramatically in interpreting the signal most familiar to him—the signal, which, since the beginning of his training three years ago, has always meant shock. As the clicking begins at once a second he freezes with forelegs stiffly extended and with signs of respiratory distress. In fact, he duplicates his reaction to the just preceding difficult negative signal, metronome 72. At the end of 10 seconds the sound of metronome 60 is terminated by the usual shock to the right foreleg. However, Robert's reaction to this mild unconditioned stimulus is quite unusual. He leaps violently upward with both forelegs in the air but then immediately resumes a tense pose. (Liddell, 1956:10)

Liddell and his associates studied many different procedures for elaborating neurotic behavior. However, in general, the conditioning procedures he used were for the most part limited to monotonous and repetitious discrimination tasks, typically involving 20 trials a day, 5 days a week, over the course of several months. Their theoretical account of experimental neurosis emphasized the importance of monotonous repetition and restraint (i.e., loss of control) as the crucial factors involved in the production of neurotic disturbances. They argued that, under conditions of experimental restraint, the mere repeated elicitation of aversive excitatory and inhibitory reflexes was enough to result in the development of experimental neurosis. Further, they found that simply restraining a previously trained sheep in the experimental harness (an apparatus they refer to as a "psychical strait jacket") for an hour session without any stimulus presentation whatsoever was sufficient to evoke evidence of pronounced autonomic and behavioral distress. Loss of control (i.e., exposure to uncontrollable and inescapable events) plays an integral role in the experiments of Liddell, which support the view that control over vital events is of critical importance for the elaboration and maintenance of adaptive behavior and vice versa. Mineka and Kihlstrom discuss the role of control and predictability in Liddell's experiments at length:

> Initially Liddell's group attributed experimental neurosis to a variety of neuroendocrine changes. Later, however, Liddell offered an interpretation very much in accord with our own, noting that the domesticated animal already lives under conditions of considerable restraint—a condition that is exacerbated by the exigencies of the laboratory experiment. Restraint, or loss of control, in either situation alone may be disturbing to the animal, and the two in conjunction are likely to be even more stressful. Liddell often emphasized that laboratory experiments which did not involve restraint of movement (as did the Pavlovian harness), such as insoluble mazes, did not produce experimental neurosis. (1978:265)

Liddell noted that many of the animals he tested exhibited vigorous efforts to break free when they were first placed into the experimental harness. These initial efforts to escape were regularly followed by a sudden lapse into a tense state of resignation. Younger animals accepted exposure to loss of control more readily than older ones. In older animals, the *freedom* reflex appeared to be more persistent and unyielding than in the more compliant and flexible younger ones. Liddell

described a 1-year-old billy goat that unremittingly continued to struggle and butt while attached to the training harness, making him useless for experimental purposes. Similarly, Pavlov reported a case involving an outgoing and friendly dog that strongly rebelled against restraint in the harness. However, he gradually overcame the dog's reactivity by reciprocally inhibiting the freedom reflex with the elicitation of another more salient reflex incompatible with continued struggling—eating. Pavlov strongly emphasized the adaptive importance of the freedom reflex:

> It is clear that the freedom reflex is one of the important reflexes, or, if we use a more general term, reactions, of living beings. This reflex has even yet to find its final recognition. In James' writings it is not even enumerated among the special human "instincts." But it is clear that if the animal were not provided with a reflex of protest against boundaries set to its freedom, the smallest obstacle in its path would interfere with the proper fulfillment of its natural functions. (1927/1960:12)

The repeated and inescapable stimulation of escape was considered by Liddell to be the causal locus of neurotic elaboration in his experiments. This viewpoint is consistent with more contemporary theories in which loss of control over significant biological events is considered instrumental in the generation of various behavioral disturbances, like learned helplessness and post-traumatic stress disorder, for example. The animals in Liddell's experiments appear to give up psychologically and thereby predispose themselves to the development of neurotic symptoms and their elaboration under the influence of repeated stimulation of aversive emotional reactions and the chronic habituation of the orienting response. Under conditions of fearful or aversive stimulation where an animal's control over the situation is impeded, and the orienting response habituated through persistent and monotonous elicitation, a growing sense of insecurity and heightened distress occur together with increased arousal and various dysfunctional efforts to adjust. Some of the more pronounced symptoms that he observed in experimentally distressed animals included hyperirritability, restlessness, insomnia, bizarre postural compulsions, dysfunctional reflex movements, eliminatory disturbances, and a tendency toward self-isolation when with conspecifics.

A study of reactive hypertension in dogs provides some suggestive evidence linking the chronic inhibition of the freedom reflex with increased stress and irritability. Wilhelm and colleagues (1953) found that highly trained and conditioned dogs exhibit a much more extreme blood pressure response to trivial stimulation (entry of a stranger, strange noise in the kennel, and change in routine) than less-well-trained counterparts. The authors speculated along with Liddell that repetitive and monotonous inhibitory training and conditioning is itself stressful and neurotogenic. In a study assessing the effects of stress occurring during guide-dog training, *stress-prone* and *non-stress-prone* guide dogs were evaluated (Vincent and Mitchell, 1996). The researchers found that stress-prone dogs tended to exhibit significantly higher blood pressure readings when compared with non-stress-prone dogs, suggesting that temperament factors play an important role in the physiological expression of stress. These observations raise many questions with regard to training methodology and the various possible side effects resulting from excessive and boring inhibitory conditioning. In addition, the adverse effects of stressful training appear to depend on a dog's temperament and the dog's inclination toward reactive autonomic arousal.

One of the experiments performed by Liddell (1964) generated unusual and dramatic results. The objective of the study was to compare the effect of maternal contact on neurosis-inducing conditioning in twin goats. Siblings at 3 weeks of age were exposed to repeated leg flexion training in the presence of a dimmed-light CS: every 2 minutes, the light in the experimental room was dimmed for 10 seconds, followed by the presentation of mild shock. Twenty such trials were carried out daily over the course of training. The twins were stimulated identically, except one was kept with its mother during testing while the other was left alone.

Several remarkable outcomes resulted

from the foregoing procedure. The twin conditioned in the presence of its mother learned to flex its leg as a kind of trick and did not develop the collateral emotional and behavioral disturbances associated with experimental neurosis. In contrast, the yoked twin, undergoing simultaneous conditioning in a separate room, became more reactive and upset as conditioning proceeded. Eventually, the isolated twin became immobile as though restrained in an invisible Pavlovian harness and subsequently exhibited many symptoms of experimental neurosis.

The foregoing experiment is an interesting confirmation of Gantt's effect-of-person theory. The twin conditioned in the presence of its mother was somehow protected from the ill-effects of the training procedure. Liddell observed an unexpected outcome of this series of experiments: all of the isolated twins died within a year (many within a few months) of various diseases, while the twins that were trained in the presence of their mothers survived into adulthood.

Experiments involving dogs performed by Liddell's group were carried out but not very often, as indicated by their lack in the literature. James (1943) utilized a conditioned avoidance response involving strong shock delivered to the foreleg of a German shepherd. The dog's leg had been weighted down so that, to avoid shock, the dog had to lift 30 pounds. The result was "total flight and escape behavior ... signaled in the kennel by the entrance of the experimenter rather than a specific signal in the laboratory (1943:117). After several months of rest, the first CS presented to the dog resulted in such a massive panic reaction that he broke out of the harness restraining him (Broadhurst, 1961). Cook (1939) reported a study by Drabovitch and Weger (1937, in French), who used a somewhat similar method as that described by Liddell. The dogs were trained to flex the left hind leg in response to a bell that was followed by shock. Once the flexion action occurred under the signalization of the bell alone, the experiment was modified in a way reminiscent of Yerofeyeva's experiment discussed earlier. Now, instead of attaching the electrode to the left hind leg, it was attached to the front left leg. The bell was rung repeatedly but without the delivery of shock. After three daily experimental sessions involving this arrangement, one of the dogs became quite agitated and on day 4 exhibited continuous convulsions of the left hind leg throughout the testing period.

A second dog involved in their study that had been exposed to leg flexion training over the course of 2 years was given a month-long break. During this period of rest, the dog's cage mate was removed and taken to the laboratory at the normal times he had been tested in the past. When the resting dog was tested after a month, he responded with unexpected and intense withdrawal reactions and convulsions of the left hind foot, a reaction that gradually generalized to the right hind leg as well. The combined convulsions resulted in the dog not being able to stand. Gradually, the dog became reactive as soon as he entered the laboratory situation, exhibiting a high degree of generalized arousal and withdrawal efforts. The researchers speculated that the daily excitement and distress of losing his cage mate may have adversely affected the dog's response to testing by "supercharging" centers controlling conditioned flexion. Although this explanation is not very appealing, the experiment does emphasize the potential inimical effects of separation distress on the elaboration of behavioral disturbances.

MASSERMAN: MOTIVATIONAL CONFLICT THEORY OF NEUROSIS

Jules H. Masserman (1943) devised several methods for inducing neurosis in cats, dogs, and monkeys. These procedures depended on what he called a *principle of uncertainty* and the collision of mutually incompatible appetitive and aversive motivational states. In the prototypical experiment, cats (although dogs were sometimes used as well) were first trained to perform a simple instrumental response to obtain food. The food-deprived animals were individually placed into an experimental compartment that contained at one end a partially closed box with food in it. The food could be easily obtained by prying open the lid. Once the cats had learned how to obtain food, a new contingency was intro-

duced. Access to the box now required that the animals wait for the presentation of a specific combination of light and sound stimuli before approaching. Finally, the cats were trained to turn on the light and sound stimuli by depressing various disk-shaped manipulanda before advancing to the box containing food.

Induction of Neurotic Conflict

After several months of such training, a critical experimental element was introduced. Upon having performed the preliminary requisite responses and just before ingesting the food delivered as reinforcement, the cat was exposed to a blast of compressed air or mild electric shock delivered to its paws. The startled cat immediately retreated from the food box and refused (temporarily) to approach it again. Eventually, however, the cat's fear subsided enough to allow it to approach the container once more. After several "safe" trials, the cat was again exposed to the delivery of unannounced mild shock or air blast. After two to seven trials involving such unpredictable aversive stimulation, the cats began to exhibit various signs of disturbance and abnormal patterns of behavior. These symptoms included an accelerated heart rate, increased blood pressure, piloerection, trembling, irregular breathing and asthma, extreme startle reactivity, irrationally fearful behavior, gastrointestinal disorders, persistent salivation, sexual impotence, persistent diuresis, and epileptic and cataleptic seizures. In addition, some compulsive tendencies also appeared, including persistent restlessness, pacing, and various repetitive behaviors. One of the few dogs exposed to Masserman's procedure appeared to have developed a superstitious behavior pattern as a result:

> Peculiar "compulsions" emerged, such as restless, elliptical pacing or repetitive gestures and mannerisms. One neurotic dog could never approach his food until he had circled it three times to the left and bowed his head before it. Neurotic animals lost their group dominance and became reactively aggressive under frustration. In other relationships they regressed to excessive dependence or various forms of kittenish helplessness. In short, the animals dis-

played the same stereotypes of anxiety, phobias, hypersensitivity, regression and psychosomatic dysfunctions observed in human patients. (Masserman, 1950:41)

These symptoms were not restricted to the experimental setting only but generalized into "the entire life of the animals and persisted indefinitely" if left untreated.

Masserman believed that the collision of mutually incompatible motivations and the evocation of approach-withdrawal conflict was of central importance to the development of neurotic behavior. However, this interpretation of neurosis has been strongly criticized by Wolpe (1958), whose experiments consisted of two general procedures for producing neurotic disturbances in cats (see Chapter 6). One group of cats was exposed to a series of inescapable shocks after a period of adaptation to the training situation; a second group was exposed to a procedure that was similar to that used by Masserman. Wolpe found a close resemblance in the behavior of both groups of cats regardless of the procedure used, suggesting to him that the motivational conflict hypothesis proposed by Masserman was wrong. According to Wolpe's interpretation, the traumatic presentation of inescapable shock alone is sufficient to produce phobic reactions and the various neurotic sequelae observed by Masserman.

One critical difference between Wolpe's experiments and those of Masserman appears to have been overlooked: the exact timing of shock. In Wolpe's experiment, shock was delivered just before the pellet was reached, whereas, in Masserman's experiment, shock was delivered just as the animal took the food into his mouth. This difference of timing appears to have a pronounced effect on the development of behavioral disturbances in dogs [see below and Lichtenstein (1950)]. To determine the relative significance of these various timing factors and to test the motivational conflict hypothesis, Smart (1965) devised a replication of Masserman's experiment in which shock was delivered at different times relative to the presentation of food. The 30 cats in Smart's experiment were divided into three groups: (1) In the preconsummatory group, shock was delivered while

the cat was opening the lid of the food box but before eating the food. (2) In the consummatory group, shock was delivered 1 second after the food was taken in the cat's mouth. (3) In the shock-alone group, shock was delivered at least 30 seconds after any preconsummatory or consummatory behavior. Smart found that the timing of shock added little to the course of behavioral disturbances exhibited by the cats. He concluded that appetitive-aversive conflict plays no significant role in the induction of experimental neurosis, thus supporting Wolpe's contention that aversive stimulation alone is sufficient to produce such behavioral disturbances.

Although Smart's study represents a serious challenge to the conflict hypothesis, Seward (1969) noted that the experiment suffers a procedural shortcoming. The level of shock used by Smart is severe (3.5 mA AC for 1 second); perhaps, argues Seward, "strong enough to suggest that any differences among his groups may well have been hidden by a 'ceiling effect.' Whether an intensity of shock could be found that would make cats neurotic if used as punishment but not if used separately remains to be seen" (1969:433). In addition, it should be noted that the motivational conflict hypothesis is backed by other forms of evidence not addressed by Smart's study. Most significant in this regard is Masserman's finding that behavioral disturbances were significantly attenuated by diminishing the intensity of one of the conflicted elements involved. For example, if a cat was fed (either manually or forcibly tube fed) prior to exposure to the experimental situation, neurotic symptoms were significantly reduced. Lastly, the motivational conflict hypothesis is not entirely falsified by Smart's investigation. He did not demonstrate that internal conflict was entirely absent at the moment of shock in the three groups involved. Various conflict reactions involving the freeze-flight-fight system are a natural and likely response to unpredictable and uncontrollable aversive stimulation regardless of whether it occurs in the presence or absence of appetitive stimulation. Actually, it would appear to be very difficult to control for the influence of motivational conflict in situations involving the presentation of unpredictable and uncontrollable aversive stimulation. Even though the cats belonging to the shock-alone group were not shocked in the presence of food, they were nonetheless under the influence of emotional and behavioral activities incompatible with shock at the moment of its delivery.

Treatment Procedures

Masserman (1950) employed a variety of treatment strategies to relieve the behavioral disturbances he had produced in cats. Although prolonged rest in a home environment was effective in some animals, the symptoms quickly recovered after the animals returned to the laboratory, even though they were not exposed to additional experimentation. One treatment method that proved effective was the so-called *environmental press*, in which a hungry cat was mechanically pressed toward an especially appetizing food item (salmon pellets spiced with catnip). At the point of highest tension, the cat "suddenly lunged for the food; thereafter they needed less mechanical 'persuasion,' and finally their feeding-inhibition disappeared altogether, carrying other neurotic symptoms with it" (Masserman, 1950:42).

Another method studied involved gentle persuasion and guidance. In this case, the cat was first encouraged to take food from an outstretched hand while outside of the compartment, then to take food while inside the compartment, and so forth, until the cat would once again open the box on its own accord. Through repeated exposure and practice, the food-inhibited cat was gradually persuaded to eat from the food dispenser. This method of therapy appears to have worked especially well with cats possessing a dependent and a trusting attitude toward the experimenter. Masserman argues that the procedure is analogous to *transference* in human psychotherapy, where a patient is encouraged to form a dependent and trusting relationship with a therapist. The therapist in turn navigates the patient through the therapeutic process of conflict resolution until the patient is able to function more effectively on his or her own. This method was particularly effective with some cats that even learned to toler-

ate the blast of air without exhibiting any apparent signs of fear. In some cases, the air blast appears to have become a positive CS for the presentation of food (Masserman, 1950).

Masserman also studied *modeling* as a method for reducing fear of the feeding apparatus. Neurotic cats were paired with naive counterparts and permitted to observe them eat without experiencing aversive consequences. Initially, the observing cats cowered as food was presented but gradually became more confident and finally advanced toward the food dispenser on their own and ate. Masserman found *vicarious extinction* (as he called it) to be the least reliable of the various treatment strategies that he employed. In conclusion, he recommends an eclectic treatment program in which a combination of various therapeutic procedures is incorporated.

In addition to the aforementioned behavioral techniques, Masserman also explored the use of various pharmacological and psychiatric interventions, like electroshock therapy. Under the influence of alcohol, barbiturates, or narcotics, the cats appeared to be more relaxed and responsive. The neurotic symptoms (at least temporarily) were abated under the influence of such medication. Interestingly, despite a natural aversion toward alcohol, neurotic cats treated with alcohol developed a preference for it over other nonalcoholic drinks—a preference that persisted until the cat's underlying neurotic condition was resolved with behavior therapy. Electroconvulsive shock affected cats in a similar way as drug therapy, except that such treatment also resulted in pronounced and permanent disintegration of behavioral and cognitive functioning and capacity.

Lichtenstein's Experiments

P. E. Lichtenstein (1950) performed a similar series of experiments with dogs and obtained results consistent with those reported by Masserman. In Lichtenstein's experiments, 14 dogs were trained to eat from a box containing pellets of food while restrained in a conditioning harness. Once they had been habituated to this situation and were eating freely, a 2-second 85-volt AC shock was applied to their forepaws. The dogs were divided into two groups. Group 1 received shock simultaneously with the presentation of food in the pattern of classical conditioning. Group 2 dogs received shock while they were actively eating the food (a punishment paradigm). The criterion for food inhibition was determined by the refusal of food during three sessions of training (60 refused presentations of food). Dogs belonging to group 1 received considerably more shocks (23 to 29) to reach the criterion level, whereas those belonging to group 2 reached a stable food inhibition within one to three shock presentations.

The symptomatology and resulting sequelae exhibited by dogs were very similar to those observed by Masserman in cats. In addition to exhibiting many of the same autonomic symptoms previously listed, other significant symptoms included increased aggression, hyperactivity, and depression. Lichtenstein observed that dogs generally followed one of two distinct patterns: increased excitation or inhibition (catalepsy). Some dogs exhibited tremors and tics—symptoms that are frequently comorbid with compulsive disorders (Leonard et al., 1993). One dog—M88—exhibited an intense activity shift while observing other dogs being fed. M88 also engaged in nearly continuous barking and rapid whirling while confined in his home cage. In general, a noticeable increase in fighting and barking was observed in dogs exposed to the procedure. In addition to increased fighting behavior, increased aggression toward the experimenter was also observed. One dog, a female named F74, reportedly bit the experimenter several times on his hands and wrists on the first day in which her eating response was fully inhibited:

> F74 appeared well adjusted and quiet until the first day of complete failure to eat in the stock. Upon being removed form the stock she bit the experimenter upon the hands and wrists several times and could not be quieted. When removed to her cage she paced in an agitated manner and was aggressive with her cage mates. Although she had not been observed to fight at all previously, there was now scarcely a

day when she was not reported to have attacked her cage mates. (Lichtenstein, 1950:23)

In Masserman's experiments, shock appears to have been presented at "the moment of food taking," causing the cat to drop the food from its mouth and retreat from the apparatus. According to Lichtenstein, this difference is significant with regard to the production of anxiety and the experimental inhibition of feeding. As previously discussed, he compared the results of the two procedures and found that the most dramatic and lasting results occurred when shock overlapped the act of eating. His experiments suggest the possible existence of a conflict intensification gradient as choice nears the critical nexus between opposing motivations (Seward, 1969).

Experimental Neurosis and Social Dominance

Masserman and Siever (1944) studied the dynamic influence of experimental neurosis on social dominance and aggressive behavior in cats. In these experiments, several previously trained cats were matched in dyads and evaluated for relative dominance by their ability to compete for and control access to food. The dyads were placed into an experimental chamber with a single bit of food for which they had to compete. As a result of such competition, a winner emerged that controlled future access to food, with the loser deferring on subsequent trials when food was presented. Using this method, three groups of four cats each were organized according to a linear dominance hierarchy. The dominant cat of each group was then exposed to the neurosis-inducing procedure previously discussed. A fourth group was exposed to a separate preparation in which one cat of a paired dyad was trained to manipulate a switch but prevented from obtaining the subsequent reward before the food was eaten by the other cat.

According to Masserman and Siever, hierarchically organized cats rarely engaged in agonistic behavior among themselves over food. Instead, the subordinate simply stayed away while the dominant cat was working the switches or eating. Aggression was regularly observed only under two conditions: (1) when cats of equal dominance status were paired together (e.g., when the alpha cat of group 1 was paired with the alpha of group 2 or 3), or (2) when the alpha cat was exposed to neurotic conflict and inhibition by aversive inhibitory training of appetitive behavior. After such training, the alpha will usually allow the subordinate to eat but will still attack the subordinate between trials.

The researchers found some interesting results derived from the experimental conditions defined for group 4, in which the trained cat could produce the reward but could not obtain it before the paired conspecific had eaten it. Both cats had been previously trained to operate the switch and were free to play either the role of operator or observer in the experiment. Several variations emerged:

1. In cases where the operator was dominant, the operator would attack the observer and prevent the observer from eating.
2. Some cats developed a cooperative strategy between themselves in which they alternated roles, but this did last beyond 10 to 24 trials, when one of them became parasitic on the other.
3. A "worker-parasite relation" developed in which one cat worked the switch while the other observed and ate. One rather clever cat found that if he depressed the switch several times, he could obtain some food by rushing to the food pan before the observer ate it all.

Although both animals had equal access and opportunity to operate the switch or observe and obtain the reward, the role of operating the switch usually proved obligatory for the more submissive of the two cats. Even though the submissive worker never received food while the dominant cat was present, he nonetheless happily operated the switch for a time as though finding some substitutive satisfaction or intrinsic reward in the operation of the switch itself. Eventually, however, this parasitic relationship broke down, with the submissive cat finally quitting:

Under such conditions, however, this arrangement broke down, and both animals, even after two days of self-starvation, would lie about the cage deigning to manipulate the signals for the others' benefit. Under these circumstances if one of the animals were removed, the other would, in most instances, proceed promptly to manipulate the switch again for her own feeding; however, some animals seemed to have been so frustrated by the proceeding that a variable amount of individual retraining was necessary before the manipulative pattern was reestablished. (Masserman and Siever, 1944)

Previously acquired instrumental behavior appears to be spontaneously depressed under the influence of stratified social relations in an appetitive-learning situation. This outcome is rather maladaptive when considering that the cats involved could have adopted other more mutually advantageous adjustment strategies. For instance, both of the cats could have simply taken turns operating the switch and eating alternately or the more dominant of the two might have simply taken over both operating the switch and controlling access to food. In the case of appetitive learning, the dominant and submissive cats appear bound to highly specific and rigid roles associated with their status. Under the contingencies of reinforcement described in Masserman's experiment, it is incumbent upon the more submissive animal to emit the requisite instrumental response while the more dominant observer obtains the reward.

Logan (1971) found a similarly dysfunctional outcome in the case of rats trained to avoid or escape shock. A linear dominance hierarchy was determined by pairing rats in various combinations and exposing the dyads to shock. The procedure involved confining paired rats in a small cage and then exposing them to a series of brief shocks until one of them attacked (dominant) and the other submitted (submissive). The rats were then exposed to various training regimens in which some were taught to avoid or escape shock by turning a wheel. Logan reported the following results: (1) If two naive rats (regardless of their status) are paired together in an avoidance-training situation, neither of them is able to learn the required response. (2) If one of them has been previously trained, then avoidance responding will continue *provided the rat is subordinate.* (3) If both rats have been previously trained to turn the wheel to avoid shock, then the rate of responding is depressed when they are placed together and exposed to usual avoidance signals. (4) Under such circumstances, the submissive rat emits most of the escape-avoidance responses, while the dominant rat initiates most of the aggressive responses elicited by shock.(5) The cooperative participation of paired rats depends on their relative dominance ranking: the more dominant the rat, the more unlikely it will respond during signaled avoidance trials. (6) The initiation of an aggressive behavior and its direction also depend on relative dominance ranking, with the more dominant individual initiating more aggressive interactions toward the more submissive conspecific.

An interesting finding of both studies was a depression of learned behavior occurring when dominant and submissive conspecifics are paired together in the same situation. In Masserman's appetitive context, the dominant cat refused to work in the presence of the submissive cat even though the former was very hungry and capable of performing the requisite response. Similarly, under conditions of avoidance training, the dominant rat, even though well trained and able to perform the requisite avoidance response, refused to do so but instead depended on the more submissive of the dyad, whose ability to avoid shock was compromised by the threats and attacks of the more dominant rat. The result was a vicious circle in which the dominant rat became more and more aggressive toward the subordinate, impeding its ability to avoid shock and thereby stimulating the delivery of more aggression by the more dominant rat:

> The phenomenon of paired-avoidance decrement coupled with aggression is certainly not adaptive. If a dominant S "knows" the avoidance response that is required, it would be reasonable to expect him to "take charge" and protect both itself and the submissive animal. Or even if the submissive S is required to make the response, it might reasonably do it in time to avoid shock rather than waiting to escape it. (Logan, 1971:196)

FRUSTRATION AND NEUROSIS: THE THEORIES OF MAIER AND AMSEL

Maier's Frustrative Theory of Abnormal Fixations and Compulsions

Masserman viewed the causes of neurosis from the perspective of conflict or the evocation of pathological fear and anxiety. He did not examine explicitly the implicit role of frustration. Norman R. F. Maier (1961) performed a series of experiments with rats to explore the effect of frustration on the development of neurotic behavior. Simply stated, Maier's studies involved training rats to perform a visual discrimination between two cards, one having a black circular shape on it and the other a white one. The rats were trained to jump from a platform located several inches away. Jumping to the positive card resulted in food and safety. The negative card, however, was latched in such a way that choosing it would cause the rat to be bumped on the nose and to fall off the apparatus onto a cloth net suspended below. The rats readily learned to discriminate between the positive and negative cards. The next step involved randomly latching the cards so that the rats could no longer make reliable discriminations before jumping. The result was that most rats soon quit jumping. To prompt them to jump, Maier employed various aversive means, like shock or a burst of air, or he directly prodded them with a stick. This resulted in the rats jumping and developing a variety of persistent fixations and preferences toward one position or the other. Even when the discrimination task was returned to its original solvable form, the rats persisted in their abnormal fixations over hundreds of trials.

Maier's experiment placed the rats in a situation of *inescapable* and insoluble conflict. The rats are conflicted between the punishing effect of banging into latched uninformative discrimination cards or receiving aversive stimulation for not jumping (an avoidance-avoidance conflict)—that is, aversive stimulation is inescapable. Some of Maier's results anticipate parallel findings in Seligman's learned-helplessness experiments. Like Seligman's helpless dogs, Maier's rats persisted over hundreds of trials in their position fixations and failed to learn. The rats appeared unable to abandon their compulsive fixations and to learn alternative, more adaptive escape responses. Also, anticipating Seligman, Maier was able to overcome the effect of inescapable punishment only by forcibly blocking fixated responses and then guiding perseverating rats into performing an easy alternative escape response. Rats learned within 20 trials of directive training to go to an open window for food and safety. Afterward, the positive card was placed in front of the location and the rehabilitated rats quickly learned to associate it with safety regardless of position. This procedure anticipates in many ways the in vivo exposure and response prevention techniques currently used in the treatment of compulsive disorders and phobias.

Unfortunately, as suggestive as Maier's findings are, his experimental design is seriously flawed, possibly confounding frustrative persistence with a negatively reinforced escape response. Under the conditions described by Maier, the fixated pattern might easily be interpreted as the result of a learned escape response evoked by aversive prodding. Maier's experiments appear to have failed to control for this possibility.

Amsel's Frustrative Effects: Response Potentiation and Persistence

Abram Amsel investigated the effects of frustration on behavior. *Frustration* is postulated as an underlying emotional factor that invigorates behavior when it is confronted with obstacles or deterrents blocking the attainment of some desired goal. This general formulation is strikingly similar to Pavlov's aforementioned description of the freedom reflex. The first and foremost response of most animals when confronted with frustration is to press harder toward the thwarted goal. Amsel refers to this drive postulate as *persistence* and the invigoration it causes as the *frustration effect*, which can be readily seen in many situations involving extinction. Typically, a previously successful behavior exposed to extinction procedures is exaggerated in form and repeatedly emitted in an effort

to secure reinforcement. Amsel quantified the frustration effect by training rats to run down a long runway at the middle and end of which they would find a goal box containing food. Once the behavior of running to both goal boxes was well established, food was no longer provided at the midway point, requiring that the rats continue along to the end of the runway before being rewarded. Frustrated animals responded by running more quickly than nonfrustrated controls (fed at both sites) (Amsel and Roussel, 1952). These studies demonstrate that behavior is strengthened and invigorated by mild frustration.

Amsel (1971) contrasted resistance to extinction with persistence, stressing that persistence is a more inclusive and general concept. *Persistence* holds equally well for behavior occurring in the presence of frustrative nonreward as it does for behavior enduring after punishment. Persistent behavior occurs despite frustration and pain—but why? Many experiments have demonstrated that partial or intermittent reinforcement renders behavior more resistant to extinction, whereas behavior maintained on a continuous schedule is prone to weaken rapidly when reinforcement is withdrawn. One way to understand this difference is to suppose that conditioned emotional reactions to frustration have become internal cues associated with periodic interruption of regular reinforcement. The animal learns that persisting in the presence of such cues will finally result in final satisfaction. Frustrative internal cues current at the moment of satisfaction are conditioned as secondary reinforcers while antecedent cues become discriminative stimuli for frustrative effort. Over the course of training under partial reinforcement, the aversive hedonic qualities of frustration are either counterconditioned (by being linked with eventual satisfaction) or habituated by repeated evocation during nonreinforced trials. Under these conditions of learning, the stimulus complex (external and internal cues) signaling frustration actually evokes, potentiates, and covertly reinforces frustrated behavior under the maintenance of partial reinforcement.

The persistence of behavior in the presence of pending punishment relies on the development of what may aptly be termed *learned courage.* Given the presence of a sufficiently desirable outcome, an animal may endure intense aversive stimulation in order to acquire it. Amsel described experiments by Miller (1960) that found an increased production of persistence or "courage" in rats that had been gradually exposed to shock to obtain a food reward. Following gradual exposure to increasing intensities of shock, preexposed rats displayed an abnormal persistence in the presence of shock over that exhibited by controls. Another situation in which persistence is likely to occur is when the probability of shock is low and the value of the concurrent reward high—that is, when the reward is sufficiently desirable to offset the threat of punishment. The latter formulation results in a cost-benefit calculation in which the risk of responding is compared with the benefits of responding (i.e., the animal appears to gamble).

Persistence is common among dogs especially when considering nuisance behaviors. Many owners inadvertently place undesirable behavior on an intermittent schedule of reinforcement while gradually escalating punitive efforts to suppress it. Begging dogs may frustratively persist in spite of periodic punishment, knowing from previous successes that the owner will eventually cave in to their demanding antics. Frustrative perseveration is frequently observed in behavior motivated by attention seeking (like jumping up and barking). The owner may facilitate such unwanted behavior by periodically allowing it to occur without appropriate punishment. Amsel states the situation very succinctly: "Persistence depends on inconsistent treatment of consistent behavior" (1971:59).

LEARNED HELPLESSNESS

The next major step in the history of experimental neurosis took place in the laboratory of Martin E. P. Seligman, who, with his coworkers, discovered that dogs exposed to traumatic inescapable shock showed signs of neurotic elaboration and disintegration on cognitive, emotional, and motivational levels of organization (Seligman and Maier, 1967; Maier et al., 1969).

Experimental Design and Procedures

Subjects were small dogs of unknown origin that were divided into three groups: escape trained (ET), yoked control (YC), and control (C). The ET group was exposed to escape training involving shock applied to the foot pads of the hind feet while restrained in a Pavlovian hammock. Flat panels located on either side of the dog's head would immediately terminate shock if pressed by side-to-side movement of the dog's head. The YC group, which was simultaneously exposed to identical conditions and stimulation but was not able to escape shock by moving the panels, was exposed to 64 traumatic inescapable shocks occurring every 90 seconds (average) for a duration dependent on the speed and pattern of ET's escape responding, for a total of 226 seconds of shock overall. The ET group could terminate the traumatic shock with the appropriate press of the fitted panels. The C group received no escape training. The following day, all three groups were exposed to escape-avoidance training in the presence of a visual CS (turning off of lights in a conditioning compartment) 10 seconds continuously prior to the delivery of shock. The required avoidance response was jumping over a hurdle (adjusted to the height of the dog's shoulder) into an identical adjacent compartment. A dog that jumped as the light was turned off could avoid shock altogether. All subjects were exposed to 10 trials of escape-avoidance conditioning.

Results

Both the ET and C groups readily learned the shuttle-box avoidance response. The YC (helpless) group, however, exhibited great difficulty in mastering the required behavior. Most of the helpless dogs failed to escape shock by jumping over the barrier when tested. Instead of making an effort to jump, they displayed intense panic reactions followed by impassivity—they simply laid down and whimpered on a wire grid of pulsating shock. As testing proceeded, they made no effort to escape at all. A striking outcome of Seligman's experiment was that inescapable shock had dramatic negative and interfering effects on postshock learning. Even when helpless dogs occasionally succeeded in jumping over the barrier, they were unable to benefit from these successes on subsequent trials. Besides failing to initiate purposeful efforts to escape shock and learning from their experience, Seligman described several other prominent characteristics associated with learned helplessness: (1) time course (after a single exposure to uncontrollable shock, most dogs recovered within 24 hours but failed to recover after repeated exposure), (2) lowered competitiveness (aggressiveness) and general vitality; (3) development of a negative cognitive set (a belief that nothing can be done, i.e., environmental events are independent of action), and (4) loss of appetite (an outcome also associated with pathological stress).

Seligman theorized that the disruption of escape-avoidance learning and collateral symptoms of helplessness were caused by the affected animal's lack of voluntary control over the traumatic event rather than the event itself. Although trauma is a necessary condition for helplessness to occur, it is causally insufficient in itself to produce the effect. Both ET and helpless dogs received identical treatment, except that the ET dogs were shocked under conditions that they could control. For learned helplessness to occur, the event must be both traumatic and outside the subject's control. Subsequent experiments with a variety of animal species have uniformly supported Seligman's conclusions. The theory has enjoyed widespread acceptance and represents a leading animal model for reactive depression and, more recently, post-traumatic stress disorder (PTSD) (Van der Kolk et al., 1985: Foa et al., 1992).

Immunization and Reversibility

Seligman originally believed that learned helplessness was a transient effect, with recovery occurring within 24 to 48 hours. Two exceptions conflicted with this general observation: (1) dogs receiving multiple sessions of inescapable shock exhibited protracted signs of helplessness, and (2) animals raised under laboratory conditions tended not to recover from the helplessness effect. He speculated

that the likely cause for this difference could be attributed to past experiences with controllable trauma. Laboratory-reared dogs were more naive (never having been exposed to escapable traumatic events) than the dogs of "unknown" origins that he had used. The latter group had come from backgrounds that may have included exposure to escapable traumatic handling. To clarify the effects of past exposure to controllable shock, Seligman performed a series of experiments on rats and found that naive adult rats did not recover over time from the effects of inescapable shock. Another group was trained to escape shock and then exposed to inescapable shock. Previous exposure to escapable shock appears to have *immunized* the escape group against the effects of learned helplessness (Seligman, 1975). Helplessness studies on weanling rats exposed to inescapable shock have demonstrated persistent interference effects lasting into adulthood. Weanling rats exposed to the immunizing effect of escapable shock did not exhibit learned helplessness when exposed as adults to inescapable shock. In fact, immunized rats did slightly better on escape-avoidance tasks as adults than did nonshocked controls (Hannum et al., 1976).

Reversing the helplessness effect was possible only by physically forcing the dogs over the shuttle-box barrier. Dogs had to be physically prompted to jump over the barrier for as many as 20 to 50 trials before they began responding on their own. After directive exposure was carried out, helpless dogs began responding like normal ones (Seligman et al., 1968).

Family dogs habitually exposed to unpredictable/uncontrollable punishment are at risk of developing disturbances associated with the learned-helplessness disorder. Traumatic punitive events involving excessive startle reactions or physical pain, which are poorly coordinated with identifiable avoidance cues or response options, meet the operational criteria of inescapable trauma. The occurrence of such interaction is particularly common in cases where punishment takes place long after the event, or when it is applied out of anger. Under these conditions, the owner should be careful not to punish but to think through a plan based on sound behavioral practice to change the offending behavior.

Another key consideration is to avoid the application of traumatic or highly threatening punishment altogether. Dogs exposed to excessive punishment will never reach their full potential but rather are bound to grow gradually callous to their owner's abusive treatment, appearing not to feel punishment by their lack of responsiveness it. In fact, helpless dogs appear to develop an endorphin-mediated analgesia stimulated by uncontrollable trauma (Drugan et al., 1985). On a cognitive level, helpless dogs have simply learned to take punishment but not to benefit from it. They have fallen victim to a negative learning set that prevents them from responding appropriately under compulsion, perhaps believing that anything they might attempt to do will only fail.

More recently, Sonoda and colleagues (1991) demonstrated that interference effects paralleling those of learned helplessness can be obtained under conditions of uncontrollable appetitive training involving the non-contingent acquisition of food. The interference effects observed adversely affected cross-motivational learning involving shock-escape training. They performed a series of experiments with rats in which three groups were exposed to various conditions of control or loss of control over the acquisition of food. Initially, all of the rats were exposed to a continuous schedule of reinforcement for lever pressing. The rats were then divided into three experimental groups. One group was exposed to additional training under both an FR 5 and then, on the following day, an FR 20 schedule of reinforcement. A second group (the loss-of-controllability group) was yoked to the first group, so that these rats received food on a schedule independently of what they did or did not do with respect to lever pressing. Finally, the third group was given the same number of pellets earned by the first and second groups but en masse in their cage. The various rats were then exposed to a simple escape-training situation (shuttle box) in which they had to jump over a barrier to escape shock. Interestingly, the rats exposed to the loss of controllability contingency proved unable to learn

the shuttle-escape task. This result is consistent with the cognitive interference effects exhibited by dogs exposed to uncontrollable shock:

> The important difference between the contingent rats and the loss-of-controllability rats is whether or not a food outcome occurred when no target response was given. Food never occurred for the response-contingent rats when no target response was given, whereas food occurred when the loss-of-controllability rats lost the contingency between a target response and a food outcome. Therefore, the loss-of-controllability rats lost the contingency between a target response and a food outcome. Hence, the interference effects in the present two experiments suggest that the cognition of the contingency between a response and an outcome is an important factor in governing an organism's behavior. (Sonoda et al., 1991:274)

POST-TRAUMATIC STRESS DISORDER

Dogs, like children in our society, are exposed to a high risk of trauma and abusive treatment, predisposing both victims to develop various debilitating behavioral and psychological symptoms. It has been estimated that some 3 million children are annually exposed to significant trauma caused by domestic abuse or violence. Perhaps as many as one-third of these children will eventually require mental health interventions of some form or another as a result of these early experiences (Schwarz and Perry, 1994). A recent estimate by the U.S. Advisory Commission on Child Abuse and Neglect stated that some 2000 children are killed annually through child abuse or neglect in the United States, and that an additional 140,000 are seriously injured. Similar estimates are not available for dogs, but one can assume that untold suffering is also inflicted on dogs by insensitive or brutal family members in equal or greater numbers.

PTSD is precipitated by unpredictable life-threatening trauma that may or may not result in actual physical injury. The ordinary symptoms of the disorder in dogs include some or all of the following: (1) increased sensitivity to startle (hypervigilance) and the exhibition of disproportionate levels of generalized or irrational fear, (2) increased irritability and hyperreactivity, (3) a tendency to behave in impulsive and explosive ways in association with increased affective lability (mood swings), (4) the presence of hyperactivity, (5) a tendency to behave aggressively under minimal provocation, (6) a strong tendency toward social isolation and avoidance, (7) a lack of normal sensitivity to pleasure and pain (anhedonia) or numbing, and (8) depressed mood. These symptoms are usually long-lasting and frequently fail to improve spontaneously over time without intervention.

After the inundation of his laboratory during the Leningrad flood of 1924, Pavlov reported that some of his dogs had developed intense behavioral inhibitions and the loss of conditioned-reflex activity:

> During the terrific storm, amid the breaking of the waves of the increasing water against the walls of the building and the noise of breaking and falling trees, the animals had to be quickly transferred by making them swim in little groups from the kennels into the laboratory, where they were kept on the first floor, all huddled up together indiscriminately. All this produced a very strong and obvious inhibition in all the animals, since there was no fighting or quarrelling among them whatever, otherwise an unusual occurrence when the dogs are kept together. After this experience some of the dogs on their return to the kennels showed no disturbance in their conditioned reflexes. Other dogs—those of the inhibitable type—suffered a functional disturbance of the cortical activities for a very considerable period of time, as could be disclosed by experiments upon their conditioned reflexes. (1927/1960:313)

During testing a week later, one of the traumatized dogs was found to have lost several previously well-conditioned reflexes, appeared abnormally restless, and remained anorexic even after 3 days of food deprivation. Several efforts were made to reverse the adverse effects of the flood, including having an experimenter present with the dog during testing (effect of person)—a procedure that proved very successful. Apparently, the smell of the experimenter had been conditioned as an olfactory cue, since the presence of his clothing (placed out of sight) was sufficient alone to restore the conditioned reflexes. After 47 days

of "therapy," normal reflex activity was obtained. However, evidence of long-term deficits was identified:

> A year elapsed after the flood, and during this time we carefully protected the dog from every kind of extraordinary stimulus. Finally in the autumn (of 1925) we were able to get the old reflex, even to the bell. But after the very first time the reflex began gradually to decrease, although it was employed only once a day; and at last it disappeared entirely. At the same time all the remaining reflexes suffered, now temporarily vanishing, now passing into various hypnotic phases ranging between the waking state and sleep although in this dog the latter state was never fully attained. (Pavlov, quoted in Gantt, 1944:29)

Gantt (1944) reported a similarly catastrophic event involving 15 dogs housed in the kennels of his laboratory at Johns Hopkins. The dogs had escaped their kennels and wandered on several floors of the building until being discovered by the night watchman. As a result of the escapade, several of the dogs had suffered various wounds, some as the result of fighting among themselves while other injuries resulted from the watchman's club. The dogs' individual responses to the traumatic event depended on their temperament type, with stable dogs being only slightly affected by the experience. Gantt explicitly recognized a linkage between the breakdown of dogs under traumatic stress and the variable effects of war conditions on soldiers (i.e., *war neuroses*).

More recently, Seligman's learned-helplessness hypothesis has been critically evaluated with respect to its usefulness as an animal model for the study of PTSD (Foa et al., 1992). As just discussed, the experience of unpredictable and uncontrollable traumatic shock is associated with a variety of dysfunctional reactions in dogs: learning deficits, decreased motivation and operant depression, the development of a negative cognitive set, decreased sensitivity to pain, and reduced social status (dominance ranking)—all symptoms found in PTSD.

The behavioral effects of learned helplessness have been traced to underlying noradrenergic pathways stimulated by inescapable trauma. In particular, the locus coeruleus (a tight grouping of norepinephrine (NE)-producing neurons located in the pons) has a wide distribution of radiating projections extending throughout the nervous system, including the limbic system, cerebral cortex, cerebellum, and hypothalamus (Van der Kolk et al., 1985). The locus coeruleus plays a central role in the modulation of autonomic arousal during freeze, fight, or flight reactions (i.e., the general defensive response to threat). For example, cats exposed to a threatening dog or another cat that has been hypothalamically stimulated to exhibit rage display a twofold to threefold increase in locus coeruleus firing rates, as well as phasic bursts of neuronal discharge that correspond in time to the threats made by the dog or stimulated cat (Levine et al., 1990). NE is the primary neurotransmitter involved in the mediation of global fear and panic reactions. Under stressful conditions of acute or chronic fear, NE turnover is increased and gradually depleted, resulting in a reduced ability to respond adaptively with appropriate escape or avoidance responding to aversive stimulation. Increasing evidence suggests that sensitization of the catecholamine receptors associated with the locus coeruleus results in behavioral changes, like hypervigilance, irritability, anxiety, and increased autonomic reactivity (Schwarz and Perry, 1994). It has been theorized that threat-sensitized neuronal connections render the normally adaptive alarm reaction dysfunctional in two opposing directions, corresponding to the positive and negative symptomatology of PTSD: (1) hypervigilance and generalized activation of the alarm-threat system, and (2) hyporeactivity and avoidance—a general deactivation of normal adaptive responses toward threatening events.

Dogs exhibiting signs of PTSD are frequently described as appearing abused, mistrusting, aloof, unpredictable, aggressive (frequently toward one human sex more than another), hyperreactive, or hyporeactive, and frequently such dogs are very resistant to training. Since PTSD appears to develop as the result of unpredictable and uncontrollable traumatic experiences, it is important that dogs be exposed to training that emphasizes event predictability and control. The successful training of such dogs depends on a program of highly predictable and controllable learning events based on reward-based and affectionate training. In some cases, a combination of forced exposure or graduated counterconditioning may be necessary to reduce maladaptive social or environmental fears and to restore a more confident and outgoing attitude.

CONFLICT AND NEUROSIS

The experimental study and description of conflict was an important area of research for Neal E. Miller. Conflict occurs when incompatible responses compete simultaneously for expression, resulting in varying degrees of behavioral disturbance: "Conflicts can distract, delay, and fatigue the individual and force him to make maladaptive compromise responses. In fact, clinical studies demonstrate that severe conflict is one of the crucial factors in functional disorders of personality" (Miller, 1971:3). According to Miller, behavioral competition between alternative courses of action occurs in two general ways: unstable equilibrium and stable equilibrium. *Unstable equilibrium* is a common state of affairs involving brief hesitation but not much conflict. For example, when forced to choose between two alternatives, such as vanilla or chocolate ice cream, one might momentarily hesitate, but quickly decide to choose one or the other of the flavors depending on one's preference. *Stable equilibrium* is much more problematic in terms of choosing between alternatives. Acting upon one choice may produce effects that either inhibit its completion or excite the expression of the incompatible response competing for expression.

Three basic forms of behavioral conflict have been identified and described in operational terms by Miller:

1. *Approach-avoidance conflict* occurs when the behavioral goal is both attractive and aversive.
2. *Avoidance-avoidance conflict* occurs when behavioral alternatives are both in some way aversive, something akin to being placed "between a rock and a hard place."
3. *Approach-approach conflict* occurs when

two behavioral alternatives are nearly equally attractive and difficult to choose between. In contrast to the other two forms of conflict described, approach-approach conflicts are usually influenced by an unstable equilibrium. As soon as one or the other of the alternatives is approached, the attraction of the other is diminished, thus preventing problematic conflict.

The amount of conflict expressed by an animal depends on the influence of four fundamental factors:

1. *Approach gradient* refers to the tendency of approach behavior to increase as the animal gets closer to the goal.
2. *Avoidance gradient* refers to the tendency of avoidance behavior to intensify as the animal comes into closer proximity to the avoided object.
3. *Approach-avoidance strength differences* refer to the finding that the avoidance gradient tends to be steeper than the approach gradient—that is, the strength of avoidance behavior increases more rapidly than approach as the animal draws near the object of approach or avoidance.
4. *Approach-avoidance drive differences* refer to the effects of variable drive states resulting from increased deprivation or aversive stimulation and their influence on approach-avoidance behavior.

Miller tested these basic principles and various predictions deduced from them by directly measuring the amount of force exerted by rats while exposed to conflict. This was accomplished by running a line and pulley from a measuring device and attaching it to a harness fitted to a rat. This procedural arrangement provided an objective means for quantifying conflict while the rat pulled away from an aversive stimulus or pulled toward an attractive one. Behavioral conflict has also been measured in terms of the disruptive effects it exerts over previously learned behavior, and various interference effects it has over species-typical motivation and behavior patterns have been assessed. Other measures of conflict include physiological changes occurring in the body of the animal, especially

those typically associated with biological stress, such as cardiovascular (blood pressure and heart rate) changes. Also, a variety of tests have been devised to measure biological markers released into the blood and other bodily fluids (cerebrospinal fluid, urine, and saliva). Of particular interest in this regard is cortisol alterations and various metabolites resulting from the breakdown of specific neurotransmitters believed to be associated with stress.

Animals conflicted between approach-avoidance options experience varying degrees of stress, depending on the nature of the choices involved. The emotional concomitants associated with such stressful conflict are *anxiety* and *frustration*, both of which can be highly adaptive and useful to animals as sources of motivational impetus to act when under the influence of less than optimal conditions. The commonsense belief that a small amount of anxiety or frustration is conducive to efficient learning and behavioral change has been verified both by laboratory study and by practical experience. However, as has been shown in many of the preceding studies, excessive amounts of anxious or frustrative arousal may impair normal functioning and evoke varying degrees of disturbance and behavioral disorganization. Under natural conditions, conflict is often precipitated by aversive or attractive events that are poorly predicted (anxiety) or uncontrollable (frustration). Numerous studies have demonstrated the debilitating effect of unpredictable and uncontrollable events on the cognitive and behavioral functioning of dogs and other animals. In combination with other sources of stress, such as monotonous and overly restrictive environments (e.g., excessive crate confinement), boredom, insufficient exercise, inadequate sensory stimulation, and other similar adverse influences that place excessive demands on a dog's adaptive capabilities, persistent conflict is a significant source of behavioral maladaptation.

Expectancy: Prediction and Control

A useful operational way to conceptualize anxiety and frustration is to define them in terms of event predictability and controllability. According to this interpretation, *anxiety* occurs in situations where an aversive stimulus is impending, and a dog can act to control it, but the exact moment of its occurrence is not well predicted by the available conditioned stimuli. *Frustration* occurs in situations where available outcomes (e.g., various rewards or ways to escape or avoid aversive stimulation) are well predicted but not under an animal's control.

Unpredictability results in training situations in which the CS is as likely to occur contiguously with the US as it is not to occur—that is, the respective occurrences of the US and CS are independent of one another. This relationship can be described in terms of probability (p): p (US/CS is present) = p (US/CS is absent). Uncontrollability occurs in training situations where reinforcement is as likely to occur as it is not, regardless of what the dog does—that is, the occurrence of reinforcement (S^R) is independent of what the animal does (R). Again, this relationship is described in terms of probability: p (S^R/R occurs) = p (S^R/R does not occur). In this case, the response is equally likely to result in the presentation of reinforcement as it is to result in the omission of reinforcement—that is, overall, the available reinforcers occur independently of the response. Seligman and coworkers (1971) described a two-dimensional representation of event unpredictability and uncontrollability in terms of their relative probability (Fig. 9.3). These relationships are graphically illustrated in terms of classical and instrumental *training spaces.* Figure 9.3 shows that the diagonal of each training space represents event independence, whereas the ordinate and abscissa represent varying degrees of probability existing between the occurrence of the represented events.

Mineka and Kihlstrom (1978) argued that the various forms of experimental neurosis previously discussed (Pavlov, Gantt, Masserman, and Liddell) result from the presentation of biologically significant events that occur on an unpredictable and uncontrollable basis. They have stressed the importance of this sort of analysis for the adequate description of anxiety and depression:

These considerations of predictability and controllability may allow future investigators to spell out some of the possible relationships between anxiety and depression in terms that are more adequately operationalized than those used in the past. Environmental events must in principle be either predictable or unpredictable and either controllable or uncontrollable, generating four possible combinations of predictability and controllability [see the foregoing classical/instrumental interactions]. Moreover, an organism may often not be able to find the correct coping response necessary to gain control; hence, events that are in principle controllable may be perceived as uncontrollable. (1978:269)

Anxiety states that fit these formal criteria can be readily observed in many everyday situations. Anxiety is present to some extent under any set of circumstances in which control is available but the significant event cannot be well predicted—that is, a dog knows what to do and is free to do it but does not know when to do it. Frustrative situations involve circumstances where a dog knows what to do and when to do it but cannot perform the behavior. These definitions of anxiety and frustration are further explored later in this discussion.

Locus of Neurotogenesis

Classical and instrumental learning phenomena are usually treated experimentally as though they functioned independently of one another. In fact, though, most learning involves the participation of both paradigms. This collaborative interaction is particularly evident in the case of attentional behavior. Attention represents a virtually seamless orchestration of classical and instrumental learning mechanisms. An important function of attention is to provide a filtering and organizing interface or gateway between an animal and the surrounding environment. This attentional interface is supported by a sensitive and complex neural substrate that is vulnerable to the influence of adverse negative stimulation impinging on it. As the result of overstrain stemming from excessive or adverse stimulation, this attentional interface

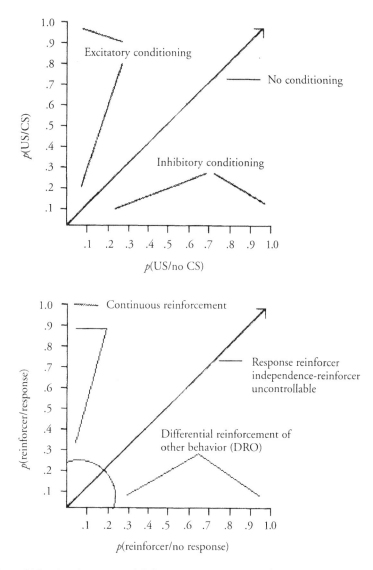

FIG. 9.3. Classical (above) and instrumental (below) contingency "spaces" describing event predictability and controllability. CS, conditioned stimulus; US, unconditioned stimulus. After Seligman et al. (1971).

may break down or become dysfunctional. External influences that strain attention (sometimes to the breaking point) are difficult discrimination tasks, monotonous and repetitive stimuli, and all variety of stressful unpredictable and uncontrollable events.

Attention is here tentatively proposed as the local site of disturbance in neurotic breakdown. Unfortunately, experimental research in this area is seriously lacking, but many findings—for example, the experiments of Broadbent (1958)—support the view that attentional activities are susceptible to adverse influences. An attentional locus of neurotogenesis is implicated by many of the characteristics of experimental neurosis, particularly the failure of an animal to perform previously learned discriminations. Clearly, without the ability to focus attention, select relevant information, and filter out irrelevant stimulation, an animal is rendered a helpless victim to the flux of chaotic events surrounding him.

Many psychiatric conditions appear to reflect an underlying defective attentional mechanism. In the case of schizophrenia, for example, patients appear unable to select and filter out relevant from irrelevant stimuli or to focus attention normally. The result is gross disorganization of behavior and cognition. Many theorists have viewed attentional disturbances as the core deficit in schizophrenia (Cohen and O'Donnell, 1993). Evidence of attentional deficits is frequently reported in the case of affective disorders like major depression and mania—symptoms that parallel in many ways the inhibitory and excitatory excesses exhibited by animals with behavioral disturbances induced experimentally. Interesting in this regard is the finding that patients suffering major depression do not find situations and stimuli associated with past reinforcement rewarding as they may have in the past. This is also a common feature of experimental neurosis in which hungry dogs or cats will refuse food, display generalized "negativism," and fall into unproductive cataleptic states.

In the case of experimental neurosis, the normally adaptive attentional and response-organizing mechanisms (impulse control) appear to be taxed beyond functional limits by overstrain or disorganized stimulation. According to this theory, the disruption of attentional mechanisms interrupts the normal chain of events that move from sensory stimulation to choice/response-organizing functions serving purposive behavior (i.e., the inventory of classical and instrumental behavioral possibilities). The emotional and behavioral result of neurotic breakdown (i.e., the failure to predict and control significant events) is a variety of affective disorders (especially those involving anxiety and depression), cognitive dysfunctions, and the appearance of disorganized and maladaptive behavior. These debilitating symptoms in turn further impact and adversely influence attentional functions.

Understanding how the absence of predictability and control impacts on behavior requires some consideration of the choice-making or impulse-control process. All learning involves making choices and inhibiting others, whether in the case of complex decisions or primitive attentional preferences—choices are made. At the most primitive level, this ability to choose takes the form of choices between responding and not responding (i.e., between inhibition and excitation). The way choices are made differs significantly between classical and instrumental learning paradigms. In the case of classical conditioning, choices are made with regard to attending to specific stimuli and contextual cues rather than others. This selective attention is determined by the comparative significance of the available stimuli and the animal's current motivational state or disposition to learn (Broadbent, 1958). Such attentional choices require the participation of various relevant cognitive functions, including various expectancies and interests (motivational factors), vigilance, and sustained searching activities operating on the external and internal environment.

Instrumental choices, on the other hand, take place according to general volitional rules and hedonic preferences for available outcomes. Obviously, classical and instrumental learning work together; in fact, as just noted, it is hard (or perhaps not possible at all) to differentiate the two learning orientations on the level of attention and choice. Instrumental choices are motivated by a drive to secure and control preferred outcomes, that is, the approach-acquisition of positive events (e.g., affection, food, and play) or the escape-avoidance of aversive ones (e.g., rejection, withdrawal of food, and isolation).

Under optimal conditions, classical and instrumental adjustments supply a progressive sense of security and regularity between an animal's needs of survival and the environment's ability to provide for them. This is accomplished (in part) by an animal's ability to predict and control the occurrence of significant events. Under stressful and neurotogenetic circumstances, such control is rendered independent of an animal's volition and ability. As a result, dogs might choose to escape from the uncontrollable situation and search for one more conducive to their needs. If all of their efforts to escape are blocked, or if their efforts only result in equally uncontrollable alternatives, then the situation becomes both uncontrollable and inescapable. This outcome may ensue even in situations where productive (i.e., controllable) alternatives exist, but an animal is unable to perceive them as such. Such loss of instrumental control is initially associated with increased levels of frustration and even more determined efforts to gain control over the difficult situation. If the occurrence of significant events still remains independent of the dog's intensified efforts, then various degrees of perseveration, regression, or frustration-motivated aggression may be exhibited. Under extreme circumstances involving aversive stimulation occurring in uncontrollable/inescapable situations, the result may include regressive fixations (Maier) or helplessness (Seligman).

Locus of Control and Self-Efficacy

Two areas of behavioral cognitive research that have some potential bearing on this aspect of neurotogenesis are locus of control (internal versus external control) expectancies proposed by Rotter (1966, 1975) and the self-efficacy expectancies postulated by Bandura (1977). Although both theories were originally articulated in terms of human learning and reinforcement theory, the researchers' findings are relevant to animal learners as well. According to Rotter's theory, the effectiveness of reinforcement depends to some extent on the organism's perception of a causal connection or contingency between its behavior and the occurrence of the reinforcing event—that is, animals must perceive that they somehow control the reinforcing event in order for it to be fully effective as a reinforcer.

But it is possible that an animal might receive regular reinforcement as the result of the emission of some behavior but not *recognize* a causal contingency between the two events—is such recognition of control over reinforcement necessary for instrumental learning to take place? That is, does the pigeon need to *know* that its key pecking con-

trols the delivery of grain. Also, consider the situation where the contingency of reinforcement is confused or mistaken. In this case, the animal correctly believes that some behavior or other that it emits is controlling the delivery of reinforcement, but, in fact, has wrongly identified which one. Can one legitimately say that the organism controls the occurrence of reinforcement in such cases or is this a case of "deluded" behavior? According to Rotter's theory, it is not enough for the behavior to be followed by reinforcement in the traditional sense of a simple *stamping-in* process; in addition, the animal must *perceive* the existence of a causal relationship between its behavior and the occurrence of reinforcement. Under natural conditions, these sorts of dilemma are largely mitigated by the centrally motivated and intentional character of learning in which the animal strives to control vital events like the acquisition of food and the escape-avoidance of danger.

Rotter argues that learners (*externals*) who perceive the presentation of reinforcement as resulting from forces outside of their control may not perceive their efforts (even when successful) as actually controlling reinforcement but rather attribute their success to external factors (e.g., the trainer's fancy). In contrast, learners who perceive that their efforts are instrumental in the obtainment of reinforcement will be more likely to feel in control of the occurrence of reinforcement and be less likely, therefore, to conclude prematurely that some difficult but, nonetheless, controllable situation is uncontrollable. Such individuals may be less prone to develop a variety of maladaptive disturbances. In addition, it is reasonable to assume that *internals* would be more resistant to the aversive effects of unpredictable and uncontrollable stimulation than *externals*. Further, animals guided by expectancies derived from internal control—that is, perceiving the occurrence of reinforcement as depending on their own efforts—will likely possess a stronger general belief or expectancy that their efforts will eventually be successful in controlling a difficult situation, while an externally driven counterpart may just give up.

Bandura's concept of self-efficacy is of some value in terms of this general problem.

Bandura defines *self-efficacy* as an expectation or "conviction that one can successfully execute the behavior required" (1977:193) to obtain a desired outcome regardless of whether or not the person is actually able to perform the necessary activity. The self-efficacy theory assumes that environmental events affect behavior indirectly via the mediating agency of efficacy expectations (Fig. 9.4). These efficacy expectations are influenced by a wide range of factors, including the success or failure of past learning experiences (i.e., outcome expectancies) and physiological states. If Bandura's self-efficacy theory is correct, then some procedure or other may be devised to *immunize* the organism against the debilitating effects of uncontrollable events by training it to believe that its efforts will eventually succeed in spite of the most adverse circumstances.

A dog's expectations regarding its abilities to control significant events are affected by a variety of factors, including its past training history. Dogs that have been relatively successful as learners will be more likely to interpret training situations as being predictable and controllable. This disposition to see things as predictable and controllable (or vice versa in the negative case) is an outcome of what Harlow (1949) has termed a *learning set* or, more specifically, a higher-order expectancy about future learning events. Such positive generalized expectancies are most likely to develop under the influence of highly controlled and formal training situations such as obedience training where the

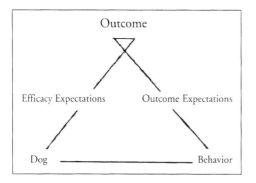

FIG. 9.4. Efficacy and outcome expectations provide complementary influences on learning.

contingencies between stimulus, response, and reinforcement are highly defined and reliable.

(*Please note that henceforth the terms* classical *and* instrumental *are often replaced with the synonyms* respondent *and* operant *in order to improve readability, and with no other purpose intended.*)

Defining Insolvable Conflict

The foregoing discussion provides a framework for developing a formal and functional definition of insolvable conflict. This is an important task, since conflict is crucial to many contemporary models of maladaptive behavior. Although the term *insolvable conflict* is frequently used, its operational definition is rather too vague to be of much use as a scientific term. It is my contention that insolvable conflict and maladaptation are elaborated from the attentional collision of unpredictable and uncontrollable events. Mere isolated respondent unpredictability (anxiety) or isolated instrumental uncontrollability (frustration) are not independently sufficient to produce insolvable conflict and to disrupt attentional organization. Insolvable conflict occurs only in cases where intense levels of respondent anxiety collide with equally intense levels of instrumental frustration, thus overstraining normal attentional and choice-making activities and causing them to become progressively disorganized and dysfunctional.

Within the general framework just outlined, classical and instrumental learning activities interact within a matrix of event predictability/unpredictability (P/–P) and outcome controllability/uncontrollability (C/–C). These interactive axes form two continua: one between anxiety and frustration and another between elation (optimism) and depression (helplessness) (Fig. 9.5). Under normal conditions in which classical and instrumental functions operate smoothly, the locus of activities rests somewhere in the center of these opposing continua, resulting in adaptive behavior and homeostatic adjustment.

These two primary classical and instrument axes cross and divide the matrix into

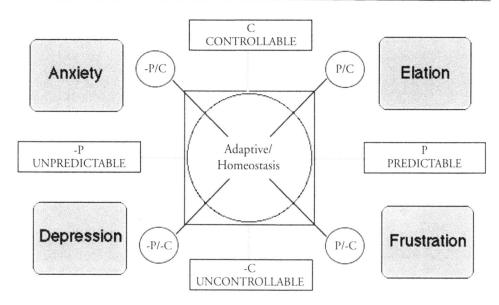

FIG. 9.5. Problematical or insolvable conflict occurs in one of two general ways: (1) when events are highly predictable but not adequately under the animal's control when they happen to occur (P/C–), or (2) when the animal has a high degree of control over the event but cannot predict when it is going to happen ((P/C). When respondent and operant events are either both unpredictable and uncontrollable (–P/–C) or highly predictable and controllable (P/C), the result is helplessness, on the one hand, and elated confidence, on the other. Neither helplessness nor elated confidence is associated with conflict. Functional disturbances corresponding to extroverted neuroticism (see above) occur in the anxiety-elation-frustration half of the matrix, whereas disturbances associated with introverted neuroticism occur in the half of the matrix bounded by anxiety-depression-frustration. Under normal conditions, all four of the above influences (anxiety, elation, depression, and frustration) contribute constructively to an animal's adaptation and homeostatic equilibrium (central area).

two equal sides—one side designated controllable and predictable, and the other designated unpredictable and uncontrollable. Four respondent-operant interactions are possible between predictability (P)/unpredictability (–P) and controllability (C)/uncontrollability (–C):

1. –P/C (unpredictable but controllable)   Anxiety
2. P/C (both predictable and controllable)   Elation/optimism
3. –P/–C (both unpredictable and uncontrollable)   Depression/helplessness
4. P/–C (predictable but uncontrollable)   Frustration

Note that the respondent-operant axis involving anxiety and frustration runs in a direction in which predictability improves as control declines. One would predict from this model

that anxiety (–P/C) is most intense when the event is highly controllable but its occurrence unpredictable. Further, maximal frustration (P/–C) occurs when the event is highly predictable, but uncontrollable. The respondent-operant axis between elation (P/C) and depression (–P/–C) promotes optimism on the one hand and helplessness on the other. Optimism occurs if the event is both highly predictable and controllable, whereas helplessness follows if the event is both unpredictable and uncontrollable. In the case of the elation/depression axis, elation emerges as an outcome of the reciprocal improvement of predictability and control as a unit. In contrast, depression is directly related to the reciprocal decline of predictability and control as a unit.

Figure 9.6 diagrammatically represents the necessary respondent-operant components required to generate problematical or insolvable

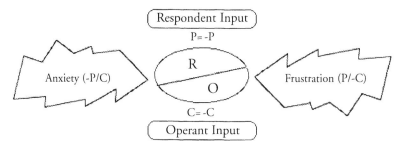

FIG. 9.6. Diagram illustrating the respondent/operant interactions required to produce problematical or insolvable conflict. Note that both operant and respondent influences produce conflict around a shared axis. Conflict is a composite of anxiety (respondent contribution) and frustration (operant contribution).

conflict. Notice that the respondent input is as unpredictive as it is predictive ($P = -P$). Likewise, the operant output is equally likely to control the event as it is not to control it ($C = -C$). This situation represents a true insolvable conflict because neither a choice based on respondent predictability nor a choice based on instrumental probabilities will succeed in resolving the dilemma. Under conditions of intense conflict with the arousal of fright-flight-fight mechanisms or exposure to strong conflicting approach-avoidance emotions, predisposed and genetically prepared dogs may experience a neurotic disturbance potentially capable of disabling attentional functions and the entire respondent-operant system. It should be kept in mind from the foregoing model that conflict takes place along a shared axis compounded of both respondent and operant components.

In the case of the respondent-operant axis between elation (optimism) and depression (helplessness), a number of interesting and paradoxical predictions can be made. When a dog is exposed to a pattern of unpredictable and uncontrollable events ($-P/-C$), the conditioned outcome is depression or helplessness. Having been reduced to a helpless state and then exposed to stimulus events and response outcomes occurring on a highly predictable and controllable basis, the model predicts that insolvable conflict will ensue— that is, the animal will not know what to do. On the surface, this outcome may seem paradoxical and unlikely, yet there is a great deal of experimental support for it in the literature of learned helplessness. After exposure to

inescapable-uncontrollable traumatic shock, helpless dogs exhibit a wide range of post-traumatic cognitive and behavioral deficits. For instance, if such dogs are consequently exposed to controllable training situations, most of them fail to learn even simple avoidance responses—responses that would have been very easy for them to learn prior to the helplessness-inducing trauma. Helpless dogs appear paralyzed, requiring direct and forceful physical prompting to escape the shock; left on their own, such dogs often just sit down and stoically accept the pain. The net result of helplessness is a collision of incompatible expectancies resulting in insolvable conflict precipitating various degrees of dysfunction within both respondent and instrumental systems.

The foregoing model also predicts conflict when dogs are exposed to a learning history in which stimulus events have been uniformly predictable and controllable. Dogs exposed to such contingencies of optimism (P/C), when subsequently exposed to uncontrollable and unpredictable conditions, should also fall victim to insolvable conflict. One might intuitively predict that such confident dogs, having known nothing but behavioral success, would go on working at the problem and only quit after expending a great deal of persistent effort and having tested out and exhausted every option. The model predicts instead that certain dogs, especially under the pressure of traumatic or intense emotional arousal, will exhibit strong signs of internal conflict and be far less flexible than dogs exposed to a more natural environment of probabilities. The occurrence of such conflict may be obtainable only under carefully controlled conditions, but the potential detriment of either extreme should be kept in mind when developing a training system or rearing practice.

The foregoing discussion underscores the importance of predictable and controllable environmental stimulation for the attainment of healthy emotional and behavioral development. In the absence of orderly information, attentional abilities and learning become progressively dysfunctional and behavior inevitably disorganized. Further, it is evident that various debilitating cognitive, emotional, and somatic effects are evoked by the perception that significant environmental events are unpredictable and uncontrollable. Stimulus events that are unusually intense or traumatic, monotonously repetitive, long enduring, or poorly differentiated from other stimuli evoking opposing responses—all of these sorts of stimuli are productive of stress and potentially result in the elaboration of behavioral disturbances and learning disorders. However, provocative events that are unanticipated (i.e., unpredictable) are particularly prone to produce a biological stress reaction. Beerda and colleagues (1998), for example, tested dogs under a variety of stress-producing conditions, using noxious stimulation. They found that saliva cortisol levels (a sensitive indicator of stress) became elevated only when noxious stimulation (e.g., intermittent sound blasts, shock, a falling bag, opening an umbrella, or physical restraint) was presented on an unpredictable basis. Noxious stimulation that was presented in a predictable fashion still caused the dogs tested to become restless, cower, and shake, but the stimulation did not induce a cortisol stress response.

Pavlov placed tremendous importance on the role of conflict and emotional distress in the development of neuroses. The studies under his supervision demonstrated the importance of clearly defined CS events and the need for a matching correspondence between a dog's moment-to-moment motivational state and the behavioral demands placed upon it. Successful adaptation depends on the development of a fluid correspondence or interface between an animal's expectations about the environment and the confirmation of these expectancies—that is, the acquisition of reliable information about what will occur and knowing what to do (and how to do it) just in case such and such occurs. These experiences result in dogs becoming progressively attuned and responsive to the social and physical environment's demands and pressures without experiencing undue distress, anxiety, or frustration. According to Pavlov, the habitual production of stressful conflict contributes a large measure to the etiology of behavioral disorders in humans and animals, especially in animals prone to neurotic elaboration [e.g., those possessing highly excitable (choleric) or inhibitable (melancholic) temperaments].

These observations underscore the importance of providing dogs with adequate instrumental control over significant events, as well as the inherent dangers of situations in which such control (and predictability) is compromised. Such situations may produce excessive and pathological demands upon dogs to adjust, precipitating the expression of disorganized and dysfunctional behavior. These effects are especially deleterious in the case of overly excitable dogs, unable to control impulses without extreme exertion and difficulty, and overly inhibited dogs, unable to act effectively even under the modest and routine demands of daily life.

Although the pronounced symptoms of behavioral disintegration described in the laboratory are rarely met with in family dogs, many canine behavioral disturbances and compulsions may be attributed to the regular occurrence of events that are unpredictable and uncontrollable. This is especially true in those cases where stimulus events evoke highly emotional and persistent conflicts. From the foregoing observations, one can conclude that remedial training for such dogs should include an effort to identify such sources of conflict and to provide the dogs with consistent and well-organized instructional activity. Behavioral training is beneficial; it makes explicit and constantly reiterates the reliability of significant events, a process that helps dogs to recover their self-confidence and to develop an expectancy that the environment is predictable and controllable.

NEUROSIS AND THE FAMILY DOG

Many everyday situations generate potentially harmful psychological conflicts and distress. For instance, routine disciplinary interaction often lacks sufficient clarity, predictability, and controllability. Further, training signals are not always carefully differentiated from one another. This lack of clarity sets the groundwork for confusion and unproductive training.

Many owners believe that their dog understands words in a way similar to how humans understand language. The urge to attribute humanlike learning and language abilities to dogs is a strong tendency, one that has attracted the noncritical support of many adherents. The belief that dogs can understand language has led some individuals to devise various means to teach them how to communicate symbolically. For example, Elisabeth Mann-Borgese (1965), the daughter of the German novelist Thomas Mann, developed a system that she thought would give dogs the ability to communicate their needs and intentions. The dogs were trained to use a typewriter especially designed for the purpose. Her efforts, as one might guess, were not very successful. Arli, an English setter, the most successful of the dogs she trained, pecked out what appears to be nothing more than meandering and nonsensical "poetry" organized by chance. What is most significant about Mann-Borgese's effort was the use of rather sophisticated instrumental training methods that she developed and used to teach her dog how to type and pick letters on cue. With regard to her other more elevated goals, however, no experimental evidence exists supporting the belief that dogs can learn to use a symbolic language in a way comparable to humans. Although her efforts failed with respect to the use of language in dogs, they did anticipate more recent and successful language learning studies in nonhuman primates.

In the case of dogs, the verbal "messages" they understand are distinctively nonconceptual in nature, being more concrete than abstract or symbolic; further, they are acquired through an associative-contextual learning process rather than a conceptual-symbolic one. Associative learning allows dogs to form a variety of connections between vocal signals and other signals, actions, and emotions having more immediate significance and meaning to them (e.g., visual gestures, physical prompts, and tonal variations of the voice).

Ideally, the differential application of tones of voice associated with reward and tones of voice associated with punishment should mediate a precise "dialectical interface" between the trainer and dog. Confusion is prone to develop when training signals are not consistently differentiated or applied. The ordinary quality of verbal exchange between humans is monotonal. This tendency often slips into the manner in which the owner attempts to communicate with his or her dog, sometimes blurring vital tonal distinctions between reward, command, and reprimand signals. When attractive and aversive signals are vague or lack explicit tonal differentiation, the potential for confusion or internal conflict between the opposing motivations stimulated by the signals involved is increased.

Similarly, when dogs are punished as the result of following an appropriate command (or rewarded for not responding), opposing expectations are likely to collide destructively. As unlikely as this sort of situation may sound, the habit of such punishment is actually very common among inexperienced dog owners. A familiar situation involving such inappropriate punishment can often be seen during recall training. In this case, dogs are sometimes punished only after they finally come or allow themselves to be caught by the exasperated owners. In other situations, dogs may be punished for coming too slowly. Such punitive interaction not only results in unnecessary stress and conflict but also progressively ruins a dog's willingness to come when called. Many persistent recall problems (unwillingness, hesitation, or slowness) can be analyzed along similar lines of improper punishment. Finally, such punishment sets up difficult-to-reverse internal conflicts about approaching when called (approach-avoidance and avoidance-avoidance conflicts), doing great damage to a dog's readiness to cooperate and thereby perpetuating a vicious cycle of frustration and ineffectual punishment.

Most dog owners at one time or another engage in the practice of noncontingent punishment (see Chapter 8). This problematic habit is especially prevalent in the mismanagement of separation anxiety and with puppies provided too much liberty before they are ready for it. A typical scenario might involve an owner coming home to find that the dog had been destructive in the owner's absence. Angered by the dog's misbehavior, the owner takes him to the spot or article and punishes him. Over time, such punitive interaction may escalate as the owner becomes progressively convinced—and more determined than ever—that the dog is acting spitefully. Alternately, on those occasions when the owner comes home and finds no sign of the offending behavior, the owner is likely to shower the reformed dog with affection and compensatory reassurance. Interpreting this turn of events to mean that the treatment had caused the dog to improve its attitude, the owner may feel justified in using the spurious cure. Before too long, though, the hiatus of good behavior will inevitably break down again, setting the stage for another series of futile punitive homecomings.

The interpersonal dynamics of noncontingent punishment can be analyzed in terms of experimental neurosis. During the foregoing greeting pattern, the owner is a provider of both attractive stimulation (approach) and aversive stimulation (avoidance) on a contingency not clearly predictable or controllable by the dog. Some days the owner returns home to punish the dog severely, whereas on others (when no evidence of destructiveness is found) the owner offers the dog affection and reassurance. The problem is that neither case is well defined by antecedent signals. The dog does not know which outcome is most likely to occur on any given occasion; neither does the dog know what to do in order to control it—that is, the greeting sequence is both unpredictable and uncontrollable.

The greeting situation is especially problematic because of the intensity of emotional conflict involved. Most dogs are very enthusiastic about seeing their owners after a long absence. The active emotions are intensely affectionate and seek reciprocation—that is, the expectant dog anticipates an equally friendly reply in kind. Instead, his sociable efforts are met with an unexpected and aggressive assault, resulting in a collision of violently opposed and conflicted emotions (structurally similar to Wolpe's and Masserman's procedure reviewed earlier). From the perspective of experimental neurosis, the collision of opposing and mutually incompatible emotional reactions predisposes the dog to develop neurotic conflict. The above homecoming exchange is especially injurious to an emotionally unstable or separation-distressed dog. Carried out over several weeks or months, such interaction may result in the elaboration of neurotic symptomatology, ranging from bizarre approach-avoidance greeting displays to extreme overarousal and hyperactivity. Additionally, affected dogs may exhibit numerous ontologically immature (regressive) displacement activities, compulsive submissive urination, exotic patterns of sham guilt, heightened insecurity, and exaggerated attention-seeking needs. Perhaps most importantly, such treatment contributes to the development of various cognitive generalizations about the unpredictability-uncontrollability of the owner's behavior, thereby planting the seeds for even greater adjustment problems.

REFERENCES

Amsel A (1971). Frustration, persistence, and regression. In HD Kimmel (Ed), *Experimental Psychopathology: Recent Research and Theory.* New York: Academic.

Amsel A and Roussel J (1952). Motivational properties of frustration: I. Effect on a running response of the addition of frustration to the motivational complex. *J Exp Psychol,* 43:363–368.

Astrup C (1965). *Pavlovian Psychiatry: A New Synthesis.* Springfield, IL: Charles C Thomas.

Bandura A (1977). Self-efficacy: Toward a unifying theory of behavior change. *Psychol Rev,* 84:191–215.

Beerda B, Schilder MBH, van Hooff JARAM, et al. (1998). Behavioural, saliva cortisol and heart rate responses to different types of stimuli in dogs. *Appl Anim Behav Sci,* 58:365–381.

Broadbent DE (1958). *Perception and Communication.* New York: Pergamon.

Broadhurst PL (1961). Abnormal animal behavior. In HP Eysenck (Ed), *Handbook of Abnormal Psychology: An Experimental Approach.* New York: Basic.

Cohen RA and O'Donnell BF (1993). Attentional dysfunction associated with psychiatric illness. In RA Cohen, YA Sparling-Cohen, and BF O'Donnell (Eds), *The Neuropsychology of Attention.* New York: Plenum.

Cook SW (1939). A survey of methods used to produce experimental neurosis. *Am J Psychiatry,* 95:1259–1276.

Drabovitch W and Weger P (1937). Deux cas de névrose expérimentale chez le chien. *C R Acad Sci (Paris),* 204:902–905.

Drugan RC, Ader DN, and Maier SF (1985). Shock controllability and the nature of stress-induced analgesia. *Behav Neurosci,* 99:791–801.

Foa EB, Zinbarg R, and Rothbaum BO (1992). Uncontrollability and unpredictability in post-traumatic stress disorder: An animal model. *Pyschol Bull,* 112:218–238.

Gantt WH (1944). *Experimental Basis for Neurotic Behavior: Origin and Development of Artificially Produced Disturbances of Behavior in Dogs.* New York: Paul B Hoeber.

Gantt WH (1962). Factors involved in the development of pathological behavior: Schizokinesis and autokinesis. *Perspect Biol Med,* 5:473–482.

Gantt WH (1971). Experimental basis for neurotic behavior. In HD Kimmel (Ed), *Experimental Psychopathology: Recent Research and Theory.* New York: Academic.

Gray JA (1971). *The Psychology of Fear and Stress.* New York: McGraw-Hill.

Gregory RL (1987). *The Oxford Companion to the Mind.* New York: Oxford University Press.

Hannum RD, Rosellini RA, and Seligman MEP (1976). Learned helplessness in the rat: Retention and Immunization. *Dev Psychobiol,* 12:449–454.

Harlow HF (1949). The formation of learning sets. *Psychol Rev,* 56:51–65.

Hebb DO (1947). Spontaneous neuroses in chimpanzees: Theoretical relations with clinical and experimental phenomena. *Psychosom Med,* 9:3–16.

James WT (1943). The formation of neurosis in dogs by increasing the energy requirements of a conditioned avoiding response. *J Comp Psychol,* 36:109–124.

Keehn JD (1986). *Animal Models for Psychiatry.* London: Routledge and Kegan Paul.

Kurstin IT (1968). Pavlov's concept of experimental neurosis and abnormal behavior in animals. In MW Fox (Ed), *Abnormal Behavior in Animals.* Philadelphia: WB Saunders.

Leonard HL, Lenane MC, and Swedo SE (1993). Obsessive-compulsive disorder. *Child Adolesc Psychiatr Clin North Am,* 2:655–667.

Levine ES, Litto WJ, and Jacobs BL (1990). Activity of cat locus coeruleus noradrenergic neurons during the defense reaction. *Brain Res,* 531:189–195.

Lichtenstein PE (1950). Studies of anxiety: I. The production of a feeding inhibition in dogs. *J Comp Physiol Psychol,* 43:16–29.

Liddell HS (1954). Conditioning and emotions: An account of a long-range study in which neuroses are induced in sheep and goats to clarify how irrational emotional behavior originates and ultimately to indicate how it may be prevented. *Sci Am,* 190:48–57.

Liddell HS (1956). *Emotional Hazards in Animals and Man.* Springfield, IL: Charles C Thomas.

Liddell HS (1964). The challenge of Pavlovian conditioning and experimental neuroses in animals. In J Wolpe, A Salter, and LJ Reyna (Eds), *The Conditioning Therapies: The Challenge in Psychotherapy.* New York: Holt, Rinehart and Winston.

Logan FA (1971). Dominance and Aggression. In HD Kimmel (Ed), *Experimental Psychopathology: Recent Research and Theory.* New York: Academic.

Lynch JJ and McCarthy JF (1969). Social responding in dogs: Heart rate changes to a person. *Psychophysiology,* 5:389–393.

Maier NRF (1961). *Frustration: The Study of Behavior Without a Goal.* Ann Arbor: University of Michigan Press.

Maier SF, Seligman MFP, and Solomon RL (1969). Pavlovian fear conditioning and learned helplessness: Effects on escape and avoidance behavior (a) the CS-US contingency and (b) the independence of the US and voluntary responding. In B Campbell and RM Church (Eds), *Punishment and Aversive Behavior.* New York: Appleton-Century-Crofts.

Mann-Borgese E (1965). *The Language Barrier: Beasts and Men.* New York: Holt, Rinehart and Winston.

Masserman JH (1943). Experimental neuroses and psychotherapy. *Arch Neurol Psychiatry,* 49:43–49.

Masserman JH (1950). Experimental neurosis. *Sci Am,* 182:38–43.

Masserman JH and Siever PW (1944). Dominance, neurosis, and aggression. *Psychosom Med,* 6:7–16.

Miller NE (1960). Learning resistance to pain and fear: Effects of overlearning, exposure, and reward exposure in context. *J Exp Psychopathol,* 60:137–145.

Miller NE (1971). Experimental studies of conflict. In *Neal E. Miller: Selected Papers on Conflict, Displacement, Learned Drives, and Theory.* Chicago: Aldine-Atherton.

Mineka S and Kihlstrom JF (1978). Unpredictable and uncontrollable events: A new perspective on experimental neurosis. *J Abnorm Psychol,* 87:256–271.

Patton RA (1951). Abnormal behavior in animals. In CP Stone (Ed), *Comparative Psychology.* Englewood Cliffs, NJ: Prentice-Hall.

Pavlov IP (1927/1960). *Conditioned Reflexes: An Investigation of the Physiological Activity of the Cerebral Cortex,* GV Anrep (Trans). New York: Dover (reprint).

Pavlov IP (1941). *Lectures on Conditioned Reinforcement,* Vol 2: *Conditional Reflexes and Psychiatry,* WH Gantt (Trans). New York: International.

Rotter JB (1966). Generalized expectancies for internal versus external control of reinforcement. *Psychol Monogr Gen Appl,* 80:1–28.

Rotter JB (1975). Some problems and misconceptions related to the construct of internal versus external control of reinforcement. *J Consult Clin Psychol,* 43:56–67.

Schwarz ED and Perry BD (1994). The post-traumatic response in children and adolescents. *Psychiatr Clin North Am,* 17:311–326.

Seligman MEP (1975). *Helplessness: On Depression, Development and Death.* San Francisco: WH Freeman.

Seligman MEP and Maier SF (1967). Failure to escape traumatic shock. *J Exp Psychol,* 74:1–9.

Seligman MEP, Maier SF, and Geer JH (1968). Alleviation of learned helplessness in the dog. *J Abnorm Psychol,* 3:256–262.

Seligman MEP, Maier SF, and Solomon RL (1971). Unpredictable and uncontrollable aversive events. In FR Brush (Ed), *Aversive Conditioning and Learning.* New York: Academic.

Seward JP (1969). The role of conflict in experimental neurosis. In B Campbell and RM Church (Eds), *Punishment and Aversive Behavior.* New York: Appleton-Century-Crofts.

Smart RG (1965). Conflict and conditioned aversive stimuli in the development of experimental neurosis. *Can J Psychol/Rev Can Psychol,* 19:208–223.

Sonoda A, Okayasu T, and Hirai H (1991). Loss of controllability in appetitive situations interferes with subsequent learning in aversive situations. *Anim Learn Behav,* 19:270–275.

Thomas T and DeWald L (1977). Experimental neurosis: Neuropsychological analysis. In JD Maser and MEP Seligman (Eds), *Psychopathology: Experimental Models.* San Francisco: WH Freeman.

Van der Kolk B, Greenberg M, Boyd H, and Krystal L (1985). Inescapable shock, neurotransmitter, and addiction to trauma: Toward a psychobiology of post traumatic stress. *Biol Psychiatry,* 20:314–325.

Vincent IC and Mitchell AR (1996). Relationship between blood pressure and stress-prone temperament in dogs. *Physiol Behav,* 60:135–138.

Wilhelm CM, McGuire TF, McDonough J, et al. (1953). Emotional elevations of blood pressure in trained dogs. *Psychosom Med,* 115:390–395.

Windholz G (1994). *Psychopathology and Psychiatry: Ivan P. Pavlov (Readings).* New Brunswick, NJ: Transaction.

Wolpe J (1958). *Psychotherapy by Reciprocal Inhibition.* Stanford: Stanford University Press.

10

Human-Dog Companionship: Cultural and Psychological Significance

The dog, i.e. the domestic wolf, was the first creature with which man got on to intimate terms, or that got on to intimate terms with him, and which in the course of thousands of years became uniquely intensified. No other animal stands in such intimate psychological union with man as the dog, which has almost become his master's thought-reader, reacting to his faintest changes of expression or mood.

> H. HEDIGER, *The Psychology and Behavior of Animals in Zoos and Circuses* (1955/1968)

THEORIES OF PET KEEPING

WHY DO people keep pets? Although the answer may seem obvious to anyone who has ever enjoyed the company of a dog, the question has been taken up as a serious scientific problem and answered in a variety of different ways. One of the earliest efforts to investigate the human-dog bond was carried out by W. Fowler Bucke (1903), who surveyed 2804 children, asking them about their attachment and reasons for preferring companionship with dogs over other pet animals. The result is a fascinating inventory of childhood attitudes, feelings, and thoughts about dogs. Bucke's analysis moves from an assessment of the child's motivations to the broader implications of the dog's domestication and close social affiliation with humans, concluding, "The dog has been, and is, a great force in the development and natural education of the child and the race" (1903:509). Another early study was performed by Lehman (1982), who collected data from 5000 child respondents to determine how they spent their time playing. Children of various ages were asked to respond to a series of questions regarding their daily play activities. He found that boys tended to spend more time interacting with dogs than girls did, with both groups showing a steady decline in the amount of time spent playing with pets (both dogs and cats) as they matured.

The study of what Bucke referred to as *cynopsychoses* would remain fallow and suffer neglect over the next several decades. During the past 20 years or so, however, this evident disregard has gradually given way to a renewed interest in the scientific study of human-dog interaction (Fogle, 1981; Katcher and Beck, 1983; Anderson et al., 1984; Serpell, 1986/1996; Bergler, 1988; Rowan, 1988). The contemporary reasons and rationale given for keeping dogs are nearly as varied and numerous as the many breeds comprising the canine family. Further, the general circumstances and motivations that guided early humans to capture and tame protodogs as pets remain subject to a great deal of speculation. These problems have generated a wide variety of hypotheses ranging from the existence of a universal human need for companionship with animals (Messent and Serpell, 1981) to theories based on domestic affiliations that developed (more or less) accidentally after the capture of wild animals. According to this latter group of theories, potential prey escaped the larder by becoming objects of affection (Hediger, 1955/1968; Zeuner, 1963; Scott, 1968; Clutton-Brock, 1977). Understanding why humans kept pet dogs in the distant past and understanding the current motivations that continue to foster the relationship have tremendous welfare implications. Many theories have been promulgated to help explain the human tendency to care for animals as pets, but none are conclusive—perhaps there is no single answer or simple formula. A brief summary follows of three prominent contemporary theories addressing the motives underlying the primal urge to keep animals as pets.

Savishinsky

Joel Savishinsky (1983) analyzed the urge to keep pets by contemporary primitive peoples on various levels of function and purpose. He concluded that while the widespread urge to keep pets might represent a plausible foundation for domestication, only rarely does pet keeping result in lasting intimacy, bonding, and controlled breeding in captivity. According to his observations, there exist several shortcomings inherent to the "pet-keeping urge" when considered as the primary motive for domesticating wild animals. Pets among tribal people are frequently kept only for a short period; they are often abused, poorly fed, and are frequently allowed to die, once the captor's curiosity is satisfied. Savishinsky argues that even though primitive peoples may catch and confine wild animals for amusement or various other short-term purposes, such activities provide little support for the hypothesis that such interests in wild animals precede or result in protodomestication. He warns that the term *pet keeping* should be applied with caution to foraging and hunting societies, especially if one wishes to employ it in the same sense as it is used to describe pet keeping among modern people.

Serpell

An opposing view of pet keeping among tribal peoples has been elaborated by James Serpell (1986/1996, 1987), who concedes that tribal children may expose their animal pets to varying degrees of neglect, abuse, mutilation, or even death resulting from play activities like "target practice," but argues that this attitude does not frequently extend to adults who display genuine affection toward their pets, caring for them in a manner not dissimilar to the way they care for their own children. He identifies two primary motivations underlying the urge to keep domestic animals: companionship and all other purposes like play, food, and status. He found that pet keeping in many tribal cultures is largely independent of economic or other practical concerns. Pets are maintained for the simple pleasures derived from their company and the satisfaction felt in caring for them. Even among those tribal people (e.g., Hawaiians) who kept dogs for food, personal pets were rarely slaughtered and not "without loud protest from the owner."

Yi-Fu Tuan

Yi-Fu Tuan, in *Dominance and Affection: The Making of Pets* (1984), analyzed the urge to keep and domesticate pets from the perspective of an enhanced sense of power. The ultimate significance of pet keeping according to Tuan is intertwined with a more fundamental urge to dominate and control nature. To domesticate is to dominate, control, and modify an animal according to human interests and design. Although the earliest intentions motivating domestication cannot be explicitly demonstrated, Tuan argues that the main motivations from early antiquity through the modern period for keeping and breeding dogs were largely utilitarian. These functions included hunting and guarding roles, but many other uses of dogs can be found, ranging from pest control to shepherding. The modern view of pet keeping based purely on affection and companionship became possible only with the advent of industrialization and the widening schism between humans and nature. As dogs became progressively divorced from a practical function, they could be more often conceptualized and used solely as an object of affection and play. The emergence of modern pet keeping brought with it conflicting urges and sentiments between dominance and benevolence, between cruelty and affection, and between ownership and friendship. The history of pet keeping is one of glaring incongruities and antitheses spawned by these conflicts inherent to pet ownership, training, and breeding.

The stories of Kipling and Aesop quoted below draw upon an idealist's vision of domestication (service, protection, and devotion), tempered by a rather cynical perspective on the whole arrangement. Collectively, these stories provide a unique insight into the psychology of domestication, revealing the perennial pros and cons of domestic existence for dogs and, by analogy, civilized existence for us. Together, they finely sum up our affectionate bond with dogs without evading the darker shadow of cruelty and domination inherent to the domestication process itself:

> Then the Woman picked up a roasted mutton-bone and threw it to Wild Dog, and said, "Wild Thing out of Wild Woods, taste and try." Wild Dog gnawed the bone, and it was more delicious then anything he had ever tasted, and he said, "O my Enemy and Wife of my Enemy, give me another."
>
> The Woman said, "Wild Thing out of the Wild Woods, help my Man to hunt through the day and guard this Cave at night, and I will give you as many roast bones as you need. ...."
>
> Wild Dog crawled into the Cave and laid his head on the Woman's lap, and said, "O my Friend and Wife of my Friend, I will help your Man to hunt the day, and I will guard your Cave." (Kipling, 1982)

Kipling's idealized vision contrasts sharply with the sense of loss and sacrifice attendant to domestication emphasized by Aesop in the fable *The Dog and the Wolf*:

> A Gaunt Wolf was almost dead with hunger when he happened to meet a Housedog who was passing by. "Ah, Cousin," said the Dog. "I knew how it would be; your irregular life will soon be the ruin of you. Why do you not work steadily as I do, and get your food regularly given to you?"
>
> "I would have no objection," said the Wolf, "if I could only get a place."
>
> "I will easily arrange that for you," said the Dog; "come with me to my master and you shall share my work."
>
> So the Wolf and the Dog went towards the town together. On the way there the Wolf noticed that the hair on a certain part of the Dog's neck was very much worn away, so he asked him how that had come about.
>
> "Oh, it is nothing," said the Dog. "That is only the place where the collar is put on at night to keep me chained up; it chafes a bit, but one soon gets used to it."
>
> "Is that all?" said the Wolf. "Then good-bye to you, Master Dog."
>
> Moral: "Better Starve Free Than Be A Fat Slave."

From Aesop's perspective, the loss of freedom is the greatest forfeiture made in exchange for domestic security. His fable is obviously an anthropomorphic metaphor, perhaps revealing more about human compromise and loss of dignity to civilized existence than it does about the dog's loss of autonomy in nature.

According to D. G. White (1991), the dog is a living metaphor that is closely associated with threshold points or boundaries between wild and domestic life. This role is symbolically embodied in the dog's almost universal association with the domestic threshold or doorway of the home. White notes that the dog is essentially related to human endeavor at the boundary or threshold between "night and day or between indoors and outdoors; or it constitutes a moving periphery, enclosing the herd that it guards from savage predators (often its cousins, wolves) or human rustlers, or providing a moving horizon between nature and culture as it pursues wild game, running ahead of its master, the hunter, who follows in its bark" (White, 1991:14–15). The long domestic association bringing humans and dogs together has been a mutually transforming symbiosis that has had a profound influence on human cultural and social evolution:

> This cohabitation with a great and changing variety of the Canidae, dating from neolithic times, has no doubt played a significant role in the rise of *homo sapiens* to dominance over our planet, in the human transformation of environment into world. ... We cannot overestimate the importance of this relationship to the "humanization" of the human species. Over the past ten to twelve thousand years, as we have completed our biological evolution through development of culture—an evolution parallel to that of the child in its formative years, when prenatal biological development is completed through acculturation—we humans have grown up with dogs at our sides. (1991:13)

These observations are echoed by J. Allman's (1999) emphasis on the mutual support and success enjoyed by the human and canid species in their close association together. He has speculated that early humans migrating from Africa some 140,000 years ago may have achieved a distinct advantage by capturing and domesticating protodogs. As this founding population spread north, the protodog's strengths as an ally may have given these early migratory ancestors of modern humans added powers and a competitive advantage over other human populations who were supplanted by their advances. Considering the recent findings of Wayne and his colleagues (see Chapter 1), who place the dog's domestication back to over 100,000

years ago, this theory of close contact between protodogs and humans has some considerable plausibility. Over the millennia, dogs and humans have complemented one another's existence, perhaps as White points out, with the dog leading the way at the horizon between culture and nature. W. M. Shleidt (1999) agrees with White's suggestion that humans and dogs have had a mutual and pronounced biological and cultural transformative influence on one another. He argues that it was the pastoralist herding pattern of wolves preying on reindeer during the last Ice Age that humans emulated and ultimately succeeded in adopting for their own with dogs at their side. As a result of this close association from such an early date, humans and canids experienced a coevolutionary process resulting in their mutual domestication and adaptation to one another. Both humans and canids appear to have undergone similar paedomorphic and other general morphological changes, including reduced physical stature and brain size. As discussed in Chapter 1, the dog's brain size is approximately 25% to 45% smaller than the wolf's brain. Similarly, the human brain has been shrinking over the past 35,000 years from an average of approximately 1450 grams to a current average weight of 1300 grams (Martin, 1990). This evidence suggests the possibility that similar evolutionary forces were concurrently operating on both humans and dogs, thereby producing similar effects on each species. Obviously, the human-dog relationship has exerted a tremendous biological, cultural, and psychological influence on human development, yet the way it all came about remains shrouded under a primordial veil that only begrudgingly and rarely gives us a glimpse into the mystery of our long relationship with the dog.

FORMING THE ANCIENT BOND

What is the basis for the universal appeal of dogs as companions? While the primeval impulse to keep dogs was certainly utilitarian to some extent, practical incentives alone cannot explain our perennial attachment and fascination. What else may have motivated early humans to capture and domesticate the ancestral dogs remains an unanswered and, perhaps, an unanswerable question. The nature of this early bond is likely to remain largely a mystery, since prehistoric human motives are impossible to verify scientifically. Despite the paucity of evidence, several authors have attempted to shed light on the situation by offering their best guesses. Juliet Clutton-Brock (1981), for example, speculated that early humans probably found familiar parallels in the social order of wolves, making interaction between the two species more easy and natural. Both species brought to the relationship analogous behavioral and social tendencies. Both species are cooperative hunters that form extended family relationships, with each possessing similar social structures and behavior patterns conformed to meet the needs of hunter-family groups. These various similarities provided a biological foundation for a close kinship and exchange between humans and dogs:

> The process of taming probably began at least 12,000 years ago but how much has changed in the actual relationship between man and dog in the period it is difficult to assess. It may be that in fact there is very little difference and the relationship is much the same now as it was at the end of the Ice Age. This is because the remarkable kinship and powers of communication that exist between human beings and dogs today have developed as an integral part of the hunting ancestry of ourselves and the wolf. It is a biological link based on social structures and behaviour patterns that are closely similar because they evolved in both species in response to the needs of a hunting team, but which endure today and have become adapted to life in sophisticated, industrial societies. (Clutton-Brock, 1981:34)

As hunters, primitive humans and wolves pursued large prey over open and wooded terrain, exerting tremendous physical and mental energy to accomplish their hunting goals. The result was the development of a high degree of physical strength and intellectual sagacity. Further, hunting was carried out as a group-coordinated and organized activity that required a high degree of social communication and cooperation. Desmond Morris (1967) suggested that the early hunter-gatherer people and the wolf may have been competitors originally, but gradually human hunters recognized the many advantages that the wolf had to offer, including valuable predatory herding and driving instincts, as well as the possession of more sensitive hearing and smelling abilities—all useful in the tracking, locating, and seizing of prey. Although it is doubtful that early humans made much organized use of the wolf's hunting skills (Zeuner, 1963), once domestication was under way it is likely that such use occurred, anticipating the conscious selective breeding of various hunting specialists, for example, gaze and scent hounds, pointers, retrievers, and terriers.

As pointed out by Clutton-Brock, the affinity between people and dogs depends on several shared behavioral and social dimensions conducive to mutual adaptability and interspecies harmony. Perhaps the most important of these factors is the reciprocal ability of humans and dogs to form strong interspecies social attachments with one another. J. P. Scott (1958) studied the social behavior of dogs in detail (as discussed in Chapter 2), isolating several critical or sensitive periods associated with social attachment occurring early in the dog's ontogenetic development. During the ensuing socialization process, strong bonds are formed that persist throughout a dog's life. If a puppy is removed from littermates prior to the onset of the socialization period, the puppy will tend to form rather exclusive attachments to humans, becoming progressively fearful or aggressive toward conspecifics as an adult. The socialization effect produces a profound impact on a dog's social identity (species recognition) and social preferences.

One widely held theory of domestication suggests that wolf pups may have been taken from their mothers and reared by humans in an effort to tame them. Studies of captive wolves have shown pronounced taming effects resulting from such early socialization, especially if the pups are taken from their mothers before the onset of the socialization period and raised in close association with people. Young and Goldman (1944/1964) collected numerous reports concerning the taming and practical use of wolves by both Native Americans and settlers. The authors noted early on that the best benefits of socialization occur when socialization is initiated shortly after a pup's eyes open. John Fentress (1967) successfully socialized a hand-reared wolf named Lupey from 4 weeks of age—an age considered questionable by many authorities for the successful socialization and taming of a wolf. Lupey was very affectionate and playful toward both humans and dogs but unpredictable or predatory toward small animals. He killed his first chicken by the time he was 13 weeks of age. Although involved in several incidents where intense threat and defensive displays were exhibited, Fentress did not report any serious attacks occurring during his 3 years of observations, underscoring the important role of familiarity, affection, and trust for the inhibition of aggressive behavior.

J. H. Woolpy and B. E. Ginsburg (1967), who analyzed in detail the dynamics of the socialization process between humans and wolves at various ages and periods of social development, found that the incipient development of fear from week 6 or 7 onward competed with successful socialization efforts. However, once socialized, wolves exhibit "all the attitudes and mannerisms of a very friendly dog." The researchers discovered that even adult wolves could be rehabilitated if patiently handled through four gradual stages of progressive socialization: (1) escape, (2) avoidance, (3) approach-aggression, and (4) friendly or socialized interaction. During initial contact, unsocialized wolves become highly emotional, exhibiting various escape efforts, signs of autonomic arousal [panting, salivation, pupillary changes (dilation), urination, and defecation], and various postural signs of fear (crouched posture, tail tucked between the rear legs, and trembling). After approximately a month of passive contact, the wolf may begin to relax somewhat but still not accept the approach of the handler. The next stage begins with the wolf making more active approaches sometimes involving biting on clothing, rubbing up against the handler, and the acceptance of petting. This stage is frequently associated with intense threat displays and a strong risk of attack, requiring special precautions and procedures to overcome. After several months of regular contact, the wolf may begin to solicit and reciprocate friendly exchanges involving licking, mouthing, and tail wagging. The benefits of socialization depend on the animal gradually learning to cope with a persistent fear of the unfamiliar.

AFFECTION AND FRIENDSHIP

Although differences of opinion exist regarding the role of companionship and intimate bonding during the early stages of domestication, clearly the contemporary urge to keep dogs as pets involves some constellation of emotional interests like intimacy, play, companionship, and security—perhaps in some cases even offering an ersatz relationship in lieu of satisfying human company. Unlike human relationships with other domestic animals, the social and psychological bond between people and dogs is profound and complex. Although very different biological entities, humans and dogs share a closeness and affinity that have linked the two species in close friendship over many thousands of years and have carried each other to every corner of the globe. Konrad Lorenz, obviously moved by his heartfelt compassion for dogs, wrote of the affectionate bond between humans and dogs in the most touching terms:

> To love one's brother as one does oneself is one of the most beautiful commands of Christianity, though there are few men and women able to live up to it. A faithful dog, however, loves its master much more than it loves itself and certainly more than its master ever can be able to love it back. There certainly is no creature in the world in which "bond behavior," in other words personal friendship, has become an equally powerful motivation as it has in dogs. (1975:x)

Following along a similar vein of analysis, Boris Levinson (1961, 1969) emphasized that the most important function of dogs in human families is a psychological one, providing a resource for nonjudgmental acceptance and affectionate exchange. In psychological terms, dogs play the role of a safe *transitional object* hovering between fantasy and reality, providing a mediating conduit for the expres-

sion of wishes, fantasies, and aggressive impulses (unfortunately often making dogs a
target for mental and physical abuse). According to Marcel Heiman, "The dog may be
considered a descendant from a totem animal
used by man in his development and useful
to him in the process of civilization. It is
noteworthy that *the dog's psychic apparatus, in
its fundamental features, seems to conform to
that of man.* ... The domesticated animal, in
particular the dog, is for civilized man what
the totem animal was for the primitive. The
dog represents a protector, a talisman against
the fear of death. ... By displacement, projection, and identification, a dog may serve as a
factor in the maintenance of psychological
equilibrium" (1956:584, italics added). In the
view of many psychoanalytically oriented
psychologists, our attitudes and feelings
about animals are an expression of unconscious strivings and repressed components of
the self.

Similarly, Samuel Corson and his associates (1977) suggested that the dog's appeal
rests mainly on its ability to give love and
tactile intimacy while remaining a perpetually
dependent and innocent object of our care
and affection. Perhaps, though, there is an
even more important factor to consider: the
dog's native ability to inspire in us a sense of
play and frivolity. Dogs yield to the willing
and receptive participant permission to become childlike and revel in the joyful release
of play and momentary self-abandonment,
revealing the "wonderful secrets having to do
with the great dog art of living abundantly
and happily in the present tense regardless of
circumstances" (Boone, 1954:74).

THE EFFECT OF PERSON

Clearly, an intuitive or empathetic faculty
plays a role in deciphering and interpreting
such signalization, whether between dogs and
humans or between dogs and other conspecifics. For example, tail wagging is a commonly relied upon social signal for determining an animal's degree of positive social
intention. In fact, the signalization expressed
by tail wagging is virtually universal among
domestic mammals. Kiley-Worthington
(1976) studied various situations in which

tail wagging occurs in domestic animals (pigs,
cattle, goats, horses, dogs, and cats) and
found a strong concurrence of tail wagging in
these different mammalian species occurring
under similar stimulus situations. The dog's
social response to familiar versus unfamiliar
persons is clearly differentiated by tail position and movement. Rappolt and colleagues
(1979) found that dogs approached their
owners with a lowered and actively wagging
tail. Strangers, on the other hand, were approached more ambivalently with the tail
wagging in a more subdued manner and held
at a higher position, especially as the stranger
moved into close contact.

Other observers have noted that some
people appear to be inherently more attractive and calming to dogs, whereas others are
more repulsive and agitating. Wolves apparently prefer contact with female humans over
males, the latter of whom they are more suspicious and wary (Fox, 1980). Lore and
Eisenberg (1986) found that, during social
approach tests, male dogs advanced toward
female subjects more readily than they did
toward male subjects. However, female dogs
willingly approached and made friendly contact regardless of the subject's gender. The
causes of this differential social response are
not fully understood, but the effect of person
can have a calming or disruptive effect on a
dog, depending on the individual making
contact. Social "chemistry" may play an important role in the etiology of behavioral
maladjustment and the development of some
behavior problems. Many trainers and behaviorists have anecdotally noted that occasionally a persistent behavior problem spontaneously improves simply by placing the dog
in a new home.

W. Horsley Gantt (1972) (see Chapter 9)
discovered that dogs experience significant
cardiovascular changes as the result of petting. These so-called *effects of person* are reciprocal between humans and dogs. Vormbrock
and Grossberg (1988) confirmed earlier findings by Katcher (1981) that petting a dog
causes a lowering of blood pressure in human
subjects. In the Vormbrock and Grossberg
study, blood pressure and heart rate were
measured under three different conditions:
while subjects were petting a dog, while pet-

ting and talking to a dog, and while talking to the experimenter. They found that the subjects experienced a significant lowering of blood pressure and heart rate while petting the dog, opposed to an increase while talking to the experimenter. Interestingly, lower heart rates were observed in subjects while either touching or talking to the dog, but, paradoxically, became higher when both touching *and* talking to the dog. Friedmann and colleagues (1980) found that coronary patients that have companionship with a dog (or other pet) enjoyed a significant prognostic advantage over patients not possessing a dog. Corson and coworkers (1977) studied the benefits of pet-facilitated psychotherapy, claiming improvement in patients who failed to respond to traditional therapy alone. Corson and Corson also studied the effects of pet dogs on the well-being of geriatric patients and isolated several therapeutic benefits presumed to stem from close interaction with dogs:

> Pet animals, and especially dogs, offered nursing home residents (including mentally retarded individuals) a form of nonthreatening, nonjudgmental, reassuring nonverbal communication and tactile comfort and thus helped to break the vicious cycle of loneliness, helplessness, and social withdrawal. Pet animals acted as effective socializing catalysts with other patients, residents, and staff and thus helped to improve the overall morale of the institution and create a community out of detached individuals. (1981:170)

Although there appears to be a clear psychological and physiological benefit derived from companionship with animals, the scientific studies thus far carried out are largely of a nongeneralizable statistical variety, many of which provide only limited validation for the hypothesized beneficial therapeutic effects of animal companionship (Wilson and Netting, 1983; Barba, 1995). Barba (1995) reviewed the human-animal interaction literature and found serious procedural shortcomings, with over 25% of the authors inappropriately generalizing beyond the sample parameters of their studies. Further, controlled experimental studies are unfortunately rare in the human-animal interaction literature. Of those controlled studies that do exist, few show a strong benefit derived from animal companionship and, unfortunately, those that do show benefit often suffer procedural shortcomings that undermine their validity. Beck and Katcher (1984), for example, were able to find only six controlled studies—none of which showed evidence of the "dramatic" results commonly observed in case reports.

There can be little doubt that companionship with dogs can provide significant benefit for people in the home, institution, and other walks of life, but the official acceptance of a therapeutic role for dogs will hinge on the development of replicable statistical studies and controlled experimental investigations. Claims not justified by data-based findings do nothing to support the future development and more widespread use of dogs in clinical and institutional settings. What is needed is unbiased and procedurally sound studies that place animal-assisted therapy on a more firm foundation of science.

WHEN THE BOND FAILS

Dogs enjoy a close association with people all around the world, playing many diverse roles ranging from family pet to guide dog for the blind. Despite the ubiquitous and affectionate affinity between humans and dogs, the relationship is filled with paradox and irony. A short survey of a few pertinent statistics reveals that human love for dogs is overshadowed by a disturbing display of indifference and outright cruelty.

The United States is the world leader in dog ownership. The Pet Food Institute (PFI) (1999) estimates that approximately 57.6 million dogs live in America, with 37.8% of all households keeping at least one dog. A survey conducted by the American Veterinary Medical Association (AVMA) puts the U.S. dog population at 52.9 million (AVMA, 1997)—up by approximately 400,000 since their last survey in 1991. American dog owners lavish affection and expensive care on their pets, spending approximately $5.6 billion (PFI, 1999) on food alone each year to keep their canine companions well nourished and another $7 billion to keep them healthy (AVMA,1997). According to the updated *US Pet Ownership and Demographic Sourcebook*

(AVMA, 1997), these expenses are on the rise, with the average cost of veterinary care climbing from $132 per dog-owning household in 1991 to $187 per household in 1996. Interestingly, between 1991 and 1996, the cost of veterinary care for the dog has risen by $2.08 billion, even though the mean number of veterinary visits for dogs has actually declined by 3.5% over the same period.

Indifference and Irresponsibility

Although dog owners can be generous and loving, they can also be equally selfish and cruel, frequently treating their pets with heartless disregard and insensitivity—if not outright contempt. Family dogs often fall victim to a "throw away" mentality adhering to their property status. A telling study reported by Line (1998) collected data on domestic animals relinquished to the Animal Humane Society in Minneapolis, including 20,903 dogs and puppies. Among some of the most common reasons given for surrendering dogs to the shelter were "moving," "no time," "too energetic/needs training," "responsibility is too much," and "needs more attention." In total, these reasons represent 42.6% of the causes given by respondents for relinquishing their pet dogs to the shelter. Similar statistics were reported by Salman and colleagues (1998), based on data from 12 U.S. animal shelters showing that 54.5% of respondents gave reasons related to housing or lifestyle issues. The American Humane Association (Nassar and Fluke, 1988) estimates that between 10.3 and 17.2 million dogs enter the shelter system each year. Of these, only 19% are placed in new homes, with the remainder being either redeemed by their owners (15%) or euthanized (66%). Anderson (1992) found during a survey of North Carolina shelters and humane organizations that approximately 76% of all dogs entering a shelter are euthanized, with only 18% being placed in new homes. The fate of the fortunate ones that find a home is not free of risk. Arkow and Dow (1984) found that dogs obtained from animal shelters were relinquished at a much higher rate (42%) than dogs acquired from other sources, suggesting the possibility that some behavior problems may be recycled through the shelter system. A rather disturbing finding reported by Arkow and Dow comes from Colorado Springs, CO. In that community, they estimated that 40% of the resident dog and cat population annually changes homes. Further, it was reported that the community shelter euthanizes 10% of the dog and cat population each year. According to the Humane Society of the United States, approximately 20 million unwanted or abandoned pets (dogs and cats) die annually as the result of euthanasia, exposure, starvation, or trauma. The picture is disconcerting, since it appears to indicate that dog ownership is perceived in terms of convenience rather than commitment and responsibility. Salman and coworkers (1998) found that only 4% of the surrendered dogs had been sent to obedience classes and a mere 1.2% had received professional training. The absence of obedience training appears to represent a strong risk factor for relinquishment. Another disturbing finding reported by Salman and associates is that a full third of the relinquished dogs had never been to a veterinarian. These statistics testify to a pronounced element of insensitivity and neglect, perhaps even institutionalized cruelty, toward companion animals—a sad and bitter culmination to our long history and friendship together.

Role of Behavior Problems

Another common and serious obstacle in the way of satisfying and affectionate companionship with man's best friend is behavior-adjustment problems. Estimates vary widely with respect to the incidence of behavior problems in dogs. A random sampling of 711 dog owners carried out at the University of Pennsylvania revealed that approximately 42% of the respondents answered "Yes" when asked, "Does your dog engage in any behavior which is a problem for you?" (Voith et al., 1992:265). The most common complaints were aggression, elimination, vocalization, destructive behavior, ingestive, running away, disobedience, and fearful behaviors. Other studies have reported much higher percentages of dog owners experiencing behavior problems with their dogs. For example, Adams and Clark (1989) found that 86% of

105 dog owners randomly interviewed in public places (Perth, Australia) reported at least one behavioral complaint. Similar numbers were reported by Campbell (1986), who found that 87% of 1422 dog owners indicated that their dog exhibited at least one behavior problem. The most common problems were jumping up on people, barking, begging, jumping on furniture, digging, destructive chewing, and fears (noises). In another survey (reported in Sigler, 1991) of veterinary clients, 90% of the respondents said they would like to improve their dog's behavior. From these studies, it is probably safe to conclude that the vast majority of dogs exhibit some need for behavioral training at some point in their lives as the result of a behavior problem. Hart and Hart noted in this regard that "behavioral problems in dogs and cats are so common that it is perhaps unusual to have a pet with no problems" (1985:vii).

Behavior problems are not only a nuisance, they are also a serious risk to the welfare of dogs, representing a leading cause for relinquishing the family dog to the uncertain fate of the shelter or to euthanasia (King, 1991). Some authorities claim that approximately 50% to 70% of all dogs euthanized in the American shelter system are surrendered as the direct result of a behavior problem (Sigler, 1991). Others have cranked the estimate of the number of dogs euthanized in the shelter system up to 11 million each year in shelters, with more than half of them being euthanized as a direct result of a behavior problem (Burghardt, 1991; Landsberg, 1991). Overall (1997) estimated that at least 7 to 8 million animals die in shelters each year because of a behavior problem, with an equal or greater number of animals being euthanized in private veterinary practice for similar reasons. Also, Reich and Overall (1998) claim that "abnormal or problem behaviors kill more pets annually in the U.S. than do infectious, metabolic, and neoplastic disease combined." These estimates are especially distressing when one considers that only half of 1% of the cat, dog, and horse owners utilized veterinary behavioral counseling in 1996 (AVMA, 1997), suggesting that behavioral intervention may be an underutilized treatment modality, with many veterinarians simply opting to euthanize the problem pet.

Recently, however, these numbers and estimates have been challenged by more carefully collected and analyzed statistical data, suggesting that considerable "overkill" may be present in the foregoing assessments (Line, 1998; Salman et al., 1998). Of the reasons given by owners for surrendering their pet dogs, behavior problems amounted to less than 30% (Line, 28%; and Salman, 26%), with a small percentage of these dogs being relinquished because of aggression toward people (Line, 3%; and Salman, 9.8%). These findings are consistent with those of Arkow and Dow (1984), who analyzed the results of a questionnaire sent out to several animal shelters across the country. Over 900 respondents were asked a series of questions regarding their reasons for giving up their dogs. Arkow and Dow found that 26% of the respondents had decided to surrender their dogs as the result of a behavior problem. Taken together, these data would suggest that far fewer than 50% to 70% of those dogs entering the shelter system are euthanized as the result of a behavior problem, as previously reported by several authors. In a study sponsored by the National Council on Pet Population Study and Policy (NCPPSP), data from four shelters located in different regions of the United States were collected, showing that, of 3415 animals surrendered to the participating shelters, 12% of their owners noted a behavior problem as a reason for their relinquishment (Anonymous, 1997).

In sum, these statistical trends suggest that far fewer dogs and cats are being euthanized because of behavior problems than had been previously estimated. Rowan (1992) estimated conservatively that the actual numbers involved are probably far smaller, with between 2 and 6 million animals (dogs and cats) being euthanized in the United States every year. After carefully analyzing the available statistics, he concluded that the statistical methods used to assess the euthanasia data are inadequate, resulting in what he referred to as a "statistical black hole." An effort is currently under way, led by the NCPPSP, to remedy this situation by collecting and analyzing pet population and demographic information in a more controlled and systematic manner. Perhaps, in the near future, more reliable information will become available to estimate the extent of the problem realistically. The bottom line is that a vast number of dogs die every year as the result of various behavior problems, but no one really knows for sure exactly how many dogs are involved.

Undoubtedly, a significant source of conflict and tension is caused by behavior problems, but despite these negative by-products of dog ownership many families and individuals opt to keep their problem dogs rather than surrender or euthanize them. Voith (1981a) found that a leading factor informing the final decision whether to keep or to get rid of a dog was the degree of affectionate attachment between the owner and dog. Of 100 cases (dogs and cats) involving serious behavior problems, 55% of the owners cited affectionate attachment as the primary reason for keeping their dog. Another 16% noted a humanitarian obligation, whereas many others claimed that they never viewed getting rid of the dog or cat as a possible consideration (Voith, 1981b). In another study, Voith (1984) found that 99% of over 700 respondents regarded their dog as a family member.

These findings emphasize the importance of early and effective intervention. It is reasonable to assume that the longer a behavior problem is permitted to persist, the more likely it is that the owner's affection for the dog will be negatively impacted. A family can invest just so much patience and tolerance before giving up on a beloved dog that has developed a serious behavior problem. Waiting until the dog bites before recommending training or behavioral counseling may be too late. It is imperative, therefore, that breeders, groomers, veterinarians, and other professionals involved with dogs be watchful for early signs and refer clients for training or behavioral counseling before it is too late.

PSYCHOANALYSIS AND THE HUMAN-DOG BOND: CONFLICTS AND CONTRADICTIONS

As already discussed, Tuan emphasized the conflicting urges of dominance and affection, cruelty and kindness, and other similar opposing motivations underlying the human urge to keep dogs as pets:

> In its long association with humans the dog has become diversified to an extraordinary degree, perhaps more so than any other animal species. Moreover, in the Western world at least, the dog is the pet par excellence. It exhibits uniquely a set of relationships we wish to explore: dominance and affection, love and abuse, cruelty and kindness. The dog calls forth, on the one hand, the best that a human person is capable of—self-sacrificing devotion to a weaker and dependent being, and, on the other hand, the temptation to exercise power in a willful and arbitrary, even perverse, manner. Both traits can exist in the same person. (1984:102)

Understanding the nature of these motivational conflicts and how they impact on the human-dog bond is of considerable importance. Much of this literature is admittedly speculative and often difficult to defend on scientific grounds; however, notwithstanding these various shortcomings, the information provides a valuable philosophical texture and backdrop for viewing some pathological and destructive facets of human-dog interaction.

Domestic dogs often grow up within a circle of privileged status existing somewhere between a toy and a child. Under such conditions, normal boundaries are often suspended on both behavioral as well as psychological levels, allowing dogs a great deal of behavioral latitude. Psychologically, the suspension of boundaries between the owner and dog permits an introjective process, whereby the dog is internalized as an ideal transitional object of affection (Levinson, 1961). This *enmeshment* results in an interspecies projection of meaning and emotional content. Introjective possession of the dog and the resultant projections tend to promote a relationship that is decidedly one-sided, selfish, immature, unrealistic, and dysfunctional, all ostensibly aimed at providing the dysfunctional owner with some degree of psychological equilibrium.

No relationship is ideal and, as problems emerge, some owners choose denial rather than face the facts. Others view the dog's behavior in less than ideal terms, attributing to it characteristics such as spitefulness, stubbornness, stupidity, and other convenient anthropomorphic interpretations. Under the influence of such confusion and irrationality, owners are prone to experience a variety of interactive problems with dogs (O'Farrell, 1997). As time passes, these dysfunctional dynamics may both polarize and profoundly distort an owner's perception of a dog. In addition, some owners may unconsciously approve and unwittingly perpetuate the very behavior problems they are seeking to eradicate. Heiman addressed this general issue, describing a patient he treated whose symptoms mirrored many of the problems she observed in her dog:

> In another session, two factors became clear: the patient's ambivalence toward the dog's behavior and the degree to which she and the dog formed a psychological unit. The patient recognized that she unconsciously approved of the very acts of the dog that she tried to curb. Thus she unconsciously permitted the dog to act toward her as if the dog were himself a child, and she were her own mother at that time. Here we see clearly the strength of the aggression acted out through identification with the dog. (1956:575)

Constance Perin (1981) has written a probing psychological analysis of the inherent contradictions and emotional conflicts observed in the American attitude toward the family dog. She divides dog owners into one of two general categories: the *responsible* and the *negligent*. The intention of her study was to isolate contributory factors underlying the development of these two styles of dog ownership. She argues that the dog is the conflicted object of an idealized love compounded with anger and infantile memories of a forever lost "once in a lifetime" bond between the infant and the mother. The dog is a symbol of superabundant intimacy informed with a paradoxical sense of profound loss, separation, and isolation—a schism that must be reached across and closed through social bonding with a biologically (and symbolically) distant companion. Instead of representing the dog as a surrogate child, Perin argues that the dog is more proximately characterized as an ideal parent from whom we receive "complete and total love," "undying

fidelity," and "nonjudgmental acceptance":

> We are, speaking symbolically, the children of our dogs. Our species difference further signifies that ultimate yielding of our parental ties and, in growing up, our coming to terms with our separateness. The Anglo-American bond with dogs is, I will try to show, a symbol of the most fundamental properties of human existence as our culture has come to understand it. (1981:79)

Later in her essay, she writes,

> Our relationship to dogs symbolizes our own fidelity to human continuity, biological and emotional. The meanings that this symbol makes available renew people's trust in one another. They help to make society possible. (1981:87)

At the core of this relationship is a universal existential crisis comprised of a psychic constellation of insecurity, anger, and longing resulting from the loss of the primal union with the mother. The ambiguous attitudes of idealization, affection, and cruelty displayed by negligent dog owners reflect a psychic imbalance and distortion maintained under the influence of repressed feelings of disappointment and anger emanating from this original loss and separation from the protective and loving parent. Heiman also noted similar dynamics in his patient and her various attitudes toward her mother, child, and dog:

> Just as the patient was about to move to the country for the summer, she discovered she was pregnant. Because of her anxiety, we agreed that she come for treatment once a week. Separation again mobilized great amounts of anxiety in her. Separation from the representative of mother meant death for the patient; thus the birth of the baby, separation from mother, being castrated, were equated with death. Whenever the patient identified herself with the dog and displaced her own unconscious wishes onto him, she spoke alternately of the dog and her baby. Her child was also identified with the mother. Her ambivalence about separation and attachment was expressed toward mother, baby, and dog. (1956:575)

According to Perin, these ambivalent and conflicted feelings are unconsciously projected onto the dog as a symbolic parental object, resulting in a perpetual cycle of love and cruelty (often unconsciously and obscured with denial). A kind of asexual Oedipal complex appears to be played out, with the dog serving as both the beneficiary of affection and the innocent childlike victim, cyclically destroyed, resurrected, and renewed.

The result of these ambivalent feelings of the owner is internal conflict and the inability to respond appropriately to the dog's behavior. Such owners tend toward extremes of unduly loving their dogs or wanting to kill them; as a result, they are often unable to do anything at all. One is inclined to suspect that herein lies the cause of the striking lack of assertiveness among some owners of dominant-aggressive dogs. It should be noted that these same people are, more often than not, very successful and aggressive competitors in their own professional fields. In some of these cases, there might exist a history of abuse and an established frame of reference correlating love and affiliation with violence, thereby shedding light on the willingness of some owners to tolerate their dog's frequent threats and actual biting. Heiman remarks poignantly on this matter:

> When the patient had adequately worked through her preoedipal relationship with her mother, the dog apparently had served its function. The dog was given to her mother, as an unmarried girl sometimes relinquishes her illegitimate baby. ... The dog helped maintain the patient's emotional equilibrium. A mother's use of a young child to act out a sadomasochistic conflict is destructive to the child, and mobilizes intense guilt in the mother; displaced to an animal, the consequences are comparatively harmless. (1956:578)

One must wonder how harmless such dynamics of displacement are for dogs, both in terms of their emotional equilibrium and physical safety. The use of dogs as outlets for negative emotions seems to have had a fairly widespread acceptance during this general period of time. In a rather bizarre and unsettling report exploring the psychosocial benefits of dog companionship for children, Bossard seriously recommended that dogs be used as ready objects for such hostile personal needs as releasing pent-up ego frustration and gratification:

> If things have gone wrong, and you feel like kicking some one, there is Waldo, waiting for you. If you have been ordered about by the boss all day, you can go home and order the dog about. If mother has made you do what you did not want to, you can now work on the dog. Long observation of children's behavior with domestic animals convinces me that this is a very important function. Often the child has been the victim of commands, "directives," shouts, orders, all day long. How soul-satisfying now to take the dog for a walk and order him about! This is a most therapeutic procedure. (1944:411)

Besides using dogs as cathartic objects for aggressive feelings, Bossard also promoted the use of family dogs for sex education, arguing that "the external physical differences of sex can be seen, identified, and discussed, without hesitation or inhibition on the part of either parent or child" (1944:411). Unfortunately, this sort of pedagogy may, in addition, facilitate abusive handling and treatment when children are left alone to investigate on their own. Recommendations like those of Bossard neglect to appreciate that dogs are feeling victims, albeit silent and forbearing, until at last they are pushed to the limits of tolerance, with the all-too-familiar devastation for both the child and dog.

Rynearson (1978) presented a series of relevant case histories involving human-animal companionship and the dynamics of pathological attachment. In one of these cases, an opposite situation to that just described, was reported involving a daughter, mother, and shared dog. In this case, the patient, who had just suffered a quarrel with her "borderline" psychotic mother, killed herself and her dog. The quarrel stemmed from the mother's demand for full custody of the dog from her daughter "because she wasn't loving him enough." The daughter became enraged and forcefully threw her mother out of the house and then proceeded to kill the dog and herself. Rynearson argues that, in most cases, interaction and attachment between humans and companion animals is harmonious and complementary; in cases involving pathological attachment and "displacement," however, two primary psychical functions may be served:

> (1) *Sustaining projective identification.* In "anxiously attaching" oneself to and "compulsively caring" for the pet, one can simultaneously and vicariously gratify a vulnerable part of the self without risking interpersonal involvement. The pet is symbolically imbued with the warm, trusting, and unconditional caring that magically nurtures the regressed, insatiable craving of the human for closeness. This degree of involvement occurs in patients with limited ego strengths and recapitulates the regressed mother-infant attachment dynamic.
>
> (2) *Symbolic intermediary.* The pet may become the focus of complicated displacement between conflicted humans [triangulation]. In a family where various members mutually distrust attachment the pet may serve as an attachment figure through which they can indirectly interact attachment. The pet becomes a trusting participant in a drama of distrust, sometimes ending in sacrifice. (1978:553–554)

It is fair to assume that, under certain circumstances, contact with dogs may be employed by some individuals as a psychological crutch used to help manage the individuals' personal emotional conflicts and anxiety. The resultant inconsistent interaction, including the application of punishment or reward based largely on the owner's shifting moods and psychological needs, has been implicated as a possible factor in the development of displacement activities in susceptible dogs (O'Farrell, 1997).

COMMUNICATING, RELATING, AND ATTACHMENT

The ease with which humans and dogs interact and socially bond depends on a shared substrate of sociobiological similarities and the ability to exchange socially significant information. The organization of such exchange is mediated by a variety of intention signals expressed through communicative facial gestures and bodily postures understood by both species. Galton emphasized the vital role played by interspecific communication and empathy in the process of domestication:

> The animal which above all others is a companion is the dog, and we observe how readily their proceedings are intelligible to each other. Every whine or bark of the dog, each of his fawning, savage or timorous movements is the exact counter part of what would have been the man's behavior, had he felt similar emotions. (1883:262)

Humans and dogs do share a surprisingly similar repertoire of affectionate and agonistic behavior patterns associated with appeasement and dominance contests (Eibl-Eibesfeldt, 1971). Although not without imperfections, humans and dogs communicate their intentions fairly well to one another and are able to mutually adjust accordingly to the demands expressed. Many et-epimeletic (care seeking) and epimeletic (caregiving) behavior patterns exhibited by people and dogs share homologous features. Both humans and dogs are dependent as young on a mother for nursing, warmth, and protection; they exhibit similar distress vocalizations when cold, hungry, or separated from siblings or maternal contact; and they exhibit a long developmental period involving playfulness. People and dogs share a strong tendency to coordinate their activities together. Allelomimetic (group-coordinated) behavior is a shared feature of both human and canine social organization. Schenkel (1967) has provided a descriptive analysis of the wolf's social displays and signals with respect to social rank and agonistic intention (Fig. 10.1). All of these considerations certainly play a role in the formation of the human-dog bond and the ability of humans and dogs to mutually communicate their intentions and needs.

What Is Communication?

A great deal of the discussion thus far and much of what follows concerning the bond between humans and dogs hinges on effective interspecies communication. What precisely does it mean to communicate with a dog? On a most basic level, communication can be defined as the reciprocal exchange of information between two or more individuals. Most animals possess a complex and flexible repertoire of expressive behaviors used to convey significant biosocial information to

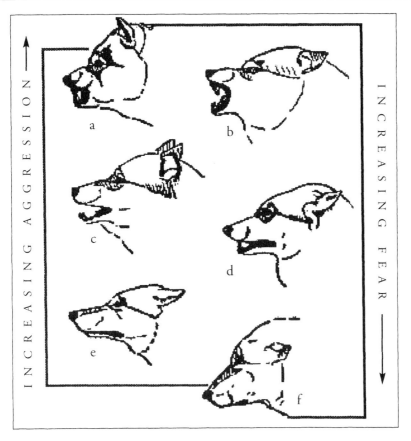

FIG. 10.1. Various emotional expressions of the wolf: (a) strong threat, (b) threat with uncertainty, (c) weak threat with increasing uncertainty, (d) weak threat with fear, (e) anxious submission, and (f) suspicion/uncertainty. After Schenkel (1967).

one another. A communicative exchange consists of at least three components: a sender, a reciprocating receiver, and a signal. The sender emits a signal to effect some change in the attitude, mood, or behavior of the receiver. The receiver confirms receipt of the information by sending an appropriate reply, indicating to the sender whether his or her message served its intended function. These species-typical displays are composed of various facial changes and bodily movements, odors, vocalizations, and tactile contacts that are organized to convey specific information between the sender and receiver. Besides the obvious function of communicating a message, expressive social behavior also exercises an important modulatory effect over emotion and mood. The purposes served by commu-

nication extend to all vital interests, but those of most particular concern here are those subserving social behavior.

Communication and the Regulation of Social Behavior

Most social behavior is mediated by communicative exchange with some assumed purpose, although it is not always obvious or apparent what that purpose might be. In highly social animals like dogs, communicative exchange serves to regulate social interaction between group members while facilitating cooperative behavior vital to the group's survival interests. The efficient coordination of cooperative behavior depends on the constant and reciprocal exchange of information between members. In wolves, a complex repertoire of threat and appeasement signals has evolved to regulate dominant-subordinate relations within the pack's hierarchically stratified social structure (Schenkel, 1967). Many of these agonistic displays are evident in the dog's behavior, reflected both in the way dogs interact with other dogs (intraspecific) and with human companions (interspecific). Besides socially stratifying and distancing signals, dogs possess a variety of affiliative signals employed to enhance social unity and affectionate exchange between group members. The greeting ritual and play bow are typical examples of socially affiliative and affectionate social expressions.

Agonistic and affiliative exchange serves many regulatory functions over the social behavior of dogs. These social communication systems reflect a highly influential social motivational substrate composed of a dyad of opposing and complementary drives (dominance and affection) that together simultaneously stratify and unify group members.

In an early effort to understand and appreciate the dog's social communication system, Darwin (1872/1965) described and cataloged many of the typical social displays exhibited by dogs. Communication systems evolve as the result of persistent social pressures placed on animals from generation to generation to conform to the greater social group or perish. Many of these expressions are innately programmed and reciprocated without much voluntary control or deliberation, but many are modified and organized by the influence of experience. Among the most conspicuous (i.e., distinctive and clear) social expressions are those associated with threat and appeasement (Fig. 10.2). Numerous exaggerated and subtle facial and postural changes are configured to express exact moment-to-moment motivational changes and intentions. The effects of these signals on the receiver depend on the *law of stimulus summation,* with each heterogeneous element expressed during agonistic displays being added together to determine or quantify the degree

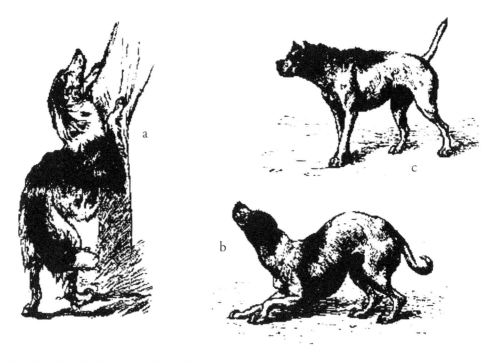

FIG. 10.2. Darwin observed and described many of the ways that dogs communicate social intention, ranging from active and passive submission (a and b) to offensive threat (c). From Darwin (1872/1965).

of imminent threat (Leyhausen, 1973). During a strong threat, dogs stand tall on their toes with hackles raised, ears erect, and tail held stiffly up. The body is tense, with the eyes singularly focused on the target, holding it transfixed with a steady and unwavering gaze. Under conditions of increasing threat, dogs retract the upper lip back and up to unsheathe the front incisors and large canines. This snarling action is often followed by a menacing low growl in immediate preparation for attack. These messages are received by subordinates and reciprocated with a parallel pattern of opposing submission displays or escalating reciprocal threat displays. If subordinates submit, the submission displays correspond in kind and quantity to the threat presented, following what Darwin called the called the *principle of antithesis*. The posture of subordinates is characterized by a diminution of size and strength, often with a lowering of the head and body toward the ground. The body tends to lean back and away from an aggressor, with ears pressed back and tail carried tightly between the legs. Some submissive dogs "grin," lick nervously, or vocalize in a high-pitched whine or yelp when they are challenged. Under conditions of increasing threat, a subordinate may cower to the ground or roll over into a lateral recumbency and expose the belly. Some dogs, especially puppies, may urinate as an ultimate act of deference. In cases where intense fear is also involved, dogs may release the anal glands. Although subordinates will not lose sight of a dominate challenger, they will carefully avoid making direct eye contact during the challenge. The forward and direct position of dominant dogs often intersects subordinates from the side, forming an agonistic-T shape in which the head of the more dominant animal may be jutted over the shoulder of the subordinate.

A dog's motivational status and intention are communicated through its expressive behavior. Anticipating what a dog is going to do next depends on properly identifying and interpreting these signals. Expressive behavior is typically compounded of conflicted intentional elements mirroring competing emotional states. Lorenz (1966) analyzed the fa-

cial threat and appeasement displays of dogs, finding that most agonistic facial displays are a composite of conflicting expressive intentions variably polarized along an aggression-fear continuum (Fig. 10.3). In fact, all threat displays, falling short of actual attack, are composed of both aggression and fear; otherwise, as Lorenz points out, aggressive dogs would simply attack without hesitation. Likewise, completely fearful dogs would just run away. Consequently, varying degrees of aggression and fear can be observed in the facial expressions of threat. A motivational analysis of these facial expressions reveals a dog's relative degree of threat and the dog's pending intentions. In Figure 10.3, the drawings at the top and bottom right-hand corners represent an imminent threat. The dog's expression depicted in the top right panel shows very little fear (the dominance aggressor), and the dog is prepared to attack without any further notice. The one located at the bottom right corner shows an example of an unstable equilibrium in which intense fear and escalating aggression collide (sharp-shy or *angstbeiser*) and, if pressed any further, the dog depicted here would certainly attack, especially if unable to flee from the situation. The dog in the center panel exhibits an equal amount of fear and aggression held in a conflict of stable equilibrium and, unless further provoked or intimidated by the local stimulus, will remain relatively stable between the two opposing motivational tendencies of aggression and fear.

These expressive motivational analyses clearly show that aggression and fear exercise a reciprocal modulatory (excitatory-inhibitory) effect on agonistic behavior. They indicate that moderate levels of fear may provide a beneficial influence on moderately strong aggressive impulses, whereas excessive fear in the presence of strong aggressive arousal may produce an undesirable dysregulatory effect—fear biting. In the case of aggressive behavior occurring without fear (e.g., dominance aggression), efforts to suppress it with punitive strategies that rely solely on the inhibitory effects of fear may only cause the aggressor to fight back even harder. In both instances, if the owner is unsuccessful, the

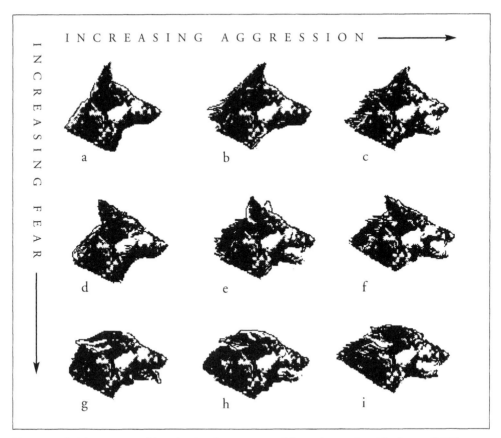

FIG. 10.3. Facial expressions of dogs showing the interaction of fear and aggression. After Lorenz (1966).

dog's behavior is instrumentally reinforced by escape-avoidance (defensive aggression) or positive reinforcement (offensive aggression).

In addition to facial expression, body posture and tail carriage are accurate indicators of a dog's changing moods and intentions. A stiff and erect tail indicates dominance and confidence, whereas a tail held low or between the legs shows fear and insecurity. The wag of a dog's tail has a wonderful and poetic range, giving the dog the means to fully express its emotional life or lack thereof. From elation to despair, the wagging tail tells all. Affection and enthusiasm are expressed through the dog's wagging and wiggling ear-to-rear smile. Similarly, at moments when high expectations are dashed by unanticipated disappointment, one can see the immediacy and sensitivity of a dog's expressive tail telling all that needs to be known about the

dog's sorrowful dejection. Darwin tells an amusing story about a large dog he once owned that was especially fond of long walks. Sometimes as they set out on a walk, Darwin would stop by his hothouse to check the plants he was studying at the time. As a result, the dog learned to anticipate a frustrating delay as they approached the greenhouse, a letdown that immediately caused him to fall from a state of elated excitement into a cheerless flop. Darwin coined the expression "hothouse face" to capture the dog's striking change of mood and expressiveness:

> His look of dejection was known to every member of the family, and was called his *hothouse face*. This consisted in the head drooping much, the whole body sinking a little and remaining motionless; the ears and tail falling suddenly down, but the tail was by no means wagged. With the falling of the ears and his

great chaps, the eyes became much changed in appearance, and I fancied that they looked less bright. His aspect was that of piteous, hopeless dejection; and it was, as I have said, laughable, as the cause was so slight. (1872/1965:60–61)

Although a happily wagging tail usually indicates a friendly intention, a wagging tail in the context of obvious threat is not to be trusted. Many highly aggressive and experienced dogs may actually look forward with some happy anticipation about the prospects of an aggressive contest or may experience some degree of conflict about the developing situation. A tail held high with a tight rapid wag is never to be trusted. The friendly, confident tail wag is a loose sweeping movement from side to side with various expressive undulations and shifts of direction. The friendly wag extends from the base of the tail, often including expressive bodily movements of the dog's rump as it twists side to side or tends to curl to one side or the other. In addition to providing visual signals, the tail wag may facilitate the transmission of various olfactory cues emanating from the anal and supracaudal glands (the latter is not present in all dogs).

In some common situations where dogs exhibit exaggerated tail wagging, the behavior may reflect a state of frustration or approach-avoidance conflict (Kiley-Worthington, 1976). During greetings, for example, a dog's locomotor tendency to move excitedly about is frustrated since it would carry the dog away from the object of affection and the benefits derived from staying close. Frustrated locomotion results in the expression of excited tail wagging, often including the dog's whole rear end. With regard to approach-avoidance conflict and tail wagging, such behavior is most characteristic of the subordinate in the presence of a more dominant figure, suggesting a pacifying function. Since fearful approach is usually characteristic of a subordinate animal, Kiley-Worthington concludes that tail wagging can be interpreted as indicating friendly intentions; but, as already noted, while this assessment is generally true, not all tail wagging invariably indicates friendly intentions. The expressive carriage of the tail provides the observer with valuable

information about the dog's emotional state and eminent intentions (Fig. 10.4), but such information must be interpreted relative to other significant signals and the context in which they occur.

Cutoff Signals

An important social modulatory signal used by dogs to postpone or break off agonistic conflict is the so-called *cutoff* signal first described by Chance (1962). Such movements are often composed of escape intentions (turning the head/body to the side or closing the eyes), et-epimeletic intentions (quick nervous licking), or displacement activities (yawning). The cutoff action has been referred to as a compromise movement by Tinbergen and defined by him as a "movement caused by ambivalent motivation ... between two conflicting movements" (1964:216). In the case of agonistic encounters, the cutoff is an expressive compromise between fighting and fleeing. One apparent function of the cutoff movement is to suspend sensory contact momentarily with the arousing stimulus, thereby breaking off stimulation that might otherwise evoke a fight, while still avoiding a chase attack if the animal should attempt to run away. Besides the relaxing effects these signals have on the animal exhibiting them, they appear also to influence the opponent to reciprocate in kind, leading to a mutual compromise. Leyhausen had this pacifying function in mind when he wrote about these secondary effects of cutoff actions:

> Such behavior, however, indicates that, on the one hand, an animal is not prepared to yield but also that, on the other, it is not for its part in an aggressive mood. Such a gesture of severing contact contains an offer of peace as well as a warning to the other not to push matters to the limit, and this is the effect it often produces, i.e., in many animals there are appropriate receptive IRMs [innate releasing mechanisms]. (1973:304–305)

The cutoff signal is not a submissive gesture but an opportunity to call a draw and walk away without further conflict and potential injury to the contestants.

Occasionally, a wolf will expose its neck to

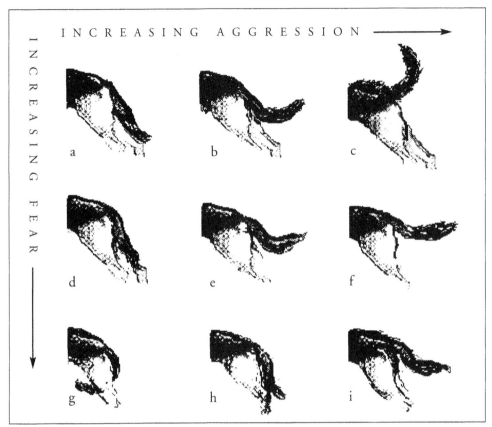

FIG. 10.4. Tail carriage showing the interaction of fear and aggression in dogs. In combination with expressive facial displays and posture, the carriage of a dog's tail communicates the dog's emotional state and behavioral intentions.

a rival as a ritualized agonistic movement. Konrad Lorenz (1966) has argued that both dogs and wolves present the neck as a submissive appeasement gesture, a ritualized expression of nonaggression in which the weapons (teeth) are turned away from the opponent while the most vulnerable part is exposed to the opponent. Schenkel (1967) has argued that this interpretation is flawed, insisting that it is always the *submissive* animal whose teeth are nearest the exposed neck of the dominant—not vice versa. The posture is not submissive but a confident taunt and challenge to an overly ambitious subordinate. According to Schenkel, what Lorenz viewed as a submissive posture is actually a threat display and challenge exhibited by a dominant, not subordinate, animal. Rather than representing a submissive intent, the exposed

neck posture is more likely a statement to the effect "I'm not much interested in fighting you right now; but, nonetheless, go ahead, I dare you to make a move." Fox (1969) has emphasized the pacifying effect of the neck display, arguing that the movement is not presented by the dominant wolf as a challenge or dare, but rather it is offered as a pacifying or calming movement intended to curtail the subordinate's agonistic adventure before it escalates into a more serious conflict. Finally, Scott claims that he has never observed a subordinate dog expose its neck as an act of deference to a dominant aggressor; instead, the subordinate is much more likely to assume a defensive and self-protective posture: "Instead of the jugular vein, the dominant dog is most likely to be presented with a mouthful of snapping teeth" (1967:379).

Effect of Domestication on Social Communication

As the result of domestication, many morphological and behavioral changes have occurred that have altered the dog's ability to communicate through facial and bodily expressions. Many of these changes have resulted from genetic alterations in the direction of relative immaturity or physical and behavioral *paedomorphosis*. Dogs never fully mature but remain in most respects at a developmental stage resembling that of a juvenile wolf. Frank and Frank (1982) have argued that the process of domestication proceeds along various paedomorphic lines, with selective pressures yielding prolonged immaturity and various corresponding behavioral changes. In the transformation from *lupus* to *familiaris*, wolves lose many of the well-defined agonistic rituals that ordinarily promote close and cooperative social interaction. They note that "the wolf's highly predictable dominance ritual has disintegrated into an assortment of independent behavioral fragments" (1982:519). However, not only have dominance displays undergone change, submission displays have also degenerated under the influence of domestication: "His submission responses have likewise lost much of their adaptive function and, consequently, their behavioral integrity and social significance; a domestic dog on his back is more probably soliciting attention than initiating submission or responding to domination" (1982:519). In the place of clearly defined and unambiguous signals has arisen a collection of generalized signals that promote social promiscuity through exaggerated care-seeking behaviors, various active and passive submission fragments, and the perpetuation of a juvenile tolerance for varied and close social contact. In comparison with the wolf's highly organized and integrated social structure, the dog appears disjointed, confused, unpredictable, and fragmented.

Besides these general effects of domestication, breed-specific changes have affected the dog's social behavior in many ways. Selective breeding has altered developmental rates, behavioral thresholds for the display of dominant and submissive behavior, behavioral tendencies and temperament traits, social bonding, and trainability. Goodwin and colleagues (1997) attempted to quantify the domestic dog's divergence from the lupine archetype and communication system based on morphological changes, bodily gesture and posture, and facial expression. Their study demonstrates that the dog's ability to communicate has gone through significant change as the result of domestication, at least insofar as human observers are concerned. Among the breeds compared, dogs whose appearance most resembles the wolf (e.g., German shepherd and Siberian husky) exhibited a corresponding greater number of wolflike signals exhibited during agonistic interactions than did dogs whose appearance was deemed dissimilar to wolves (e.g., cavalier King Charles spaniel, Norfolk terrier, and French bulldog). Among wolves, these signals are used to modulate agonistic interactions and to prevent an escalation of aggression. One would assume, therefore, that in dog breeds without an effective agonistic signaling system that they would be more prone to engage in conspecific aggression, but this does not appear to be the case. The authors speculate that dogs have a much higher threshold for aggression and, consequently, they do not require the more intricate social communication devices exhibited by wolves. Also, dogs may rely on more subtle communication devices for the management of agonistic behavior that remains to be more fully elucidated.

THE QUESTION OF ANIMAL AWARENESS

Viable social communication between humans and dogs implies that there exists some degree of conscious awareness or, at least, empathetic sensitivity mediating the exchange, but does a genuine sense of empathy or self-awareness exist in the mind of the dog or is such a supposition a projection of human imagination? The fact that dogs and people enjoy each other's company and form lasting affectionate bonds raises several important questions: Do dogs have a private personal experience analogous to human consciousness? Do dogs experience feelings similar to those of their keepers? Is there an evolutionary continuity of conscious experience shared by both species? A negative response to any of these questions would greatly diminish the worth of the social bond existing between the two species. Concluding that dogs lack conscious awareness and empathetic sensitivity would imply that the social exchange is one-sided (at least in terms of conscious awareness and empathy)—a kind of social onanism rather than a true relationship in the usual sense of the word.

The Western philosophical tradition equates consciousness with the ability to use language. According to this view, *knowing* and *thinking* depend on a shared language through which knowledge and thought are exchanged and confirmed or denied. The presence of consciousness is attributed to someone based primarily on the existence of such language-mediated exchange. However, language-based exchange alone can hardly prove beyond all shadow of doubt that consciousness actually exists in others as it does in oneself. The phenomenon of consciousness is preeminently a private experience whose existence is hard to define or prove to exist. We can only "guess" or assume that consciousness exists in other people (or animals) by inference from our own personal experience of consciousness and the world. But just because we cannot *prove* that others are conscious in the same sense that we are, it hardly follows that we are therefore logically compelled to deny or seriously question the reality of their consciousness. On the contrary, the shared or public nature of consciousness is not questioned at all, but we all proceed with our affairs as though others are approximately as self-aware and conscious as we are and motivated in a similar manner—at least, until we discover evidence to the contrary.

Although it would seem reasonable to apply a similarly pragmatic paradigm to the study of animal awareness and cognition, the notion of animal awareness is highly controversial. The rejection of animal awareness arose within the context of the Judeo-Christian tradition and, in particular, Cartesian rationalism, which explicitly denied the existence of animal awareness. According to

Descartes, animals are no more than animated organic automatons, programmed like a machine to perform and function as they do without conscious awareness or rational intent. An animal's appearance of conscious deliberation and sensitivity is an illusion on the same order as that exhibited by a mechanical robot. Describing the Cartesian perspective, John Passmore writes, "What we hear as a cry of pain is of no more significance than the creaking of a machine," and continues,

> These teachings, it should be observed, were more than metaphysical speculations. They had a direct effect on seventeenth-century behavior as manifested, for example, in the popularity of public vivisection, not as an aid to scientific discovery but simply as a technical display. "They administered beatings to dogs with perfect indifference," so La Fontaine, a contemporary observer, tells us, "and made fun of those who pitied the creatures as if they had felt pain. ... They nailed poor animals up on boards by their four paws to vivisect them and see the circulation of the blood which was a great subject of conversation." (1975:204)

The resistance to the idea of attributing consciousness to dogs or other animals is complex. Our cultural resistance to the idea probably rests more on moral and ethical grounds than it does on scientific or philosophical ones. If we attribute awareness and sensitivity to animals of a similar kind and extent to our own experience, we are then thrust into an uncomfortable moral dilemma stemming from the various uses we make of animals (Carson, 1972). To subjugate, kill, or experiment on an animal that is unaware of its plight is ethically very different from performing the same actions on a fully sentient and sensitive being. Together with the attribution of awareness to animals comes an ethical imperative that may be simply too hard for many of us to accept or one that is perceived to be economically untenable. Whatever the case may be, by concluding and accepting that animals are endowed with a private experience or self-awareness comparable to our own, we are brought face to face with a moral crisis that would revolutionize how we view and treat animals under our care.

Understandably, given what is at stake, the debate surrounding the existence or nonexistence of animal awareness is sometimes a heated one. This state of affairs is unfortunate, since, as Donald Griffin (1981, 1984, 1992) has argued for many years, animal awareness and cognition should be approached with the same cool scientific scrutiny and systematic study that other natural phenomenon are investigated. For such study to proceed, though, one must first concede that animal awareness and cognition might exist to some degree—otherwise there is no object of study. The burden of proof then shifts to an examination of the extent to which animal awareness exists based on accepted scientific criteria and standards.

Historically, the study of animal awareness and cognition has been almost fully neglected, but new interest in the subject has appeared with the publication of a series of important books and articles by Griffin and others (Regan, 1983; Walker, 1983; Burghardt, 1985; Bekoff and Jamieson, 1996). Griffin (1981) has attempted to develop a scientific basis and discipline (*cognitive ethology*) for the study of animal awareness. He has argued strongly in favor of an "open" mind with regard to the hypothetical existence of consciousness and subjective self-awareness in animals:

> If we take for granted that our own mental experiences are real and significant, it seems more likely than not that because the central nervous systems of other animals are basically similar, they will share with our brains the capability of making possible at least some kinds of mental experiences. To conclude that nothing of the kind ever happens requires that we postulate an unparsimonious qualitative distinction between human brains and all those others that seem to have such similar structural and functional properties. (1981:167)

Temple Grandin (1995) has suggested that animal awareness and *thinking* be viewed as a kind of perceptual activity based on direct sensory information and memories. Human thinking is distinguished from animal thinking by the reliance of human thinking on symbolic representations and abstract concepts. According to this viewpoint, dogs, somewhat akin to the thinking style of artists or musicians, consider things primarily in terms of their immediate sensory significance (e.g., smells, sounds, sights, and tactile sensations), relevance to the animal's current motivation state, and associated memories brought to the situation. Awareness poises the animal for effective action within the context of a changing environment.

In the early 1930s, Otto Tinklepaugh (1934) warned comparative psychologists not to fall victim to what he termed a widespread and growing anthropomorphic phobia. He observed that many researchers in their fear of appearing anthropomorphic have arbitrarily renamed and redefined animal behaviors so as not to be accused of anthropomorphism. In Tinklepaugh's opinion, this subterfuge is "comparable to differentiating between the 'sweating' of a monkey and the 'perspiring' of man." He continues,

> Other investigators, for similar reasons, have avoided stating their honest convictions concerning the behavior they have observed. The purposes of science demand accurate observation, accurate description, and, where possible, logical interpretation. Though all interpretation is subject to modification or even to reversal, no one is in as good a position initially to evaluate the various factors that enter into an investigation, and to interpret the results, as is the collector of the data. The anthropomorphic phobia has no place in scientific psychology. (1934:507)

Cognition Without Awareness

Despite Tinklepaugh's encouragement, most behavioral scientists have found it expedient to exclude notions like *animal awareness* and *animal minds* from their investigations but without necessarily denying that they exist. For the most part, this rejection is justified simply because such phenomena do not yield amiably to controlled manipulation and direct measurement. Furthermore, the addition of an intervening variable like *consciousness* offers little theoretical advantage to their studies but does add considerably to the complexity of the subject matter. This appears to be exactly the position that Niko Tinbergen adopted, writing that although "the ethologist does not want to deny the possible existence of subjective phenomena in animals, he claims that it is futile to present them as causes, since they cannot be observed by scientific methods" (1951/1969:5). According to Tinbergen, the study of subjective states (e.g., hunger, fear, anger, and sleepiness) is the domain of physiologists—not psychologists. Apparently, what is needed is an operational definition of consciousness formulated in experimental terms and the intellectual freedom to study it without suffering the accusation and stigma of anthropomorphism.

Recent trends in animal behavior research have turned toward the careful analysis of cognitive functions but without necessarily agreeing about the existence of animal awareness or what that might mean (Vauclair, 1996). In the study of animal behavior and learning, the existence of animal awareness is often implied (but not explicitly articulated or even presumed by researchers) as a precondition for adaptational adjustment between the organism and the environment. This is especially evident in cases where adaptation depends on cognitive functions like prediction, expectation, and choice between alternative courses of action—cognitions implying the existence of conscious deliberation.

As already discussed in detail (see chapters 6 and 7), many leading contemporary learning theorists have adopted various *cognitive* hypothetical constructs in an effort to make theoretical sense of their experimental findings. Robert Rescorla (1988), for instance, has found that many acquisition and extinction phenomena involving classical conditioning cannot be adequately understood in terms of the traditional Pavlovian conventions alone but require the additional implementation of various cognitive constructs in order to be fully explained. Classical conditioning is not merely the mindless connecting of a conditioned stimulus (CS) with an un-

conditioned stimulus (US), so that the CS gradually comes to elicit a response similar to the one elicited by the US. In addition to the mere physiological effects and stimulus-response associations obtained by pairing the CS with the US, an animal also learns about various interdependent *relationships* between CS and US. According to this viewpoint, classical conditioning is a cognitive or *mental* activity aimed at securing a viable and continuously updated environmental interface and adaptation.

This general line of reasoning conforms with the cognitive emphasis suggested by the pioneering learning theorist Edward Tolman (1934). In opposition to the majority of early behaviorists, Tolman proposed that learning be studied experimentally from a cognitive perspective. He suggested that animal learning be studied as an interpretive and purposive activity taking place within a cognitive field of "sign-gestalt expectations." As might be expected from the foregoing, interest in Tolman and other gestalt theorists (e.g., Piaget) have enjoyed a recent resurgence of attention, especially among comparative psychologists.

Empathy and Awareness

The subtle social communication occurring between humans and dogs seems to imply that there exists a shared cognitive or empathetic substrate mediating, assessing, and evaluating mutual intentions and meaning, as well as deliberating on different possible courses of action based on parallel appraisals and emotions experienced by the affected communicators. That is, meaningful communication would appear to require an internally represented and empathetic experience of the other. Grandin (1995) has emphasized the importance of such empathetic identification for the ethologist attempting to connect with and truly understand an animal under observation and study.

The mammalian limbic system has been identified as the area of the brain evolved to interpret and experience emotion, making it a likely area where social learning, bonding, and affectional attachment take place. Paul MacLean (1986) found that mammalian maternal behavior, separation-distress vocalization, and play are organized at the level of the cingulate gyrus, an important part of the limbic system. The cingulate gyrus is the structural dividing line between the reptilian and mammalian brains. Furthermore, it is reasonable to assume that a brain system involving the cingulate gyrus provides the common neural matrix for empathetic exchange and reciprocal attachment between mammals, especially between humans and dogs. The functional and morphological similarity of this neural structure may determine the potential depth and range of social bonding between mammals. The analogous behavior and intention apparent between humans and dogs is not necessarily an anthropomorphic conceptualization but a profoundly experienced similarity based on an instinctual need for closeness, nurture, care giving and receiving, emotional expression, and play.

K. J. Shapiro (1990) proposed that the communication gap between humans and dogs can be bridged by a method he calls *kinesthestic empathy*. In a paper presented at the American Psychology Association Convention in Atlanta in 1988, he took a radical departure from the conventional rejection of anthropomorphic speculation and espoused a *phenomenological method* for assessing the experience of others, including the other as experienced by dogs:

> A kinesthetic empathy, consisting of the meaningful actual or virtual imitation or enactment of bodily moves, is possible. It is possible because we both have living, mobile, intending bodies. ... Empathy is the direct apprehension of the intent, project, attitude, and experience of the other. ... More generally, I can also directly apprehend your or a dog's project, purpose, or anticipated intent. ... Empathy is a general access to the intended world of the other. (1990:191)

According to Shapiro, empathy does not depend on inference, form, analogy, self-identification, or "body complementarity" with the object of empathy; rather, empathy occurs as the result of "a moment in which I, if only focally, forget myself and directly sense what you are experiencing." Unfortunately, Shapiro's method raises many questions and problems that he fails to address adequately,

especially with respect to the control of empathetic errors due to anthropomorphism and cultural biases influencing ones empathetic perceptions.

MYSTICISM

Some authors and poets have attempted to extend interspecific communication and empathy beyond the scientific realm to the level of spiritual union and identity—what Rilke has termed *inseeing*:

> I love inseeing. Can you imagine with me how glorious it is to insee, for example, a dog as one passes by. To insee (I don't mean inspect, in which one immediately comes out again on the other side of the dog, regarding it merely, so to speak, as a window upon the humanity lying behind it, not that)—but to let oneself precisely into the dog, the place in it where God, as it were, would have sat down for a moment when the dog was finished, in order to watch it under the influence of its first embarrassments and inspirations and to know that it was good that nothing was lacking, that it could not have been better made. ... Laugh though you may, dear confidant, if I am to tell you where my all-greatest feeling, my world-feeling, my earthly bliss was to be found, I must confess to you: it was to found time and again, here and there, in such timeless moments of this divine inseeing. (Quoted in Woloy, 1990:47)

These efforts reveal both the potential benefits, as well as the excesses, of the foregoing *empathetic method* described by Shapiro. J. Allen Boone (1939, 1954), an early proponent of the method, has described a visionary process of empathetic exchange between him and the dog Strongheart, a famous police dog and canine actor. He recounts his discovery, writing in *Kinship with All Life*,

> What made our silent conversations so easy and so rewarding was the invisible Primary Factor that was responsible for the entire activity. In order to understand this deeply hidden secret, it is important to know that what actually went on in those communion sessions of ours was not the hit-or-miss exchange of thoughts between the "larger and more important brain of a human" and the "smaller and less important brain of a dog." Not at all. Brains as such had no more to do with it than ribs. And that something had all the love of the

boundless Mind of the Universe moving back of it and in it and through it.

Neither Strongheart nor I was doing any communicating as of ourselves. Neither of us was expressing himself as an original thinker or an independent source. On the contrary, we were being *communicated through* by the Mind of the Universe. We were being used as living instruments for its good pleasure. The primal, illimitable and eternal Mind was moving through me to Strongheart, and through Strongheart to me. Thus I came to know that it moves through everything everywhere in a ceaseless rhythm of harmonious kinship. (1954:76)

The evident experience of harmony and silent interpenetration between Boone and Strongheart reaches ecstatic proportions. Boone believed that he had formed with Strongheart a spiritual conduit for directly experiencing the sacred rhythms of nature:

> Thus did Strongheart and I share in that silent language which the Mind of the universe is constantly speaking through all life and for the greater good of all life. Thus did we make use of that wondrous inner route from mind to mind and from heart to heart. Thus did we cross each other's boundaries, only to find that there were no boundaries separating us from each other, except in the dark illusions of the human senses. (1954:80)

Boone thought that he had discovered a dormant potential for interspecies communication and understanding. The relationship consequently established between himself and Strongheart was full of meaning, vitality, and urgency. According to Boone, a contemplative link is always available and accessible through earnest and sincere recognition of the fundamental equality of human and dog existence—a recognition and experience that is fully obtained at any moment through the vehicle of a pure and sincere heart or what Shapiro refers to as "the direct apprehension of the intent, project, attitude, and experience of the other" (1990:191).

In the 1930s, Boone lived in a period of social and economic turmoil in which the world seemed to be falling apart. His personal search for meaning took him on a journey around the world. During this odyssey,

he composed his *Letters to Strongheart*—an outpouring of love and respect for his lost friend who had died. An important goal of the book was to place the dog's cultural role and purpose into a new perspective. For Boone, the dog was a salutary spiritual influence, perhaps our only hope of coming to our senses before destroying ourselves. In his estimation, the dog embodied the perfected traits of nobility, sincerity, devotion, unselfishness, strength, honesty, and pure enthusiasm for life. In essence, the life of the dog is a poetic expression of profound virtue and meaning:

> He composes a poem by turning himself into a poem, from the tip of his nose to the tip of his tail. The human writes poetry. The dog lives poetry. And who among us, in a Cosmos in which so much of reality has yet to be discovered, is qualified to say whether the human or the dog method of self-expression is nearer the ultimate of reality. (1939:111)

For Boone, "good poetry is any dog doing anything." Beyond the dog's physical form and materiality, Boone believed existed a spiritual essence waiting silently to guide our edification and improvement.

While traveling in Japan, he had the opportunity to attend a tea ceremony. At the conclusion of tea, he asked the tea master how one might find the greatest satisfaction in life. The host replied, "By disciplining one's self, and learning to live divinely in small as well as great things." Boone then asked the master to describe some of the characteristics of the superior life. The list of attributes included various qualities and traits, such as love, contentment, unselfishness, appreciation, loyalty, sincerity, simplicity, frugality, gratitude, self-control, the capacity for small enjoyments, serenity, honesty, poise, genuineness, courage, sympathy, tolerance, understanding, good manners, strong observation, strength with gentleness, unselfish attitudes, dignity, and the ability to be interested in people and things for their own sakes and not for personal return. Boone further inquired of the master what would one be called who possessed all of those characteristics. The master replied that such a person would be regarded as an *enlightened one*. A Japanese guest having tea with Boone then asked him whether he had ever known such a person. Boone confirmed with a nod that he had, and the following dialogue between the two ensued:

> "An American?" he queried, enthusiastically.
> "Only by adoption," I told him. "His name is Strongheart."
> "An Indian!" he exclaimed like a puzzled child.
> "No," I said, "most people call him a dog." (1939:88)

The dog is a familiar image in Buddhist mystical symbolism and philosophy, especially those teachings belonging to the Zen sect, and Boone's koanlike comment would have surely produced a strong impression on those present. Even in Japan today, the Zen initiate is frequently tested with a koan that has a dog as the subject of consideration. In fact, the most famous koan of all is the one based on the story of the 9th-century Chinese Zen master Chao-chou (or Joshu) in Japan. Joshu was asked by a petitioning monk whether dogs possessed a Buddha nature; the Master replied without hesitation, "Mu." The word *Mu* is variously translated as "no" or "nothing," but this literal interpretation fails to convey the term's intended meaning or the various spiritual nuances associated with it in this context. Joshu's reply is not a simple denial of the dog's Buddha nature, nor can it be interpreted as an empirical statement about dogs. In fact, Joshu's Mu is intended to defy and defeat rational understanding and explanation. Instead of thinking about the koan's rational meaning, seekers are urged to abandon reason and approach it with their whole being (like Boone's dog poet), not relying on intellectual support or guidance. The meaning of Mu is attained only after exhaustive internal search and meditation. Gradually, through the influence of rigorous training and self-control, and provided that the seekers are able to forget the self, they are brought face to face with Mu as a direct revelation. This state of mind transcends the ordinary web of appearances and dualistic individuation, and moves into a realm of nondifferentiation where both denial and affirmation are equally meaningless. A realm where dog and seeker are no longer two, but one embraced by the all-encompassing Mu. Here, the seeker dissolves into the dog, dog into seeker, dog and seeker into Mu, and Mu into the quietude of emptiness. This transformation and intercommunication between human and dog is more or less the central theme of Boone's spiritual quest.

Michael Fox (1980), a prominent animal behavior researcher, veterinarian, and psychologist confides that he experienced the wolf, not only as the object of scientific research and analysis but also as a "teacher and mirror" guiding him to a higher understanding of himself and mediating a closer relationship with nature. He felt that this inner recognition and heightened awareness was given to him through a mystical union with the wolf but only after the arbitrary barriers separating him from the wolf were dissolved and replaced with a direct intuitive vision and apprehension of the wolf as a living being—a soul: "Man and wolf are not only of one earth, but they are also of one essence" (1980:4). The outcome of this visionary experience for Fox was the birth of an empathetic kinship with the wolf and a "common ground within the essence of life."

Despite the discomfiture that such ideas may cause some scientifically inclined readers, dogs and other animals have served and continue to serve an important spiritual function in the psychic life of modern humankind. Whether such a spiritual function played a role in the early bonding process between humans and dogs during primitive times is not clear, although it is known that dogs were frequently buried with their owners, ostensibly serving as guides into the spirit world. Shamans of living tribal cultures often make use of helping spirits in the form of wolves or dogs, as well as other animals (Eliade, 1964). Before setting off on their ecstatic journey, Chukchee and Eskimo shamans turn themselves into wolves—a transformation that enables them to move freely through the depths and heights of nature. The shamanic experience is not intrinsically different from the foregoing testimony of Boone and Fox: the animal as a helping spirit mediates a more profound union with nature and oneself. According to Jungian analyst Eleanora Woloy (1990), dogs provide modern humankind with a vital contact point with nature. Under the dehumanizing influence of alienation—isolated from both nature and one's instincts—dogs offer a comforting source of reunion on both levels. In addition to practical considerations, the ancient covenant between humans and dogs served both a symbolic and mythical function, embodying the ideals of faithfulness, devotion, trust, love, protection, and cooperative submission for the greater good.

Dog Devotion: Legends

The close bond between people and dogs has been the perennial subject of poetic and literary idealization throughout history. One of the most poignant examples of this literature comes from an ancient Hindu text, the *Mahabharata* (Mally, 1994). Purported to be the oldest dog story, it recounts the celestial journey of a Brahmin king and his dog to heaven. The spiritual passage is filled with strife and danger, with the old Brahmin losing all of his earthly friends and family along the way—all except for his faithful dog. When at last he reaches his destination and stands before the portals leading to ultimate liberation and bliss, Indra appears before him and blocks the way:

> The celestial doors were opened for him, but his weary, long suffering, and steadfast old hound might not enter! Yudishthira saw within the walls the glories of Heaven; he saw, too, the faithful, gaunt dog cowering at his feet and gazing pleadingly up into its master's eyes; the king's heart was torn with longing and gratitude.
>
> "O Wisest One, Mighty God Indra!" he cried, "this hound hath eaten with me, starved with me, suffered with me, loved me! Must I desert him now?"
>
> "Yea," declared the God of Gods, Indra, "all the joys of Paradise are yours forever, but leave here your hound."
>
> Then exclaimed Yudishthira in anguish.
>
> "Can it be that a god can be so destitute of pity; Can it be that to gain this glory I must

leave behind all that I love? Then let me lose such glory forever!"

And Yudishthira turned sadly toward his forlorn dog. But the mighty Indra called to him again.

"Do you not understand? The creature is unclean; it would defile the altar fires of Paradise! Know this indeed: into Heaven, such cannot enter."

The Brahmin king could not be persuaded to abandon his dear friend but proclaims the injustice of leaving his devoted dog behind after all the many travails they had suffered so long together. The supplicant king would not betray his innocent dog even if it meant losing eternal bliss. Instead, he turns away, saying "Farewell, then, Lord Indra. I go and my hound with me." Just as he speaks these words, the dog is transformed into the god Dharma (Justice), who proclaims,

> "Behold, son, you have suffered much! But now, since you would not enter Heaven lest your poor dog should be cast away, lo! there is none in Paradise shall sit above you! Enter. Justice and Love welcome you."

In Homer's depiction of the reunion of Odysseus with his old dog Argos, the warrior king, after a 20-year absence, finds his neglected dog Argos near death "half destroyed with flies" and lying prostrate on a dung heap. In spite of the many intervening years, and the dog's weakened state, Argos still recognizes his master hidden under the cloak of a beggar. The old dog, mirroring his master's plight, collects his last bit of strength "to wag his tail, nose down, with flattened ears," but collapses before he can reach his master's hand. Odysseus wipes away a tear as his old friend dies in disgrace. Plutarch tells a similarly moving story that further underscores the Greek's appreciation of the dog's special attachment and devotion to humans. During the Persian War, all able Athenians were recruited and forced to leave their families to fight the invading Persian forces:

> When the whole city of Athens were going on board, it afforded a spectacle worthy of pity alike and admiration, to see them thus send away their fathers and children before them, and, unmoved with their cries and tears, pass

over into the island. But that which stirred compassion most of all was, that many old men, by reason of their great age, were left behind; and even the tame domestic animals could not be seen without some pity, running about the town and howling, as desirous to be carried along with their masters that had kept them; among which it is reported that Xanthippus, the father of Pericles, had a dog that would not endure to stay behind, but leaped into the sea, and swam along by the galley's side till he came to the island of Salamis, where he fainted away and died, and that spot in the island, which is still called the Dog's Grave, is said to be his. (*Plutarch's Lives: Themistocles*)

Many other examples of extraordinary devotion and attachment leading up to modern times could be recounted, but a particularly noteworthy one in this regard is the story of an Akita: Hachi-ko (Coffman, 1997). The story tells how the dog routinely greeted his owner (a professor at Tokyo University) at 3:00 PM every afternoon at the Shibuyu subway station. One fateful day, however, the dog waited in vain, since the professor had suffered a fatal stroke while at school that day. Undaunted, the determined Hachi-ko went back to the station day after day to await the belated return of his lost master. As a result of his extraordinary fidelity and determined steadfastness, Hachi-ko became a Japanese cultural icon during his lifetime (1922 to 1934), with visitors coming from all over the country just for the opportunity to pet the famous dog. A bronze statue was erected in his honor bearing testimony to his devotion and long vigil. After 9 years of waiting, the dog finally collapsed and died of old age at the base of the statue dedicated to his memory.

CYNOPRAXIS: TRAINING AND THE HUMAN-DOG RELATIONSHIP

Michael Fox (1979) has identified and described various functions served by dogs and the corresponding relationships formed between humans and dogs as a result of those roles. The interactions between humans and dogs range from indifference to close companionship and a heightened sense of responsibility or stewardship. These roles and values

are organized within a hierarchical system that moves from an object-oriented exploitive relationship to an appreciation of dogs for their own sake, a level of interaction that Fox refers to as *transpersonal relatedness*. On the transpersonal level, dogs are appreciated for what they are rather than for the emotional or utilitarian gratification that they might provide. At the lowest rung of this hierarchy are dogs exploited for some utilitarian purpose such as a family pet for children or dogs specifically trained for practical purposes. Under the heading of utilitarian-exploitation, Fox includes dogs used for laboratory research as well as dogs trained for work (e.g., hunting, shepherding, guarding, pulling, search and rescue), competitive uses (e.g., conformation, agility, obedience), military and police dogs, and service dogs of all kinds. Most of these various roles and functions include both exploitive purposes and emotional dependencies which the dogs are expected to serve. On the level of transpersonal relatedness, dogs are valued for their intrinsic worth—not for some remote purpose. In addition to valuing dogs for their own sake, Fox emphasized the importance of a heightened sense of responsibility, the highest level of interaction, which he refers to as stewardship. *Stewardship* refers to a refined concern for a dog's well-being and quality of life based on an appreciation of the dog from the perspective of transpersonal relatedness.

Obviously, there exist many purposes for which the dog's behavior is modified by training, ranging from utilitarian interests to improved household manners. Aside from practical considerations, a central goal of the training process is to enhance the human-dog relationship by promoting interactive harmony and interspecies appreciation, while at the same time striving to raise the dog's quality of life, that is, the trainer assumes the responsibility of stewardship in his or her dealings with a dog. Behavioral intervention that emphasizes these values is here referred to as *cynopraxis*. The term is composed of two Greek roots: cyno (*kunos*) or "dog" and praxis (*prassein*) "to do." *Praxis* refers to the application of theoretical knowledge for some practical purpose. In the present context, it refers to the application of ethology, learning theory, and supporting areas of scientific research (e.g., neurobiology) to the humane management and control of dog behavior. However, these characteristics only provide a partial picture of the meaning and character of praxis and the cynopraxic process.

Aristotle used the term *praxis* in the *Nicomachean Ethics* (Irwin, 1985) with three interdependent meanings that have relevance for understanding cynopraxis as a canine behavioral art. Praxis is voluntary and goal directed, regulated by informed and rational choice, and performed as an end in itself. According to Aristotle's teachings, virtuous action (voluntary, rational, and an end in itself) inevitably results in *happiness*. Similarly, cynopraxic intervention strives to attain harmonious and *joyful* coexistence between humans and dogs through a similar triadic scheme of intervention. Central to this purpose is the exercise of effective behavioral control and management, which is attained through actions guided by rational purposiveness. Herein lies the importance of science and sound practice for the cynopraxic trainer and counselor. However, to achieve these goals, the cynopraxist, in addition to exercising rational objectivity and ethical restraint, embraces subjective sensibilities that infuse the cynopraxic arts with a distinctive *feeling* dimension. Finally, the cynopraxic process is an end in itself, insofar as there are no training goals or objectives for cynopraxists that exist beyond the attainment of interactive harmony between human and dog.

Cynopraxic intervention takes place within the context of a family-pack system and home, with the express purpose of improving the human-dog relationship and the overall quality of a dog's life. Although the cynopraxic process operates under the preemptive constraints of scientific behavior theory, it strongly emphasizes the value of *subjective* and *dynamic* factors that influence the formation and maintenance of the bonding process. Consequently, in addition to generalizable *data*, cynopraxists address highly individualistic or *intimate* (Lat. *intimus* or "inmost, deepest") influences that contribute to

the intensification of the human-dog bond. Specifically, cynopraxis embraces and promotes the value of play, esthetic sensitivity, emotive-cognitive empathy, intuition, compassion, and ethical constraints; that is, subjective attributes that are shunned by a strictly scientific analysis. In effect, cynopraxis places scientific knowledge into the perspective of a humane and *feeling* art, with the explicit and self-limiting goals of fostering social harmony and well-being through informed training and counseling. Achieving these ends may require that some minor or major modification of a dog's behavior and surroundings takes place, but such modifications are justified only to the extent that they serve these dual cynopraxic purposes. Cynopraxists view behavioral adaptation as an epigenetic process involving various biobehavioral predispositions interacting with learning experiences (e.g., development, socialization, and training)—all taking place within the context of a social relationship and home environment. Consequently, behavior adjustment problems are analyzed in terms of their functional significance and relation to a dog's relative ability or failure to form satisfying relationships or to occupy a common domestic environment harmoniously with human or other animal companions. In general, the cynopraxic arts address dog behavior problems as obstacles blocking the way to the formation of a more satisfying and joyful human-dog life experience and interspecies appreciation. Although the establishment of control is often necessary and desirable, behavioral control for the sake of domination or for the sake of objectives harmful to the dog or degrading to the human-dog bond is inconsistent with cynopraxic philosophy. Cynopraxic trainers are distinguished by an attitude of composure (mental and physical), presence, and sincerity of purpose that informs their actions—personal qualities that mediate connectedness with the dog and facilitate the bonding process. Cynopraxic intervention guides behavioral change through the augmentation of affection, communication, and trust.

The perennial bond between humans and

dogs has always involved some balance of companionship and work. Cynopraxists recognize and appreciate the importance of cooperative activity between humans and dogs; however, training activities that place a utilitarian purpose or objective above the human-dog relationship or employ dogs in activities that threaten their safety and welfare fall outside of the cynopraxic scope of practice. Practical dog training for competition, entertainment, service, or work may conflict with cynopraxic interests, depending on the specific purposes of such training and other considerations associated with such activities. Obedience training, in the sense of the Latin root, *oboedire*, or the act of "listening to," exercises a profound mediating influence between humans and dogs. The locus of obedience training resides within a shared human-dog moment of intensified attention and recognition of each other, with the purpose of promoting mutual understanding, cooperation, and refinement of interaction. Obedience training, as such, is an instrumental cynopraxic tool for enhancing interactive harmony and appreciation. From the cynopraxic point of view, training and the bond formed as a result of training are coextensive and mutually dependent on each other. In total, the training process begins and ends as a celebration of the human-dog bond and its actualization. However, practical dog training that strives to establish control for the sole purpose of dominating a dog or in order to exploit its labor and services is demeaning and destructive of this unique bond and its potential. In essence, such training exploits the bond in order to achieve remote purposes or objectives beyond it, a process that is ultimately alienating for both trainers and dogs. Under the influence of such training, dogs are gradually transformed into tools or weapons, while the trainers run the risk of losing their moral center in the process. Further, when a dog's services are no longer needed or useful, it may be "officially" stripped of life and sentiency (the very characteristics that made its training possible in the first place), thus degrading it to the status of an inanimate object or piece of surplus equipment unworthy of special care or protection beyond that given to other things that have become obsolete or useless.

A military working dog, for example, typically forms a profound connection with its handler as a result of training, but this training may also require that the dog learn to perform tasks that add nothing to the bonding process or to the dog's quality of life. In fact, such dogs are often deliberately exposed to danger and harm as a direct result of performing the services for which they are trained. The following examples will help to clarify some of these concerns. During World War II, Russian war dogs were trained to run under enemy tanks with explosives strapped to their backs. These dogs were transformed into living bombs by exploiting their affection and trust. Not only are the dogs at risk of danger and harm, so is the fundamental bond between the handlers and the dogs. Reportedly, Nazi SS were trained side by side with a companion German shepherd. At the conclusion of the grueling 12-week course of training, the soldier, to receive his coveted stripes, had to kill his canine comrade by breaking its neck. Presumably, this cruel practice proved that the soldier's allegiance to the Nazi cause was held above his affection and loyalty to his dog (Arluke and Sanders, 1996). Arguably less premeditated and diabolic, but nonetheless following a similar vein of insensitivity, during the abrupt and chaotic evacuation of military forces from Vietnam in 1973, American soldiers were ordered to leave their scout dogs and sentry dogs behind to fend for themselves against an encroaching enemy. These remarkable dogs, who had served nobly and saved many lives, were abandoned as disposable military equipment, with little more official recognition than that given to a jeep or tent peg. Handlers and dogs alike suffered greatly as a result of this inhumane policy.

As noted above, cynopraxic training and counseling take place within a context consisting of a social relationship and a shared home environment. In contrast, the laboratory study of animal behavior is first and foremost the study of *caged* behavior, occurring under the influence of various experimental deprivations and manipulations. In most studies, an animal's relationship with an experimenter is either nonexistent or minimized, and there is rarely little genuine consideration given for the animal subject's quality of life. All *effects of person* and other external influences from the environment are assiduously controlled and excluded as much as possible, so that the specific stimulus-response variables under observation can be measured against an experiential backdrop that is common to all animal subjects. Under the sterile social and environmental conditions of the laboratory, observations are made with little or no reference to an animal's relationship to the experimenter or to the surrounding environment outside of the experimental chamber. These methodological considerations represent cardinal distinctions between the experimental study of dog behavior and cynopraxis. Whereas behavioral scientists experimentally evaluate various hypotheses about how behavior is organized, perhaps hoping to discover fundamental laws in the process, cynopraxists mediate between dogs and owners under the relatively uncontrolled circumstances of a home environment in order to facilitate interactive harmony. Whereas scientists seek "truth" and lawful relations governing animal behavior, cynopraxists strive to attain the simple joys and benefits resulting from the enhancement of the human-dog bond.

A procedural strength of experimental science has been its objective neutrality with respect to its subject matter and findings. In the case of animal studies, the resulting distance between scientists and their animal subjects has often been the target of ethical criticism. When studying inanimate and insentient life, one is not obliged to consider the feelings and distress wrought by one's experimental manipulations. This is not the case, however, when experimenting upon animals, which appear to experience pain and deprivation in a way that is not too dissimilar from our own experience of such things. Consequently, when performing experiments on animals, a researcher's otherwise laudable objectivity runs a risk of attracting the humane critic's scorn and insinuations, suggesting that the scientist's "objective distance" is just a shallow excuse for insensate aloofness and cruelty. This sort of accusatory attack is unfair but does emphasize the need for scientists to perform their research in the most humane ways possible and to consider the welfare of their animal subjects by minimizing the stress and pain to which they are exposed during experimentation. Cynopraxic trainers and counselors recognize the practical value of science but also recognize its inherent ethical and esthetic limitations. Although scientific knowledge is of great importance for effective intervention (insofar as it promotes informed and rational interventions), cynopraxists are bound by empathetic, esthetic, and ethical constraints to apply such knowledge for the actualization of the human-dog relationship and to promote the dog's well-being.

REFERENCES

Adams GJ and Clark WT (1989). The prevalence of behavioural problems in domestic dogs: A survey of 105 dog owners. *Aust Vet Pract,* 19:135–137.

Allman JM (1999). *Evolving Brains.* New York: Scientific American Library.

American Veterinary Medical Association (1997). *U.S. Pet Ownership and Demographic Sourcebook.* Schaumberg, IL: AVMA, Center for Information Management.

Anderson DG (1992). The control of pet over-population. *Vet Technol,* 13:119–123.

Anderson RK, Hart BL, and Hart LA (1984). *The Pet Connection: Its Influence on Our Health and Quality of Life.* Minneapolis: University of Minnesota.

Anonymous (1997). Top 10 reasons for relinquishment identified. *JAVMA,* 210:1256.

Arkow PS, Dow S (1984). The ties that do not bind: A study of the human-animal bonds that fail. In RK Anderson, BL Hart, and LA Hart (Eds), *The Pet Connection: Its Influence on Our Health and Quality of Life.* Minneapolis: University of Minnesota Press.

Arluke A and Sanders CR (1996). *Regarding Animals.* Philadelphia: Temple University Press.

Barba BE (1995). A critical review of research on the human/companion animal relationship: 1988–1993. *Anthrozoos,* 8:9–15.

Beck AM and Katcher AH (1984). A new look at pet-facilitated therapy. *JAVMA,* 184:414–421.

Bekoff M and Jamieson D (1996). *Readings in An-*

imal Cognition. Cambridge: MIT Press.

Bergler R (1988). *Man and Dog: The Psychology of a Relationship.* Oxford: Blackwell Scientific.

Boone JA (1939). *Letters to Strongheart.* New York: Prentice-Hall.

Boone JA (1954). *Kinship with All Life.* New York: Harper and Row.

Bossard JHS (1944). The mental hygiene of owning a dog. *Ment Hyg (Arlington, VA),* 28:408–413.

Bucke WF (1903). Cyno-psychoses: Children's thoughts, reactions, and feelings toward pet dogs. *J Genet Psychol,* 10:459–513.

Burghardt GM (1985). Animal awareness, current perceptions, and historical perspective. *Am Psychol,* 40:905–919.

Burghardt WF (1991). Behavioral medicine as a part of a comprehensive small animal medical program. *Vet Clin North Am Adv Comp Anim Behav,* 21:207–224.

Campbell WE (1986). The prevalence of behavior problems in American dogs. *Mod Vet Pract,* 67:28–31.

Carson G (1972). *Men, Beasts, and Gods: A History of Cruelty and Kindness to Animals.* New York: Charles Scribner's Sons.

Chance MRA (1962) An interpretation of some agonistic postures: The role of "cut-off" acts and postures. *Symp Zool Soc Lond,* 8:71–89.

Clutton-Brock J (1977). Man-made dogs. *Science,* 197:1340–1342.

Clutton-Brock J (1981). *Domesticated Animals from Early Times.* Austin: University of Texas Press.

Coffman C (1997). Hachi-ko: A primer in loyalty. *Dog Kennel,* 2:38–40.

Corson SA and Corson EO'L (1981). Companion animals as bonding catalysts in geriatric institutions. In B Fogle (Ed), *Interrelations Between People and Pets.* Springfield, IL: Charles C Thomas.

Corson SA, Corson EO'L, Gwynne PH, and Arnold LE (1977). Pet dogs: A nonverbal communication link in hospital psychiatry. *Comp Psychiatry,* 18:61–72.

Darwin C (1872/1965). *The Expression of the Emotions in Man and Animals.* Chicago: University of Chicago Press (reprint).

Eibl-Eibesfeldt I (1971). *Love and Hate: The Natural History of Behavior Patterns.* New York: Holt, Rinehart and Winston.

Eliade M (1964). *Shamanism: Archaic Techniques of Ecstasy.* Princeton: Princeton University Press.

Fentress JC (1967). Observations on the behavioral development of a hand-reared male timber wolf. *Am Zool,* 7:339–351.

Fogle B (1981). *Interrelations Between People and Pets.* Springfield, IL: Charles C Thomas.

Fox MW (1969). The anatomy of aggression and its ritualization in Canidae: A developmental and comparative study. *Behaviour,* 35:243–258.

Fox MW (1979). The values and uses of pets. In RD Allen and WH Westbrook (Eds), *The Handbook of Animal Welfare: Biomedical, Psychological, and Ecological Aspects of Pet Problems and Control.* New York: Garland STPM.

Fox MW (1980). *The Soul of the Wolf.* New York: Lyons and Burford.

Frank H and Frank MG (1982). On the effects of domestication on canine social development and behavior. *Appl Anim Ethol,* 8:507–525.

Friedmann ES, Katcher AH, Lynch JJ, and Thomas SA (1980). Animal companions and one year survival of patients after discharge from a coronary unit. *Public Health Rep* 95:307–312.

Galton SF (1883). *Inquiries in to Human Faculty and Its Development.* London: Macmillan.

Gantt WH (1972). Analysis of the effect of person. *Cond Reflex* 7:67–73.

Goodwin D, Bradshaw JWS, and Wickens SM (1997). Paedomorphosis affects agonistic visual signals of domestic dogs. *Anim Behav,* 53:297–304.

Grandin T (1995). *Thinking in Pictures and Other Reports from My Life with Autism.* New York: Vintage.

Griffin DR (1981) *The Question of Animal Awareness: Evolutionary Continuity of Mental Experience.* New York: Rockefeller University Press.

Griffin DR (1984). *Animal Thinking.* Cambridge: Harvard University Press.

Griffin DR (1992). *Animal Minds.* Chicago: University of Chicago Press.

Hart BL and Hart LA (1985). *Canine and Feline Behavioral Therapy.* Philadelphia: Lea and Febiger.

Hediger H (1955/1968). *The Psychology and Behavior of Animals in Zoos and Circuses,* G Sircom (Trans). New York: Dover (reprint).

Heiman M (1956). The relationship between man and dog. *Psychoanal Q,* 25:568–585.

Irwin T (1985). *Aristotle: Nicomachean Ethics.* Indianapolis, IN: Hackett.

Katcher HA (1981). Interactions between people and their pets: Form and function. In B Fogle (Ed), *Interrelations Between People and Pets.* Springfield, IL: Charles C Thomas.

Katcher AH and Beck AM (1983). *New Perspective on Our Lives with Companion Animals.* Philadelphia: University of Pennsylvania Press.

Kiley-Worthington M (1976). The tail movements of ungulates, canids and felids with particular reference to their causation and function as displays. *Behaviour*, 56:69–115.

King M (1991). Throwaway animals. *Anim Agenda*, May:12–20.

Kipling R (1982). *Just So Stories*. Garden City, NJ: Doubleday.

Landsberg GM (1991). The distribution of canine behavior cases at three behavior referral practices. *Vet Med*, 86:1011–1018.

Lehman HC (1928). Child's attitude toward the dog versus the cat. *J Genet Psychol*, 35:67–72.

Levinson BM (1961). The dog as a "co-therapist." *Ment Hyg (Arlington, VA)*, 46:59–65.

Levinson BM (1969). *Pet-Oriented Child Psychotherapy*. Springfield, IL: Charles C Thomas.

Leyhausen P (1973). The biology of expression and impression. In BA Tonkin (Trans), *Motivation of Human and Animal Behavior: An Ethological View*. New York: Van Nostrand Reinhold.

Line S (1998). Factors associated with the surrender of animals to the urban humane society. Convention Notes, Proceedings of the 135th Annual Convention of the American Veterinary Medical Association (AVMA), Baltimore, MD, July 25–29, 1998. Schaumberg, IL: AVMA.

Lore RK and Eisenberg FB(1986): Avoidance reactions of domestic dogs to unfamiliar male and female humans in a kennel setting. *Appl Anim Behav Sci*, 15:261–266.

Lorenz K (1966). *On Aggression*. New York: Harcourt Brace Jovanovich.

Lorenz K (1975). Forward. In MW Fox (Ed), *The Wild Canids: Their Systematics, Behavioral Ecology and Evolution*. New York: Van Nostrand Reinhold.

MacLean PD (1986). Culminating developments in the evolution of the limbic system: The thalamocingulate division. In BK Doane and KE Livingston (Eds), *The Limbic System: Functional Organization and Clinical Disorders*. New York: Raven.

Mally EL (1994). *A Treasury of Animal Stories*. Edison, NJ: Castle.

Martin R (1990). *Primate Origins and Evolution: A Phylogenetic Reconstruction*. Princeton: Princeton University Press.

Messent PR and Serpell JA (1981). An historical and biological view of the pet-owner bond. In B Fogle (Ed), *Interrelations Between Pets and People*. Springfield, IL: Charles C Thomas.

Morris D (1967). *The Naked Ape*. New York: McGraw-Hill.

Nassar R and Fluke J (1988). *Shelter Reporting Study*. Denver, CO: American Humane Association.

O'Farrell V (1997). Owner attitudes and dog behaviour problems. *Appl Anim Behav Sci*, 52:205–213.

Overall K (1997). *Clinical Behavioral Medicine for Small Animals*. St Louis: CV Mosby.

Passmore J (1975). The treatment of animals. *J Hist Ideas*, 36:195–218.

Perin C (1981). Dogs as symbols in human development. In B Fogle (Ed), *Interrelations Between People and Pets*. Springfield, IL: Charles C Thomas.

Pet Food Institute (1999). PFI Fact Sheet. Washington, DC: Pet Food Institute.

Rappolt GA, John J, and Thompson NS (1979). Canine responses to familiar and unfamiliar humans. *Aggressive Behav*, 5:155–161.

Regan T (1983). *The Case for Animal Rights*. Berkeley: University of California Press.

Reich M and Overall K (1998). Abstract: Paper presentation. AVSAB, Baltimore, MD.

Rescorla RA (1988). Pavlovian conditioning: It's not what you think it is. *Am Psychol*, 43:151–160.

Rowan AN (1988). *Animals and People Sharing the World*. Hanover, NH: University Press of New England.

Rowan AN (1992). Shelters and pet overpopulation: A statistical black hole. *Anthrozoos*, 5:140–143.

Rynearson EK (1978). Humans and pets and attachment. *Br J Psychiatry*, 133:550–555.

Salman MD, New JG, Scarlet JM, and Kass PH (1998). Human and animal factors related to the relinquishment of dogs and cats in 12 selected animal shelters in the United States. *J Appl Anim Welfare Sci*, 1:207–226.

Savishinsky JS (1983). Pet ideas: The domestication of animals, human behavior, and human emotions. In AH Katcher and AM Beck (Eds), *New Perspective on Our Lives with Companion Animals*. Philadelphia: University of Pennsylvania Press.

Schenkel R (1967). Submission: Its features and function in the wolf and dog. *Am Zool*, 7:319–329.

Schleidt WM (1999). Apes, wolves, and the trek to humanity. *Discovering Archaeol*, 1:8–10.

Scott JP (1958). Critical periods in the development of social behavior in puppies. *Psychosom Med*, 20:42–54.

Scott JP (1967). The evolution of social behavior in dogs and wolves. *Am Zool*, 7:373–381.

Scott JP (1968). Evolution and domestication of the dog. *Evol Biol*, 2:243–275.

Serpell JA (1986/1996). *In the Company of Animals: A Study of Human-Animal Relationships.* New York: Cambridge University Press (reprint).

Serpell JA (1987). The influence of inheritance and environment on canine behavior: Myth and fact. *J Small Anim Pract,* 28:949–956.

Shapiro KJ (1990). Understanding dogs through kinesthetic empathy, social construction, and history. *Anthrozoos* 3:184–195.

Sigler L (1991). Pet behavioral problems present opportunities for practitioners. *AAHA Trends,* 4:44–45.

Tinbergen N (1951/1969). *The Study of Instinct.* Oxford: Oxford University Press (reprint).

Tinbergen N (1964). The evolution of signaling devices. In W Etkin (Ed), *Social Behavior and Organization Among Vertebrates.* Chicago: University of Chicago Press.

Tinklepaugh OL (1934). "Gifted" animals. In FA Moss (Ed), *Comparative Psychology,* 483–510. New York: Prentice-Hall.

Tolman EC (1934). Theories of learning. In FA Moss (Ed), *Comparative Psychology,* 367–408. New York: Prentice-Hall.

Tuan Yi-Fu (1984). *Dominance and Affection: The Making of Pets.* New Haven: Yale University Press.

Vauclair J (1996). *Animal Cognition: An Introduction to Modern Comparative Psychology.* Cambridge: Harvard University Press.

Voith VL (1981a). Attachment between people and their pets: Behavior problems of pets that arise from the relationship between pets and people. In B Fogle (Ed), *Interrelations Between People and Pets.* Springfield, IL: Charles C Thomas.

Voith VL (1981b). Profile of 100 animal behavior cases. *Mod Vet Pract,* 62:483–484.

Voith VL (1984). Human/animal relationships. In RS Anderson (Ed), *Nutrition and Behavior in Dogs and Cats.* New York: Pergamon.

Voith VL, Wright JC, Danneman PJ, et al. (1992). Is there a relationship between canine behavior problems and spoiling activities, anthropomorphism, and obedience training? *Appl Anim Behav Sci,* 34:263–272.

Vormbrock JK and Grossberg JM (1988). Cardiovascular effects of human-pet dog interactions. *J Behav Med,* 11:509–517.

Walker S (1983). *Animal Thought.* London: Routledge and Kegan Paul.

White GW (1991). *Myths of the Dog-Man.* Chicago: University of Chicago Press.

Wilson CC and Netting FE (1983). Companion animals and the elderly: A state-of-the-art summary. *JAVMA,* 183:1425–1429.

Woloy EM (1990). *The Symbol of the Dog in the Human Psyche: A Study of the Human-Dog Bond.* Wilmette, IL: Chiron.

Woolpy JH and Ginsburg BE (1967). Wolf socialization: A study of temperament in a wild social species. *Am Zool,* 7:357–363.

Young SP and Goldman EA (1944/1964). The Wolves of North America: Parts 1 and 2. New York: Dover (reprint).

Zeuner FE (1963). *A History of Domesticated Animals.* London: Hutchinson.